HEALTH AND HUMAN DEVELOPMENT

PUBLIC HEALTH YEARBOOK 2013

HEALTH AND HUMAN DEVELOPMENT
JOAV MERRICK - SERIES EDITOR –
NATIONAL INSTITUTE OF CHILD HEALTH AND HUMAN DEVELOPMENT,
MINISTRY OF SOCIAL AFFAIRS, JERUSALEM, ISRAEL

PUBLIC HEALTH YEARBOOK 2013

JOAV MERRICK
EDITOR

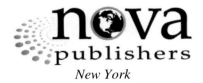

nova publishers
New York

NOTICE TO THE READER

The Publisher has taken reasonable care in the preparation of this book, but makes no expressed or implied warranty of any kind and assumes no responsibility for any errors or omissions. No liability is assumed for incidental or consequential damages in connection with or arising out of information contained in this book. The Publisher shall not be liable for any special, consequential, or exemplary damages resulting, in whole or in part, from the readers' use of, or reliance upon, this material. Any parts of this book based on government reports are so indicated and copyright is claimed for those parts to the extent applicable to compilations of such works.

Independent verification should be sought for any data, advice or recommendations contained in this book. In addition, no responsibility is assumed by the publisher for any injury and/or damage to persons or property arising from any methods, products, instructions, ideas or otherwise contained in this publication.

This publication is designed to provide accurate and authoritative information with regard to the subject matter covered herein. It is sold with the clear understanding that the Publisher is not engaged in rendering legal or any other professional services. If legal or any other expert assistance is required, the services of a competent person should be sought. FROM A DECLARATION OF PARTICIPANTS JOINTLY ADOPTED BY A COMMITTEE OF THE AMERICAN BAR ASSOCIATION AND A COMMITTEE OF PUBLISHERS.

Additional color graphics may be available in the e-book version of this book.

Library of Congress Cataloging-in-Publication Data

ISBN: 978-1-63321-095-0

Published by Nova Science Publishers, Inc. † New York

CONTENTS

INTRODUCTION

Joav Merrick, MD, MMedSci, DMSc[1,2,3,4]*

[1]National Institute of Child Health and Human Development
[2]Health Services, Office of the Medical Director, Division for Intellectual and
Developmental Disabilities, Ministry of Social Affairs and Social Services, Jerusalem
[3]Department of Pediatrics, Hadassah-Hebrew University Medical Center,
Mount Scopus Campus, Jerusalem, Israel
[4]Kentucky Children's Hospital, University of Kentucky,
Lexington, Kentucky, United States

In this Public Health Yearbook 2012 we will touch upon several public health topics like community capacity building, global health and health promotion.

Charles-Edward Amory Winslow (1877-1957) the American bacteriologist and public health expert defined public health or population health, as

> "...the science and art of preventing disease, prolonging life and promoting physical health and efficacy through organized community efforts for the sanitation of the environment, the control of community infections, the education of the individual in principles of personal hygiene, the organization of medical and nursing services for the early diagnosis and preventive treatment of disease, and the development of the social machinery which will ensure every individual in the community a standard of living adequate for the maintenance of health...to enable every citizen to realize his or her birthright and longevity" (1).

Winslow already in the early years the 20th century found that for the successful implementation of assuring a healthy population there must be a need for community involvement "...through organized community efforts"

This was prior to the establishment of the terms, *community capacity building* or *community-based participatory research*, that in order to prevent disease and promote health, the role of the community in achieving this mission of public health was essential. In this

---

* Correspondence: Professor Joav Merrick, MD, MMedSci, DMSc, Medical Director, Health Services, Division for Intellectual and Developmental Disabilities, Ministry of Social Affairs, POBox 1260, IL-91012 Jerusalem, Israel. E-mail: jmerrick@zahav.net.il.

Yearbook you will find two sections of community building with state of the art research with many questions such as:

Specifically, how do we develop shared governance in our partnerships? How do we serve as leaders and contributors? How do we engage in dialogue with the varied stakeholders who often believe another department or agency needs to take on the responsibility of addressing the public health issue? By learning the skills and principles necessary to help our target communities build their capacity to improve the health of their residents, only then will we make great strides towards achieving national, as well as global, health benchmarks.

The World Health Organization defines health promotion "as the process of enabling people to increase control over and to improve, their health". It moves beyond a focus on individual behaviour towards a wide range of social and environmental interventions, but discussions on how to define health promotion already emerged in the 1970s from the Lalonde report in Canada, which contained a health promotion strategy "aimed at informing, influencing and assisting both individuals and organizations so that they will accept more responsibility and be more active in matters affecting mental and physical health".

Health promotion and health service using socio-ecological approach has been effective to promote mental, physical health, improve social functioning and social support in a range of population group. Socio-ecological approach addresses the importance of the interaction between individual level characteristics, families, institutions, and community support to promote health to optimal level.

In this Yearbook you will find evidence to demonstrate the central concepts of health promotion around resilience at individual and organisation and system level as important to children's and youth quality of life, their learning outcomes, benefit employees' performance and health outcome, and chronic disease, dental student stress, depression and anxiety, and dental patients' knowledge about treatment and their health outcomes.

REFERENCES

[1]   Winslow CEA. The untilled field of public health. Modern Med 1920;2:183-91.

SECTION ONE - BUILDING COMMUNITY CAPACITY

In: Public Health Yearbook 2013   ISBN: 978-1-63321-095-0
Editor: Joav Merrick   © 2014 Nova Science Publishers, Inc.

Chapter 1

LESSONS LEARNED FROM BUILDING AN INFRASTRUCTURE FOR COMMUNITY-ENGAGED RESEARCH

Calpurnyia B Roberts, PhD[*,1]*, Ruth Browne, MPP, MPH, ScD*[2]*,*
Tracey E Wilson, PhD[3]*, Kweli Rashied-Henry, MPH*[1]*,*
Nicole Primus, MPA[1]*, Raphael Shaw, MPH, MD*[1]*,*
Humberto Brown[2]*, Ferdinand Zizi, MBA*[4]*,*
Girardin Jean-Louis, PhD[4]*, Clinton Brown, MD*[4]*,*
Yvonne Graham, RN, MPH[5]* and Marilyn Fraser-White, MD*[2]

[1]Brooklyn Health Disparities Center, Brooklyn, New York, United States of America
[2]Arthur Ashe Institute for Urban Health, Brooklyn, New York, United States of America
[3]Department of Community Health Sciences, School of Public Health, SUNY Downstate Medical Center, Brooklyn, New York, United States of America
[4]Department of Health Sciences, SUNY Downstate Medical Center, Brooklyn, New York, United States of America
[5]Office of the Brooklyn Borough President, Brooklyn, New York, United States of America

ABSTRACT

Before community-based participatory research (CBPR) can commence an infrastructure needs to be established whereby both academic researchers and community members can participate in CBPR as equitable partners throughout the research process. Objectives: We describe the key principles of the Brooklyn Health Disparities Center (BHDC), a community-academic-government partnership, to guide the development for an infrastructure to support, increase, and sustain the capacity of academics and community members to engage in CBPR to address cardiovascular health disparities in Brooklyn,

* Correspondence: Calpurnyia B. Roberts, PhD, SUNY Downstate Medical Center, 450 Clarkson Drive, Brooklyn, New York 11203, United States. E-mail: Calpurnyia.roberts@downstate.edu.

New York. Methods: The guiding principles of the BHDC consist of 1) promoting equitable and collaborative partnerships 2) enhancing research capacity and 3) building/sustaining trust. Delphi survey, youth summer internship programs, and workshops were among the tools utilized in enhancing community capacity. Results: Several lessons were gleaned: design programs that are capable of building trust, skills, capacity, and interest of community members concomitantly; be flexible in terms of the priorities and objectives that the partners seek to focus on as these may change over time; and build a groundswell of local advocates to embrace the research and policy agenda of the BHDC.

Keywords: Community-based participatory research, health disparities, minority health, partnerships

INTRODUCTION

In the United States, conventional research has contributed to overall improvements in health outcomes and longevity; yet, health disparities between racial/ethnic and socioeconomic groups continue to persist (1).

There is a growing interest and support for more comprehensive and participatory approaches to reduce health disparities that takes into account social determinants of health, such as community-based participatory research (CBPR) (2-4).

CBPR involves both the academic researchers and members of a community participating as equal partners in all aspects of the research process in order to address a health concern (5). Cultivating successful CBPR partnerships can facilitate the reduction of health disparities by enhancing the identification or refinement innovative research questions (6), discovery of local barriers in order to enhance recruitment of study participants (7,8) and dissemination of health information (6).

Centers of Excellence sponsored by the National Institute for Minority Health and Health Disparities are responsible for making advances towards ameliorating the health of underserved populations and ultimately eliminating health disparities in part by building research capacity. Thus, Centers of Excellence are in a pivotal position to use CBPR to alleviate health disparities and provide academic researchers (i.e., faculty, residents, and students) and community members with opportunities to collaborate in community-engaged research initiatives. However, before such initiatives can commence it is strongly suggested that an infrastructure be established whereby both academic researchers and community members understand the intricacies of CBPR from shared decision making, cultural competency, research methods, health disparities, to social determinants of health (9).

The Brooklyn Health Disparities Center (BHDC) is funded through a Centers of Excellence P20 mechanism. Established in 2004 in Brooklyn, New York the BHDC seeks to improve minority and new immigrant health thereby eliminating cardiovascular health disparities in Brooklyn, where rates of cardio-metabolic risk factors: heart disease, hypertension, diabetes, and HIV are higher than national levels, and are among some of the highest in the United States (10).

The BHDC resulted from the mutual collaboration between a community-based organization (Arthur Ashe Institute for Urban Health), an academic institution (SUNY Downstate Medical Center), and a government entity (Brooklyn Borough President's Office)

after a needs assessment was completed by the Brooklyn Borough Office in 2003 to evaluate whether a health disparities center in Brooklyn was essential. AAIUH is a community-based organization that collaborates with community members to design, incubate, and replicate neighborhood-based interventions that address health conditions that disproportionately affect minorities. SUNY Downstate Medical Center is the only academic medical center institution in Brooklyn.

In this article, we detail the three key principles employed by the BHDC to build an infrastructure that supports the development of community-driven research between these partners and the Brooklyn community: 1) promote equitable and collaborative partnerships 2) enhance research capacity and 3) build and sustain trust. We also highlight the traditional and unique methods implemented to expedite these principles followed by a summary of the intermediate outcomes and lessons learned. Our experience can serve as a developmental guide to create an infrastructure that supports multidisciplinary partnerships and capacity building with a goal of eliminating health disparities using CBPR.

Principle #1: Promote equitable and collaborative partnership

First, in order to enhance community capacity an equitable and collaborative partnership was solidified (4,5). AAIUH and SUNY Downstate Medical Center have worked together for nearly twenty years, and have had an on-going association with the Office of the Brooklyn Borough President. Thus, a rapport existed, and the formation of the BHDC signified a deeper commitment. To ensure that equity and collaboration are promoted within the BHDC, several strategies are employed: 1) agree on decision-making responsibilities 2) share resources and 3) receive additional guidance from two advisory bodies.

Sharing decision-making responsibilities has been invaluable to the creation and sustainability of the BHDC

Early during the formation of the BHDC, an explicit consensus on the rules of governance was reached. The leadership of the overall BHDC is shared between an appointed SUNY Downstate faculty member, the Chief Executive Officer of the AAIUH, and the Deputy Borough President. The two institutional entities (SUNY and AAIUH) have an equal vote in the decision-making activities at the BHDC, which includes decisions regarding fiscal matters, grant applications, selection of projects, hiring of staff, and membership selection into the BHDC. In addition, each of the Center's four cores (e.g., Administrative, Research, Research Education/Training, and Community Engagement) is led by a representative from the academic and community arms, which enhances collaboration across the partners. While the Brooklyn Borough President's Office is not involved in the day-to-day decision making, the Deputy President of Brooklyn provides oversight and direction by including the BHDC on various strategic committees in Brooklyn, such as the Health Advisory Committee and the Public Health Funding Task Force, which have given the BHDC the opportunity to address community well-being, foster collaborations, and exchange information. The active dual decision-making within the BHDC has increased the capacity of individual researchers collaborating within the BHDC to lead and function as a unit. Further, it has enabled the BHDC to strengthen and expand collaborations within the center and across the Brooklyn community. For instance, the BHDC surveyed faculty members to gain a sense of whether they participate in CBPR studies. The information collected was incorporated into a grant to increase the use of CBPR at SUNY Downstate Medical Center.

Partners of the BHDC offer resources through organizational support and/or expertise
SUNY Downstate provides organizational support for the BHDC by assisting in necessary infrastructure and oversight to ensure appropriate and timely management of all post-award processes in compliance with institutional, state, and federal guidelines and requirements. These areas encompass, but are not limited to verification of allowable costs, financial reporting, responsible conduct of research, protection of human subjects, and progress reports. Institutional support for BHDC is additionally given by SUNY in the form of four key commitments: 1) Space Allocations 2) Supplemental funding for research, training, and outreach activities 3) In-kind Personnel (e.g., Administrative and Faculty) and 4) Library Access. The community partner, AAIUH, offers nearly twenty years of expertise in developing behavioral interventions to meet the health needs of urban racial/ethnic and immigrant populations (culturally competent services, improved access, health promotion, disease prevention, and early diagnosis and treatment of disease) (11-13); creating minority student training models for those pursuing careers in the health sciences; and long-standing relationship with the community. The Deputy President for the Brooklyn Borough avails her staff, including members of the Communication Department, in particular the policy analysts in education and youth advocacy who offer insight into grant submissions and strategic collaborations. The Borough President's Office has also provided the BHDC an outside venue for community meetings and trainings.

Sharing leadership and resources recognizes the unique leadership, expertise, and accountability that each partner brings to the BHDC. It also demonstrates commitment and buy-in into the BHDC. The BHDC equitable partnership model has resulted in several major accomplishments. For example, the BHDC received support through a P20 funding mechanism from the National Center of Minority Health and Health Disparities (NCMHD) in 2009. Through this funding mechanism, the BHDC has been enabled to renew its commitment to address health disparities by sponsoring training workshops in CBPR for CBO leaders and their staff; host seminars; and educate underrepresented teen minorities about health disparities and community-engaged research. National Heart, Lung, Blood, and Institute funding was obtained for health disparities research training and career development of underrepresented minority (URM) junior faculty.

In addition to the internal leadership, the overall operation of the BHDC is guided with the assistance of two advisory bodies
Since 2006, a Program Advisory Committee (PAC) and Community Advisory Board (CAB) have proffered an overall view of the progress of the BHDC (Figure 1). The members give advice on the vision, direction, and research methods implemented at the BHDC.

The PAC consists of six members who each have extensive experience in working in the areas of health disparities, diverse populations, immigrant health, community outreach, and governance using various approaches including CBPR (14-24). The PAC meets with the BHDC Executive Committee quarterly and offers recommendations on the fiscal direction taken by the Center. Importantly, the PAC also handles any disputes between the principal investigators that fail to reach a consensual solution.

Considering that the main goal of the BHDC is to reduce health disparities, community-based organizations (CBOs) that either deliver health and social services or specialize in ameliorating social determinants of health (e.g., food access and racism) to residents in Brooklyn were recruited to participate on the CAB. The fourteen CBOs on the CAB were also recruited to reflect the ethnic/cultural diversity of Brooklyn (e.g., African-Americans, Caribbean-Americans, Arab-Americans, Latinos, and White-Americans). The CBOs were identified through existing partnerships with the AAIUH and by recommendations from the Brooklyn Borough President's Office. The CAB convenes with the BHDC executive committee at least quarterly. Given the CAB members close connection with the Brooklyn community, the CAB has been able to assist in providing advice about the research projects, especially the cultural framing of the interventions, delivery of health messages to their constituents, and assist in recruiting additional community partners to participate in the health initiatives sponsored by the BHDC. The CAB members, in addition to the AAIUH staff, voice community concerns and are considered partners in the BHDC. Memorandum of understanding (MOU) were created to designate the roles, duties, and commitment of the partnership at each stage of the developmental process.

Over the years, the PAC and CAB have made significant contributions, including providing input and feedback on the construction of a logic model and synthesis of a *Research and Policy Agenda*. Creating the logic model was an opportunity for the CAB members to offer suggestions for the direction of the BHDC and to learn about this technique, as most of the CAB members were not familiar with this technique. The *Research and Policy Agenda* details high-priority health concerns identified by our CAB members through an iterative process involving the Delphi Survey. These activities enabled the BHDC to be responsive to our community and refine previous hypotheses. For example, the identification of the health concerns in Brooklyn resulted in the expansion of the research goals of the BHDC to include HIV in addition to cardiovascular diseases as an area of interest. The information gleaned from this initiative is being utilized in guiding grant submissions and project development.

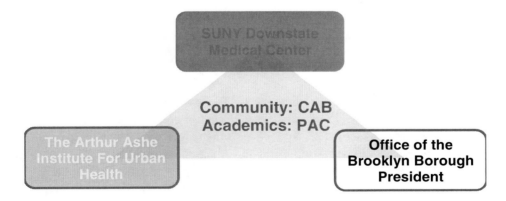

Figure 1. The Brooklyn Health Disparities Center (BHDC) is a multi-disciplinary partnership between an academic (State University of New York Downstate Medical Center), community-based (Arthur Ashe Institute for Urban Health), and a government entity (Office of the Brooklyn Borough President). CAB = Community Advisory Board; PAC = Program Advisory Committee.

Principle #2: Enhance community capacity to engage in research

BHDC is actively encouraging the use of community oriented participatory approaches by conducting capacity building targeted to faculty at SUNY Downstate and community members in Brooklyn. Specifically, capacity building at the BHDC was implemented through raising awareness about health disparities, executing CBPR training workshops, and aiding CBOs in preliminary data collection by focusing on aspects of community capacity, such as community participation, leadership, skills, resources, sense of community, and community values (9). These particular activities were implemented in order to build on community strengths, and enable our community members to be equitable partners in data collection, interpretation, and other aspects.

First, an emphasis was made on increasing the awareness and understanding of health disparities among academics

Although there is active health disparities research at SUNY Downstate, we held several events in order to enhance the knowledge of faculty, staff, and students about minority health, health disparities, and cultural competency. Moreover, these events were a means to inform the research community at SUNY on the utility and expertise of corroborating with community members to conduct research. A summit was organized in 2004 entitled "Bridging Healthcare Disparities: Getting Healthy and Living Well in the Black Community." Between 2005 and 2006 a monthly health disparities seminar series and a cultural competency curriculum regarding clinical education was presented monthly university-wide. The seminar series was punctuated by two annual events: a Health Disparities Symposium and a summer program for minority junior investigators (i.e., "Program to Increase Diversity among Individuals Engaged in Health-Related Research"). Attendance in the series was broad, and included medical residents, students, and faculty in all disciplines. Other activities included community forums and town hall meetings, such as: "Taking Action Against Cardiovascular Disease in Communities: A Training for Service Providers" and "Eliminating Disparities in Cardiovascular Care and Outcomes: Best Practices".

In collaboration with our CAB members, a bi-annual workshop was hosted in 2010 and 2011 to encourage the use of CBPR

The purpose of the workshops was to build the capacity of our community partners and SUNY researchers to engage in CBPR through co-learning. Two community leaders from twenty-two CBOs in Brooklyn, including the CAB members, were invited to attend four CBPR training workshops. SUNY researchers within the Public Health School and Medical Department were also invited. The first two workshops were designed to educate the participants on concepts relevant to CBPR including: "Program Evaluation", "Building Strategic Partnerships", "Policy and Advocacy using Evidence-Based Research", and "Research Methodology and Granting Writing". The next two workshops covered topical issues and methodologies intended to further elucidate CBPR, such as social determinants of health and power mapping. Another important feature of the workshops involved multiple CAB members presenting with their academic or government partner on a previously implemented CBPR project that they had conducted. The activities informed and empowered community and academic partners about the steps involved in conducting CBPR and the importance of developing trust and equitable partnerships. It was also a training opportunity for some of the staff affiliated with the BHDC. From the workshops, the majority of community members learned new skills related to CBPR that they could use in the future (84%) and that could assist them in developing collaborations with academics to pursue CBPR partnerships.

Community capacity building was also been actively sought through training a summer internship for high school students
In 2010 and 2011, the BHDC executed a four-week summer program to train a total of 80 underrepresented minority high school students in Brooklyn about health disparities through course work and a practicum experience. The practicum provided an opportunity to strengthen community capacity to engage in CBPR as it enabled the CBOs to gather preliminary data that could be used for future research projects. The interns assisted the CBOs with either a literature view; geographic mapping of diseases and/or resources; survey design and implementation; or focus groups/in-depth interviews for three days a week during the afternoon. A total of seventeen different CBOs participated, including organizations affiliated with the CAB, in 2010 and 2011. Each CBO hosted on average 2 students. Training high school students in CBPR has helped multiply the effectiveness of the BHDC in achieving community cohesion, increasing the potential for CBPR projects to be initiated, and assisting young students in their quest for higher education in research and medicine. Over 70% of the participating CBOs as indicated in a post-survey evaluation were able to use information from the summer projects to advance their work. For instance, preliminary data gathered by interns at the Arab-American Family Support Center was used to submit a CBPR grant proposal spearheaded by the AAFSC and a BHDC Post-doctorate fellow. Data collected by interns at Make the Roads New York (MRNY) assisted the organization in preparing a publication "Rx for Safety" as part of their pharmacy campaign to include translations on prescription medication (25). In collaboration with staff from the BHDC, the data was also incorporated into a community-engaged grant proposal submission to the Sociological Initiative Foundation. Diaspora Community Services plans to use information from a needs assessment to provide comprehensive sexual health services to neighborhood adolescents, create a community plan, and apply for future funding.

Principle #3: Building and sustaining trust with community-based organizations

As a part of building community capacity, trust needs to be continually garnered. Over the years, the BHDC has built trust in the community and within the partners by sharing leadership with community leaders, capacity building at the academic and community level, and recognizing the expertise and richness of the community as described in Principles #1 and #2. Specifically, trust is has been fostered between AAIUH, SUNY Downstate, Brooklyn Borough President's Office, CAB and PAC members, and the wider Brooklyn community through on-going involvement in the activities sponsored by each of these groups.

Staff of the BHDC have joined coalitions, attended outreach events, co-sponsored events, participated in grant submissions, and disseminated information about CBO sponsored events to others. For example, the Post-Doctoral Fellow at the BHDC is a member of the Brooklyn Partnership to Drive Down Project Diabetes Coalition sponsored by the Greater Brooklyn

Health Coalition and CAMBA to address the disproportionate high prevalence of type 2 diabetes and obesity in Central and East New York, Brooklyn. The Post-Doctoral fellow contributed to the needs assessment and social media campaign. BHDC provided in-kind support for the Caribbean Health Disparities Summit hosted by one of the CAB organizations. These joint activities have been invaluable in engendering a familiarity/comfort amongst partners, common interests, reciprocity, and co-learning.

INTERMEDIATE OUTCOMES

The aforementioned principles developed and implemented over the past several years have been critical in achieving numerous intermediate outcomes, which will facilitate the development of CBPR projects. These intermediate outcomes include being responsive to the research interests of the community, identifying researchers at SUNY Downstate Medical Center to conduct CBPR, increasing the capacity of CBO leaders and academics to participate in CBPR, and fostering several community-academic collaborations. In addition, the health disparities curriculum for the high school students was integrated into a science and math after-school program, the Health Science Academy located in Brooklyn. Notably, from these activities, the BHDC has established itself as a committed and trusted partner with the community it serves.

Concerning the CBOs, an evaluation was conducted after the two workshops and the summer program by an outside evaluator to provide an overview of the effectiveness of the BHDC in increasing the capacity of community organizations to participate as equitable partners in community-engaged research. The seventeen organizations surveyed strongly agreed that the information provided over the years increased their knowledge of community health issues and will use the newfound knowledge and skills to bring about change in the community (Figure 2). In addition, the CBOs overwhelming expressed a willingness and freedom to speak openly and honestly at the BHDC meetings; bring up new ideas; and have a sense of ownership in the BHDC accomplishments.

Lessons learned

Several valuable lessons were gleaned during this formative process. These lessons revolved around partnership development, capacity building, and establishing/maintaining trust.

Partnerships
In order to continue strengthening relationships among the partners and the community members it is pertinent to have flexibility in terms of the issues and objectives that the partners want to concentrate on because these priorities may change over time. Through regularly scheduled evaluation and tracking efforts we were able to accomplish this. Moreover, changes in the focus of the partners may lead to changes in the financial plans. Thus, the budget and other resources should be adjustable in order to allow for these unexpected changes.

Although BHDC hosted various seminars and workshops to endorse the use of CBPR by our academic partners, and several CBPR projects have ensued, more work is needed to integrate our academic partners. Our academic partners communicated interest in using the CBPR approach, but expressed that they had too many competing interests and obligations. In order to facilitate their engagement on CBPR projects, faculty members were invited to be Co-Investigators on several community-engaged grant applications written by investigators affiliated with the BHDC. In addition, the BHDC submitted a federal grant to prepare URM junior faculty in CBPR through a didactical and practicum experience.

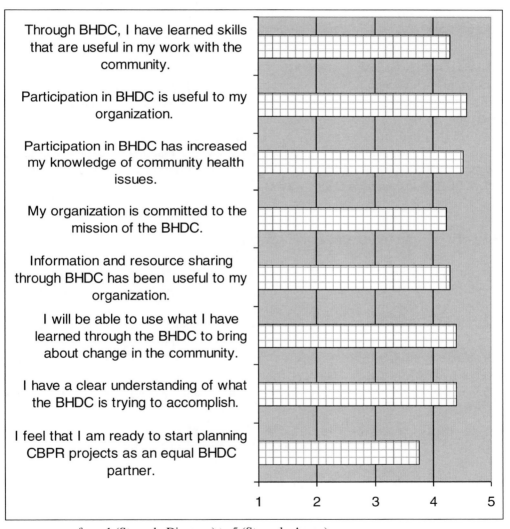

Responses range from 1 (Strongly Disagree) to 5 (Strongly Agree).

Figure 2. Mean responses concerning knowledge, commitment, and research skills among community-based organization leaders who have collaborated with the Brooklyn Health Disparities Center, New York, New York (n=17).

Capacity building

The amount of time required to adequately cover the CBPR material at the training workshops was a concern. Considering that CBOs are overtaxed, the workshops were designed to be only half-a-day. As a result, numerous topics were covered in a short amount of time. Attendees at the workshops thought this was cumbersome and suggested that more than two half-day workshops should be offered per year or that the workshops be extended by several hours. Also, the PAC advised that the center build a groundswell of local advocates to embrace our shared agenda and use this influence to leverage greater institutional support.

Some of the initial activities at the BHDC have diminished, such as the seminar series. While the seminars are less frequent, the information from the seminars have been integrated into the curriculum for the URM junior faculty trainees. BHDC staff members are also proactively involved in making oral and poster presentations at SUNY Downstate during campus events, which highlight the work of the BHDC and serves as a means of recruitment.

The relations between BHDC and the CBOs were strengthened because we were able to connect through the common interest of investing in our youth. Combining the workshops and internships programs provided needed data for CBOs while concomitantly exposing the youth to research and additional career opportunities and building trust between partners. Through the workshops and student internships, BHDC has been able to increase the research capacity of CBOs to engage in CBPR with academics.

Trust between partners and community

Despite our best efforts to retain staff and personnel, we have learned over the years that there is a need for a sustainability plan within the BHDC to respond to changes in staffing and other resources. In addition, it is important to recognize that frequent transition in staff occurs within the CBOs. Trust can be maintained by generating a plan whereby newcomers are given an overview of the mission of the BHDC, the history, accomplishments, and objectives at the meetings and/or through reading material. The information can be reinforced by having experienced members reach out and informally speaking with the newcomers. A communication plan will allow relationships to evolve while sustaining trusting relationships.

CONCLUSION

While there are no absolutes in how to proceed in developing CBPR oriented projects, the principles presented have proven to be beneficial in guiding the BHDC during this formative process to develop and maintain a multidisciplinary partnership, educate all partners, and build trust. These activities have taken years to engender and have allowed the development of new community-driven projects that are responsive to the community needs while at the same time addresses issues of importance in clinical practice and health disparities research.

Upcoming funding activities are based on the priorities identified from the community over the upcoming years. Earlier in 2011, the BHDC submitted a national grant to the NIMHD in order to implement interventions focused on reducing HIV and cardiometabolic risk factors (i.e., sleep apnea) among Blacks in Brooklyn using a CBPR approach. In addition, the scope of the grant includes: 1) collaborating with local CBOs to develop their own community-engaged initiatives 2) provide CBPR training and educational opportunities to high school, undergraduate, and master's students with CBO leaders as mentors 3) institutionalize conference series on health disparities and CBPR in Brooklyn 4) assess the Center's technical assistance 5) evaluate measures of power and shared decision making and 6) launch evidence-based policy and advocacy initiatives.

These principles should prove useful to other community-academic-government partnerships interested in building the capacity of individuals and CBOs to engage in research as equitable partners in order to improve individual and community health and ultimately reduce health disparities.

ACKNOWLEDGMENTS

We acknowledge the National Center on Minority Health and Health Disparities P20MD005092 for funding these projects. We extend gratitude to the members of our community advisory board and other community based organizations for their participation in the workshops and the BHDC Youth Summer Internship Program. We also acknowledge the support of the program advisory committee and the Brooklyn Health Disparities Center partners: Arthur Ashe Institute for Urban Health, SUNY Downstate Medical Center, and the Office of the Brooklyn Borough President.

REFERENCES

[1]   Harper S, Lynch J, Burris S, Davey Smith G. Trends in the black-white life expectancy gap in the United States, 1983-2003. JAMA 2007;297(11):1224-32.

[2]   Mercer SL, Green LW. Federal funding and support for participatory research in public health and health care. San Francisco: Jossey-Bass, 2008.

[3]   Minkler M, Wallerstein N. Community based participatory research for health. San Francisco: Jossey-Bass, 2003.

[4]   WK Kellogg Foundation Evaluation Handbook. Battle Creek; 1998.

[5]   Israel BA, Schulz AJ, Parker EA, Becker AB. Review of community-based research: assessing partnership approaches to improve public health. Annu Rev Public Health 1998;19:173-202.

[6]   Lindenmeyer A, Hearnshaw H, Sturt J, Ormerod R, Aitchison G. Assessment of the benefits of user involvement in health research from the Warwick Diabetes Care Research User Group: a qualitative case study. Health Expect 2007;10(3):268-77.

[7]   Sung NS, Crowley WF, Jr., Genel M, Salber P, Sandy L, Sherwood LM, et al. Central challenges facing the national clinical research enterprise. JAMA 2003;289(10):1278-87.

[8]   Macaulay AC, Commanda LE, Freeman WL, Gibson N, McCabe ML, Robbins CM, et al. Participatory research maximises community and lay involvement. North American Primary Care Research Group. BMJ 1999;319(7212):774-8.

[9]   Baker EA, Motton FL. Methods in Community-Based Participatory Research for Health. San Francisco: Jossey-Bass, 2005.

[10]   Ritzel S. Report Card on Brooklyn's Health. In: Center SDM, editor. Brooklyn, 2001.

[11] Brown N, Naman P, Homel P, Fraser-White M, Clare R, Browne R. Assessment of preventive health knowledge and behaviors of African-American and Afro-Caribbean women in urban settings. J Natl Med Assoc 2006;98(10):1644-51.

[12] Browne R, Vaughn NA, Siddiqui N, Brown N, Delmoor E, Randleman P, et al. Community-academic partnerships: lessons learned from replicating a salon-based health education and promotion program. Prog Community Health Partnersh 2009;3(3):241-8.

[13] Wilson TE, Fraser-White M, Feldman J, Homel P, Wright S, King G, et al. Hair salon stylists as breast cancer prevention lay health advisors for African American and Afro-Caribbean women. J Health Care Poor Underserved 2008;19(1):216-26.

[14] Andrulis DP. Community, service, and policy strategies to improve health care access in the changing urban environment. Am J Public Health 2000;90(6):858-62.

[15] Andrulis DP. Moving beyond the status quo in reducing racial and ethnic disparities in children's health. Public Health Rep 2005;120(4):370-7.

[16] Andrulis DP, Brach C. Integrating literacy, culture, and language to improve health care quality for diverse populations. Am J Health Behav 2007;31 Suppl 1:S122-33.

[17] Andrulis DP, Siddiqui NJ, Gantner JL. Preparing racially and ethnically diverse communities for public health emergencies. Health Aff (Millwood) 2007;26(5):1269-79.

[18] Bayne-Smith M, Fardy PS, Azzollini A, Magel J, Schmitz KH, Agin D. Improvements in heart health behaviors and reduction in coronary artery disease risk factors in urban teenaged girls through a school-based intervention: the PATH program. Am J Public Health 2004;94(9):1538-43.

[19] Mays GP, Hesketh HA, Ammerman AS, Stockmyer CK, Johnson TL, Bayne-Smith M. Integrating preventive health services within community health centers: lessons from WISEWOMAN. J Womens Health (Larchmt) 2004;13(5):607-15.

[20] Gany F, Dobslaw R, Ramirez J, Tonda J, Lobach I, Leng J. Mexican urban occupational health in the US: a population at risk. J Community Health 2011;36(2): 175-9.

[21] Gany FM, Gonzalez CJ, Basu G, Hasan A, Mukherjee D, Datta M, et al. Reducing clinical errors in cancer education: interpreter training. J Cancer Educ 2010;25(4):560-4.

[22] Gany F, Trinh-Shevrin C, Aragones A. Cancer screening and Haitian immigrants: the primary care provider factor. J Immigr Minor Health 2008;10(3): 255-61.

[23] Gany FM, Shah SM, Changrani J. New York City's immigrant minorities. Reducing cancer health disparities. Cancer 2006;107(8 Suppl):2071-81.

[24] Gany FM, Herrera AP, Avallone M, Changrani J. Attitudes, knowledge, and health-seeking behaviors of five immigrant minority communities in the prevention and screening of cancer: a focus group approach. Ethn Health 2006;11(1):19-39.

[25] Rx for Safety: Establishing Standards for Clear and Accessible Prescription Medication. New York City: Make the Road; 2011.

Submitted: January 02, 2012. *Revised:* February 01, 2012. *Accepted:* February 03, 2012.

In: Public Health Yearbook 2013
Editor: Joav Merrick
ISBN: 978-1-63321-095-0
© 2014 Nova Science Publishers, Inc.

Chapter 2

LEARNING TO USE TENSION TO CREATE SUSTAINABLE PARTNERSHIPS FOR RESPONSIVE POLICY AND PRACTICE IN THE HEALTH SECTOR

Dianne McCormack, RN, PhD*,
Dawn Marie Buck, BSc, MHSc
and Bonnie McGraw, RN, BN

Department of Nursing and Health Sciences, University of New Brunswick, Saint John, New Brunswick, Extra-Mural Program/Community Health Centres, Horizon Health New Brunswick, Saint John, New Brunswick and Community Development, St. Joseph's Community Health Centre, Saint John, New Brunswick, Canada

ABSTRACT

Partnership development between universities and communities is gaining support through multi-partner funding initiatives, interprofessional education, and expanded practice teams. University and community partnerships combine scientific knowledge often based in academia and community wisdom grounded in community relevance to address practical and long term solutions to health issues. One partnership model "Partnership model: Living inventory of engagement" that evolved from a university-community partnership steers diverse partners from multiple disciplines to collaborate in order to address the concerns of citizens. This model links two dominant health models, primary health care and determinants of health, in a conceptual framework. Exemplars that are composites of the lived experience of partners from within the health sector demonstrate the model and the effectiveness of using tension to facilitate the engagement process and solution generation. An environment where partners focus on the work of the partnership and not the environmental context is preferred.

---

* Correspondence: Professor Dianne McCormack, RN, PhD, Department of Nursing and Heath Sciences, University of New Brunswick, POBox 5050, Saint John, New Brunswick, Canada. E-mail: dianne.mccormack@unb.ca.

Keywords: University-community partnerships, partnership model, tension, reciprocal capacity building, health care models

INTRODUCTION

University and community partnerships combine scientific knowledge often based in academia and community wisdom grounded in community relevance to address practical and long term solutions to broad environmental and health issues. Bringing people together from diverse disciplines requires the development of an effective partnership where partners respect, listen, share expertise, and learn from each other. The key to maintaining a partnership is learning to successfully work through the tensions within the engagement process so that all partners are aware of the broader and sometimes different issues partners are addressing within their respective disciplines. Partners are motivated to gain knowledge about the expertise of partners and are challenged to use a multi-perspective lens when considering issues of common interest.

Within the health care sector, there is general acceptance that outcomes for clients improve when stakeholders work in partnership (1). Governments, funding agencies, and professional societies have endorsed initiatives, such as, adopting interprofessional education (2-3), funding multi-partner research (4) and expanding practice teams (5,6).

The purpose of this paper is to describe the utility of a partnership model that evolved from a university-community partnership. The development of this model is described elsewhere (7). In this paper, partnership classifications categories are described, health care delivery models are compared, and the importance of naming, expecting, and using tension is discussed, and the environmental context is explored. When using tension, growth and creativity occurs both within the partnership and for each partner. Tension is defined as a strain that generates differences amongst partners; presenting an opportunity for partners to engage in reciprocal learning. When tension is embraced and not perceived negatively as conflict or a barrier to overcome, partners are challenged to think differently and to move toward continued growth and development. Partners are encouraged to venture outside their "comfort zones" to a new space where creative and effective solutions are found. Exemplars that are amalgamated composites of the lived experiences of the authors demonstrate that tension is a positive concept in the engagement process.

Partnership classification categories

There are many adjectives that describe the attributes or the specific expectations that define a particular partnership. To prevent any language blurring that could potentially create misunderstanding, partnership attributes are classified into categories and exemplars are used to demonstrate the defining elements of each category. When partners from many disciplines collaborate, language clarity sets the stage for mutual understanding.

In intradisciplinary - also named unidisciplinary or intraprofessional - members share the same discipline and may have similar values and philosophies even though they may have diverse skills and expertise (8,9).

For example, three nurses who work at a Community Health Centre have the common focus of promoting health for all clients who live in a predominately low socioeconomic environment. One nurse may specialize in issues of chronic disease and computer literacy; another may have a specialized interest in diabetes; while another may be involved in school health with a special interest in promoting the health of all children living with chronic illnesses.

Even though the common threads of chronic illness and compromised living environments underlie each of their interests, each nurse has a specific skill set and brings a unique perspective to the intradiscipline team goal of addressing the health concerns of community clients. The collaboration between these three nurses is grounded in a primary health care philosophy with a health determinant lens that emphasizes safety and security, and access to accurate and timely health information.

In pluridisciplinary partnerships, members from different disciplines practice their profession independently (8). In some situations, partners may even share the same physical space. However, there is no sharing of goals even though partners may see the same clients or may consult the expertise of the other without any commitment to apply the wisdom gained. For example, Community Health Centre staff, possibly including a nurse, social worker, and occupational therapist, and case workers from the Department of Social Development (Income Assistance) may provide services and guidance to the same client but never meet to problem solve with the client or even communicate insights gleaned or progress achieved with each other.

Multidisciplinary partners come from different disciplines and function independently but share a common goal (8-10). For example, a community may come together to offer a breakfast program for children - spiritual leaders may contribute food, school staff may offer physical space, while nutritionists may develop well balanced menus. All of these activities are conducted independently but a common goal to ensure a healthy breakfast for children is realized.

Interdisciplinary or interprofessional partners represent different disciplines but pursue a common goal or purpose together; perspectives are shared, common understanding between partners is reached, symmetry of power is nurtured, and shared decision-making is maintained (8,9). For example; a teacher, nurse, police officer, business owner, and librarian come together to conduct a community health needs assessment based on the determinants of health framework. The community owns the data and through town hall meetings concerns are prioritized and action plans are developed – everyone is invited to participate and every person gains.

Another example is reflected in the coming together of officials from all three levels (municipal, provincial, national) of government, community members, business leaders, city police, and Community Health Centre staff to address the common purpose and daunting task of reducing poverty. This team sets out to build awareness of the depth and scope of poverty in the city, to engage community members experiencing poverty so that the lived experience of poverty can be understood, and to build individual and community capacity using a social justice approach to ensure a "hand-up" approach to realizing equity.

PARTNERSHIP CHALLENGES WITHIN THE HEALTH SECTOR

The notion of partnering is accepted and expected within health care teams who provide care, conduct research, or develop education programs Despite this emerging climate of defining, describing, and initiating partnerships within the health care sector, complications arise from work organization disconnect, work culture diversity, and differences in perspectives and ideologies. Yet models of care that integrate the concept of partnership as depicted in the Primary Health Care Model and the Determinants of Health Model receive limited attention, while the dominant model of care, the Biomedical Model, presents limited opportunity for partnership and at the very best supports the development of multidisciplinary partnership. Reviewing the conceptual basis of these models of care will reveal that the acceptance of the biomedical model as the dominant model makes tension an expected ingredient within health care partnerships.

Biomedical model

The philosophical underpinnings of the biomedical model are grounded in scientific principles explicated by Descartes in the 17th century (11,12). This way of thinking creates a reductionist view of the world; reducing complex phenomena such as the human body to its simplest parts (11-14). By examining the physical indicators of diagnostic tests and observations, diagnoses are made and subsequently treated using accepted protocols (15-17). Through medical intervention, the body's physiological functioning is restored. The focus of care within this model is confined to the physical aspect of the body and is orchestrated by collecting information so that the source of the problem can be identified and treated or fixed (11,15,18,19).

Within the biomedical model, curing dominates all other actions (20) and health problems are viewed in the context of pathology (12,14,21-26). There is an underlying assumption that each health problem or challenge has a specific cause that can be discovered and treated using specialized regimens (11,12,22-23). Health care providers are the experts in health care and they develop the goals and direct the treatment plan (21,23). Health care recipients are expected to comply with the treatment plan (23).

According to Raphael, Bryant and Rioux (27): "Governmental, public, and the media's concerns are firmly entrenched within a medical model of health whereby the body is a machine that is either running well or in need of repair....The allocation of government spending to the health care system, research activities, and disease foundations reflects this commitment to the medical model" (p113). Despite this persistent endorsement of the biomedical model, at the beginning of the 21st century, this model is viewed "increasingly as incompetent and deficient" (11). Because the narrow focus of the model limits the efficacy with which the model can address health issues such as chronic illnesses and diverse life stressors (14,19,28-31), a living paradox has been developed for partners within the health care sector. This situation is further compounded by more informed health care recipients who are taking an interest in being active, rather than passive, partners in health care (11,32).

Primary health care model

The World Health Organization (WHO)(40) defined primary health care as:

> ...essential health care based on practical scientifically sound and socially acceptable methods and technology made universally accessible to individuals and families in the community through their full participation and at a cost the community and the country can afford to maintain at every stage of their development in the spirit of self-reliance and self-determination.

Inherent within this definition of primary health care are five guiding principles that must be implemented simultaneously (34,35). These principles delineate the attributes of this model of health and direct the actions of health care providers and clients. Each principle has equal importance; the order in which the principles are discussed is irrelevant.

The principle of essential health care includes promotive, preventive, curative, rehabilitative, and supportive health services (33), developing appropriate community resources to reflect the needs of community members. Another principle, accessibility, is defined by the WHO (33) as having health care "geographically, financially, culturally and functionally within easy reach of the whole community" (p58). This principle specifies that citizens must have access to services or resources that can be used to promote health. The principle of socially acceptable, scientifically sound and affordable delivery methods and technology "directs that methods, techniques and equipment be scientifically proven, be in keeping with the accepted cultural values of the community, be affordable, and be able to address adequately a known health challenge" (34). This principle dictates that efficiency and effectiveness of interventions be assessed.

Key to the success of primary health care is the principle of full community participation (35). Clients are active partners in care. Health care providers are consultants who enable clients to promote their health to a higher level. This way of working with citizens is quite a power shift from the previous way of working together within the biomedical model (32,35,37). The principle of intersectoral collaboration extends full community participation to include involvement from all sectors in society.

Intersectoral collaboration includes clients, health professionals, economists, politicians, housing experts, social workers, traditional healers and others (35,38). It is inclusive of all persons whose actions influence the health of the population. Within the biomedical model approach to health care, there is evidence of multidisciplinary activity amongst health care providers, but there is minimum involvement of clients and the involvement of people from sectors outside of health is random.

Extensive changes are required within the infrastructure of the health care system so that acceptable communication channels can be developed and a team effort legitimized. The primary health care model embraces inclusiveness and places the responsibility of health on the agenda of all sectors as well as individual citizens (33-35,37,39-44).

Determinants of health model

In the determinants of health model, all psychosocial risk factors and socioeconomic risk conditions are considered when determining health status (27,45-47). The socioeconomic conditions provide the context for personal health factors to be developed or be constrained. Key health determinants include; income and social status, social support networks, education, employment and working conditions, physical environments, biology and genetic endowment, personal health practices and coping skills, healthy child development, health services, gender, cultural, and social environment (27,45,46,48-50). These factors do not influence health in isolation but are interconnected and when combined create an overall influence on health (46,51-54).

The success of the determinants of health model is dependent upon collaboration between and within sectors (45,55). Health care providers are responsible for assessing the health needs of citizens, making appropriate referrals, and engaging in advocacy, but the political will of the country must embrace collaborative teams if partnering between sectors is an expected goal (56). Interestingly, collaboration between sectors is identified as one of the five principles of the primary health care model. Having all stakeholders investing in the health of the nation is likely to create improved health status. Therefore, it is imperative that networks be developed to enable the sharing of ideas and resources across sectors. Maintaining the integrity of the sector and even disciplines within the sector must be assured if the blending or sharing of resources is to be accepted (57-59). The intersectoral approach to working together suggests that all policies are health policies and all human activity contributes to health (18,27,37).

In summary, health care providers may approach partnership from any one of the models described above with most entering the partnership with a distinct hybrid model developed from adopting aspects of each model. In this environment of pluralistic models, diversity reigns. Generally, when diversity is embraced, understanding and decision making is enhanced and partnerships are positioned to develop creative answers to complex problems. However, the overwhelming acceptance of the biomedical model facilitates the adoption of group think or the acknowledgment that conflict must be resolved whereby creative energy is diminished and an environment that harbors tension is created. The challenge is to discover a process that embraces tensions so that responsive practice and policy is engendered. A Partnership Model: Living Inventory of Engagement was developed to answer this challenge (7).

A PARTNERSHIP MODEL: LIVING INVENTORY OF ENGAGEMENT

The Partnership Model: Living Inventory of Engagement is grounded in the philosophy of primary health care but incorporates a determinant of health lens. The tenets of the model embrace social justice including equal access, partnership participation, shared power, effective communication, intersectoral collaboration, and being responsive to the essential needs of the community (7). Using the analogy of a house to describe the Partnership Model:

Living Inventory of Engagement, the primary health care model is the foundation of the house and the determinants of health model describes the different rooms within the house.

This Partnership Model: Living Inventory of Engagement takes on the shape of a spiral where lessons learned are carried forward and influence the next turn in the spiral (7). Because feedback is expected and anticipated at all points in the spiral, new members can enter into the spiral at any time. Therefore, the partnership is continually open to new ideas, members, questions, or resources. Ideally, the needs of the partners are aligned with the needs of the whole community and unanswered questions fuel and sustain the partnership while new ideas are expected, invited, and encouraged.

Partnerships are cultivated through developing trust, building confidence, demonstrating mutual respect, ensuring equal opportunity, and so on (7). The intentions, expertise, and expected rewards of each partner are understood. Generally, partners enter into a partnership when goals or questions requiring solutions indicate that diverse knowledge and skills are needed, making the uniqueness each partner brings to the partnership an asset. In all likelihood this diversity will also create tension for the partners. The continued development of the partnership is spurred through using this tension while being attentive to reciprocal capacity building so that each partner gains from being actively involved in the partnership.

Tension and partnership

When individuals with unique strengths and assets engage in therapeutic, professional, or social interactions, tension should be expected. Partners, then, have two options, 'use tension or 'avoid tension'. The following exemplars illustrate the benefits of using the Partnership Model: Living Inventory of Engagement. One exemplar demonstrates that partners who use tension are successful in addressing partnership goals; while another exemplar reveals a situation where tension is not used and opportunities to generate solutions are missed.

Use tension

Learning to use tension requires consistent partners who are committed to using a team approach to pursue a common goal, are issue focused, and are interested in making communication open and transparent (7). Paying attention to building trust and mutual respect, utilizing partner expertise to move the partners toward reciprocal capacity building, and desiring a positive change through social action, guide the partners through the tension (7).

Exemplar grounded in experiential knowing. Health providers at a Community Health Centre were called to action when it became clear that some individuals accessing health care service at the Community Health Centre could not manage their diabetes because of financial matters. Government policy that responded to this need was very restrictive and many individuals were falling through the cracks. Even though the Community Health Centre had experts who gather community wisdom through community development, other partners with expertise in policy development, poverty, and diabetes management were sought. See figure 1. Nine partners, representing different organizations and/or programs, were invited by health care providers from the Community Health Centre to a meeting to discuss this issue.

Even though different disciplines from different organizations were represented, all supported the goal: To identify an avenue to influence government policy. An interdisciplinary or interprofessional partnership was in the making.

Each community partner brought different expertise to the discussions. The combined wisdom generated multiple perspectives and knowledge was gained from the diverse experience within the partnership. The complexity of the issue unfolded through shared knowledge and reciprocal learning. The new knowledge gained enabled partners to construct the problem so that defining attributes of the problem were specific to the needs of clients and described the barriers that emerged when clients attempted to manage their diabetes while living in financial distress. Even though partners were diverse, the common philosophical belief in social justice and willingness to activate the role of advocacy was identified. Government policy was not responsive to the needs of those individuals who experience diabetes and financial hardships. Many of these citizens, particularly the working poor, were excluded by the current policy.

Valuing reciprocal learning and using open communication strengthened the partnership and enhanced the practice of all partners. To identify possible action steps, a brain storming exercise was conducted.

All members were expected to openly express their ideas and to ask questions. Questions concerning effective communication strategies and responsibilities for advocacy were discussed. Open communication allowed partners to feel less frustrated and more action orientated.

To ensure equal opportunity to participate, a number of meetings were teleconferenced to a distant site and communication was enhanced by maintaining and circulating minutes. The idea of partnering in order to advocate for more responsive policy was empowering for the partners which led to new knowledge being generated.

Ideas for policy alternatives and raising public awareness were defined. The partners selected to raise awareness about this issue through a letter writing campaign, a production of a video, and arranging to hold meetings with members of the legislature. There was a unified voice concerning the action plan but tension surfaced when senior management of the regional health authority joined the partnership and questioned the authority of the partnership to raise this matter directly with government. This response created tension for the newly developed partnership and challenged partner commitment to the project.

The tension arose from the need to allocate more time and resources in order to respond to the concerns raised by the new partner. New questions were generated. Were there others methods for partners to advocate for diabetic clients experiencing financial hardship? Could the partners work with senior management to discuss alternative communication strategies? Was more knowledge required to inform senior management of the issue?

Even though some partners were uncomfortable addressing this issue with senior management, it was decided that the tension could best be addressed by inviting senior management to a meeting to discuss different perspectives. The open discussion resulted in reciprocal learning. The partnership gained a better understanding of the problem and the importance of using appropriate channels of communication. Together, the partners gained better appreciation of the need to give voice to, and advocate for, a client group who were not having their health concerns addressed. Multiple presentations addressing this issue were made to the hospital board, to Members of the Legislative Assembly, and at a regional meeting of the Canadian Diabetes Association.

By working through the tension a positive outcome was realized. A partner from this interdisciplinary partnership was invited by government to sit on a newly formed Government Task Force on Diabetes - new responsive policy is in the making and reciprocal capacity building is continuing. Using tension strengthened the partnership and moved the partners towards the achievement of their goals.

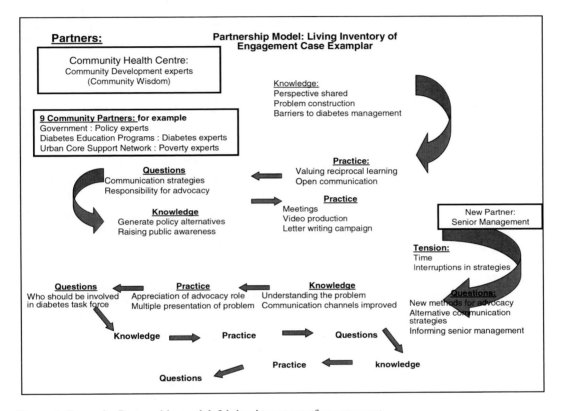

Figure 1. Example: Partnership model: Living inventory of engagement.

Avoid tension

Although working though tension to achieve a common goal has many benefits for developing improved and relevant programs and policies, partners may decide to avoid tension; choosing not to invest time and energy in examining the causes of tension. Subsequently, the source of the tension is not addressed even though partners may continue to pursue the common goal of the partnership.

This avoidance of tension can result in being stuck and unable to move towards more collaborative programs in practice or more relevant policies. This inaction protects the status quo which might be the hidden goal for some partners; allowing them to continue with existing services and protocols rather than examining and responding to the changing needs of clients. The partnership is likely to be challenged further when existing programs are provincially mandated. The appealing smooth road of continuing the same practice or supporting the current policy appears more promising than taking the more challenging bumpy roads of changing practices and policies to respond to client and community needs.

Exemplar grounded in experiential knowing. A high school principal asked community health care providers to develop a coordinated comprehensive program to address the physical, mental, and emotional health needs of students. This request brought health care providers from many disciplines together. Service delivery mechanisms currently employed, roles of individual health care providers, mandates endorsed by the health care providers involved, and communication processes were challenged. Tension was experienced as differences concerning confidentiality, student and parental consents, shared documentation and assessment tools, overlapping roles and responsibilities, and physical location of service delivery arose. These tensions created obstacles as the interdisciplinary partnership was developing. Some of the partners chose to avoid the tension and present support for current practice; enabling these partners to dismiss the request from the school principal and defend the status quo - a mandated service delivery model for all high schools.

The principal, however, was not easily deterred by provincial health department mandates and policies and refused to give up on the idea of providing coordinated primary health care services for students. The school had one goal: To improve health services for students. The school team aligned themselves with other stakeholders who might have interest in promoting the health of high school students. The principal and guidance counselor presented the goal to the Parent Student Support Council and to regional family physicians. These stakeholders supported the identified goal. The principal and his team were encouraged by the positive response.

For some health sector partners, this support from other partners and a focus on student health issues helped them to invest time in addressing the tensions. Other potential health sector partners continued to struggle with the idea of changing current practice and continued to avoid the tension.

The next strategy utilized by the principal and his team focused on identifying physical space that was neutral for all health providers. Because the high school was selected for all meetings, the workplaces of health providers who were promoting the maintenance of independent silos rather than collaborative practice was avoided. This strategy highlighted that physical location had the potential to create a positive environment for partners to begin collaboration. However, tensions continued to be avoided and some partners insisted on maintaining departmental mandates; making the development of communication processes haphazard and the goal for coordinated health services for students unattainable.

The tension created from differences regarding shared charting and universal student consent were not addressed and continued to undermine the work of the partnership. The traditional communication pattern of referral was continued, reciprocal capacity building was avoided, and policy remained only partially responsive to the needs of students. Tensions between partners resulted in coalitions being built around two factions – one wanting to be more responsive to student health needs, the other, supporting the status quo.

This lack of collaboration between partners caused conflict. Partners spent time and energy "putting out fires" while the underlying reasons for the tension were avoided. This inaction resulted in increased tensions at personal, professional, and organizational levels. Even partners from other sectors including education, justice, and social services did not understand why coordinated health care and communication patterns were not being improved for students. All interested stakeholders and potential partners had become immobilized by the tensions.

Clearly, having a strong champion but avoiding tension resulted in unresponsive stagnated policies continuing and the development of interdisciplinary partnerships to improve student access to evidence based health practice did not happen. The best choice for collaborative action remained limited to multidiscipline partnerships that were protected by restrictive policies and supported by the status quo. The optimal goal of coordinated student health services was not achieved. This approach to avoid tension was not helpful and would not be supported if the partnership had been guided by the previously described Partnership Model: Living Inventory of Engagement.

THE ENVIRONMENTAL CONTEXT OF PARTNERSHIPS

The environmental context in which the partnership develops has the potential to nurture the partnership or hinder its development. Although environmental conditions often fuel tension and partners implementing the Partnership Model: Living Inventory of Engagement benefit from the reciprocal learning generated from tension, the purpose of the partnership gets lost when partners are required to repeatedly focus on environmental conditions. Therefore, an environment where partners focus on the work of the partnership and not the environmental context is preferred. Developing partnerships need to pay particular attention to physical space, and work organization including time, work flexibility, and funding in the formative stage of the partnership. Each of these environmental aspects are interconnected but are described separately.

Physical space

Partners need to develop a sense of belonging that goes beyond being committed to a common goal. The need to feel at ease fosters one's ability to participate. Therefore, community practice environments need to be located in a space where the more vulnerable partners feel comfortable. Initially this space may be seen by some partners as inconvenient and unfamiliar. For example, even though business partners may find meeting at a soup kitchen uncomfortable, individuals living in poverty may be immobilized in a board room setting. Accepting discomfort for business partners might create a positive environment for adding the experienced voice of citizens who live in poverty. Community settings such as schools and community centres have the potential to provide physical space where partners can feel at ease and actively contribute to the partnership.

When programs and partners are asked to share space it is important that there is a philosophical match between the partners. Partners with aligned mandates are likely to benefit from reciprocal capacity building. For example, if mental wellness is a priority of the partnership, offering space to programs addressing mental health concerns is advantageous. Collaboration and teamwork can be enhanced when partners share space and compromised when partners are geographically separated. In the latter situation, communication networks need to be attentive that dialogue processes create reciprocal learning.

Work organization

Time. Partnership development, team building, and collaboration require an investment of time (7). When engaging in community development and advocacy work, reciprocal capacity building is expected, making an investment of time likely. When partners are committed to investing and honoring time, transparency in time obligations, readiness to participate, and expectations that require specific skill sets to complete the work of the partnership make these commitments explicit. Taking the extra time for questions to be raised bring issues to the surface so that partners have an opportunity to identify and address tensions. For that reason, time expectations need to be discussed as the partnership is forming.

As the incidence of chronic disease increases, clients in the health sector will benefit from an investment in time from an interdisciplinary team committed to sharing expertise and being responsive to client need (1). Adding clients to the interdisciplinary team compounds this investment of time. However, responsive practice is enhanced and the benefits of learning from the process are integrated.

Work flexibility

The barriers that may prevent partners from fully participating might be related to the organization of work within individual partner environments. For example, when advocacy is necessary, partners need to not only invest time but also have autonomy or work flexibility to organize work schedules so that the goal of the partnership can be achieved in a timely fashion. Work environments that embrace continuous learning and a culture for social action, enable partners to stretch with a purpose - work outside the box.

Funding

Tensions can develop in health sector partnerships when one partner is seen as well-funded and the other is not. For example, partners from the medical or treatment system have proportionally the greater majority of the funds within the health sector. While partners who work in illness prevention, health promotion, or community development initiatives must submit proposals to gain access to funding or engage in fundraising initiatives. In populations where there is a high incidence of poverty, access to health care services may be compromised due to costs related to childcare, transportation, and medication. These situations may require partners from illness prevention, health promotion, or community development to advocate for changes in fee structures that extend beyond the health sector yet they have limited funding to support this work.

In summary, a responsive environment for offering and developing health services must address space to meet and work together, flexibility in work schedules, adequate funding, and time to journey through the process of partnership engagement. Many services, traditionally available in hospital settings, might benefit from being situated in community spaces where there is greater potential for the active involvement of clients who need access to the service. Active client participation can result in reciprocal capacity building for clients and providers. However, this shift in physical space may generate a number of questions concerning roles, confidentiality, leadership, and so on. For example, providing employment, mental health, and sexual health services within a resource centre for youth creates a one stop shopping choice for youth while providing partnership opportunities for providers. In working with and embracing the ideas of youth, the health and social care professionals reexamine not only the available services but also how services are offered so that more appropriate practice delivery models and relevant policies can emerge. As well, new partners might be leveraged so that new services are created. Even though coordinated health related practices are likely to achieve better outcomes,(1) tremendous tensions are likely to be generated by providers from diverse disciplines. If the Partnership Model: Living Inventory of Engagement is used as a guide, these tensions have the potential to strengthen and further promote the work of the partnership enabling collaborative interdisciplinary team action.

CONCLUSION

Health policy furnishes a template for health services and health funding. This template generally reflects the conceptualization of the health concept within the dominant health model of the day (55,60). The consultative nature of health policy development is dependent on the health model directing the process. In the last half of the 20th century, three health models direct health policy, programs, and services. Each of these models conceptualize partnering differently as do providers who adopt either of these models or a hybrid conceptualization of two or even all three of the models. In view of this situation, health environments are ripe for tension.

The dominant health model that best supports partnering is the primary health care model. This model includes intersectoral partnerships with clients, within a context of social justice. The Partnership Model: Living Inventory of Engagement is grounded in the philosophy of primary health care and is presented as a mechanism to facilitate the collaboration of health care providers. Partners guided by the Partnership Model: Living Inventory of Engagement are expected to connect, to gain an understanding of the diverse perspectives of all partners, and to work together in a nonhierarchical way; valuing and integrating the expertise of each partner into the partnership. Each situation presents an opportunity to understand both the parts and the whole.

Because partners who are guided by the Partnership Model: Living Inventory of Engagement are directed to generate new questions, any essential health care need or health determinant that is significant to the partners may be addressed. The exemplar examining diabetes management while living in financial distress demonstrates the utility of the model.

When partners expend energy to avoid tension, as in the exemplar describing a coordinated comprehensive program to address the physical, mental, and emotional health needs of high school students, the creative energy generated by the tension that could have been applied to the work of the partnership is lost. Instead, energy is directed towards maintaining the status quo that is self-serving and not in the best interest of individuals or the community for which the practice or policy is designed. Because most issues related to health is complex, the usual practice to address each separately culminates in an unsatisfactory response. Citizens experience these issues as an integrated whole or as one entity.

When partners capitalize on the energy created by tension emerging from differences, opportunities are presented to develop responsive policy, engage clients, and create best practices. Partners who accept tensions as opportunities and embrace reciprocal capacity building accept that all partners are important in reaching effective solutions. Together, these partners create an openness to listen, to learn from each other, and to be transformed. Partners grow, learn, and create by building on the expertise that others bring to the partnership, and in the process complex issues are resolved, partnership connections and commitments are strengthened and responsive practice and policies are developed. When partners name or make explicit their gain – new knowledge, skills, and so on - the partners remain engaged and willing to invest in the partnership. When members of the health care sector embrace interdisciplinary partnerships, access will be enhanced as every door will be the right door for clients.

REFERENCES

[1]   Health Council of Canada. Teams in action: primary health care teams for Canadians. 2009. Accessed 2010 Feb 18. URL:http://www.healthcouncilcanada.ca/teamsinaction.pdf

[2]   Canadian Interprofessional Health Collaborative. Interprofessional education and core competencies: literature review 2007. Accessed 2008 June 15. URL:http://www.cihc.ca/resources-files/CIHC_IPE-LitReview_May07.pdf

[3]   Canadian Interprofessional Health Collaborative. Curricula approaches from 20 Health Canada funded IECPCP projects. 2008. Accessed 2008 Dec 10. URL:http://www.cihc.ca/resources-files/CIHC_IPE-LitReview_May07.pdf

[4]   McCaffrey L. The history of the community-university partnership for the study of children, youth, and families. Edmonton, AB: McCaffrey Consult, Health Res Eval, 2007.

[5]   Barrett J, Curran V, Glynn L, Godwin M. CHSRF Synthesis: Interprofessional collaboration and quality primary healthcare. 2007. Accessed 2008 June 10 URL:http://www.chsrf.ca

[6]   Canadian Nurses Association. Interprofessional collaboration. 2005. Accessed 2006 Mar 06. URL:http://www.cna-nurses.ca/CNAdocuments/pdf/publications/PS84_Interprofessional_Collaboration_e.pdf

[7]   McCormack D, Buck D-M, McGraw B. A partnership model evolves from a living inventory of engagement. Can J Nurs Leadersh 2010;23(4):61-80.

[8]   Lessard L, Morin D, Sylvain H. Understanding teams and teamwork. Can Nurse 2008;104(3):12-3.

[9]   MacIntosh J, McCormack D. Partnerships identified within primary health care literature. Int J Nurs Stud 2001;38:547-55.

[10]   Davies L, Ring, L. Building better teams: a toolkit for strengthening teamwork in community health centers. Toronto, ON: Ass of ON Health Centers, 2007.

[11]   Longino CF. Beyond the body: an emerging medical paradigm. Am Demogr 1997;19(12):14-8.

[12]   Shaver JF. A biopsychosocial view of human health. Nurs Outlook 1985;33(4):186-91.

[13]   Black HK. Jake's story: a middle-aged, working-class man's physical and spiritual journey towards death. Qual Health Res 2001;11(3):293-307.

[14]   Sim J. The concept of health. Physiother 1990;76(7):423-8.

[15]   du Pre A. Communicating about health: current issues and perspectives. Toronto, ON: Mayfield Pub, 2000.

[16]   Robertson A. Shifting discourses on health in Canada: from health promotion to population health. Health Promot Int 1998;13(2):155-66.

[17]   Simmons SJ. Health: a concept analysis. Int J Nurs Stud 1989;26(2):155-61.

[18]   Evans RG, Stoddart GL. Producing health, consuming health care. In: Evans RG, Barer ML, Marmor TR. Why are some people healthy and others not? NY: Aldine de Gruyter,1994.

[19]   Glouberman S. Social inequality - Aristotle's insight. Ottawa, ON: Can Policy Res Networks, 2000.

[20]   Strobe M, Schut H. The dual process model of coping with bereavement: rationale and description. Death Stud 1999;23:197-224.

[21]   Davis DR, Jansen GG. Making meaning of alcoholics anonymous for social workers: myths, metaphors, and realities. Social Work 1998; 43(2):169-83.

[22]   Hoke B. Promotive medicine and the phenomenon of health. Arch Environ Health 1968;16:269-78.

[23]   Potash HM. Assessment through the dialectic: the necessary forgotten link. J Pers Assess 1999;72(2): 185-9.

[24]   Treloar LL. People with disabilities - the same, but different: implications for health care practice. J Transcult Nurs 1999;10(4):358-64.

[25]   Tripp-Reimer T. Reconceptualizing the construct of health: Integrating emic and etic perspectives. Res Nurs Health 1984; 7:101-9.

[26]   Wilder M, Fischer S, Brunner A. Development of a questionnaire for quantitative assessment in the field of health and human rights. Soc Sci Med 2002;55:1725-44.

[27]   Raphael D, Bryant T, Rioux M. Staying alive: critical perspectives on health, illness, and health care. Toronto, ON: Can Scholars Press, 2006.

[28]   Helman CG. Limits of biomedical explanation. Lancet 1991;337(8749):1080-84.

[29]   Mann JM. Health and human rights. Br J Med 1996;312(7036):924-5.

[30]   Newbold KB. Problems in search of solutions: health and Canadian Aboriginals. J Commun Health1998;23(1):59-73.

[31]   White MA, Johnstone AS. Recovery from stroke: does rehabilitation counselling have a role to play? Disabil Rehabil 2000; 22(3):140-3.

[32]   McCormack D. An examination of the self-care concept uncovers a direction for healthcare reform. Can J Nurs Leadersh 2003;16(4):48-62.

[33]   World Health Organization. Declaration of Alms-Ata. Geneva: WHO, 1978.

[34]   MacIntosh J, McCormack D. Primary health care: interpreting the concept. Info Nurs 1994;25(1):10-1.

[35]   MacIntosh J, McCormack D. An integrative review illuminates curricular applications of primary health care. J Nurs Educ 2000;39(3):116-23.

[36]   McElmurry BJ, Keeney GB. Primary health care. In: Fitzpatrick JJ, Stevenson JS. Annual review of nursing research. New York: Springer, 1999:241-68.

[37]   Davidson P, MacIntosh J, McCormack D, Jones E. Primary health care: a framework for policy development. Holist Nurs Pract 2002;16(4):65-74.

[38]   Munro M, Gallant M, MacKinnon M, Dell G, Herbert R, MacNutt G et al. The Prince Edward Island conceptual model for nursing: a nursing perspective of primary health care. Can J Nurs Res 2000;32(1):39-55.

[39]   Barnes D, Eribes C, Juarbe T, Nelson M, Proctor S, Sawyer L, et al. Primary health care and primary care: a confusion of philosophies. Nurs Outlook 1995; 43(1):7-16.

[40]   Collado CB. Primary health care: a continuing challenge. Nurs Health Care 1992;13(8):408-13.

[41]   Farley S. The community as partner in primary health care. Nurs Health Care 1993;14(5):244-9.

[42]   Shoultz J, Hatcher PA. Looking beyond primary care to primary health care: an approach to community-based action. Nurs Outlook 1997;45(1):23-6.

[43]   Shoultz J, Hatcher PA, Hurrell M. Growing edges of a new paradigm: the future of nursing in the health of the nation. Nurs Outlook 1992;40(2):57-61.

[44]   Shoultz J, Kooker BM, Sloat AR, Hatcher PA. Four ways to teach primary health care in a changing world. Int Nurs Rev 1998;45(6):187-91.

[45]   Federal, Provincial, and Territorial Advisory Committee on Population Health. Strategies for population health: investing in the health of Canadians. Ottawa, ON: Health Canada, 1994.

[46]   Health Canada, Population and Public Health Branch. The population health template: key elements and actions that define a population health approach. Ottawa, ON: Health Canada, 2001.

[47]   World health Organization. Closing the gap in a generation: health equity through action in the social determinants of health. Geneva: WHO, 2008.

[48]   Health Canada. Towards a common understanding: clarifying the concepts of population health. Ottawa, ON: Health Canada, 1996.

[49]   Public Health Agency of Canada. Health status indicators. 2010. Accessed 2010 Jan 14. URL: http://www.phac-aspc.gc.ca/ph-sp/determinants/determinants2-eng.php#status

[50]   Public Health Association of Canada. What determines health? 2003. Accessed 2003 Oct 24.URL: http://www.phac-aspc.gc.ca/ph-sp/determinants/index-eng.php

[51]   Hamilton N, Bhatti T. Population health promotion: an integrated model of population health and health promotion. Ottawa, ON: Health Canada,1996.

[52]   McKague M, Verhoef M. Understandings of health and its determinants among clients and providers at an urban community health centre. Qual Health Res 2003;13(5):703-17.

[53]   O'Hara P. Social inclusion health indicators: a framework for addressing the social determinants of health. Edmonton, AB: Edmonton Social Planning Council, 2006.

[54]   Richmond CAM. Ross NA. The determinants of First Nation and Inuit health: a critical population health approach. Health Place 2009;15:403-11.

[55]   MacKay L. Changing approaches to health: The history of a federal/provincial/ territorial/advisory committee. Ottawa, ON: Canadian Policy Research Networks, 2001.

[56]   Pender L. The federal role in health promotion: under the radar. In: O'Neill M. Pederson A. Dupere S. Rootman I. Health promotion in Canada. Toronto ON: Can Scholars Press, 2007:92-105

[57]   Anderson JM.. Immigrant women speak of chronic illness: the social construction of the devalued self. J Adv Nurs 1991;16:710-7.

[58]   Boydell KM. Goring P. Morrell-Bellai TL. Narratives of identity: re-presentation of self in people who are homeless. Qual Health Res 2000;10(1):26-38.

[59]   Snow DA. Anderson L. Identity work among the homeless: the verbal and avowal of personal identities. AJS 1987;92:1336-71.

[60]   Kisilevsky S. Groff P. Nicholson C. The health gradient challenge: a new approach to health inequities. Ottawa, ON: Canadian Policy Research Networks, 2000.

Submitted: January 03, 2012. *Revised:* February 01, 2012. *Accepted:* February 03, 2012.

In: Public Health Yearbook 2013
Editor: Joav Merrick

ISBN: 978-1-63321-095-0
© 2014 Nova Science Publishers, Inc.

Chapter 3

LESSONS LEARNED FROM NATIONAL AND INTERNATIONAL IMPLEMENTATIONS OF SAFECARE®

Jenelle R Shanley, PhD*, Megan L Graham, MPH,
John R Lutzker, PhD, Anna Edwards-Gaura, PhD,
Daniel J Whitaker, PhD, and Shannon Self-Brown, PhD
National SafeCare Training and Research Center, Institute of Public Health,
Center for Healthy Development, Georgia State University, Atlanta, Georgia,
United States of America

ABSTRACT

Child abuse and neglect is a persistent public health concern, and wide-spread implementation of evidence-based interventions is needed. Dissemination of evidence-based parent training programs to address child maltreatment is in a nascent stage, however. Some guidance exists on how to approach implementation efforts to build community capacity to address this, but those involved in implementation encounter many challenges. This often requires "thinking on your feet" to address each issue as it occurs and examining the after-effects to ensure the problem has been resolved. SafeCare is an evidence-based program disseminated nationally and internationally. Throughout various SafeCare implementations, a multitude of challenges have occurred and several solutions have been applied. The purpose of this paper is to discuss six emerging themes from lessons learned and the strategies used to address them in building community capacity to address child maltreatment. This paper is intended to serve as guidance for other implementation efforts to minimize challenges and increase effective implementations of evidence-based programs.

Keywords: Implementation, evidence-based program, child maltreatment, SafeCare, parent training

---

* Correspondence: Jenelle R Shanley, PhD, Assistant Professor, Faculty of Institute of Public Health, Center for Healthy Development, Georgia State University, PO Box 3995, Atlanta, GA 30302 United States. E-mail: jshanley@gsu.edu.

INTRODUCTION

Child maltreatment, which includes abuse and neglect, is a major public health concern. In the United States (US) in 2009, the rate of substantiated maltreatment was 10.1 victims per 1,000 children (1). Neglect is the most common form of child maltreatment in the US, with over three-quarters (78%) of cases involving neglect. Child maltreatment disproportionately affects younger children, with one-third of victim cases of maltreatment involving children under age four in 2009 (1).

The US Centers for Disease Control and Prevention recognizes child maltreatment as a public health problem that affects the physical and mental health of children and adults (2). The economic and societal burden associated with child maltreatment is extraordinary, an estimated $100 billion per year in the US (3), which includes judicial, social service, foster care, and medical/mental health costs. Costs are not only immediate, as adverse childhood experiences, such as child maltreatment, are linked to high-risk behaviors in adults such as smoking, drug and alcohol abuse, as well as chronic diseases such as cancer and heart disease, contributing significantly to healthcare and societal costs (4-5). Clearly, early prevention and intervention efforts are needed to circumvent these negative outcomes, and dissemination of evidence-based parent training programs is a vital step towards developing community-based programs to address this significant public health concern.

The good news is that several behavioral parenting programs exist, and have been shown in rigorous trials to reduce child maltreatment (6-8). One such program is SafeCare, an evidence-based program (EBP) for parents with children birth to five years old (9). SafeCare is unique as it addresses three areas associated with child abuse and neglect: parent-child interactions, child health, and home safety. Parents are taught to: 1) increase positive interactions with their children; 2) effectively identify symptoms of childhood illness and make proper health care decisions; and 3) identify and eliminate home safety hazards. Each of the three modules is typically conducted in 6 weekly sessions, resulting in about 18 sessions for program completion. SafeCare is built on the premise that teaching parents and having them practice positive interaction skills and appropriate responses to illness and home hazards will reduce the incidence of child maltreatment.

SafeCare has shown to be an effective parenting intervention for at-risk families and families with substantiated maltreatment. Each SafeCare module has undergone rigorous single-case studies to evaluate the effectiveness of each intervention module (10-13). Further, several clinical trials document the positive short and long-term impact of SafeCare, and its predecessor, Project 12 Ways, on families and reduction of future reports of child maltreatment (7, 14-15). The most significant study to date was a statewide trial in the Oklahoma child welfare system, in which over 2,200 families were followed for an average of six years. In survival analyses, SafeCare reduced the likelihood of child maltreatment recidivism by 26% compared to services as usual (7). Studies are currently underway to broaden SafeCare's reach and reduce training and implementation costs, including establishing a hybrid of SafeCare with Parents As Teachers and utilizing technology enhancements.

With increased demand for SafeCare training, the National SafeCare Training and Research Center (NSTRC) was established in 2007 with funding from the Doris Duke Charitable Foundation. NSTRC's objectives include providing national and international training and implementation of SafeCare, and conducting ongoing research to strengthen its impact on preventing child maltreatment. The SafeCare training program at NSTRC includes three levels of training: home-visitor (provides SafeCare to families), coach (performs fidelity monitoring and support), and trainer (conducts training within the organization). Each SafeCare site must have a coach who conducts routine fidelity monitoring and support of home visitors and receives direct support from NSTRC trainers for the first year of implementation. Sites can opt to establish their own SafeCare Trainers after a minimum of one year of successful implementation to sustain or expand their SafeCare program. This model of implementation is based on the premise that providing local agencies with expertise and capacity to self-sustain SafeCare operations is one way to promote long-term, affordable, and sustainable operations.

As with any EBP, SafeCare training and implementation is a process, not an event. It requires several essential components and key players as implementation moves from exploration to long-term program sustainability. Fixsen and colleagues' literature review describes several drivers of the implementation process (16). This review provides an excellent foundation for structuring implementation processes; however, many challenges will still be encountered. The Kaufman Best Practices project identified several potential barriers to implementing EBPs in child welfare service settings, including funding, willingness of agencies and providers to uptake new EBP, and the disparity between research and clinical practice (17). Many other authors have also identified individual, organization, and systems-level factors that can affect implementation (18-21).

This paper describes several lessons learned in establishing SafeCare nationally and internationally, and what we have done to overcome those challenges. We describe major six themes that have emerged and the strategies used to overcome them in subsequent implementations.

LESSONS LEARNED

Lesson 1-All aboard

Like the adage, "It takes a village to raise a child," it takes a variety of individuals to create a successful implementation. Before implementation begins, NSTRC collaborates with a training agency to determine who will be involved in and impacted by the implementation process. This includes those who will be conducting the service with families as well as individuals who will be supporting them, including administrative staff, supervisors, agency heads, referral sources, and funding agents. Research shows it is necessary to have organizational and systemic buy-in at all levels to support a successful implementation (22).

Prior to the onset of implementation (i.e., before training), NSTRC faculty conduct an orientation to provide a foundational understanding of the program, the goals, the targeted population, and anticipated outcomes. This sets the stage for encouraging investment in the success of the program and a team approach to problem-solving. This initial orientation has been effective for reducing confusion, answering questions about the implementation process, and provide an opportunity for all involved to collaboratively work out anticipated concerns or challenges to a successful implementation.

For example, with a recent SafeCare implementation, we conducted an orientation that involved over 40 individuals, including the 6 trainees. This involved a multitude of professionals from various levels of the organization. A question was raised about how to provide to families resources that are directly related to SafeCare topics (e.g., safety items, first aid kits). NSTRC and site staff discussed past solutions that had been implemented as well as possible new solutions and resources. In the end, trainees and supervisors decided to compile a list of resources with which they would follow-up regarding possible donations of supplies for families.

Another issue that is facilitated by the orientation process is discussion of appropriate referrals. This is best discussed with providers, supervisors and stakeholders responsible for family referrals. Without appropriate referrals, implementation efforts are often disrupted or halted because of insufficient or inappropriate referrals. For example, one SafeCare agency referred families who had significant pressing concerns, such as parental substance abuse, that needed to be addressed prior to initiating SafeCare. By educating referral sources about SafeCare, providers were able to more carefully screen families and provide referrals likely to begin and complete the program. By discussing issues, such as funding, referrals, and unique site concerns, during the orientation phase of implementation, we are able to improve agency's readiness prior to workshop and field training, and as a result minimize problems as providers begin SafeCare with families.

Lesson 2–Start small and slow

Often sites are in a hurry to implement prior to ensuring readiness. This can be for many reasons: eagerness to implement, funding for training that must spent before a particular date, or pressure from the top of their organization. Ideally, training dates should not be set until the readiness process has been thoroughly explored. However, practical realities sometimes dictate otherwise; entities sometimes have funds that must be expended by a certain date or else lost or returned to the funder, and thus the choice is sometimes to proceed with a premature implementation or no implementation. NSTRC works with agencies to maximize implementation benefits while minimizing burdens on agencies, but implementation efforts are frequently impacted by these logistical restraints reducing ideal implementation.

Additionally, sites can often be eager to "go big," by training a large number of providers within their agency. We recommend starting small for several reasons. Starting with a smaller number of trainees allows a site to test how SafeCare implementation will work for their specific agency and to work out issues that arise with referral sources, workload demands, coaching processes, and other issues before expanding an implementation. Problems such as these are much easier to resolve on a small versus a large scale. Starting small may also allow an implementation site to choose 'early adopters' within their agency, or individuals who are interested in and enthusiastic about trying a new model. This maximizes the chances for early successes, which can in turn lead to later successes as early adopters can assist other providers with the model (21). An example of this in a very successful implementation was a county wide rollout of SafeCare in San Diego, CA. To begin the rollout, 12 providers from several agencies were selected to be part of an initial "seed" team that would receive training in SafeCare and begin the implementation process. At the end of the one year period of coaching and support, a few of the top performers from the seed team were selected to be trainers and coaches for other staff and several other San Diego-based agencies. A key to this model working was funding from the United Way of San Diego to train the seed team, and for the seed team to train and support others. This "cascading diffusion" model is being replicated in several California counties with federal funding, and has been used in other implementations as well (23).

Lesson 3-Get it in writing

Documenting details about the implementation process and expectations of providers, support personnel, and agency heads is proving to be an important part of SafeCare implementation. While these verbal encounters with individuals at various levels of the organization are beneficial, confusion frequently arises as the implementation process unfolds, and complementing verbal communication with written communication is necessary.

NSTRC has developed documents that provide an outline of key SafeCare implementation processes. Certification documents highlight requirements for home visitors, coaches, and trainers. Further, there is a wealth of information posted on our website (www.nstrc.org) and flyers are available documenting the implementation process. In addition, NSTRC is now developing documents that highlight roles and expectations of home visitor, coach, trainer, and the agency, which will be discussed and signed prior to workshop training. These documents define each role (e.g., home visitor), the certification process for that role, expectations of an individual in that role, and any limitations present (e.g., home visitors without trainer-training are not able to train others in SafeCare). In addition, an agency agreement details expectations of the agency, as well as what the agency can expect of NSTRC. It is anticipated that this documentation process will clarify responsibilities and reduce confusion for the various individuals involved in the implementation process.

An example of the need for documentation emerged in the early stages of SafeCare implementation with one community agency. Following orientation, it became evident that individuals chosen by the agency to be coaches were confused about their roles as coaches, despite discussions about this during orientation. During workshop and field training it became evident that these trainees had not discussed coaching tasks with their supervisors, and they were concerned about integrating these new responsibilities within their current job duties.

We worked with the coaches and their supervisors to maximize the trainees' acquisition of SafeCare skills while minimizing the burden of the certification process with their extant work activities. With more clear documentation illustrating the duties of coaches, it is possible that this confusion would have been averted.

Lesson 4-Keep close contact

Supporting agencies from the inception to implementation is important for success (24). This involves regular communication between NSTRC and personnel at various levels of the implementation site. Across the implementation process, especially for the first year, NSTRC has routine contact with the training agency. It occurs as two levels: 1) between NSTRC faculty and agency administrators, and 2) between the NSTRC trainers or external SafeCare trainers and trainees, primarily agency coaches (who in turn have contact with the home visitors).

At the onset of implementation, communication between NSTRC faculty and agency administration largely focuses on agency readiness, including referrals, funding streams, and agency capacity to implement SafeCare. This communication tends to abate as implementation progresses and the agency becomes more skilled with SafeCare. Communication between trainers and trainees often focuses on specific implementation concerns and service to families, particularly SafeCare certification, fidelity monitoring, and support. Trainer-trainee conversations occur at several levels. At the onset of implementation, trainers have weekly individual contact with trainees, referred to as coaching sessions. Once a trainee is certified, communication becomes bi-weekly or monthly, with accompanying monthly fidelity monitoring.

Outside of individual coaching sessions, trainers routinely communicate with sites during bi-weekly team meetings and monthly agency meetings. Team meetings involve discussing program-specific challenges and successes to promote collaborative learning and a sense of pride among colleagues. These opportunities can reinforce performance of those who are doing well and provide examples of good practice amongst colleagues.

Monthly agency meetings are encouraged to further facilitate communication among agency personnel. These are especially critical early in the implementation process. This meeting provides opportunities for providers, administrators and support individuals to discuss SafeCare and relevant challenges. This provides a means for discussion about providers' performance with SafeCare and to resolve issues as needed.

Other contacts are established on an as-needed basis. With a recent international implementation, we found it beneficial to communicate bi-weekly with the organization leads. This provided an opportunity to prevent challenges and more quickly resolve issues that did arise. For example, NSTRC identified a several-month delay between training and implementation (i.e., providers seeing families) as a challenge to implementation. As a result, NSTRC trainers conducted refresher courses with trainees prior to implementing SafeCare.

Lesson 5-Certify milestones

A process imbedded within SafeCare implementation is certification and re-certification. The certification process for home visitors, coaches, and agency trainers involves a sequence of activities completed under direct support by NSTRC (or local coach and trainer once certified). This begins with several training activities (e.g., quizzes, role-plays) and is completed with fieldwork (e.g., fidelity monitoring, reliability observation). Fidelity monitoring is a key aspect of implementation effectiveness for EBTs, and thus is a requirement of SafeCare implementation (24).

Throughout the certification process, NSTRC promotes a supportive environment designed to enhance individuals' skills while providing them with opportunities to develop into successful SafeCare providers, coaches, and trainers. Positive feedback is routinely provided, as well as constructive and corrective feedback. Trainees for whom direct feedback is uncommon (i.e., audiotapes of sessions reviewed, live monitoring of initial coaching and training sessions) are at times initially apprehensive, but once they experience the collaborative, supportive process, they express less unease and more confidence in their skills. Once the certification process is complete, a process for which criteria are set that are explicated during the readiness and workshop training portions of implementation, trainees are provided with a certificate from NSTRC to represent their accomplishments.

We have bolstered our certification process by increasing the in-field requirements early in the implementation process, to offer more support and coaching in the early phases. This revised certification enhances evaluation of trainees' preparation for reduced support and more autonomy over time. With the expanded criterion, trainers anecdotally report improved confidence in the trainees they support. Similarly, trainees express increased confidence in their skills and appreciate the added support as they develop their skills.

As many of our sites mature to self-sustained implementation, we are recognizing the importance of recertification to ensure sites continue to provide SafeCare with fidelity and utilize the most updated SafeCare materials. We are developing a formal recertification process for individuals that will involve a simpler version of the certification process. In addition, we are creating an agency accreditation.

Lesson 6-Regarding international endeavors

While the lessons we have discussed so far are relevant to domestic endeavors, NSTRC has also conducted international implementations, which have unique challenges. The NSTRC has recently conducted training in the United Kingdom (UK) and Belarus. These trainings have come about from requests for more structured, evidenced-based interventions to prevent child maltreatment in international settings. To assist with this, NSTRC obtained grant funds from Georgia State University's International Strategic Initiatives Program to develop SafeCare International, a version of SafeCare adapted for international use.

The goal of our international work has been to identify the basic principles within the SafeCare curriculum, which can serve as the basis for international adaptation. For example, the SafeCare Health module implements a decision-making process to help parents decide how to care for their children when sick or injured. While the actual treatment course will vary across countries depending on the country's health care system, the basic principles underlying the decision-making process remain the same (e.g., seek emergency care). After articulating the basic principles of the health module, we revised the home visitor and parent training materials by altering or removing items that are specific to the US healthcare system to ensure that the materials instead capture cross-cultural principles (e.g., instead of prompting a parent to call 911 in a medical emergency, adapted materials focus more generally on seeking medical emergency help). Thus, the new SafeCare curriculum is comprised of basic principles that can be applied in virtually any country.

Training was requested in the UK as part of efforts there to help end cruelty to children. To date, the NSTRC has trained 30 home visitors and 9 coaches to implement SafeCare in the UK. Because of the similarities between the social service systems in the UK and the US, the implementation plan in the UK was very similar to that which typically occurs in the US, including using the same training protocols, certification procedures, and fidelity monitoring. The most notable change was to adapt the Health Module to account for the differences in the health care systems, particularly a government health program.

Training has also been conducted in Belarus to support development of new approaches to parental health, as the results of a transition from policies that resulted in institutionalization of many children. The institutionalization of children in eastern European countries in the 1970s and 80s has been documented to have had significant negative impacts on child growth and development. The new emphasis on children remaining with their families has brought demand for training and supports for parents and the organizations and individuals that serve them.

In Belarus, the major goal of the first SafeCare training was to introduce concepts of structured parenting approaches, as well as the rationale behind them, including information about child attachment, child development, unintentional injuries, and health promotion. Trainers from NSTRC will be returning to Belarus to conduct more in-depth skill training and implementation of SafeCare. While the training model will be similar, many of the training specifics and implementation processes will be different. For example, coordinators will be trained to help facilitate role-plays to account for language differences. In addition, opportunities for fidelity monitoring posttraining will be limited due to constraints on communication with sites. This work will help pilot procedures for international training that are anticipated to be implemented in other countries in the future.

While many of the same implementation factors apply in both US and international settings, in international work some become particularly prominent, such as examination of contextual issues prior to training. For example, the need to understand the political climate, the social service system within the country, and the system of health care is essential to understanding adaptations that may be needed for SafeCare. Lessons learned have also emphasized the need for flexibility, as many instances of adaptation were not identified until training took place. This has also highlighted the need for experienced, well-educated trainers, as these individuals can most easily identify situations where adaptations and instantaneous flexibility may be necessary for successful uptake and implementation.

DISCUSSION

The purpose of this paper was to discuss six themes of challenges encountered during national and international SafeCare implementation and the strategies used to overcome them. There are a variety of necessary tasks that create a smoother and more successful implementation and allow for guidance when issues arise, as they often do despite best efforts. Our aim was to provide direction to organizations and to those involved in dissemination efforts to build community capacity to address child maltreatment. Through the lessons we have encountered and the solutions we have employed, we hope to inform others to facilitate their own program implementations.

The first five themes we discussed involve broad buy-in of the implementation, starting small and being deliberate when first starting, being clear about expectations, having ongoing communication and support, and reinforcing milestones achievement. We also addressed challenges that arise from international implementation, in particular the need for flexibility in adapting content based on the contexts within the country and its individual and professional culture.

While these themes occur often in our dissemination of SafeCare, we do find that no strategy addresses all concerns, and flexibility is a continuous theme. Being flexible throughout implementation allows for easier adjustment to best suit the needs of all involved.

In addition, we are incorporating technology to facilitate dissemination and implementation of SafeCare, with the goal of improving upon our effective implementation strategies to build community capacity to address child maltreatment.

Use of technology in implementation

There are several technology advancements that can facilitate building of community capacities to address child maltreatment (25). At NSTRC, we are working on integrating technology into our current implementation efforts in order to expand reach and utility of our program, reduce training and support costs, and increase efficiency and cost-effectiveness of SafeCare. We have developed several pieces of technology that will assist with future implementations. The first is a training portal, which will assist SafeCare trainers at NSTRC and externally with monitoring trainee progress. It will track trainee milestones, allow for communication between trainers and trainees (and teams), and allow for the transfer of audio recording of sessions to be scored for fidelity. The portal will also track program data to provide ongoing evaluation.

We are developing a high-quality, interactive online training course. Currently, SafeCare training begins with an in-person workshop that is four to five days long. With the development of the online training course, our goal is to shorten the in-person workshop by providing most of the didactic content through the web course. This will reduce cost of training, and hopefully expand the reach of SafeCare.

Also, we are pursuing the use of tablet-based applications that can be used by providers to deliver and enhance SafeCare content. The tablet applications will walk the home visitor through the outline of the sessions to ensure all the steps are completed, and can be used to show videos of good parent-child interactions, and to video record and review the interactions between the target parent and child.

CONCLUSION

Implementing an evidence based program is not a simple process, and the field of implementation science is just beginning to provide data to inform best practices in implementation. Obviously, a great deal of empirical work is needed to better understand implementation processes. NSTRC is currently making strides to contribute to the implementation literature through several federally funded grants.

REFERENCES

[1]   US Department of Health and Human Services. Child maltreatment 2009. Administration for Children and Families, Administration on Children, Youth and Families, Children's Bureau. 2010. URL: http://www.acf.hhs.gov/programs/cb/stats_research/index.htm#can.

[2]   Centers for Disease Control and Prevention. Injury center: Violence prevention. 2010. URL: http://www.cdc.gov/ViolencePrevention/childmaltreatment/consequences.html

[3]   Wang CT, Holton J. Total estimated costs of child abuse and neglect in the United States. Washington, DC: Prevent Child Abuse America, 2007.

[4]   Felitti VJ, Anda RF, Nordenberg D, Williamson DF, Spitz AM, Edwards V, et al. Relationship of childhood abuse and household dysfunction to many of the leading causes of death in adults: The adverse childhood experiences (ACE) study. Am J Prev Med 1998;14:245-58.

[5]   Anda RF, Brown DW, Felitti VJ, Bremner JD, Dube SR, Giles WH. Adverse childhood experiences and prescribed psychotropic medications in adults. Am J Prev Med 2007;32:389-94.

[6]   Chaffin M, Funderburk B, Bard D, Valle LA, Gurwitch R. A combined motivation and parent–child interaction therapy package reduces child welfare recidivism in a randomized dismantling field trial. J Consult Clin Psychol 2011; 79:84-95.

[7]   Chaffin M, Hecht D, Bard D, Silovsky JF, Beasley WH. A statewide trial of the SafeCare model with parents in child protective services. ISRN Pediatr 2012; 129:509-15.

[8]   Prinz R, Sanders M, Shapiro C, Whitaker D, Lutzker J. Population-Based Prevention of Child Maltreatment: The US Triple P System Population Trial. Prev Sci 2009;10:1-12.

[9]   Lutzker JR, Bigelow KM. Reducing Child Maltreatment: A guidebook for parent services. New York: Guilford, 2002.

[10]   Lutzker S, Lutzker J, Braunling-McMorrow D, Eddleman J. Prompting to increase mother–baby stimulation with single mothers. J Infant Child Adolesc Psychother 1987;4:3-12.

[11]   Bigelow KM, Lutzker JR. Training parents reported for or at risk for child abuse and neglect to identify and treat their children's illnesses. J Fam Violence 2000;15:311-30.

[12]   Metchikian KL, Mink JM, Bigelow KM, Lutzker JR, Doctor RM. Reducing home safety hazards in the homes of parents reported for neglect. Child Fam Behav Ther 1999;21:23-34.

[13]   Tertinger DA, Greene BF, Lutzker JR. Home safety: Development and validation of one component of an ecobehavioral treatment program for abused and neglected children. J Appl Behav Anal 1984;17:159-74.

[14]   Gershater-Molko RM, Lutzker JR, Wesch D. Project SafeCare: Improving health, safety, and parenting skills in families reported for, and at-risk for child maltreatment. J Fam Violence 2003;18:377-86.

[15]   Gershater-Molko RM, Lutzker JR, Wesch D. Using recidivism to evaluate Project SafeCare: Teaching bonding, safety, and health care skills to parents. Child Maltreat 2002;7:277-85.

[16]   Fixsen DL, Naoom SF, Blasé KA, Friedman RM, Wallace F. Implementation research: A synthesis of the literature. Tampa, FL: University South Florida, Louis de la Parte Florida Mental Health Institute, National Implementation Research Network, FMHI Publication 231, 2005.

[17]   Kauffman Best Practices Project. Closing the quality chasm in child abuse treatment: Identifying and disseminating best practices: Findings of the Kauffman best practices project to help children heal from child abuse. Charleston, SC: National Crime Victims Research Treatment Center, 2004.

[18]   Aarons GA, Hurlburt M, Horwitz SMC. Advancing a conceptual model of evidence-based practice implementation in public service sectors. Adm Policy Ment Health 2011;38:4-23.

[19]   Glisson C, Schoenwald SK. The ARC organizational and community intervention strategy for implementing evidence-based children's mental health treatments. Ment Health Serv Res 2005;7:243-59.

[20]   Greenhalgh T, Robert G, MacFarlane F, Bate P, Kyriakidou O. Diffusion of innovations in service organizations: systematic review and recommendations. Milbank Quart 2004;82:581-629.

[21]   Horwitz SMC, Chamberlain P, Landsverk J, Mullican C. Improving the mental health of children in child welfare through the implementation of evidence-based parenting interventions. Adm Policy Ment Health 2010;37:27-39.

[22]   Mendel P, Meredith LS, Schoenbaum CDS, Wells KB. Interventions in organization and community context: A framework for building evidence on dissemination and implementation in health services research. Adm Policy Ment Health 2008;35:21-37.

[23]   Ogden T, Forgatch MS, Askeland E, Patterson GR, Bullock BM. Implementation of parent management training at the national level: The case of Norway. J Soc Work Pract 2005;19:317-29.

[24]   Durlak JA, DuPre EP. Implementation matters: A review of research on the influence of implementation on program outcomes and the factors affecting implementation. Am J Community Psychol 2008;41:327-50.

[25]   Self-Brown S, Whitaker D. Parent-focused child maltreatment prevention: Improving assessment, intervention, and dissemination with technology. Child Maltreat 2008;13:400-16.

Submitted: January 03, 2012. *Revised:* February 01, 2012. *Accepted:* February 03, 2012.

In: Public Health Yearbook 2013
Editor: Joav Merrick

ISBN: 978-1-63321-095-0
© 2014 Nova Science Publishers, Inc.

Chapter 4

BUILDING BETTER COMMUNITIES: SHARED LEADERSHIP AND AUTHENTIC CHANGE

Jane Ellery, PhD* and Peter J Ellery, PhD

Fisher Institute for Wellness and Gerontology and Department of Landscape Architecture, Ball State University, Muncie, Indiana, United States of America

ABSTRACT

In the mid-1990s higher education started allocating more resources toward social, ethical, and civic issues in the community, making a gradual shift toward greater campus engagement within local communities. Objective: The specific aim for this paper is to highlight previously identified characteristics of successful partnership development, tie these characteristics to a case study of a university-community partnership, and enhance the existing recommendations based on the experiences that emerged during partnership development. Study group and methods: This case study represents the development of prior ties and a working relationship between a mid-west university and several county school districts. Results and conclusions: Establishing Prior Ties and trusted relationships can facilitate community-campus partnership development important in achieving successful community-based outcomes. Additionally, expecting the community partners to identify programs and activities, focusing on the academic outcomes and allowing the community partner to receive recognition for success from the community, and serving in a mentoring role rather than an expert role may allow universities to develop useful community-campus partnerships.

Keywords: Community-campus partnerships, partnership development, case study, community development

---

* Correspondence: Jane Ellery, PhD, Associate Director and Assistant Professor Fisher Institute for Wellness and Gerontology, Ball State University, 2000 W University Ave, Muncie, IN 47306 United States. E-mail: jellery@bsu.edu

INTRODUCTION

Since the mid-1990s and Boyer's call for higher education to turn its resources toward social, ethical, and civic issues in the community (1, 2), higher education has been making a gradual shift toward greater campus engagement within local communities. Federal, state, and local resources, research indicating the value of immersive learning for students, and shifts in academic scholarly activity for university faculty have helped fuel this change in higher education's mission. Higher education institutions are engaging the community in a variety of ways including cooperative extension and continuing education programs, clinical and pre-professional practice opportunities, university directed administrative initiatives, academic outreach missions, faculty professional service, student volunteer activity, community access to facilities and cultural events, and service learning classes (3). The benefits of these community-campus partnerships have been well documented in the literature, including new insights and learning, better informed community practice, career enhancement for individuals involved in the partnership, greater public awareness of the institutions involved, improvements in the quality of teaching and student learning, increased opportunity for student employment, additional funding and access to resources and information, a more rapid internalization and adoption of change, and a more effective and efficient use of resources (4-11).

Despite these benefits, however, many communities and community organizations do not seek out or engage in partnerships with institutions of higher education. Research evaluating the usefulness of community-campus partnerships suggests that many communities have a negative perception of higher education. Many community members report that academics often use communities as a source for subjects in research or that they feel they are expected to be passive recipients of programs that those in higher education have identified as addressing their needs. Many communities also perceive that higher education representatives work in an elitist rather than a cooperative manner, fail to recognize assets that the community can bring to the partnership, do not include the community in the research process itself, and do not continue to work with the community to ensure long-term sustainability of the initiatives (3, 12, 13).

A question of trust

In many cases, community-campus partnerships fail to develop into long term working relationships or strategic alliances. From a business perspective, Tyndall notes that true strategic alliances are partnerships founded on a shared sense of obligation toward the other's welfare and a mutual trust that each partner will work toward that obligation. Each party now has a stake in the other's performance, and the risks and rewards of any venture undertaken together are shared. He also notes that successful strategic alliances can be readily recognized. Strategic alliances provide each partner with improvements in areas like total resource effectiveness and lowered business costs, and they are often characterized by terms like: purposeful (i.e., there are specific objectives to the work being done); well-defined (i.e., the roles, responsibilities, and resources required for tasks and personnel are clearly defined and established between the partners); open-ended (i.e., obligations and work commitments are ongoing and are not just contract or task bound); intentional and committed (i.e., both partners willingly and proactively commit energy and resources to establish and maintain the relationship); collaborative (i.e., both partners work together to integrate operations and information); and flexible (i.e., both partners share a commitment to orderly productive change) (14). In addition, research now suggests that inter-organizational trust is positively related to increases in the complexity, number of partnership interactions, and size of the monetary contracts shared within the partnership. Subsequent successes also further reinforce the inter-organizational trust (15, 16), strengthening the ties that already exist between partners and consolidating the partnership into an on-going strategic alliance.

Understanding inter-organizational trust in partnerships

Inter-organizational trust has been defined as the realistic expectation a partner organization will fulfill its obligations, act in a predictable manner, and respond in a fair, unselfish and responsible way (17). Researchers have also concluded that inter-organizational trust encompasses both calculative and non-calculative elements (18). In this definition, the calculative elements of inter-organizational trust relate to the costs and penalties associated with a breach in trust and the degree to which these costs and penalties exceed the gains that would be obtained through the engagement of opportunistic behaviors. This relationship between cost and gain provides a level of confidence that each partner's behavior will be both reliable and predictable (19). The non-calculative element refers to learning about the partner organization, as well as the identification and even internalization of the partner's interests and motives (20). The level of inter-organizational trust experienced in a partnership directly impacts the effects and benefits obtained from the partnership. A model depicting the relationship between inter-organizational trust and the potential benefits and effects of cooperation through partnerships has been proposed by Zhe and Ming (21) (See Figure 1).

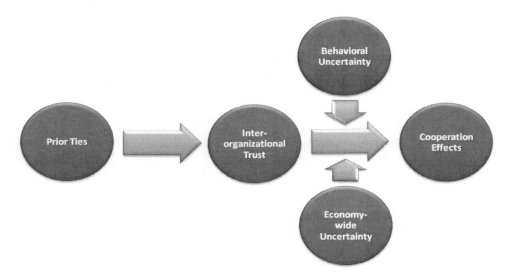

Figure 1. The Influence of Prior Ties, Behavioral Uncertainty, and Economy-wide Uncertainty on Inter-organizational Trust and the Resulting Cooperation Effects [adapted from Zhe and Ming (21)].

In this model, Prior Ties appear to be instrumental in the establishment of strong inter-organizational trust (21). Prior Ties are the personal and social relationships that members of each partnering organization have with one another prior to the establishment of a formal or business partnership. Partnerships built on already-established Prior Ties foster trust and trust-worthy behavior (22). Successful businesses highlight the importance of maintaining these social and personal relationships to ensure that the partnership remains both strong and on-going, even when partners are not currently engaged in projects together (23).

However, the relationship between inter-organizational trust and the effects or benefits obtained through cooperation appear to be complicated and also influenced by external factors. Harrigan (24) suggests that the degree to which cooperation benefits or effects will be experienced also depends on factors like behavioral and economic uncertainty. Behavioral uncertainty arises when a partner's behavior is inconsistent with the expected behavior. This inconsistency in behavior during the course of a partnership erodes inter-organizational trust and impacts the effects and benefits experienced from the cooperative effort. Economic uncertainty relates to the level of economic risk assumed when undertaking the partnership and can also impact the potential benefits and effects of a partnership. For example, changes in the economic environment during a partnership may lead to one partner being unable to meet their commitments due to financial restrictions. This would also impact the outcomes and benefits experienced as a result of the partnership.

METHODS

Faculty members affiliated with an institute at a university in the mid-west were interested in developing an experiential-based environment for students completing a minor in workplace wellness, so they contacted several local school districts to initiate conversations. The primary purpose of this initial exchange was to assess each school's interest in establishing wellness programs for their staff and to discuss the potential for university students to support this effort. These conversations helped establish important personal ties between university faculty and school employees, with both groups using the meetings to learn about each other's needs and to identify potential projects.

The initial, tangible product that the groups worked on was a grant proposal entitled TLC: Teachers Leading the Charge (TLC) toward Healthier Living. While the grant was not funded, it created an opportunity for the individuals involved in the university-school district partnership to talk about mutually beneficial projects as they worked to establish a strategic plan outlining how the employee wellness initiative could move forward. Individuals involved in the partnership began working toward employee wellness programming for the schools, and the workplace wellness minor started moving through the academic approval process.

Concerns related to childhood obesity led the federal government to mandate that all schools have local wellness policies in place by January of 2006. In response to this mandate a local, wellness-minded family foundation committed to financially supporting the development of local school wellness policies. An intern from the institute working with a wellness leader at one of the local schools helped establish a process for the partnership to use as they expanded from employee wellness programming to school wellness programming.

The Prior Ties established as a result of the employee wellness efforts allowed the partners to quickly retool and begin incorporating student wellness initiatives into the ongoing efforts.

Establishing clear goals for the partnership allowed each group to understand the benefits of cooperation. The goal for the institute was to provide outstanding, real-world educational experiences for students. The school districts initially joined the partnership to improve employee wellness. With the new federal expectation, these school districts also became interested in developing local wellness policies benefiting students and their families. To meet these identified goals, the institute assumed responsibility for managing the organization of a county-wide process for writing wellness policies, providing support personnel during the labor intensive start-up phases, and organizing personal and professional development opportunities related to school wellness. The schools participating in the project assumed responsibility for identifying wellness leaders and champions, for determining the wellness initiative activities most appropriate for their population, for deciding how and when these programs would be delivered during the school year, and for the administration and management of these programs. The local family foundation provided grants to both the university and the local schools to partially fund the efforts.

Consistent with Harrigan's finding that behavioral and economic uncertainty impact cooperation effects (24), several unplanned or unexpected situations impacted the efforts. The shift from employee wellness to developing local wellness policies as a result of a federal mandate was met successfully by all groups. This can be attributed to many factors, including the hard work and commitment of the individuals involved, the funding from the local foundation, and the prior ties that had been established.

During this same period, the economic downturn led to the university eliminating the contract faculty position that had been identified to oversee the interdisciplinary workplace wellness minor offering that started this whole process. Unfortunately, this meant that the student experiences designed into the courses did not eventuate to support the school employee wellness efforts. In two of the school districts, however, the healthcare purchasing trust returned funds in excess of the funding cap, allowing the schools to spend this money on their employee wellness initiatives. The school districts used some of the funding to hire teachers and interns to coordinate employee wellness opportunities. These efforts are still underway today, and the university-community partnership is continuously working to identify opportunities to allow students to benefit from learning in these environments. Additionally, several participating schools have been recognized through the "Healthy Hoosier School Awards" program.

RESULTS

This case study represents a successful, on-going, community-campus partnership that has expanded on a set of existing principles associated with successful, or authentic, community-campus partnerships (25). These principles involve guidelines developed from research concerning community perspectives toward community-campus partnerships.

1. A relationship that is characterized by mutual trust, respect, genuineness, and commitment exists between the partners.

2. The partners involved develop agreed upon mission statements but understand that each entity may be working toward different, but related, outcomes.
3. The partnership is built upon identified strengths and assets but also works to address areas that need improvement.
4. The power is balanced among partners, and shared resources are equitably distributed.
5. Clear, open and accessible communication between partners is an ongoing priority, including listening to each need and developing a common language.
6. Roles, norms, and processes essential to the partnership are established through input and agreement of all partners.
7. Feedback to, among, and from all stakeholders in the partnership is encouraged and respected, with the goal of continuously improving the partnership and its outcomes.
8. All partners share credit for the partnership's accomplishments.
9. The individuals involved recognize that most partnerships take time to develop and opportunities for collaboration may not be constant or ongoing.

Three additional guidelines evolved to help promote each school-community's sense of autonomy in the program development process.

1. The community partners were responsible for identifying the programs and activities to be delivered.
2. The university partners assumed a "silent partnership" role while in the school, understanding that academic recognition and exceptional student learning experiences were the primary university expected outcomes from the effort.
3. The role of the university partners was to support the work of the community partners, and the role of the community partner was to encourage change in the schools.

Each of these additional guidelines was important to the partnership process because the guidelines helped provide a greater degree of autonomy, ownership, and responsibility for the project. This enhanced the likelihood that the program would be successful and self-sustaining. Most importantly, these guidelines strengthened the partnership by establishing trust and acknowledging the community's role and contributions in the project. This was considered critical as this project was an investment in the establishment of a community-campus partnership. All of the entities involved in the partnership wanted the partnership to not only survive, but thrive, so future community-campus projects would be welcomed and undertaken with the same level of optimism and success.

DISCUSSION

The establishment of an alliance takes time and a great deal of effort to develop. While more research is needed to determine the antecedents associated with trust in a relationship or the factors that comprise a successful alliance, the activities associated with this case study suggest that the development of an alliance is possible through the following stages:

1. Initial networking – find opportunities to meet people in the community who share a similar interest in encouraging a social change. Some options to consider: attend (and possibly organize) community coalition meetings and educational offerings, offer to write a related column in the local newspaper, begin a blog and personally invite potential partners into discussions on topics related to your shared interests. Avoid using networking tools for self-promotion or the selling of professional services. Instead, use these opportunities as a way to start conversations and allow those involved to learn about each other's background experience and areas of expertise. Contributing to professional discussions and helping others without seeking return or profit shows a genuine interest in mutual success and helps establish validity as a trusted community resource.

2. Establishing Face-to-Face Time – add personal contact to the networking process. While social networks are good at developing distant relationships, personal friendships are still more easily established through personal interaction. This may have to be done through conferences and other professional meetings when potential partners are not geographically close. In all occasions, gatherings should include both social and professional interactions. Developing personal ties will help projects move from discussions into action.

3. Initiating Collaboration through Low Cost, Low Share and Low Risk Projects – once you have established "Prior Ties" through a personal relationship with the potential partner, find a small scale joint venture that will benefit both partners and that allows both partners to experience a working partnership. Doing this may help both partners develop a shared vision, a vested interest in each other's success, and a shared sense of risk as well as accomplishment. With small, low cost, low share, and low risk projects, partners can see if their administrative and management styles are well suited for a joint work environment.

4. Repeat Instructions until Alliance is Formed – as each project is successfully completed, the comfort and trust level between the two partners will continue to grow. Each partner recognizes the benefits the other offers and these benefits range from immediate income and work through continued joint ventures to support and resources during periods where both partners are engaged in activities independently of one another.

ACKNOWLEDGMENTS

Preparation for this paper and the work associated with this case study were partially funded by the Ball Brothers Foundation.

REFERENCES

[1]   Boyer EL. Creating the new American college. Chron High Educ 1994;Sect A48.
[2]   Boyer EL. The scholarship of engagement. J Public Serv Outreach 1996;1(1):11-20.
[3]   Bringle RG, Hatcher, J.A. Campus and community partnerships: the terms of engagement. J Soc Issues 2002;58(3):503-16.

[4]   Ambile TM, Patterson JM, Wocjik P. Academic-practitioner collaboration in management research: a case of cross-profession collaboration. Acad Manage J 2001;44(2):418-32.

[5]   Buys N, and Bursnall S. Establishing university-community partnerships: processes and benefits. J Higher Educ Policy Manage 2007;29:73-86.

[6]   Davies RM. Industry-university collaborations: a necessity for the future. J Dent 1996;24(1-2):3-5.

[7]   Hollis A. Co-authorship and output of academic economists. Labour Econ 2001;8:503-30.

[8]   Kellet C, Goldstein A. Transformation in the university and the community: the benefits and barriers of collaboration. J Fam Consum Sci 1999;91(2):31-5.

[9]   Kezar A. Redesigning for collaboration within higher education institutions: an exploration into the developmental process. Res High Educ 2005;46:831-60.

[10]   Landry R, Amara N. The impact of transaction costs on the institutional structuration of collaborative academic research. Res Policy 1998;27:901-13.

[11]   Mead N, Beckman K, Lawrence J, O'Mary G, Parish C, Unpingco, P, et al. Industry-university collaborations: different perspectives heighten mutual opportunities. J Syst Softw 1999;49:155-62.

[12]   Ferman B, Hill TL. The challenges of agenda conflict in higher-education-community research partnerships: views from the community side. J Urban Aff 2004;26:241-57.

[13]   Achieving the promise of authentic community-higher education partnerships: community case stories [Internet]. Seattle, WA: Community Campus Partnerships for Health; 2007 [Accessed 2010 Feb 21]. Available from: http://depts.washington.edu/ccph/pdf_files/CPS-Casestories.pdf.

[14]   Tyndall G. Strategic alliances must be true partnerships. Marketing News 1990;24:8-8.

[15]   Hitt MA, Bierman L, Uhlenbruck K, Shimizu K. The importance of resources for the internationalization of professional service firms: the good, the bad and the ugly. Acad Manage J 2006;47:385-99.

[16]   Young-Ybarra C, Wiersema M. Strategic flexibility in information technology alliances: the influence of transaction cost economics and social exchange theory. Organization Sci 1999;10(4):439-59.

[17]   Zaheer A, McEvily B, Perrone V. Does trust matter? Exploring the effects of inter-organizational and interpersonal trust on performance. Organization Sci 1998;9:141-59.

[18]   McEvily B, Perrone V, Zaheer A. Trust as an organizing principle. Organization Sci 2003;14:91-103.

[19]   Ring PS, Van de Ven AH. Structuring cooperative relationships between organizations. Strat Mgmt J 1992;13:483-98.

[20]   Lewicki RJ, Bunker BB. Developing and maintaining trust in work relationshi ps. In: Kramer RM, Tyler TR. Trust in organizations: Frontiers of theory and research. Thousand Oaks, CA: Sage Publishers, 1996:114-39.

[21]   Zhe Z, Ming J. When does trust influence cooperation effects in public-private partnerships? SAM Adv Manage J 2009;74(3):21-32.

[22]   Granovetter M. Economic action and social structure: the problem of embeddedness. Am J Sociol 1985;91:481-510.

[23]   Wolff MF. Building trust in alliances. Res Technol Manage 1994;37(3):12.

[24]   Harrigan KR. Strategies for joint ventures. Lexington, MA: Lexington Books, 1985.

[25]   Principles of good community-campus partnerships [Internet]. Seattle, WA: Community Campus Partnerships for Health; 2009. [cited 2010 Feb 20]. Available from: http://depts. washington.edu/ ccph/principles.html#principles.

Submitted: November 14, 2011. *Revised:* March 01, 2012. *Accepted:* April 21, 2012.

In: Public Health Yearbook 2013
Editor: Joav Merrick

ISBN: 978-1-63321-095-0
© 2014 Nova Science Publishers, Inc.

Chapter 5

CAPACITY BUILDING ASSISTANCE: THE 360° APPROACH AND LESSONS LEARNED

Abidemi Adelaja, MPH[*1], *Kristin Wunder, BS, BA*[1],
George Gates, MBA[1], *Adora Iris Lee, MPH, MDiv*[2],
Susan Rogers, PhD[3], *and Colin Bill, MA*[4]

[1]FHI 360 Center on AIDS and Community Health (COACH),
Washington DC, United States of America
[2]International Relief and Development, Arlington, Virginia, United States of America
[3]FHI 360, New York, New York, United States of America
[4]ETR Associates, Scotts Valley, California, United States of America

ABSTRACT

AED was funded by the US Centers for Disease Control and Prevention (CDC) to provide capacity building assistance (CBA) services targeted to strengthening health departments' internal infrastructure and service to HIV prevention community planning groups (CPGs) in all 65 U.S. jurisdictions. The AED project adopted the name CBA 360° to reflect its comprehensive approach to conducting capacity building through needs assessments, service delivery plans and implementation, and evaluation. Our approach was centered on provision of tailored, responsive assistance with clearly defined outcomes that included three primary steps: 1) in-depth needs assessment, 2) development of a tailored service delivery plan, and 3) multi-phase evaluation. Results: Our team learned several valuable lessons: 1) Established systems and protocols were important in ensuring timely response, effective reporting, and quality, 2) An in-depth needs assessment was critical to identifying the actual need(s) and creating recipient buy-in, 3) A tailored service delivery plan based on the needs assessment was the blueprint to providing relevant and appropriate services, and consistent outcome review ensured appropriate service provision, 4) Identifying the appropriate service delivery method(s) was instrumental to effectively building knowledge/skills and 5) Conducting evaluations immediately following each provided service and within 1- to 3-months following service

[*] Correspondence: Abidemi Adelaja, FHI 360 Center on AIDS and Community Health (COACH), 1825 Connecticut Avenue NW, Washington, DC, 20009 United States. E-mail: AAdelaja@fhi360.org.

completion resulted in a higher response rate and informed future services. Results show that our methods were well-received, relevant, and effective. Satisfaction and achievement of the objectives was high (4.10 out of 5); and follow-up evaluations indicated that retention and application of knowledge/skills was also high (4.02 out of 5).

Keywords: Community, AIDS, HIV, service

INTRODUCTION

The Capacity Building Assistance Program (CBA) of the US Centers for Disease Control and Prevention (CDC) helps high-risk minority individuals, organizations, and communities improve their ability to deliver effective evidence-based interventions and core public health strategies for HIV prevention. AED was funded to provide CBA services for two groups, 1) to assist health departments in all 65 US jurisdictions in strengthening their internal infrastructure and management and service to their constituents in HIV prevention, particularly community planning groups (CPGs), and 2) to strengthen CBA providers and the CDC Capacity Building Branch staff by developing and managing resources for the CBA Resource Center.

The AED CBA for health department component adopted the name CBA 360° to reflect its comprehensive approach to conducting capacity building through needs assessments, service delivery plans, training, webinars, conference calls, peer exchange, and evaluation during and following delivery of CBA services. Although the process of providing CBA appears on the surface to be straightforward, it goes far beyond a simple request-response transaction.

CBA is a complex system of quickly grasping the nature of the CBA request; learning the underlying factors that may affect service provision and outcomes; and building relationships with recipients and other stakeholders to make appropriate decisions and render the best service in the best format—all in a timely manner.

Project implementers too often get caught up in the day-to-day work of getting the job done and have little time—or make little time—to reflect on the bigger picture of successful project implementation. As the CBA 360° project drew to a close for AED, we deliberated about what we learned in delivering CBA to health departments and CPGs in the United States. In doing so, we discovered what we probably already knew—that CBA 360°'s approach offers a rich experience and practical lessons for any group that undertakes CBA. What follows are the lessons we would like to share.

METHODS

Our overall approach was grounded in the desire to achieve the CDC's overarching capacity building goal of enabling organizations to provide effective public health strategies to reduce the burden of HIV infection among at-risk populations. Health departments have a unique role in administering HIV prevention programs in that they serve a dual role – a primary location for service delivery as well as local CBA providers to the organizations they fund. Understood from our previous experience and supported by formative research conducted during initial program design, our approach was centered on provision of tailored, responsive assistance with clearly defined outcomes to be agreed upon with the recipient prior to implementation of services. The following five design tenets guided how the program responded to CBA requests:

- Conduct a needs assessment and diagnose CBA needs by communicating with recipients and other stakeholders.
- Identify appropriate and proven methods of CBA, factoring in adult learning theories, knowledge and skill retention, and sustainability.
- Identify attainable and measurable goals and objectives for the CBA response.
- Develop materials appropriate and specific for the CBA response, and gather input and feedback from target groups for future use.
- Evaluate both the process and outcome of CBA with its recipients.

In addition to our overall approach, a key factor in our response was to identify the best CBA service delivery method – resource sharing, web-based training or knowledge sharing, in-person training, or a blend of the different delivery methods. Recognizing health departments' as well as our own organization's financial resources and staff time limitations, including travel restrictions, our team was equipped to easily identify the best delivery method for the identified need(s).

Developed materials were transferred to the health department or CPG after conclusion of the CBA service for further dissemination and/or future reference to ensure transfer and sustainability of knowledge and skills within the health department and CPG.

PARTICIPANT SELECTION

The CDC developed a web-based system to triage requests for CBA services – the CBA Request Information System (CRIS). The system allowed for any agency that was directly funded by the CDC to access the system and request assistance. For organizations that did not have direct access to the system, e.g., CPGs, the health department would submit a request on behalf of the entity requesting assistance. Organizations also have the ability to request a specific provider in order to complete follow-on activities of previously-provided services. Upon receipt of a request, the CDC would review and assign a CBA provider based on the following: harmonization of the requested need and a CBA provider's funding category or area of specialization, geographic location, and the number of requests a CBA provider was currently managing, among other factors. Upon receipt of notification of a request, a provider was responsible for reviewing the request and confirming their ability to respond.

TECHNICAL INFORMATION

Excellence in CBA service is built on a foundation of collaboration, facilitated by appropriate adult learning technologies, and is regularly monitored to ensure that service is meeting recipients' needs. Each of these components was incorporated into our CBA service provision and continuously checked to ensure appropriate and effective services.

Understanding the system and/or process

The CRIS system facilitated continuity of services among the 32 funded CBA providers served as a mechanism for a larger program evaluation. It was critical to understand how this system functioned in order to develop internal systems and protocols that were responsive to the health departments' and CPGs' needs and the funder's requirements. Our team developed a detailed two-part Internal CBA Protocol, or 'checklist', to guide the implementation of CBA services from receipt of the initial request to completion and closure. A CBA Liaison was designated as a CBA Lead to serve as the request manager and a main point of contact for each request. The CBA Lead was responsible for each phase of the CBA delivery process and completion of the Protocol, and was assisted by other team members as needed.

Protocol

Part 1, or the 'checklist' component, outlined responsibilities, timelines for completion, was filled in with actual dates based on the date the request was received, and was updated after each stage of the request was complete. Protocol – Part 2 was developed to capture qualitative information from communication with CBA recipients and stakeholders as well as detailed information related to the CBA service to be delivered. After responding to the initial set of requests received, the Protocol was revised to ease the burden of reporting for the CBA Leads.

For example, CRIS requires that the delivery method(s) for services to be provided under each request be entered separately, including goals and objectives for each delivery method, expected number of participants, and expected deliverables. As a result, the Delivery Method section in the Protocol was redesigned to mimic CRIS which allowed CBA Leads to easily copy and paste information from the Internal Protocol into CRIS in a coordinated manner.

Training on CRIS was provided five months after the program began. The orientation was extremely helpful in understanding how information was to be reported and would have been even more helpful at the outset of the program. As a result, our team was able to revise the Protocol to better fit the needs of CRIS as well as our internal process for providing services to ensure consistent quality.

Needs assessment

The CBA 360°-developed needs assessment tool was revised for each recipient. After an initial call to confirm receipt of the request, the CBA recipient was asked to fill out a preliminary online needs assessment to provide basic health department and CPG background information, additional details about the request, and a list of individuals that would participate in CBA services. A more detailed call was then conducted to identify the specific need(s) and to describe the complete CBA process to the recipient. These initial steps fostered a better understanding of the CBA process and greater buy-in from the recipients.

CBA 360° found that the needs assessment uncovered the recipients' real need(s), which were typically more complex than the need described in the initial request. The team frequently discovered that in attempting to fulfill the need(s), health department staff and/or the CPG were lacking basic knowledge and/or skills that were essential to successful completion of the larger need(s).

After these supportive services were offered, the CBA recipients were able to receive more advanced training to ensure that the identified need(s) were addressed and the knowledge and skills were sustainable. This detailed needs assessment process enabled us to set realistic goals that were achievable in scope and within a reasonable amount of time.

Development of the CBA service delivery plan

An initial service delivery plan for each CBA request was drafted by the CBA recipients and the CBA Lead following a 60- to 90-minute conference call with the CBA recipient. Each plan was finalized in approximately two weeks and submitted for approval. The CBA team engaged in "group think" sessions to brainstorm ideas on the best way to respond to the request.

These sessions included identifying the true need(s), whether the request should be broken into smaller, more manageable requests, whether the plan would build recipients' capacity and skill rather than simply do the recipients' work, and the amount of time needed to complete services. Key assurances for the plan included:

- Make timeframes clear, and make sure that activities relate to a deadline. Clarity around deadlines for each action not only helped ensure timely completion of a CBA request, but also helped the recipient stay focused on the purpose and objectives of the CBA request. CBA 360° found that flexibility around deadlines and sticking to an agreed upon timeframe were important in facilitating timely completion of the CBA request and achieving objectives. CBA 360° recognized that health department staff and CPG members had competing priorities and time commitments, and designed realistic objectives with this in mind.
- Keep asking key questions: Will the action actually build the required capacity? Whose capacity is being built? Incorporating these questions into group think sessions kept us mindful that the goal of CBA was to build the organization's capacity, not just an individual's. CBA 360° learned first-hand about the daily demands placed on a health department, and that it seemed easier to step in and do the work the CBA request was meant to address. However, health departments are better served if the CBA provider and the recipients collaborate to design the service response, its deadlines, and agree upon the work the CBA provider and recipients will each complete so that skills and knowledge are transferred. Health department contacts were encouraged to include additional relevant staff or to ensure the knowledge gained is transferred to other staff.

Service provision

Lessons learned in managing and executing CBA requests have been critical. Understanding the need(s) of recipients, ensuring key stakeholders are involved, keeping people informed as CBA services progress, and staying flexible have an impact on timely, relevant CBA service provision. While each of the service delivery methods below can function independently,

CBA 360° discovered that often combining more than one delivery method to respond to requests proved valuable and effective in ensuring knowledge and skills transfer to CBA recipients.

Web-based

E-learning can open new, cost-effective opportunities for CBA, bringing together people from disparate locations through voice, video, and Internet technologies. CBA providers should understand the "learning" that e-learning should facilitate so that the e-learning vehicle is appropriate to the learning goal(s). It is also important to understand adult learning principles, especially the difference between information sharing and capacity building, to determine how much interactivity there must be for learning to occur.

When creating the service delivery plan, we learned to ask CBA recipients what "interactive" means to them, what content they expect to cover and their level of knowledge on the subject. Recipients were also asked beforehand how they plan to apply what they will learn in the webinar and asked again after the webinar for reinforcement. In addition, we determined what was better for participants to read ahead of time and what was better for interactive participation. The best way to reinforce learning is through practice, so CBA recipients were given ample opportunities to practice the knowledge and/or skills being transferred. We built the capacity of recipients to use technology by asking recipients to co-facilitate an event such as a webinar or to lead a follow-on webinar.

Face-to-face

When possible and necessary, face-to-face CBA was provided to facilitate hands-on skills building activities outlined in the service delivery plan. Providing on-site training and technical assistance allowed for more direct capacity building service provision, opportunities for providing valuable feedback, guidance, and corrective action and/or recommendations, and to assess the CBA recipient's comprehension and ability to sustain capacity that was built. As with web-based service provision, collaborating with CBA recipients, as appropriate, on face-to-face activities reinforced learning, information sharing, and capacities to implement skills learned post-CBA. Examples include assigning small-group facilitators to assist with activities and recipients contributing to the development of case studies used for role play activities.

Resource sharing

CBA 360° also provided CBA services in the form of resource sharing and information dissemination. Instead of direct CBA like a workshop, training or webinar, an organization may have requested materials, tools/instruments, and, as needed, guidance on the development of a presentation or tool/instrument. Often, CBA recipients requested resources or information as a standalone or as a follow-up to a CBA request. CBA was provided in these instances via e-mail communications or technical assistance calls with the recipient. As was the case with web-based activities, resource sharing proved a cost-effective method and provided an immediate response to recipients' need(s).

As a means of assessing the effectiveness of service provision, CBA recipients were informed that CBA 360° would monitor and analyze process, outcome, and follow-up data as part of the project's evaluation, and that CBA recipient input was strongly encouraged.

QUALITY ASSURANCE AND EVALUATION

As part of a comprehensive approach, CBA 360° developed a four-step evaluation process: 1) mid-CBA check-in; 2) individual presentation (web-based or in-person) assessment; 3) post-evaluation; and 4) follow-up evaluation. Quality assurance was reflected in all aspects of CBA 360°'s response to a CBA request, from receipt of the request to the final follow-up evaluation. To streamline our process, we created internal protocols for regular monitoring and data capture, and used this information to improve systems and services.

To ensure buy-in, new and returning CBA recipients were informed of the evaluation process and its importance to our approach. Objectives for each request, measured in the quantitative assessments (steps 2-4), were developed and agreed upon in the service delivery plan. Each step of the evaluation process is described below.

Mid-CBA check-in

The mid-CBA check-in, a brief informal telephone conversation conducted by the Evaluation Specialist with key CBA recipients, was added partway through Year 2 of the project. The purpose of the call was to give recipients the opportunity to provide feedback on services provided up to the check-in point. CBA 360° used the feedback to adjust services as needed to ensure objectives and expectations were met. The check-in was guided by the following questions: How are the CBA services that CBA 360° is currently providing to you progressing? How can CBA 360° improve our CBA service delivery to you? Are there any other comments you would like to share?

The CBA Lead identified the appropriate CBA recipient representative(s), aiming to have representation from all parties involved as appropriate (i.e., health department staff and CPG members), to complete the assessment; and shared the information with the Evaluation Specialist. Upon completion, results were shared with the CBA Lead and the other team members. This process facilitated additional brainstorm sessions to improve on-going CBA service delivery.

Individual presentation assessment

Assessments were conducted for each service delivery method (i.e., webinar or face-to-face trainings) of each request through a post-presentation survey administered via an on-line survey or paper-based tool. Five main areas – presentation objectives, planning and organization, quality, participant's overall level of satisfaction, and the effectiveness of the presentation in meeting the participant's need(s) – were assessed.

Post-evaluation

CBA 360° sought to conduct a post-evaluation with each of the key CBA recipients for each request that was completed. The evaluation assessed the planning process, achievement of the overall CBA objectives, knowledge and/or skills transfer, participants' satisfaction, and, if used, AED consultants.

Follow-up evaluation

CBA 360° initially planned to collect follow-up evaluations at 3- and 6-month intervals however; this practice was revised to 1- and/or 3-month intervals. We learned that the shorter interval increased response rates and that recipient recall was improved as less time had passed between completion of services and evaluation. Due to limited time to complete multiple evaluations, especially those receiving services for multiple requests, CBA 360° strove to complete at least one follow-up evaluation at either 1- or 3-months. The follow-up timeframe was determined by the CBA Lead based on the nature of the request.

Based on the evaluation process established, CBA 360° found the following steps to be vital in assuring quality and effective evaluation of the CBA service(s) provided:

Make sure CBA recipients are familiar with evaluation procedures to help manage expectations and elicit better cooperation. CBA recipients were familiarized with each step of the CBA assessment process—mid-CBA check-in, webinar/presentation assessment, post-CBA evaluation, and follow-up evaluations. Setting deadlines for completing the surveys and sending reminder emails were also critical in getting a sizeable response rate.

Send out evaluations immediately after the CBA event and no more than three months after completing the request. CBA 360° found that the recipient response rate to the individual presentation assessment was higher if it was prepared early so that it could be administered immediately following the presentation. The same was true for face-to-face trainings whereby a paper-based evaluation should be prepared ahead of time, and administered at the end of the training. Recipients of multiple CBAs may become confused if assessment intervals are too long following completion of a request. We learned that follow-up evaluations result in more accurate recall and receive a higher response rate from all CBA recipients when they are sent immediately after the CBA is completed and at 1-month and 3-month intervals, rather than 3- and 6-month intervals. In accordance with CBA 360°'s internal protocol, the CBA Lead immediately notified the Evaluation Specialist of plans to close the request so that evaluation instruments can be prepared in a timely manner. In addition, reminder emails to participants to complete the evaluations were found to be very helpful. Develop a systematic way to capture results and feedback and share them to improve future services. CBA 360° team members were required to keep detailed descriptions of their activities. This included information about their successes and challenges, and how these relate to the annual work plan agreed upon with the funding organization. Documenting activities on a monthly basis—with frequent referral to project goals, the work plan, and deliverables—made reporting easier, fuller, and more accurate and helped staff reflect on their work as it progressed. Capturing results and lessons learned at an early stage through mid-CBA check-ins and individual presentation assessments presented a great opportunity for reflection on services provided and mid-course adjustments, if needed. Having a dedicated staff was critical to monitor the quality of CBA delivery, conduct ongoing evaluations, and prepare required reports.

RESULTS

Scores for the quantitative assessments were derived by totaling the average scores of each assessment area and calculating an average across all assessment areas. For example, the overall post-CBA evaluation score was calculated by averaging the average scores of each of the five assessment areas. Below is an overview of the usefulness of the mid-CBA check-in, followed by the overall scores for each quantitative assessment and what each may mean for the CBA services provided by CBA 360°.

Mid-CBA check-in

CBA 360° conducted two mid-CBA check-in assessments in Year 2 of the project. As previously mentioned, this piece of our evaluation process was initiated later in the project. Overall, CBA recipients were happy to participate in the check-in, which gave them an opportunity to ask for a revision in planned service provision if needed. The check-in also served as an affirmation of their effort in the CBA services.

Individual presentation assessment

The presentation assessment yielded an overall high score of 4.01 out of 5 across all presentations conducted [N=30 across 5 assessments]. This is roughly translated to 80% achievement. CBA 360° is confident in asserting that we were able to meet the objectives set out by the CBA recipients through the webinar presentations and face-to-face trainings conducted. Table 1 details average scores for the presentation assessments that were conducted.

Table 1. Average scores for presentation assessments (N=30 across 5 assessments)

Presentation topic	Objectives	Planning	Quality	Presentation rating	Effectiveness	Overall Score
Connecting the Dots of Community Planning	4.81	3.94	-	4.50	4.00	
Survey Design	3.89	4.63	-	3.50	4.80	
The Relationship of the National HIV/AIDS Strategy to HIV Prevention Community Planning	4.00	4.67	-	4.00	4.00	4.01
Operations Committee Action Planning Workshop	3.52	3.93	3.71	3.71	3.29	
Using Available Data to Set HIV Prevention Community Planning Group Priorities	3.70	4.36	3.50	3.60	3.60	
Average Scores	3.99	4.30	3.61	3.86	3.94	

Table 2. Average scores for post-evaluations (N=42 across 7 evaluations)

CBA service	Objectives	Knowledge/ skills transfer	Consultant	Planning	CBA service rating	Overall Score
Community planning orientation	-	3.84	-	4.39	4.33	
Capacity building needs assessments	4.00	4.67	-	4.75	5.00	
Evaluating community planning process	5.00	4.75	-	5.00	5.00	
Social determinants of health	4.60	3.40	-	4.70	3.20	
Community & member participation in Community Planning Group planning process	4.00	4.20	4.25	4.44	3.50	4.19
Leadership Development for chairs, co-chairs, and co-chairs elect	3.25	2.50	3.00	3.06	2.50	
Leadership; team building	5.00	4.67	-	5.00	4.00	
Average Scores	4.31	4.00	3.63	4.48	3.93	

Table 3. Average scores for follow-up CBA evaluations (N=12 across 4 evaluations)

CBA Service	Retention of knowledge/skills	Application of knowledge/skills	Relevance of CBA service	Overall Score
Community planning orientation *(6-month follow-up)*	3.99	3.65	4.00	
Capacity building needs assessments *(3-month follow-up)*	3.61	3.50	5.00	
Evaluating community planning process *(3-month follow-up)*	5.00	4.13	5.00	4.26
Social determinants of health *(3-month follow-up)*	5.00	3.25	5.00	
Average Scores	4.40	3.63	4.75	

Post-evaluation

The post-evaluation yielded an overall high score of 4.19 out of 5 across all evaluations carried out in Years 1 and 2 [N=42 across 7 evaluations]. (Please note that the objectives measured were not assessed in the first CBA request post-evaluation because the team had very little time to prepare a response to the request.) The overall score of 4.19 indicates that CBA 360° met approximately 84% of the expectations of the CBA recipients. CBA 360° made an effort to review and share our findings with CBA recipients. When possible, supplemental services were provided to resolve unmet expectations. Findings were also shared among the CBA team in order to improve future CBA service delivery. Table 2 details average scores for the post-evaluations that were conducted.

Follow-up evaluation

The follow-up CBA evaluation yielded an overall high score of 4.26 out of 5 across all evaluations carried out in Years 1 and 2 [N=12 across 4 evaluations]. The overall score can be roughly translated to CBA 360°'s success in meeting 85% of the follow-up criterion we hoped to achieve. Retention and application of knowledge and/or skills was moderate to high at 4.40 (out of 5) and 3.63 (out of 5) respectively. Additionally, 95% of respondents felt that the services provided were relevant to their needs. Table 3 details the average scores for the follow-up CBA evaluations that were conducted.

DISCUSSION

CBA 360° found that a system for responding to and monitoring CBA requests, protocols for facilitating the management of CBA service delivery, and clear mechanisms for addressing challenges in responding to requests and assessing CBA recipient's capacity, resulted in positive feedback and achievement of program objectives. Our evaluation highlights that most CBA recipients reported an increased ability to retain and apply the knowledge and/or skills imparted in the months following the completion of CBA service delivery. These outcomes demonstrate CBA 360°'s success in ensuring the relevance of services provided by tailoring CBA services, rather than taking a "cookie-cutter" approach to CBA service delivery that does not meet the needs of the recipient.

The effectiveness of CBA 360°'s tailored approach began with the initial step of conducting a comprehensive needs assessment. The needs assessment provided a broader understanding of the recipient's current needs and capabilities and contributed to our being able to transfer knowledge and skills more effectively. Including the recipient in the development of the service delivery plan and assigning participatory roles in planned activities ensured active engagement of the recipient in the delivery of CBA activities. Including evaluation as a component of the service delivery resulted in a higher number of responses to the evaluations. Recipients were aware of the process and were prepared for the evaluations to be administered.

CBA 360°'s overall tailored and inclusive approach to conducting capacity building successfully met project and stakeholder goals as is reflected in the outcomes of the project. Implementing a structured and participatory capacity building model that incorporates monitoring systems can prove beneficial in a CBA provider's ability to deliver effective and comprehensive services that are both impactful and sustainable.

ACKNOWLEDGMENTS

This work was completed under a contract between the Centers for Disease Control and Prevention (CDC) and AED. The project closed on May 31, 2011. On July 1, 2011, Family Health International (FHI) acquired the programs, expertise, and assets for AED. The newly formed entity of FHI and AED is known as FHI 360. Funding for the CBA 360° project was provided by the Centers for Disease Control and Prevention (CDC) under Contract Number U65 PS001648-02.

Submitted: January 03, 2012. *Revised:* February 02, 2012. *Accepted:* February 03, 2012.

In: Public Health Yearbook 2013   ISBN: 978-1-63321-095-0
Editor: Joav Merrick   © 2014 Nova Science Publishers, Inc.

Chapter 6

STAKEHOLDER DIALOGUE ABOUT EVIDENCE-BASED PRACTICE: AN E-LEARNING TOOL TO FACILITATE DISCUSSION

Molly Jean Ferguson, MPH,
*Elizabeth Ryan, EdD, and Bonnie Spring, PhD, ABPP**

Department of Preventive Medicine, Northwestern University, Chicago,
Department of Family and Community Medicine, Northwestern University Feinberg
School of Medicine, Chicago, and Department of Preventive Medicine,
Feinberg School of Medicine, Department of Preventive Medicine,
Northwestern University, Chicago, Illinois, United States of America

ABSTRACT

Evidence-based practice is a cornerstone of effective health promotion for patients and populations. However, few tools have been available to train the diverse professional groups that need to collaborate to address behavioral and psychosocial problems. The Evidence Based Behavioral Practice (EBBP) project, sponsored by the National Institutes of Health, provides web-based tools that were designed as a learning resource to harmonize and upgrade the approach to evidence-based practice among a variety of stakeholders. Interactive online learning modules provide experiential training in the evidence-based practice process for individuals and communities, critical appraisal of evidence, and shared decision-making with affected parties in a health decision. A recent module, entitled "Stakeholder Dialogue about Evidence-Based Practice" was developed as a stimulus to spark discussion and perspective-taking among academics, practitioners, and community members. The module features clips of interviews with a variety of stakeholders as well as didactic commentary. Community clinicians offer candid descriptions about how trust, communication, and time impose challenges to conducting research, while conveying more favorable views about quality improvement research.

* Correspondence: Bonnie Spring, PhD, ABPP, Behavioral Medicine Director, Northwestern University
Department of Preventive Medicine, 680 N Lake Shore Drive Suite 1220, Chicago, IL 60611 United States. E-mail: bspring@northwestern.edu.

The stakeholder module affords a valuable tool to introduce academic and community partners to each other's points of view, as a way of paving the way toward successful collaboration for research to practice translation.

Keywords: Practice-based research, community-based research, evidence-based practice

INTRODUCTION

There is a growing consensus that movement towards evidence-based practices will improve accountability for health care practice and help stimulate needed development of the research evidence base. This description of the development of, and lessons-learned from, the Resources for Training in Evidence-Based Behavioral Practice (EBBP) project's module entitled Stakeholder Dialogue about Evidence-Based Practice (1) outlines an approach to upgrade EBBP across settings and professions. The approach incorporates several components: 1) defining and understanding practice-based research, community-based research, and community-based participatory research; 2) starting a dialogue among stakeholders about existing misconceptions, goals, and ideas; 3) engaging these stakeholders as collaborators in furthering research to practice translation through discussion; 4) rapid dissemination of training resources via the world wide web; and 5) dissemination of the knowledge base to a variety of stakeholders.

As a result, the EBBP team decided to create a module that educates practitioners, community-members, and researchers about one another's perspectives, misunderstandings of motivation and goals, and ways to move forward.

EBBP PROJECT DEVELOPMENT AND BACKGROUND

In 2006, the National Institute of Health's Office of Behavioral and Social Science Research (OBSSR) commissioned the Resources for Training in Evidence-Based Behavioral Practice (EBBP) project. The goal of the project is to bridge the gap between behavioral research and practice by harmonizing and upgrading the evidence-based practice approach across health professions. The EBBP Project team is comprised of a multidisciplinary Council, Scientific Advisory Board, Practitioner Advisory Council (PRAC), and a panel of expert consultants. The Council for Training in Evidence-Based Behavioral Practice includes representatives from medicine, nursing, psychology, public health, and social work. Using a team science approach, the EBBP Project identifies training gaps and creates learning resources to facilitate research to practice translation across disciplines. Professionals from the major health disciplines are collaborating to learn, teach, and implement evidence-based practice through the training website www.ebbp.org. In addition to training tools, the Council has collaborated to create the three circles diagram, depicting the Transdisciplinary EBBP Conceptual Model (see figure 1).

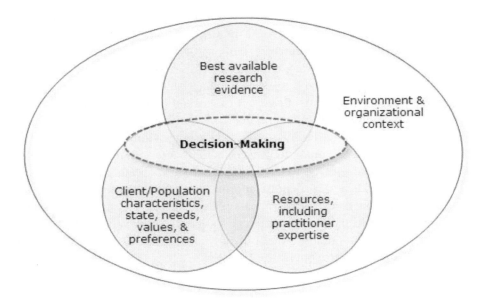

Figure 1. Transdisciplinary EBBP Conceptual Model.

The transdisciplinary EBBP model integrates the most important advances made within evidence-based practice models for social work, nursing, medicine, public health, and psychology (2). The model emphasizes the importance of shared decision-making, including the environment and organizational factors that influence feasibility in specific contexts. Evidence-based behavioral practice entails making decisions about how to promote healthful behaviors by integrating the best available evidence with practitioner expertise and other resources, and with the characteristics, state, needs, values and preferences of those who will be affected. This is done in a manner that is compatible with the environmental and organizational context. Evidence is comprised of research findings derived from the systematic collection of data through observation, experiment, the formulation of questions, and the testing of hypotheses. In addition to the three circles of EBBP conceptual model, the EBBP website is also home to nine completed training modules.

Topics include: 1) the EBBP Process module teaches users how to conduct the steps of the EBBP process with a simulated client and/or community; 2) the Searching for Evidence module teaches the strategies for choosing and using EBBP information tools; 3) the Systematic Review module teaches users how to evaluate and conduct a systematic review; 4) the Critical Appraisal module teaches about the critical appraisal and hierarchy of evidence; 5) the Randomized Controlled Trials module teaches users the basics of how to design and conduct randomized controlled trials (RCTs); 6) the Shared Decision-Making with Individual Clients module teaches users about the shared decision-making process by having them work through cases and attempt to balance the best available evidence with client preferences and resources in a clinical setting; 7) the Collaborative Decision-Making with Communities module teachers users about the collaborative decision-making process by having them work through a case from the point of view of a public health program manager working in a local health department; 8) the Stakeholder Dialogue about Evidence-Based Practice module combines didactic contact on practice-based, community-based, and community-based participatory research, along with video interviews of stakeholders discussing the barriers and facilitators to evidence-based practice; 9) the Implementation of Evidence-Based Practices module teaches learners about the implementation process through theoretical frameworks and the illustration of two real-world case examples of EBP implementation.

The EBBP website is also host to several other interprofessional training resources, including up-to-date announcements of relevant events and funding opportunities, a platform for users to upload and download syllabi on evidence-based practice, a resource library with links to articles, glossaries, and teaching tools, and a blog with contributions from experts across disciplines. The EBBP training tools were initially targeted towards graduate students across disciplines, but have evolved to target practitioners on an interprofessional level. The goal of the site is to provide a user-friendly, informative, interactive platform where students, academics, and practitioners can learn about evidence-based practice in a translational, interprofessional format. In the three years since its launch in November 2008, the site has had over 54,000 page views (almost 34,000 unique users) from 136 countries, with current traffic averaging 2,700 users per month.

METHODS

The goal of this particular module was to educate practitioners, community-members, and researchers about one another's perspectives, varying views on research and collaboration, and ways to move forward. Dr. Elizabeth Ryan, Assistant Professor and the Vice Chair for Education in the Department of Family and Community Medicine at Northwestern University's Feinberg School of Medicine identified community stakeholders. Dr. Bonnie Spring, Chair of the EBBP Council, identified Academic stakeholders through the connections she has developed at Northwestern. The identified stakeholders included clinicians, community health workers, community advocates, and academics from urban and rural settings, all of whom were willing to talk about their views about research. We utilized telephone calls or email requests to contact the interview pool and asked about their interested and willingness to participate in a recorded phone interview (30 minutes in length) and filmed in-person interview (60 minutes in length). The first round of interviews for this module by telephone, where we asked general questions to stakeholders about evidence-based practice and practice-based research, barriers to implementing evidence-based practices in their setting, and the feasibility of overcoming these barriers. We transcribed interviews and the EBBP team reviewed the transcripts and identified themes and key questions to ask in order to elicit these themes. From the telephone interviewee pool, we interviewed those stakeholders who consented on video. The EBBP team conducted these video interviews at Northwestern University and in community-based settings. We broke the resulting video content down into 60-90 second clips and grouped into themed categories. We paired the clips with didactic content on practice-based research and evidence on successful communication between researchers and practitioners/community members.

We identified themes and relevant didactic content in the next stage of developing the interactive course activities that relate to the video clips. Activities include learning about specific examples of components within the Three Circles Model of Evidence-Based Practice, definitions and examples of practice-based research, community-based research, and community-based participatory research, the components of translational research and how this is applied to practice, and exercises that allow learners to identify the pieces needed for successful partnership between stakeholders.

RESULTS

The goal of this tool is to start a dialogue between the stakeholders (e.g., researchers, practitioners, and community stakeholders) to understand each other's perspectives about research and evidence-based practice. This user-directed/exploration-oriented learning module does not dictate a forced order. Rather, learners may peruse the content that interests them most by clicking on related links to similarly themed content. Learners should be able to view all of the content in approximately one hour. Learning objectives were developed and are presented at the beginning of the module. By the end of viewing the module, learners should be able to:

- Describe practice-based research and community-based research from at least three different stakeholder perspectives.
- Compare different stakeholder perspectives on research evidence.
- Understand shared decision-making and collaboration between researchers and stakeholders in the practice and/or community.
- Describe stakeholder perspectives on practitioner, client, and community involvement in research.
- Identify barriers and facilitators to conducting research and implementing evidence-based practices in community settings, and describe the ways that different stakeholders perceive to overcome them.

Questions were broken down by themes including perceptions about different types of research, barriers to conducting research in practice and/or community settings, feasibility of overcoming these barriers, ways to motivate practitioners to participate in research, and evidence of value to practitioners. Video clips (about 60-90 seconds each) are grouped by theme in the module, so that learners can select an area of interest and view answers from a variety of stakeholders on that topic (see table 1 for summary).

Table 1. Stakeholder Summary Answer Table

QUESTION	STAKEHOLDER	ANSWER
What does research mean to you?	Community activist- urban setting	"Evidence-based practice is…really what drives what we do at the ground level, what happens in the community, and what happens among people. If we're doing work based on assumptions or a few people's great ideas, we may not know that we're doing the right thing because we're not asking the people who it's impacting and who would benefit."
	Health educator- urban setting	"Research to me means the academic efforts that are going on in our community to try to better our communities and our knowledge of the way our communities work and the way our world works."

Table 1. (Continued)

QUESTION	STAKEHOLDER	ANSWER
	Academic administrator- urban setting	"Empowerment is the key thing that I really want to emphasize with community research because it was really about the community taking a great stake into their intent and I tend to define empowerment with a kind of sense of self-determination."
How do you feel about quality improvement research?	Nurse- urban setting	"I feel that quality improvement means that you're not going to assume that you've met whatever goal. It's that you're always continuing to grow and that there are always more goals to reach, and I think that's very important."
	Physician- rural setting	"I think quality improvement research is really where it's at. Myself, I'm not really into research for novel things. I suppose I could be talked into that, but not too much. Primarily quality-based research is what is practical for my type of practice."
	Health educator- urban setting	"I think that quality-improvement research is absolutely essential in order to do what we do in the clinic. Neighborhoods change, populations change, needs change, budgets change. We need to sort of figure out constantly what our patients and what our community needs."
	Physician- urban setting	"Quality-improvement research is easily the research that I believe in the most....anybody that's been through medical school, the first thing they think of is bench research, you know working at the lab. That has no appeal to me, personally...but, a broader definition of research, talking about quality-improvement, that's what really motivates me to get involved."
How do you think patients and/or community-members feel about research?	Physician- urban setting	"I think a lot of my patients, being from an underserved community, have some reluctance about being a research subject. They certainly wouldn't want to perceive themselves that way, many people would not."
	Academic administrator- urban setting	"Community members have a lot of historical mistrust of research, especially within disenfranchised communities that may be over-researched. There's a different in how people may think of research that's conducted by...a public land grant institution, versus an institution...that is a private institution.
	Community activist- urban setting	"The community wants to do research. They may not always understand their role in research because historically, they have not been invited to participate in an equitable relationship in research. I believe it's going to take both the community learning the academic language and the academic learning the community language to make that culture shift, but the will and the interest is there."
	Academic professor- urban setting	"The research participants that we work with can be very, very nervous about research and of course there's a historical context for that...we need to be very clear with them, what will happen to the data, what the purpose of the research is, who will be there and what we'll be doing."
	Nurse- urban setting	"Most of the patients that I see are of low income and low health literacy, and I think that predominant feelings about research for these patients are negative because they are concerned that they may be manipulated to be involved in a study that might do them harm, and that it's for the greater good for someone else but not relating to themselves."
	Physician- rural setting	"My patients are fairly open to participating in it. When I have tried, on a limited basis, they have seemed open and excited to be a part of it. It makes them feel that they're assisting with progress."

QUESTION	STAKEHOLDER	ANSWER
What are some barriers to conducting research in community and practice settings?	Community activist- urban setting	"…academics come in with assumptions. People hear things in the news…and make generalizations about the people in a community or a particular population. And I think it's important for researchers to spend time observing, spend time listening, and really affirming if their assumptions are correct."
	Nurse- urban setting	"So much of my time I feel is spent working with my patients in some very basic ways to try and make sure we both know what medications they're taking, whether or not they've made certain referrals and kept them and gotten the results… as an individual in a clinical perspective, I'm not going to start up a research study from the beginning to the end. It's not going to happen for me."
What is the feasibility of overcoming barriers?	Community activist- urban setting	"If we can get presidents and deans at the universities to value and better inform academics how to go about doing this… you have to create a culture within the university that is going to motivate academics to engage communities, and give them the time and the resources do it in a meaningful way."
	Academic administrator- urban setting	"Barriers are going to exist no matter what. Part of us in public health, our role is to really find problems. I think that what motivates today's community-based researchers is that…we can empower people, and make that fine transition communication between the academics and the community. What it's going to take is a strategy to really adjust to the changing trends that exist, and be mutually engaging with each partner at the table."
	Nurse- rural setting	"Information that can be accessed as to what you're doing, why you're doing it, the benefits of it, because people have to buy into what you're doing… it is important to get that information out so there is not miscommunication, misinformation."
	Physician- urban setting	"Neither side should feel superior to the other…researchers need to come into a situation not with that false modesty, but with a real desire to partner with the organization they're working with."
What can be done to motivate practitioners to participate in practice-based research?	Academic professor- urban setting	"Motivating practitioners to participate in practice-based research is actually a lot easier than most people think. It's on their radar; they want to do it. They just need some help in figuring out which evidence-based practices and how do we get these in place. I think it's really on us now to deliver and be as conscientious as we can be to provide them with the types of tools that they really need."
	Physician- rural setting	"…it is probably difficult, but I think of course financial incentives would be helpful."
How would you like to see treatment guidelines presented so that they factor in diversity and contextual issues?	Physician- urban setting	"..when I'm evaluating treatment guidelines…I want to make sure that the research has incorporated African American patients, low-income patients, women who are younger than the typical research age. I want to make sure that those projects have incorporated the people that I work with."
	Health educator- urban setting	"I think treatment guidelines need to represent the communities in which you're working, and the needs of that community and diversity of that community."
What are the specific sources of evidence that you value?	Physician- rural setting	"…primarily I use the online resource *Up to Date*. I also use the *Prescriber's Newsletter* for things related to medications."

Table 1. (Continued)

QUESTION	STAKEHOLDER	ANSWER
	Nurse- rural setting	"…I value those which can be documented, something I can see in black and white such as test results. Something that I can use that will help me plot to the next goal or phase…something that is observable to the eye…something that is even verbally spoken I value, because many times what a patient reveals in conversation between a nurse and him/her is not the same information that gets communicated with the physician. So, those types of evidence cannot be discounted."

LESSONS LEARNED

From the interviews conducted for the Stakeholder Dialogue about Evidence-Based Practice module, there were many consistent themes that arose. First, most stakeholders saw research and evidence-based practice as not only helpful but also integral to community empowerment and advancement. However, quality-improvement research was overwhelmingly favored over "bench" or "lab" research, because of its perceived applicability to specific populations in particular settings. Practitioners generally expressed that quality improvement research was the main type of research they could see themselves conducting. Among this subset of stakeholders, those who worked in urban settings indicated that they perceived patients and community members as being weary of research because of negative historical connotations with underserved groups. However, one rural practitioner indicated that her patients were very open to research because of its contribution to helping others.

When asked about barriers to conducting research in community settings, lack of time and prevalence of incorrect assumptions on the part of academics were discussed. Increased communication, genuine partnership, incentives to practitioners, and support from academic institutions was cited as the methods most feasible for overcoming these barriers. While stakeholders expressed positive feelings about treatment guidelines, they indicated that their lack of cultural-tailoring was problematic. In particular, those practitioners interviewed from rural settings valued online open-access evidence as well as information from patients.

A primary component of the EBBP process is shared-decision making with not only other health professionals, but with the clients and communities themselves. Shared-decision making utilizes the best available evidence while engaging the patient to share in selecting and implementing a specific approach. Integrating evidence, expertise, resources and client/community preferences is the essence of shared-decision making. When engaging in community-based or practice-based research, shared decision-making between academic institutions and practitioners/communities is integral to an equitable, successful collaboration. The Stakeholder Dialogue about Evidence-Based Practice module is a free, web-based tool for a variety of healthcare stakeholders that initiates a discussion of misconceptions, misunderstands, and ways to move forward. This dialogue serves, as a way to begin to bridge the gap between a variety of stakeholders from various settings and professions, in the hopes that increased discussions will lead to more successful and comprehensive collaborations based in shared decisions.

REFERENCES

[1]   Spring B, Ferguson MJ, Carbone E, Ryan E. Online training module: Stakeholder dialogue about evidence-based practice. Evidence-based behavioral practice: Bridging research and practice 2011. Accessed 2011 Nov 05. URL: http://www.ebbp.org/training.html.

[2]   Spring B, Hitchcock K. Evidence-based practice in psychology. In: Weiner IB, Craighead WE, eds. Corsini's encyclopedia of psychology, 4th edition. New York: Wiley, 2009:603-7.

Submitted: November 15, 2011. *Revised:* January 30, 2012. *Accepted:* February 08, 2012.

In: Public Health Yearbook 2013   ISBN: 978-1-63321-095-0
Editor: Joav Merrick   © 2014 Nova Science Publishers, Inc.

Chapter 7

DRIVING EQUITY AT A COMMUNITY LEVEL: CASE STUDIES OF COMMUNITY-BASED PEER-DELIVERED HEALTH-CARE SERVICES AND PROGRAMS

Margot Lettner, LLB, BSW (Hons), Estelle Sun, BA (Hons), and Bob Gardner, PhD*

Wasabi Consulting, Toronto, Ontario and The Wellesley
Institute, Toronto, Ontario, Canada

ABSTRACT

Phase 1 of this project, reported here, is an exploratory investigation into the effectiveness of community-based, peer-delivered healthcare services and programs in a diverse urban community, the Greater Toronto Area (GTA), Ontario, Canada. Peer health workers have shown promise in working with marginalized or other hard-to-reach groups who face complex barriers to good healthcare, well-being and quality of life. Inconsistent definitions and reporting measures have made formal and comprehensive evaluation challenging. This study uses two complementary research methods: a Literature Review, and Case Studies constructed from key informant interviews at selected health and social service providers in the GTA. It analyzes where peer healthcare initiatives tend to be located, what services they provide, and how their context and design interact to determine their workability and success. It highlights the facilitators, success conditions and best practices, as well as the challenges or barriers. Peer health workers are "the best messengers" to penetrate communities that non-peers cannot. Peer models drive enriched data collection and analysis, enhanced capacity for relevant and actionable research-into-policy and practice, and innovative community collaboration and broader partnerships. Peer work experience also provides "pathways" to professional education and employment. Resourcing is difficult. Peer models take more project management time, particularly around role clarity and mentoring. Gender and remuneration are key issues.

---

* Correspondence: Margot Lettner, Associate, The Wellesley Institute and Principal, Wasabi Consulting, 10 Bingham Avenue, Toronto, Ontario, Canada M4E 3P9. E-mail: ml.wasabi@rogers.com.

The findings suggest promising directions for program development and service interventions that build community-engaged scholarship, practice and capacity; and will interest researchers, policymakers, providers and advocates aiming to drive health equity into practice.

Keywords: Peer health workers, peer workers, health ambassadors, health navigators, health promoters, health talkers, community-based health care, community-based health workers

INTRODUCTION

The Wellesley Institute, based in Toronto, Ontario, Canada is a non-profit and non-partisan research and policy institute focused on developing research and community-based policy solutions to the problems of urban health and health disparities. Wellesley commissioned this Case Study Series, Driving Equity at a Community Level: Case Studies of Community-Based Peer-Delivered Health-Care Services and Programs, in 2010 to complement a Literature Review it conducted, "The Potential of Community-Based Peer-Delivered Healthcare Services and Programs" (1). The series was envisioned in several phases, with Phase 1 focusing on peer workers in health programs and services located in the Greater Toronto Area (GTA).

Interest in peer health workers, and evidence of their practice and its outcomes among health and social service providers and their clients in the Greater Toronto Area, developed out of a series of Health Equity Roundtables facilitated by The Wellesley Institute in 2009. These Roundtables brought together about 30 service providers, policymakers, and community- and academic-based researchers as "key informants" to create an informal best practices and advocacy network in the GTA around health disparities or inequities, socio-economic determinants of health, promising directions and gaps, and enablers and barriers to change.

The emerging philosophy and practice of peer workers was one area of discussion. At the suggestion of the Roundtables, The Wellesley Institute collaboratively developed this project to "dig deeper" into how and why peer workers provide health and social services in the GTA through a parallel and complementary Literature Review/Case Study approach that looks at three key lines of experiential inquiry: how the peer-based program or service works, why it works (facilitators, success conditions or best practices), and what challenges working with this model presents (barriers). This paper reports on Phase 1 of the project.

Two notes about terms and definitions used in this project. "Peer" is a flexible term as currently used in both the literature and in practice. This project adopts the definition suggested by the literature: "the term 'peer' is defined loosely as someone from the community being served. Such a loose definition allows for varying levels of expertise, from laypersons to professionals, so long as the person possesses the identifying traits of the community" (1). Similarly, when speaking of community, the literature suggests that:

> 'Community' refers to a group of people sharing identifying common traits such as ethnicity, race, religion, location or neighbourhood, sexual orientation, past or present health concern, educational status, age, lifestyle, and life-stage. To be community-based, a service or program must take place as close to the community as possible (1).

Where necessary, this paper refers to the broader term "health and social service providers" to reflect the reality that the health and social service sectors do cross over, both in policy and practice; and that many service providers are, in fact, multi-service agencies that work across sectors, disciplines and areas of practice. Several of the eight specific programs or services studied are multi-service agencies.

A comment about the project's scope. The terms of reference were highly focused for several reasons. The project had limited resources to access and collect data among communities of practice whose existence, location, size and client reach were relatively unknown among health and social service providers in the GTA, or known primarily through ever-changing networks of community-based contacts.

As a result, Phase 1 was envisioned as a preliminary, exploratory or "pilot" research project, a starting-point to explore the discussions, promising directions and recommendations from the Health Equity Roundtables and suggest next steps for Phase 2. The case study findings reported in this paper are therefore based on data gathered from a relatively small number, eight, of community-based peer-delivered healthcare services and programs that constitute field work component of the project.

It is hoped that Phase 2 will be more research-intensive and geographically-extensive. It is also hoped that it will be developed in collaboration with a broader-based group of partners; and, from a strategic perspective, to respond to and enrich a public policy environment increasingly interested in and directed towards applied research and policy-into-practice innovations, as well as knowledge-sharing among academic and community-based researchers, practitioners, policymakers and people who use health and social services.

As the literature shows three most common kinds of community-based, peer-delivered care, the project team looked for service providers working in these areas as potential project participants/key informants: health promotion and prevention, navigation of the complex healthcare system, and comprehensive service provision. The resulting Case Studies are therefore aligned accordingly. The team added a fourth kind, community-based research/inclusion research methods, in order to capture the extensive work being done by a selection of province-wide networks to document and support awareness and practice of peer delivery (2). While it is useful to review the findings specific to each kind of care, reading across the groups highlights their common themes.

Two notes to reading this paper. The Case Studies featured are real-time histories and experiences of front-line practitioners and management, "live" experiential qualitative data. These data are therefore shown in a practice-note format where appropriate.

Finally, this paper has been edited for space from the original Research Report and Literature Review. The background or "how it works" information that gives more nuanced comparative context, as well as practical implementation and administration detail, about the eight specific programs or services studied has been highly compressed. This allows the results and discussion of the findings – "why it works" and "challenges" – to be foregrounded. Both the full Literature Review and Research Report can be read or downloaded at www.wellesleyinstitute.com (1, 3).

METHODS

A literature review was conducted to assess the potential of peer-delivered, community-based health-care services. Evaluations of peer services were reviewed, along with a deeper analysis of 15 programs that fall under the promotion, navigation, and comprehensive service delivery categories (4-17). Preference was given to Canadian programs, however compelling international cases were also included for review. The findings show enormous potential for peer-delivered services to improve health care and health outcomes among marginalized populations. Several common facilitators and barriers to program success were identified.

The field research component of this project, the Case Studies, looks at eight different health and/or social service programs or services situated in six different agencies in the GTA. The exclusive field research method used is qualitative through key informant interviews based on a standardized research instrument. Table 1 reproduces the instrument, a progressive series of factual and interpretive/opinion questions.

Participating organizations either self-identified or were invited. The primary selection criteria were: community-based organizations providing health and/or social programs or services to diverse client populations and known to support or host relatively mature peer-based delivery. Although the particulars and depth of their experience were shaped by variables of organization model, type of services, staff recruitment approaches, and communities served/catchment area and so differed, all key informants were experienced in developing, implementing and evaluating community-based peer-delivered healthcare services and programs in an urban health setting.

Secondary selection criteria ensured that key informants represented a diverse range of health and social service providers, from community health clinics providing direct service through patient drop-ins to non-profit organizations specializing in mentoring clients through diagnosis, treatment and recovery; from chronic disease to acute care expertise; from office to street health service settings.

All case studies are situated in and report on community-based peer-delivered healthcare services and programs that operate within a primarily publicly-funded, universally-accessible health and social service system, the Ontario Health Insurance Plan (OHIP) that operates within the legislative and regulatory requirements of the Canada Health Act, and its complementary federal-provincial-territorial agreements.

Key informants participated in a one-hour interview with project staff, who developed an interview instrument focused on collecting basic information about the genesis, structure, and mandate/goals of the program or service; the process the organization used to commit to and develop peer delivery; client demographics; and evaluation. Interviews were conducted in-person or by conference call. Interview notes were taken, reviewed and analyzed by the project team.

Given that the terms of reference resulted in a smaller sample size and dataset, to test consistency of findings as well as introduce a broader perspective and analysis that might suggest new lines of inquiry for a Phase 2, the Case Study data were also compared with the outcomes of the Literature Review to look for correlated, conflicting or neutral findings. This comparison also emphasizes that a core competency for working in public policy issues – whether advocacy, gathering and analyzing evidence, collaboration and partnership, strategic and operational planning, policymaking, frontline service and in-service training – is taking research-into-practice and practice-into-policy, that is, making research, policy and practice interactive.

RESULTS

The results of the comparative analysis between the findings from the Case Studies and the Literature Review are reviewed first. This analysis is then supplemented and illustrated in practice by reference to the eight case studies of actual community-based peer-delivered health programs and services that form the basis of the "live" data.

While the sample size is relatively small, representing a small selection of agencies currently working with peer-based models in active practice settings in the GTA, and the data therefore very preliminary, the results show promising directions. The findings from both the Case Studies and the Literature Review show significant correlations along key facilitators, success conditions or best practices for developing and implementing community-based peer-delivered health services that tend to locate in organizational culture and administration (open change management system, creative leadership, champions), human resource policy (flexibility, innovation), and partnerships (community-building, third-party endorsement).

The comparative findings also show significant correlations regarding key challenges or barriers in organizational culture and administration (provider, funder, regulator), human resource policy (definition of employee/staff, conventions of contracts/collective agreements), funding/resourcing (base/project funding, core/discretionary budget items) and peer worker training/ongoing mentoring.

A convergence of practice and literature

First, here are the key findings in brief from the literature. The literature shows the potential for peer-based models in health and social service delivery to contribute to positive outcomes in both client health and community development:

> Current evaluations of community-based, peer-delivered healthcare services and programs show promising results…. Of the organizations that conducted surveys about user preferences, many marginalized groups clearly state that they prefer healthcare providers who are experienced with problems they are going through….patients have a strong preference for service providers who they can trust to be accepting of them and to implicitly understand their viewpoints…with whom they share key individual traits: race, gender, religion, sexual orientation, age and life stage, cancer, street involvement and drug abuse…. Evaluations of the success of programs and services that incorporate these design principles show increases in healthy behaviour (1).

> [I]t is clear that there is enormous potential for these types of services to improve healthcare access and utilization and health outcomes…. Of the cases reviewed, existing program evaluations have documented increased client satisfaction, shorter wait times, higher screening rates, and healthier lifestyle choices, particularly among underserved and vulnerable populations (1).

Second, because peer-delivery contributes to more equitable access to care, it supports both community and individual capacity building, emphasizes and encourages information sharing, builds networks, and develops partnerships across communities (1).

Third, the literature reports there is a real gap between the intent of providers or caregivers to be "fair" when providing services to clients and client experiences of "fair treatment":

> From qualitative studies involving health service providers and members of marginalized groups, we know that despite caregivers' beliefs that they are fair and free of prejudice, their choices and treatment towards certain patients is negatively impacted by discrimination and biases. Patients from vulnerable groups consistently report feeling uncomfortable talking openly with their caregivers, feeling judged, being misinterpreted, not receiving culturally or religiously appropriate and sensitive care, and feeling embarrassed. Membership in various vulnerable or disadvantaged groups often translates into additional barriers to accessing healthcare services such as communications difficulties, logistical problems such as work and children, cultural beliefs that are at odds with utilizing healthcare services, and not having appropriate health services in close proximity (1).

Taken together, these three findings from the literature provides important context and rationale for the theory and practice of peer health workers in frontline healthcare delivery and community-based or inclusion researchers.

The literature identifies four main facilitators, success conditions or best practices that support peer delivery:

- flexibility to accommodate the dynamic needs of both peers and their communities
- paid compensation for peer workers for work done
- initial and ongoing training and support/mentoring for peers
- program/service evaluation to facilitate mature peer delivery and continuity (1)

The case study data add these two additional facilitators:

- participation by peers in program or service development, from recruitment to mentoring to monitoring
- rigorous quality assurance, again from recruitment to mentoring to monitoring (3)

Together, the literature and the case study data provide a congruent, pragmatic and promising guide to what makes peer delivery work; as key informants in the case studies emphasized, and which is reported below in greater and more operational detail, peers are "the best messengers" and penetrate more deeply into communities than non-peer workers. More significantly, the literature and this study agree on four main challenges or barriers to peer delivery:

- peer life-stage, specifically, a person's ability to adapt their own health and lifestyle to a work environment
- definition, establishment, and maintenance or breach of personal boundaries between peers and co-workers where peers are similar to the clients they serve

- marketing to marginalized communities often removed from usual ways to share information
- predominance of unstable, usually grant-based, funding that dismantles initiatives before maturity (1, 3)

The case study data add these four additional barriers:

- conflict in philosophy of service delivery between peer and non-peer workers (although training/mentoring and interdisciplinary teams mitigate this)
- organizational capacity to support customized peer needs as well as service demand and client expectations
- client preferences for credentialed professionals or specific delivery settings, e.g., individualized care instead of groups
- scaling up, i.e., to date, peer delivery and inclusion research are generally found in relatively small-scale initiatives, replicating them in larger projects often meets with institutional and funder resistance (3)

Again, when their results are integrated, the literature and the case study data provide a congruent, pragmatic and promising guide to the challenges in implementing peer delivery. A look at more specific findings from the case study data now amplifies these comparative results and further strengthens the argument for an iterative approach to research, practice and policy, both with respect to the study of peer health workers and policy research, development and evaluation in general.

Case study findings, peer-delivered health promotion and prevention

Findings from two case studies of peer-delivered health promotion and prevention programs (18-19) have been integrated and are profiled below (Case Studies: Peer Nutrition Program, Toronto Public Health, Toronto, Ontario, www.toronto.ca/health; and Breast Health Ambassadors, South Riverdale Community Health Centre, Toronto, Ontario, www.srchc.ca). The data are strong and consistent that peer-delivered services work in health promotion and prevention for these reasons:

- Peers are the "best messengers" and can penetrate into parts of communities that non-peers cannot: "it's the passion of peer workers, they have the pulse of the community, go the extra mile." Peers also demonstrate a "multiplier effect" in knowledge translation and service delivery: "First, 20 families know about breast health, then 40 know"
- Peer work translates equity into equal opportunity, e.g., people get information in a way they understand
- Quality training and coaching, e.g., be clear about the boundaries between knowing answers to questions and undertaking to find out, what to talk about and what not to discuss with participants, having peers work in pairs and with the coordinator

- Provider organization has to commit to the model and ongoing support, mentoring, quality assurance
- Informal evaluation indicates that peer work experience provides good bridging or "pathways" to professional education and employment for people in immigrant communities or who are marginalized or have low educational levels

The data are also strong and consistent that peer delivery presents these challenges in health promotion and prevention:

- Resourcing for robust and sustainable service, including funding
- Contact with hard-to-reach communities: "Those that are absent from the program's reach"
- Compensation for peer workers, viewed both as a labour market and social justice issue: "No one else volunteers their time, why should peer workers?"
- Recognition by health care system, especially in health promotion, and flexibility for less rigid service delivery models (e.g., models defined by age ranges leave people out)
- Working with peers means more work for the provider as mentor and quality overseer
- Conflict between philosophy of professionals and that of peer workers, but training can mitigate
- Unionization, but customized labour force model can mitigate
- Retention

Case study findings, navigation of the healthcare system

Findings from one case study of a national peer-delivered health system navigation program (20) are profiled below (Case Study: Willow Breast Cancer Support Canada, Toronto, Ontario, www.willow.org). The data are strong and consistent that peer-delivered services work in health system navigation for these reasons:

- Clear expectations about what the peer program is to deliver: "Define what you are and are not as a provider and your range of service"
- Appropriate and rigorous peer candidate recruitment, application and screening processes with a focus on candidate's capacity to be effective and understand the boundaries between self-care/empathy and caregiving/sympathy, to reduce the risk of harm within the program
- Structured training focused on peer practice" "Training is an equalizer…[capacity] is not about a particular intellectual package"
- Co-facilitators or "wing women" to support each peer, especially with respect to self-care, gradual introduction of peers into practice

The data are also strong and consistent that peer delivery presents these challenges in health system navigation:

- Desire to help is larger than capacity to serve, as well as ability to build that capacity and referral network that builds with it
- Working with diversity, e.g., relationship building with communities for a deeper understanding of cultural competency as well as linguistic barriers
- Liability of peer support groups is unclear, as they are not accredited and there is no "global standard" for peer work
- Resourcing for robust and sustainable service, including funding
- Resource management, e.g., development of code of conduct for peers, compensation
- Feedback, evaluation and recognition of peer workers: "It's the daily stuff...like 'how are you?' and 'what do you need?'"
- Retention, particularly where per work is driven by survivors (e.g., further diagnosis, financial instability, death)

Case study findings, comprehensive service provision

Findings from three case studies of peer-delivered comprehensive service provision (21-23) are integrated and profiled below (Case Studies: Diabetes and Urban Health Initiative, South Riverdale Community Health Centre, Toronto, Ontario, www.srchc.ca; Toronto Harm Reduction Task Force, Toronto, Ontario, www.torontoharmreduction@yahoo.ca; and Harm Reduction Urban Health Initiative, South Riverdale Community Health Centre, Toronto, Ontario, www.srchc.ca).

"Comprehensive service provision" in this project means service that crosses sectors, disciplines or areas of practice, usually involving diverse teams of laypersons and professionals serving target populations with complex needs. Harm reduction strategies, for example, may include addiction, mental health and well-being, nutrition, and community development services. The data are strong and consistent that peer-delivered services work in comprehensive service provision for these reasons:

- Peers are the "best messengers" and can penetrate into parts of communities that non-peers cannot, particularly where stigma and criminalization of behaviours are issues and trust in providers can be compromised: "The stuff they know, I don't know how else I would find out" and "The wisdom of the community will always exceed the knowledge of the expert."
- Service delivery context must be participatory to ensure relevance, i.e., developed by peers
- Clear roles and responsibilities: "We all do what we're good at"
- Services based on a "how to manage" approach, such as diabetes management, is an inadequate response; it must be co-located with a focus on health literacy and health beliefs as a broader response to chronic disease management

The data are also strong and consistent that peer delivery presents these challenges in comprehensive service provision:

- Resourcing for robust and sustainable service, including funding

- Recognition that peer models are distinct relationship-building and intervention models for work with diverse communities: "Not a buddy system"
- Resolution of the conflicted status of peer workers as "staff or clients?" e.g., what equity of relationship do peer workers have with agency employees when they also access agency services
- Communities with cultural parameters that are adverse to groups or group learning; or are only highly responsive to credentialed professionals such as doctors for information and advice, or recognize health providers along preferred lines of gender, class, and age (generally male, relatively high socio-economic status, older); or stigmatize the health issue being addressed and create misinformation as well as conflicting choices for intervention
- Access to in-service or continuing education for peer workers to strengthen referral training for co-indicated health and social issues, as well as training in crisis and case management, trauma, and mental health issues; accessing the potential of peer networks that seem loose by agency standards are still functional
- Retention of peer workers; recognition that compensation improves retention and ownership

Case study findings, community-based or inclusion research methods

Findings from two case studies of peer models as the foundation for community-based or inclusion research methods (24-25) are integrated and profiled below (Case Studies: Count Us In! Marginalized Women, Inclusion, and Stroke, Ontario Women's Health Network, Toronto, Ontario, www.owhn.on.ca; Toronto Community-Based Research Network, Toronto, Ontario, www.Toronto CBR.ca).

The data are strong and consistent that peer models work as the foundation of community-based or inclusion research methods. At the project level, peer models combined with community- or inclusion-based research methods work for these reasons:

- The lived experience of peers informs the lives of others, creates "a sense of belonging" to the community and ownership of the research
- Keeps the focus on health equity strategies and tools that are relevant to the most marginal populations and reduces their health disparities
- Benefits for peer workers: access to training, enhanced knowledge and skills, companionship of learning in peer-facilitated groups (shared experience, contacts, resources), broader work, networking and education opportunities, income: "Being in the driver's seat, not the passenger seat"

At the level of organizations and systems, peer models work for these reasons:

- Penetrate into parts of communities that non-peers cannot; bring together partners with shared values and strong credibility, as well as clear partnership agreements, terms of reference, advisory committees

- Support collaborative research partnerships and communities of practice, building capacity at the local level and increases knowledge transfer and exchange
- Enhance credibility, relevance and quality of data collection and consequent research, policy and service products: "Better results for people, providers, and policymakers"
- Benefits for organizations: increased credibility with communities, better capacity for knowledge and collaboration, better health outcomes for clients, better organizational outcomes for providers

The data are also strong and consistent that peer models present challenges when combined with community-based or inclusion research methods. At the project level, these are the challenges:

- Research team competencies in peer work, e.g., experiential understanding of equity and inclusion framework, ability to meet diversity of communities, flexibility to adapt project to changing needs, capacity to support and retain peer workers, capacity to share power among team members equitably, ability to manage enhanced expectations of research impact
- Realistic project timelines that integrate the basic requirements and outcomes of both peer and standard project management models, e.g., recruitment, training/ongoing mentoring, participation, conflict resolution, retention
- Ability of peers to have a voice broader than their own and see themselves relative to other members of their community; and confidentiality issues and protocols when inclusion researchers and participants know each other, belong to the same communities
- Designing and maintaining ongoing knowledge translation strategies and tools so resources can be adjusted as communities change; encouraging online and other dialogue can be difficult

At the level of organizations and systems, peer models present challenges for these reasons:

- Lack of informed and supportive organizational support and culture
- Still used primarily in relatively small projects; interest in and support for adaptation for larger projects, e.g., in hospitals, government, has been problematic" "Must have more than one inclusion researcher, no 'lone voice'"
- Funding for direct service delivery where inclusion researchers work with front-line providers can be difficult, as can funding for direct research costs can also be difficult, e.g., honoraria, food, transportation, meeting space, increased staff time for mentoring, dissemination and advocacy, internal and external training, childcare, interpretation
- Ethics and funding approval protocol developed principally for academic-based research, e.g., timing of approvals often precedes recruitment of peer workers, perception that community-based or inclusion research is not valid research

DISCUSSION

Promising directions: Towards a more comprehensive peer practice for Ontario.

The Literature Review and the Case Study findings from this project agree on five key outcomes of community-based peer-delivered healthcare services and programs:

- Peer health workers are the "best messengers" to, from and with communities
- Peer models drive enriched data collection and analysis, enhanced capacity for relevant and activist research-into-policy and practice, and innovative community collaboration and broader partnerships
- Peer models take more project management time and may require different project milestones and deliverables
- Resourcing, including funding, is difficult
- An emerging labour market and social justice dimension to peer models, although unintended in practice, indicates that peer work experience provides good bridging or "pathways" to professional education and employment for people in immigrant communities or who are marginalized or have low educational levels

The Literature Review and the Case Study findings also highlight the need for further research and development of practice-informed knowledge about peer health workers in these areas:

- Different "job titles" – from "peers" to "navigators" to "promoters" to "teams" – across organizations result in peer workers with different levels of expertise, training, and membership status in communities, makes assessment of "who to evaluate" difficult
- Different meanings of "peer" across communities, organizations, and program/services, makes assessment of relative "peerness" and its relationship to outcomes difficult
- High variability and customization in program/service mandates and guidelines for peer work, e.g., recruitment/selection strategies and criteria, makes assessment of "what to evaluate" difficult
- High variability in documentation of program and service demographics, e.g., peer gender, age, community membership, training/mentoring, roles, paid/volunteer, recruitment strategies, measures of satisfaction; as well as program location, size, duration, funding/resources, outcomes
- The continuation of historical gendered patterns of unpaid caring work provided by women, even in an innovative service model such as peer delivery that supports equity-based practice in marginalized communities: peers are most frequently women – even among non-gender-specified services – and their unpaid work contains labour costs in the health care system

Finally, Phase 1 of this project suggests further and more localized research directions to build a more comprehensive picture of community-based peer-delivery in Ontario's health and social programs and services:

- Moving beyond the initial GTA scope to a provincial scope to enable outreach and data collection from a cross-section of organizations that work with peer delivery models across Ontario
- Collaborating on development of a clearinghouse for Ontario-based health and social service providers at a minimum to document peer-delivered programs and services; share best practices and evaluation outcomes and recommendations; and mentor among health and social service front-line providers and management, researchers, and policymakers

ACKNOWLEDGMENTS

Financial and research support for phase 1 of the Case Study Series Community-Based Peer-Delivered Healthcare Services and Programs and the preparation of this paper was provided by The Wellesley Institute, Toronto, Ontario, Canada, www.wellesleyinstitute.com.

Table 1. Interview questions for key informant interviews

Context – Project Description
The Wellesley Institute is building an inventory of community-based, peer-delivered programs and services that advance health equity based on case studies. The initial focus of this inventory is GTA-area health and social service providers, although this lens may broaden provincially as our research progresses. Preliminary research indicates that these initiatives are often found in three service clusters: peer health promotion/education, system navigation, and community health and support. They are offered by diverse service providers under different names, e.g., ambassadors, navigators, health talkers, lay educators/advocates, facilitators.
Wellesley is interested in working towards a more comprehensive picture of where these programs and services are, what services they provide and how, and how their context and design interact to determine their workability or success. As part of Wellesley's mandate is to lead and facilitate research, policy interventions, and community engagement to shape policy change that enhances health equity for urban populations, we continue to gather evidence-based data that provides the foundation for this work. We see this particular project as filling a critical information gap in our heath equity work with public policy decisionmakers, communities, and partners.
Interview questions
1. Please briefly describe your organization.   2. Please describe how your organization supports health equity in its programs, services, projects, and/or organizational culture.   3. Based on the above description of community-based, peer-delivered programs and services that advance health equity, does your organization have any programs, services, or projects like this?   4. If yes, please describe each program, service, or project, e.g., name, what it does, how it works, client/patient profile, staff profile, delivery area, funding envelope, informal or formal evaluations.

5. What did you learn from this experience in general, e.g., what works and doesn't work to advance health equity at community, operational, and organizational/policy levels?

6. More specific to this program, service or project, what specific factors affected its outcomes? How were they facilitators or challenges to success? e.g., the impact of community partnership, fit with existing or proposed government policy or program priority, developmental phase and process (pilot or mature), access to and type of funding/other resources, support of champions or decision makers, learnings from similar initiatives, social or economic determinants of health.

7. What is your idea of "success" for this program, service, or project's advancement of health equity, and was it successful?

8. Did you informally or formally evaluate this program, service, or project? If so, what did you learn from this case study or assessment? Would Wellesley be able to review it?

9. What are you, or would you, do differently?

10. In your view, what are the best contexts and best outcomes that service providers should aim for to support advancing health equity? What complementary policy and resource supports are needed?

11. What other programs, services or projects like yours should Wellesley contact for this research?

12. Is there anything else you'd like to add to your comments? Would you like to remain involved in this research? How?

REFERENCES

[1]   Sun E. The potential of community-based peer-delivered healthcare services and programs. Toronto: Wellesley Institute, 2010.

[2]   Roche B, Guta A, Flicker S. Peer research in action. Accessed 2011 Nov 05. URL: www.wellesleyinstitute.com. uncategorized/peer-research-in-action.

[3]   Lettner M. Every service user is a service provider: A case for community-based peer-delivered healthcare services and programs. Toronto: Wellesley Institute, 2010.

[4]   McKeown D. Peer nutrition program evaluation. Toronto: City Toronto, 2006.

[5]   The early years peer outreach training curriculum for newcomer women. Accessed 2011 Nov 05. URL:http://accessalliance.ca/sites/accessalliance/files/documents/3.1%20-%20Peer%20Outreach%20Curriculum.pdf.

[6]   Karwalajtys T, McDonough B, Hall H, Guirguis-Younger M, Chambers LW, Kaczorowski J et al. Development of the volunteer peer educator role in a community Cardiovascular Health Awareness Program (CHAP): a process evaluation in two communities. J Commun Health 2009;34(4), 336-45.

[7]   Healthy women healthy communities. Accessed 2011 Nov 05. URL: http://www.mujersana.ca/index.php.

[8]   Peer health worker evaluation: A pilot project of Kitchener Downtown Community Health Centre. Kitchener: Centre Community Based Research, 2009.

[9]   Wellspring Cancer Support. Accessed 2011 Nov 05. URL: http://www.ywbc.ca/ and http://sunnybrook.ca/foundation/media/item.asp?c=1andi=436andpage=.

[10] Native sisters program. Accessed 2011 Nov 05. URL: http://www.innovations.ahrq.gov/content.aspx?id=1879.

[11] Gibson KB, Raven J, Spittal P. Evaluation of the mobile access project (MAP). Vancouver: Unpublished, 2006.

[12]   White S, Park YS, Israel T, Cordero ED. Longitudinal evaluation of peer health education on a college campus: impact on health behaviors. J Am Coll Health 2009;57(5):497-505.

[13]   WeCARE project website. Accessed 2011 Nov 05. URL: http://www.ucdmc.ucdavis.edu/cancer/Education_programs/patients/Peer_Navigator.html.

[14]   Steinberg ML, Fremont A, Khan DC, Huang D, Knapp H, Karaman D, et al. Lay patient navigator program implementation for equal access to cancer care and clinical trials: essential steps and initial challenges. Cancer 2006;107(11):2669-77.

[15]   Sherbourne Health Centre website. Accessed 2011 Nov 05. URL: http://www.sherbourne.on. ca/programs/programs.html.

[16]   The crack users project: A manual. Toronto: Street Health, 2007.

[17]   Sampaio LFR (Producer). The primary health care (APS) strategy in Brazil, 2006. Accessed 2011 Nov 05. URL:http://www.google.ca/url?sa=tandsource=webandcd=1andved=0CBUQFjAAandurl=http% 3A%2F%2Fwww.lachealthsys.org%2Fdocuments%2Fevents%2Fhonduras06%2FPrograma_Salud_Fa miliar_Brasil_ENG.ppsandrct=jandq=brazil%20family%20health%20programandei=peM1TdPYA8L qgQeorbW-Cwandusg=AFQjCNFu65u0THrpGAxlmkcY4mOe7ztyzgandsig2=D2vvL8Ik8w Gr0eEptaembAandcad=rja

[18]   Peer nutrition program. Toronto: Toronto Public Health, 2010. (interview)

[19]   Breast Health Ambassadors, South Riverdale Community Health Centre. Toronto, Ontario, 2010. (interview)

[20]   Willow Breast Cancer Support Canada. Toronto, Ontario, 2010. (Interview)

[21]   Diabetes and Urban Health Initiative, South Riverdale Community Health Centre. Toronto, Ontario, 2010. (Interview)

[22]   Toronto Harm Reduction Task Force. Toronto, Ontario, 2010. (Interview)

[23]   Harm Reduction Urban Health Initiative, South Riverdale Community Health Centre. Toronto, Ontario, 2010.

[24]   Count Us In! Marginalized Women, Inclusion, and Stroke. Ontario Women's Health Network. Interview. Toronto, Ontario, 2010.

[25]   Toronto Community-Based Research Network. Toronto, Ontario, 2010. (Interview)

Submitted: November 15, 2011. *Revised:* February 01, 2012. *Accepted:* February 09, 2012.

In: Public Health Yearbook 2013
Editor: Joav Merrick

ISBN: 978-1-63321-095-0
© 2014 Nova Science Publishers, Inc.

Chapter 8

LESSONS LEARNED IN THE DEVELOPMENT OF A CLINICAL INFORMATION SYSTEM IN AN URBAN UNDERSERVED COMMUNITY HEALTH CLINIC: A COMMUNITY PARTNERED PARTICIPATORY RESEARCH (CPPR) APPROACH

Sheba M George, PhD[*,1,2]*, David Hindman, PhD*[3]*,*
Chizobam Ani, MD, MPH[4]*, Omolola Ogunyemi, PhD*[1]*,*
Sukrit Mukherjee, MS[1]*, Ramarao Ilapakurthi, MS*[1]*,*
Mary Verma, MD[3]*, Richard S Baker, MD*[5]*, and Melvin Dayrit, MD*[6]

[1]Center for Biomedical Informatics,
Charles R. Drew University of Medicine and Science, Los Angeles,
United States of America
[2]Department of Community Health Sciences, School of Public Health,
University of California, Los Angeles, United States of America
[3]Behavioral Health Services, Comprehensive Health Center,
Los Angeles County-Department of Health Service, Los Angeles,
United States of America
[4]Department of Family Medicine, Charles R. Drew University of Medicine and Science,
Los Angeles, United States of America
[5]College of Medicine, Charles R. Drew University of Medicine and Science,
Los Angeles, United States of America
[6]Department of Family Medicine, Comprehensive Health Center, Los Angeles County-
Department of Health Service, Los Angeles, California, United States of America

---

[*] Correspondence: Sheba George, PhD, Assistant Professor, Charles R. Drew University of Medicine and Science, 1731 E. 120th Street, Los Angeles, CA 90059 United States. E-mail: shebageorge@cdrewu.edu or shebageorge@ucla.edu.

ABSTRACT

Community Partnered Participatory Research (CPPR) offers a research approach to identify and address barriers to Health Information Technology (HIT) use in underserved healthcare settings. CPPR is a form of community-based participatory research that advocates equal community and academic partnerships, an approach that is advanced as particularly suitable for physician co-leadership. This paper describes how a team of academic informatics researchers and care providers from a comprehensive community health center are using a CPPR approach to develop and eventually implement a computerized clinical information system for chronic disease management. The setting is a large, urban primary care clinic serving a mostly uninsured minority patient population. Here we describe how the twelve guiding principles of CPPR are reflected in our collaboration. We conclude with lessons learned and achievements to date.

Keywords: Community partnered participatory approach, health information technology, underserved healthcare setting, academic-community collaboration, chronic disease management

INTRODUCTION

Urban underserved communities manifest the highest burden of chronic diseases and the most challenged health care infrastructure in the United States. Improving the management and treatment of chronic diseases is an ongoing challenge for community clinics that provide care for underinsured/uninsured minority populations (1). Several strategies for improving the overall quality of care, efficiency and improving outcomes in general and especially for primary care settings in these communities have been proposed, including the recently popular chronic care model approach (2,3). This approach emphasizes health information technology (HIT) development and utilization as a core strategy for improving coordinated and decision supported care. Such HIT systems incorporate core functions that support; health information and data collection, results management, decision support, electronic communication and connectivity, patient support, administrative processes, and reporting and population based health management (4).

Diabetes Registries are a form of basic HIT systems of particular utility in resource poor settings and are the most widely used HIT in community health care settings (5,6). Chronic diseases, such as diabetes are better managed through the use of registries - electronic depositories of key clinical data on diabetic patients used to target and track high-risk patients, send reminders to patients, and provide physicians with guideline concordant care alerts and reminders – with the potential to lead to significant improvements in clinical outcomes (7). While HIT systems, such as disease registries, have the potential to improve medical care dramatically, particularly in public non-specialty primary care settings, the adoption and implementation of HIT systems in general have had less than expected success (8-11).

Community health centers, the principal providers of primary care services within the urban health care safety net system, face multiple challenges in the development and implementation of HIT. Multi-factorial influences including but not limited to (a) resource availability, (b) organizational disposition and capacity for HIT adoption and implementation,

(c) HIT systems design and adaptability (d) provider and staff perceptions of utility and (e) unintended consequences of HIT implementation all contribute to the slow rate of deployment of these systems in these settings where they are most needed (12-14). While community clinics have been identified as prime targets for the adoption of HIT innovations such as disease registries, little is known about the utilization of HIT and specifically disease registries in such settings (12,15). A recent first of its kind comprehensive survey of HIT use among California Community Clinics suggests that while 96% of the clinics have diabetes registries in place, only 31% report that all providers use the registries (6). The discrepancy between the pervasive presence and low utilization of diabetes registries in such settings suggests that significant barriers to adoption may exist.

Among several barriers to HIT access and use for underserved populations are the following: a) lack of representation of stakeholders in the determination of community needs; b) HIT applications not targeted to the particular needs of such communities and consequently not appreciated by community members; c) lack of trust by community members of HIT applications and their utility; and d) HIT developers' lack of understanding of the needs and cultures of target communities (15). Several strategies have been identified to address these barriers including policy, funding, research and education. One of the key recommendations highlighted the importance of using "... participatory action research frameworks, taking special care to involve all stakeholders in the development, conduct and leveraging of all results of research" (15).

Community Partnered Participatory Research (CPPR) offers a research approach, which addresses the barriers identified to HIT use in underserved communities. While Community-Based Participatory Research (CBPR) is the more prevalent form of participatory action research, a common shortcoming of research that is labeled as CBPR is that while research may be "based" in the community, important decisions about research questions, design and interpretation of findings tend to be controlled by the academic arm and the "community" tends to have little to no voice.(16) CPPR is a form of CBPR that "promotes equal community and academic partnership and power sharing in all phases of research, grounded in evidence-based practice as defined from academic and community perspectives, a framing of CBPR that is suited to physician co-leadership"(16). In their JAMA article on CPPR, Jones and Wells argue that for physicians, who generally experience time pressure in interactions, spending the requisite time to develop partnerships and share planning authority can be challenging. CPPR, with its emphasis on equitable and collaborative research and predictable activities, enhances the capacity of practicing physicians to engage in research activities. While Jones and Wells assume that the physicians are on the academic end of the spectrum collaborating with community members, in this project, the physicians were representative of the community, as members of a community health center collaborating with mostly non-physician and some physician academics from a university. Nevertheless, the argument made by Jones and Wells about CPPR's suitability for busy physicians balancing clinical, research and community commitments still holds.

While community can have diverse meanings ranging from a geographical area, a group with related values and norms to a community-based organization, for this project, community refers to a comprehensive health center (CHC) serving minority populations in South Central Los Angeles. This paper describes how a team of academic multidisciplinary researchers at Charles Drew University of Medicine and Science (CDU) and care provider partners from the CHC are together using a CPPR approach in order to develop, implement and evaluate a clinical information system for chronic diseases in this primary care setting. Here we present lessons learned from our process of using CPPR to develop this collaboration and achievements to date.

METHODS

Recognition of the challenges to the development and implementation of HIT in such settings and a desire to address them has led to a unique multi-disciplinary collaboration between researchers at the Center for Biomedical Informatics at CDU and clinicians at the CHC's primary care outpatient clinics (Family Medicine). This clinic provides care to a patient population that are largely minority, underserved and uninsured (70% or more of the patients lack public or private insurance). The CHC is a Los Angeles County Department of Health Services ambulatory care clinic that records approximately 13,000 annual patient visits with a patient population that is largely Latino (55%) and African American (37%). The academic team included a PhD biomedical informatician, a physician, a software developer, a networks engineer, and a medical sociologist. Clinic personnel included two physician champions, the clinic's IT director, a health psychologist as well as input from nursing personnel.

One of the issues identified in the literature related to the capacity for HIT adoption among CHCs is the software customization requirement in order for successful implementation. While customizing "off-the-shelf" applications to meet the specific needs of the client is common to many IT implementations, the unique nature of CHCs make the tailoring of such generic HIT innovations a particularly complex endeavor since most CHCs lack in-house HIT expertise (12). The Family Medicine Clinic at this CHC has attempted to utilize one such "off-the-shelf" called the Chronic Disease Electronic Management System (CDEMS) in the past for depression management. Recognition of the need for extensive customization of CDEMS was one of the factors that led to the current collaboration between CDU and this CHC. A goal of this collaboration is to develop a computerized system for managing chronic diseases in primary care settings that takes into account the socio-technical barriers to successful implementation and forges academic-community partnerships with community clinics that cater to medically underserved patients.

Table 1. Sequence of Activities for CPPR

1) Identify health issue that is a priority to community and which academic partner has capacity to address.
2) Develop a coalition of community and academic stakeholders that inform, support, share & use products.
3) Engage community through provision of information, seeking input and assessment of readiness to engage.
4) Initiate workgroup that develops, implements and evaluates action plans under a leadership council.

Though data in the current discussion are limited to a singular case study with a limited sample size, lessons learned are informative regarding the impact of local context on the implementation of HIT and the use of CPPR in such settings. Case studies are appropriate where they illustrate a phenomenon in a manner that expands existing understandings of practices that are so complex as to only be understood through practical application in the local context (17). The under-resourced and over- burdened CHC that serves the safety net patient population is indeed this sort of complex environment.

COMMUNITY PARTNERED PARTICIPATORY RESEARCH APPROACH

Table 1 outlines the steps necessary in using a CPPR approach. The CDU-CHC collaboration was established using a similar process, beginning with the identification of the need. Because this CHC has a high burden of chronic diseases, particularly diabetes (35% prevalence), developing a clinical information system to manage diabetes care was a high priority issue for them. Academic partners at the CDU Center for Biomedical Informatics had the interest and multidisciplinary capability to develop, implement and evaluate this HIT innovation. A coalition of stakeholders was formed, including senior leadership at CDU and the CHC and the working team members. The community at the CHC was engaged via presentations and meetings held with different stakeholders (medical, nursing, IT and administration) to introduce them to the project and get their input. With the "buy-in" of key stakeholders secured, the core collaboration work team, made up of eight individuals from CDU and the CHC, has met twice a month on the average for a year and a half. The academic partners have traveled eight miles for the two-hour in-person meetings held at the clinic to facilitate ease of participation for the CHC participants. To date, the team has focused most of its efforts on developing the HIT system and piloting the system before full implementation. Table 2 contains an abbreviated list of the twelve guiding principles of the CPPR approach as outlined by Jones and Wells (16).

Table 2. Twelve Guiding Principles of CPPR

1) Joint leadership
2) Written agreement
3) Regular communication
4) Transparent process understood by all participants
5) Solve problems collectively
6) Transparent process of evaluating progress/impact
7) Balance Academic and community goals
8) Financial/ in-kind support for community partners
9) Facilitate community leadership and growth
10) Understand community history and priorities
11) Respect of community values and time frames
12) Seek support and recognition from leaders of the Academic institution for CPPR & time requirements.

While the first six principles are necessary to most successful collaborations between any two groups with different goals, the last six acknowledge and attempt to compensate for the potentially different levels of power between academic and community partners.

RESULTS

Given that our community partners included physicians and other health care professionals familiar with research, we did not have to bridge a large gap in terms of their understanding of the process. However, we still struggled to find common ground to the extent that our goals for the project and the organizational structure under which we were operating were different. Below we present the results of our application of the twelve guiding principles of the CPPR approach in this collaboration.

1) Joint leadership: All our activities have been co-planned, displaying joint leadership with equal power and a spirit of cooperation. In typical community based partnership research, there can be a tendency for academic leaders to overpower community members. However, in this project, community members of the team were fairly equal to the academic side, both in terms of number, voice and power in the decision making process. The academic team members brought informatics and sociotechnical expertise and research skills to the table while the clinic's team members had both medical expertise and knowledge of local practices, workflow and care related needs. Together, each was indispensable to the development of the project and each side understood and appreciated the need for the other, which resulted in openness to joint leadership.

2) Written agreement: We did not have a specific written agreement for this project, partly because the CHC and CDU have had a long relationship of collaboration. However, on-going review and approvals were obtained from the CHC management as necessary. CDU medical students and residents train at the CHC site and some of the team members have collaborated on several other projects. While generally specific written agreements are advisable, the long history of prior interactions facilitated the collaboration without one for this project.

3) Regular communication: Regular communication has been maintained through bi-monthly meetings, regular email contact among participants and using a jointly developed procedure for agenda setting and completion. For example, the team's approach to facilitating meetings includes an agenda generated and circulated in advance by a member of the CDU or CHC team, allowing other team members to include additional items on the agenda. Meetings have been recorded and actions items delegated for follow-up purposes and to ensure productivity.

4) Transparence of process for all participants: Because of the multidisciplinary nature of this project, one of the inherent challenges was to help all participants understand the process from the different disciplinary aspects. There were computer scientists, social scientists, providers with different health care backgrounds, including medicine, nursing, and psychology. All the activities associated with the project were discussed and vetted by the group. As a result of a lot of discussion and translation across multiple disciplines, the academic and community partners were fully engaged in decision-making.

5) Solve problems collectively: A potential problem involved access to patient data to populate the registry database. While the CHC could not give CDU access to confidential patient data at the clinic because of HIPPA rules, together the partners deputized CDU staff and development efforts were conducted within the CHC's IT location. The academic partners were made non-compensated employees of the CHC, subject to all rules and regulations of CHC employee. Through open communication and creative resolution of a potential problem, the academic- community collaboration together created a legacy of problem solving strategies.

6) Transparent process of evaluating progress/impact: We have a dedicated project manager who is a member of the academic team with the primary responsibility of tracking and following-up on action plans. Regular accountability and leadership from this individual team member has helped the project team better evaluate progress, follow-up with assigned tasks, and facilitated communication between the academic institution and CHC. On-going development and implementation evaluations were conducted and reports presented by team members at the meetings for feedback and on-going modifications as necessary. Furthermore, the CHC management is considering the use of the evaluation data as a quality improvement tool.

7) Balance Academic and community goals: Balancing academic goals with the community's clinical goals has not always been easy. Despite an outstanding level of cooperation, flexibility and understanding from individual team members on both sides, delays have resulted due to external factors, such as existing policies at the clinic level and extenuating and unforeseen circumstances that created difficulties in accessing needed resources for the project. Such delays have impinged on both academic and community goals, making it particularly challenging for academic timelines.

8) Financial/ in kind support for community partners: The community partners for this project participated on their own time, taking on the project commitments in addition to their hectic clinical schedules. While they were primarily interested in the end goal of a customized and locally tailored diabetes registry to improve their patients' health care and outcomes, the CHC team members were also interested in the research goals of developing publications and grants. As such, this project also provided an avenue for primarily clinical personnel to participate actively in academic production on their clinical areas of expertise. There is a clear understanding on the part of all project members that community partners will be included in grants and other funding opportunities that may be initiated by academic partners.

9) Facilitate community leadership and growth: We facilitate community leadership and collaborative growth in the planning process through integrating the CHC's requirements and goals for care improvement and evaluation along with other academic areas of interest. We additionally involve community members in joint authorship and grant writing activities. For example, in addition to the present publication, we have successfully published another paper involving all team members (19).

10) Understand community history and priorities: Obstacles to continuing progress of the project have come from factors outside the team's purview, such as changes in the greater organizational affiliations and limitations imposed by the larger governing association of which the clinic is a part. This has led to substantial delays in meeting academic goals. In such cases, the academic team members have submitted to the community's priorities and to the past experience of the CHC team members to manage the limitations appropriately. The history of prior collaborations have allowed for academic and community team members to develop a mutual capacity to understand each other's priorities.

11) Respect of Community values and time frames: A commitment to community values and time frames has been a guiding principle that this project team continues to find challenging. It has been an extended commitment with many roadblocks and challenges along the way. Participants from both sides have been allowed to move "on and off" the bus (i.e., engage and disengage as commitments have changed) unlike other research projects. For example, when the CHC had an upcoming visit from a regulatory agency, which did not allow for active participation in development efforts, the partners together agreed to scale down activities to accommodate the temporary change in effort by the CHC team while the CDU team continued development activities.

12) Seek support and recognition from leaders of the Academic institution for CPPR and time requirements: CDU is fortunate to have a strong tradition of collaborating on research with the community since "conducting education and research in the context of community service" is part of the very mission of the institution. CPPR has been used widely in this effort, particularly in several projects engaging these methods at CDU. The vice-president of research at CDU is an active proponent of CPPR and recognizes the importance of such research approaches. Consequently, the academic team members have benefited from such recognition and support in their ability to sustain involvement in this collaboration despite many delays.

DISCUSSION

This CPPR collaboration has been useful in several ways. Below, we present the lessons learned and future directions. First, it has allowed the development of a chronic disease management system, which is more consistent with the conditions found in safety net community clinics, with the potential of being implemented in other such clinics. A public domain "off-the-shelf" registry software –Chronic Disease Electronic Management Systems (CDEMS) (12), initially used by the CHC for depression management, was found to be inadequate because it failed to meet the practice needs of the physicians in the clinic. Limitations of the CDEMS system include 1) assumptions about provider continuity of care, which were not true for this safety net system; and 2) the limitations of Microsoft Access with respect to security, lack of support for data warehousing, customization, and modularization. The new HIT system– CDU Electronic Disease Registry to Improve Chronic Care (CEDRIC) – has been tailored to the safety net clinic requirements (18). The development of CEDRIC improves upon the previous system by 1) capturing the local work practices and needs in the capabilities of the new system; and 2) using a full-fledged Relational Database Management System (MySQL) which facilitates improved security, customization, modularization and support for data warehousing. This system, designed around a point of care progress note, which will record the patient's pertinent medical information, is the key product developed to date.

Furthermore, the academic-community partnership and the CPPR approach have provided a process and the resources to the team to develop and tailor the CEDRIC registry to the specific needs of the CHC and similar safety net clinical settings. For example, while the standard CDEMS registry progress note assumes continuity of care by a primary care provider (PCP), this does not always apply for community clinic settings where there is very poor continuity since the average patient tends to see several different PCPs based on availability. Consequently, the related assumption in the CDEMS registry that the physician quality of care can be measured across patients, based on their patients' outcomes does not hold for the safety net community clinic setting. Because of the many weeks of discussion about the specific needs of the providers in relation to the registry, the academic-community team was able to identify this issue and was able to change the "off-the-shelf" registry progress note to include the PCP's identification number. Thus, we were able to identify the physician that actually sees a patient on each note to assess continuity of care, making the registry more acceptable to the providers and allaying their fears that their performance would be measured vis-à-vis patients on their panels who were not consistently under their care. In addition, the team was able to include lab tests, services and medications in the CEDRIC progress note that were part of the local practice and eliminate those that were not relevant to the setting. These adaptations to local circumstances improve the chances of participation from clinic providers in the use of the chronic disease management system.

Finally, the academic-community collaboration has provided an opportunity for communication and building relationships between academic and clinic partners. It has allowed the building of rapport and trust between team members. The CPPR approach has not only helped lay the foundation for accomplishments to date but such rapport and trust between researcher and community are a very critical component of future research products and continued collaboration in community-based participatory research.

ACKNOWLEDGMENTS

This work was supported in part by the US National Center for Research Resources (NCRR) under grant U54 RR026138-01.

REFERENCES

[1]   Dievler A, Giovannini T. Community health centers: promise and performance. Med Care Res Rev 1998;55(4):405-31.

[2]   Wagner EH, Austin BT, Von Korff M. Organizing care for patients with chronic illness. Milbank Quart 1996;74(4):511-44.

[3]   Wagner EH, Austin BT, Von Korff M. Improving outcomes in chronic illness. Managed care and chronic illness. Gaithersburg: Aspen Publishers, 1996:103-24.

[4]   Dick RS, Steen EB. The computer-based patient record: an essential technology for health care. Washington, DC: Natl Acad Press, 1991.

[5]   Epping-Jordan JE, Pruitt SD, Bengoa R, Wagner EH. Improving the quality of health care for chronic conditions. Qual Saf Health Care 2004;13(4):299-305.

[6]   The State of Health Information Technology in California: Use Among Physicians and Community Clinics. Oakland, CA: California Healthcare Foundation, 2008.

[7]   Schmittdiel J, Bodenheimer T, Solomon NA, Gillies RR, Shortell SM. Brief report: The prevalence and use of chronic disease registries in physician organizations. J Gen Intern Med 2005;20(9):855-8.

[8]   Wears RL, Berg M. Computer technology and clinical work still waiting for Godot. JAMA 2005;293:1261-3.

[9]   Harrison MI, Koppel R, Bar-Lev S. Unintended consequences of information technologies in health care--an interactive sociotechnical analysis. J Am Med Inform Assoc 2007;14(5):542-9.

[10]   Southon FCG, Sauer C, Dampney CNG. Information technology in complex health services organizational impediments to successful technology transfer and diffusion. Am Med Inform Assoc 1997;4:112-24.

[11]   Heeks R. Health information systems: Failure, success and improvisation. Int J Med Inform 2006;75(2):125-37.

[12]   Moiduddin A, Gaylin DS, Health information technology adoption among health centers: a digital divide in the making? Washington, DC: George Washington University, National Health Policy Forum, 2007.

[13]   Helfrich CD, Savitz LA, Swiger KD, Weiner BJ. Adoption and implementation of mandated diabetes registries by community health centers. Am J Prev Med 2007;33(1 Suppl):S50-8; quiz S9-65.

[14]   Fiscella K, Geiger HJ. Health information technology and quality improvement for community health centers. Health Aff (Millwood) 2006;25(2):405-12.

[15]   Chang BL, Bakken S, Brown SS, Houston TK, Kreps GL, Kukafka R, et al. Bridging the digital divide: reaching vulnerable populations. J Am Med Inform Assoc 2004;11(6):448-57.

[16]   Jones L, Wells K. Strategies for academic and clinician engagement in community-participatory partnered research. JAMA 2007;297(4):407.

[17]   Sandelowski M. What's in a name? Qualitative description revisited. Res Nurs Health 2010;33(1):77-84.

[18]   Ogunyemi O, Mukherjee S, Ani C, Hindman D, George S, Ilapakurthi R, et al. CEDRIC: A computerized chronic disease management system for urban, safety net clinics. Stud Health Technol Inform 2010;160(Pt 1):208.

Submitted: January 02, 2012. *Revised:* February 02, 2012. *Accepted:* February 09, 2012.

In: Public Health Yearbook 2013
Editor: Joav Merrick

ISBN: 978-1-63321-095-0
© 2014 Nova Science Publishers, Inc.

Chapter 9

PACIFIC CEED LEGACY PROJECTS AND LOCAL PROJECTS: CULTURALLY TAILORED PROMISING PRACTICES TO PREVENT BREAST AND CERVICAL CANCER IN THE US AFFILIATED PACIFIC ISLAND JURISDICTIONS

Angela U Sy, DrPH[*1], *Karen A Heckert, PhD, MPH, MSW*[2], *Curtis Jamison, MPH*[3], *Gregory G Maskarinec, PhD*[3], *Ahnate Lim, MA*[4], *and Lee Buenconsejo-Lum, MD*[3]

[1]School of Nursing and Dental Hygiene, Department of Nursing, University of Hawai`i at Manoa, Honolulu, Hawaii, United States of America
[2]Global Health and Community Development Committee, Health Promotion Sciences Division and Global Health Institute, Mel and Enid Zuckerman College of Public Health, University of Arizona, Tucson, Arizona, United States of America
[3]Department of Family Medicine and Community Health, John A Burns School of Medicine, University of Hawai`i at Manoa, Honolulu, Hawaii, United States of America
[4]Department of Psychology, University of Hawai`i at Manoa, Honolulu, Hawaii, United States of America

ABSTRACT

From October 2008 to September 2010, the Pacific Center of Excellence in the Elimination of Disparities (CEED) awarded 29 one year grants to projects serving Pacific Islanders in the US Affiliated Pacific Islands and Hawai`i. These projects promote culturally tailored approaches addressing cancer prevention, education, and control in the

*Correspondence: Angela U Sy, DrPH, Assistant Professor, School of Nursing and Dental Hygiene, Department of Nursing, 2528 McCarthy Mall, Webster Hall #402, University of Hawai`i at Manoa Honolulu, Hawai`i 96822, United States. E-mail: sya@hawaii.edu and ahnate@hawaii.edu.

Pacific and include promising practices documentation and sustainability plans. Pacific CEED Promising Practices and evaluation reports were reviewed, with lessons learned identified for replication, adaptation, and dissemination throughout the USAPI. Qualitative content analysis was conducted by reviewing 19 Promising Practices Reports. An inductive and thematic coding approach was employed to identify factors related to promising practices, lessons learned, and project sustainability. It was found that collaborations with community partners contributed to the successful implementation of the Pacific CEED projects by engaging community participation and promoting leadership from committed community coordinators. Thus Pacific CEED Legacy and Local Projects reveal attributes of promising approaches for implementing and sustaining culturally tailored programs, policies, and practices to prevent cancer among Pacific Islanders within their unique, resource limited communities.

Keywords: Public health, cancer, prevention, Pacific Islands

INTRODUCTION

The U.S.-Affiliated Pacific Islands (USAPI) consists of many small islands scattered over 2.5 million square miles of Pacific Ocean comparable in area to that of the continental U.S. (1). The USAPI jurisdictions are comprised of three freely associated states (the Federated States of Micronesia [FSM], the Republic of Palau and the Republic of the Marshall Islands [RMI]), two U.S. territories (American Samoa and Guam) and the Commonwealth of the Northern Mariana Islands (2). Under the Compacts of Free Association, residents of the freely associated states of the FSM, RMI, and Palau do not require visas to enter and reside in the U.S.

Most jurisdictions are economically underdeveloped with severely inadequate health and educational systems. Significant geographic barriers to healthcare in the Pacific results in poor health in these underserved communities, with life expectancies in the USAPI being 9 to 12 years shorter than that in the US (3).

Factors that contribute to health disparities in the USAPI include an insufficient number of trained health care providers and rapid cultural upheaval with economic dependence on foreign aid (4, 5). Top-down efforts employing Western solutions in these communities without considering their cultural, social and economic contexts have often created new problems (6-10). For example, the establishment of tertiary care hospitals in one urban center of each jurisdiction has increased, rather than reduced, health inequities (7).

The use of participatory methods to increase participation in problem solving and decision making by those being assisted has been recommended (6, 8, 10, 11). This ground up approach helps ensure that unique issues are appropriately identified and interpreted, that proposed strategies are culturally and resource appropriate, and that change will be adopted and sustained within the communities (6, 8, 12, 13).

Cancer in the USAPI

Cancer is the second leading cause of death in the USAPI (14). Cancers that are potentially curable such as breast and cervical cancers are found in advanced stages because a lack of resources results in inadequate prevention and screening services (15). Training to conduct prevention and screening programs is limited, and when available, often does not incorporate culturally relevant strategies (14).

A 2007 needs assessment of the USAPI revealed higher cancer prevalence and lower screening rates compared to the U.S. (14) The prevalence of cervical cancer in the Marshall Islands, with a population of 52,000, was 60.5/100,000, compared to that in the US in 2004 of 8.3/100,000 (14, 16). Guam, which has the highest standard of living of the six USAPI jurisdictions, still has low rates of cancer screening in comparison to the U.S. In 2002, 60 percent of Guam women aged 40+ had had a mammogram in the past 2 years compared to 76 percent in the U.S. Seventy eight percent of women aged 18+ in Guam had had a Papanicolaou (Pap) test in the past three years compared to 87 percent in the U.S. (14, 17).

Pacific Center of Excellence in the Elimination of Disparities

Pacific CEED is funded by the Racial and Ethnic Approaches to Health (REACH) U.S. program of the Centers for Disease Control and Prevention from 2007 to 2012. Pacific CEED aims to reduce breast and cervical cancer disparities in the USAPI through community based participatory approaches, policy and systems changes across the cancer prevention-to-care continuum. Pacific CEED's goals are to 1) provide the infrastructure to implement, coordinate, adapt, and disseminate culturally relevant, evidence-based programs toward breast and cervical cancer prevention and control; 2) implement initiatives according to the Socio Ecological Model, i.e., at organizational, community, systems, policy changes and individual levels; 3) evaluate projects and document promising practices and outcomes; 4) expand local and regional partnerships in the USAPI and at the U.S. national levels; and 5) serve as a national expert resource center on approaches to prevent breast and cervical cancer.

Pacific CEED subcontracts and awards direct grants to local projects to support changes at the various levels of the Socio Ecological Model. The remote and disparate locations of the Pacific island nations require approaches that are culturally relevant and affordable.

Local projects address change in individual knowledge, attitudes, behaviors, and skills among the island communities to promote healthy lifestyles, train providers, and increase access to resource-appropriate breast and cervical cancer screening, diagnosis and treatment and to palliative care.

Pacific CEED Legacy Projects and Local Projects

Beginning in year two of the REACH U.S. cooperative agreement in 2008, Pacific CEED has funded 29 one-year Legacy and Local Projects. Legacy grants provide startup funds to communities to initiate innovative interventions and/or to strengthen community capacity. Proposed projects must support or be associated with the Centers for Disease Control and Prevention (CDC) Comprehensive Cancer Control (CCC) Program and/or the Breast and Cervical Cancer (B&CC) Early Detection Program and address the national cancer plan(s) in their jurisdiction.

Local Projects are direct grants aimed to supplement the regional and jurisdictional CCC programs in compliance with the Pacific Region Cancer Coalition's expectation that portions of the external funding be distributed equitably among the USAPI. Local Projects fill gaps for CCC programs by providing resources and technical assistance in breast and cervical cancer prevention and control. Local projects focus on capacity building, testing innovative interventions, policy change, systems changes, formative data collection, program planning, implementation and evaluation.

METHODS

Each Legacy and Local Project submits a Promising Practices Report at the end of its one year funding period (Figure 1).

Qualitative analysis using an inductive approach was employed on the content of 19 Promising Practices Reports for the grant funding periods 2008 to 2010, comprising the first two rounds of the Legacy Projects. The content analysis and thematic coding were based on four themes: factors related to promising practices, lessons learned, themes related to project sustainability, and breast and cervical cancer prevention and control strategies. Table 1 lists the Pacific CEED Legacy and Local Projects Promising Practices Reports reviewed, year Projects were funded, and priority area addressed for the CDC funding periods September 2008 to September 2010.

RESULTS

Four Pacific CEED projects assessed key cancer issues for their respective jurisdictions (see table 1). Guam American Cancer Society (ACS), Chuuk CCC, Kosrae CCC, Guam CCC, and Yap Area Health Education (AHEC) projects were successful in identifying and training community members most appropriate to collect data collection within their respective communities. These projects were also engaged community participation in the assessment processes by their respective hard-to-reach populations who were not accessing breast and cervical cancer screening. The Guam CCC assessment of providers' awareness of the breast and cervical cancer screening (B&CC) guidelines and their training needs involved successful participation of providers in the survey with a response rate of 74%.

Facilitator Characteristics

Kosrae CCC and Yap AHEC carefully selected facilitators to train as focus group discussion (FGD) facilitators as part of their respective formative data collection to help plan their community interventions. Chuuk CCC selected students at the College of Micronesia and trained them to conduct the Youth Risk Behavioral Factor Survey (YRBS). The following were key characteristics for selecting (FGD) facilitators and note takers:

- Respected member of the community, but not intimidating (for instance a health care worker, but not a chief)
- Well-liked by the community.

- Matched by age, gender, language and/or culture of the facilitator with the focus groups depending on the topic being assessed.

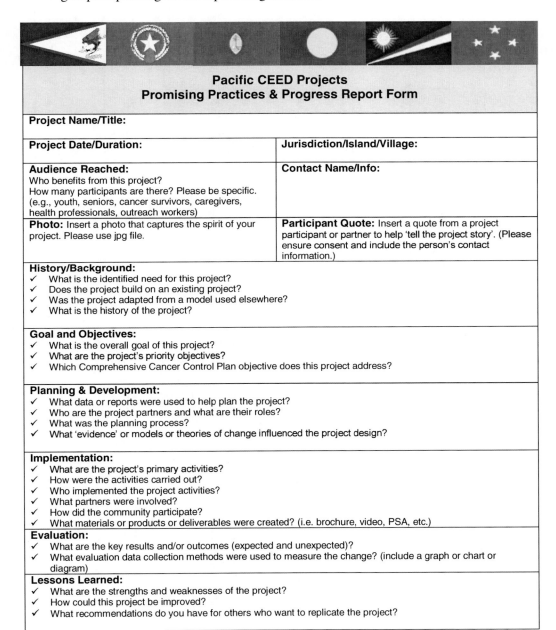

Figure 1.

The purpose of the Guam ACS FGDs was to explore cultural beliefs and practices related to seeking health information and medical care. Guam ACS did not emphasize FGD facilitator characteristics and training for the FGDs with Chuukese and Chamorro, and FGDs were not conducted in-language nor facilitated by trained members of the community.

Table 1. Legacy and Local Projects Activities Reviewed from Promising Practices Reports

Community Assessments	Organization	USAPI Jurisdiction
2008-2009		
Understanding the role of cultural hierarchy and religion in the Chuukese community: developing culturally relevant cancer education and delivery mechanisms	Guam ACS	Guam
2009 – 2010		
College of Micronesia (COM) FSM Chuuk Youth Risk Behavior Survey Training Workshop and Pilot Surveys	FSM Health	Chuuk, FSM
An Investigation of Kosraean Women's Health Seeking Behaviors & Preferences for Health Information Sources	Kosrae CCC	Kosrae, FSM
Exploring Yapese Beliefs on Death and Dying	Yap AHEC	Yap, FSM
Guam Breast and Cervical Cancer Early Detection Program: A survey to assess the new Breast & Cervical Cancer Policies and Guidelines[1]	Guam CCC	Guam
Cancer Prevention and Health Communication		
2008-2009		
Tasi le Ola (One Life): An exploration of traditional beliefs and practices to develop the Breast Cancer Prevention Radio Drama Serial	Am. Samoa CCC	American Samoa
Training in Health Communication & Focus group discussions to assess readiness for HPV vaccine	Pohnpei DOH	Pohnpei, FSM
Training on Cancer Affecting Women & Practical Solutions for Early Detection & Information Dissemination Project	Pohnpei DOH	Pohnpei, FSM
No Woman Left Behind - Enhancing Breast & Cervical Cancer Screening Skills Training	Yap DOH	Yap, FSM
Women United Together to Prevent Breast & Cervical Cancer: Healthy Lifestyles	WUTMI	RMI
2009 – 2010		
Pilot Program Geared to Develop Culturally Competent Practices against Breast and Cervical Cancer in Kwajalein Atoll	Kwajalein AHCB	Kwajalein, RMI
Pohnpei GO LOCAL Community Awareness on Diet and Lifestyle to Help Prevent Cancer[1]	Island Food Community	Pohnpei, FSM
Mutun Alu Program ('entering belief,' in Kosraen)	KKWCA	Pohnpei, FSM
Project LEARN, the Micronesian Community Network	MHAC	Hawai'i

Policy and Advocacy Projects		
2008-2009		
Mobilization of Micronesian Communities in Hawai'i for Health Equity	MHAC	Hawai'i
2009–2010		
FSM National Tobacco Policy Summit	FSM CCC	FSM
Pohnpei GO LOCAL Community Awareness on Diet and Lifestyle to Help Prevent Cancer[2]	Island Food Community	Pohnpei, FSM
Micronesian Health Advisory Coalition Interpreter/Translator Training	MHAC	Hawai'i
Guam Breast and Cervical Cancer Early Detection Program: A survey to assess the new Breast & Cervical Cancer Policies and Guidelines[3]	Guam CCC	Guam
Creation of Cancer Screening Standards for the Republic of Marshall Islands	RMI DOH	RMI
Systems Change		
2008-2009		
National workshop on Non-Communicable Diseases (NCD) to review the first five years strategic Plan and Draft the next 5 year NDC strategic implementation Plan	Palau MOH	Palau
2009–2010		
College of Health in the Ministry of Health	Palau MOH	Palau

[1] Also listed under Policy and Advocacy projects.

[2] Also listed under Cancer Prevention and Health Communications projects.

[3] Also listed under Community Assessment projects.

Rather, two senior health professionals and consultants from the Guam CCC program conducted the assessments. Additional focus groups were not conducted because the project had hoped to find facilitators through their organizational partnerships, rather than selecting and training their own facilitators as was done with the Kosrae CCC and Yap AHEC projects.

Focus Group Discussions – Community Assessment Questions

Conducting culturally relevant FGDs helped obtain information for the projects' assessments. Kosrae CCC and Yap AHEC developed questions respectful of culture and gender, and both projects included questions as to how the health profession can better serve their communities.

Assessment Surveys

The Chuuk CCC YRBS and Guam CCC B&CC provider awareness and patient surveys were at different stages of implementation. Chuuk COM recruited and completed training of youth surveyors, while Guam CCC completed the provider assessment of its new breast and cervical cancer guidelines.

Summary of Community Assessment Projects

Kosrae's formative research addressed Kosrean women's knowledge and attitudes toward breast and cervical cancer screening. Yap AHEC assessed traditional palliative care. Chuuk CCC trained college students to conduct the YRBS. Guam CCC demonstrated that a community survey with health providers on their awareness of B&CC screening guidelines can achieve a high response rate.

Guam ACS conducted two focus groups and obtained findings on culturally relevant health messages for the Chuukese community. However Guam ACS learned that additional focus groups could have been conducted had more attention been given on recruiting and training facilitators from the community.

Cancer Prevention and Health Communications

Nine Pacific CEED projects developed programs to change knowledge, attitudes, and behavior related to cancer prevention with culturally relevant health promotion and prevention activities (Table 1). The American Samoa Community Cancer Coalition (Am. Samoa CCC), Yap CCC, Pohnpei Women's Advisory Council (WAC), Kwajalein Atoll Healthcare Bureau (HCB), Island Foods Community of Pohnpei, and Kolonia Kosrae Women's Christian Association (KKWCA) projects demonstrated increases in health knowledge and behaviors related to cancer prevention among project participants.

Community Reach

Pacific CEED projects were successful in reaching their respective communities. The Island Foods Community of Pohnpei reached 30,000 community members through its radio, television, and email messages and face to face workshops. The American Samoa CCC reached 62% of 200 women sampled through the broadcasting of an original radio drama program for three weeks. The Pohnpei WAC provided community education and outreach in 56 villages through 60 trained women leaders from 19 local women's groups. The Kwajalein AHCB distributed over 3000 brochures on B&CC prevention.

Kwajalein AHCB markedly increased B&CC screening rates, which was based on the documentation of screening rates since 2005. The largest increase in B&CC screenings occurred in the same year that Kwajalein AHCB was awarded its Legacy Project. From 2009 to 2010, cervical cancer screening rate using Pap smear tests increased 500% from 78 to 502 cases.

The RMI Women United Together Marshal Islands' (WUTMI) project educated many community members on healthy lifestyles, chronic diseases, and cancer prevention. Approximately 225 participants attended five days of health education sessions while up to 500 people attended opening ceremonies, including government officials, members of business sectors, WUTMI partners, and the general public. Representatives from 23 of the 24 outer islands were provided with transportation to the events on the main island. WUTMI created and distributed 320 t-shirts, 200 handbags, and 200 key chains with health awareness messages. Most importantly, all participants were also screened for breast and cervical cancer at the local department of health.

Breast and Cervical Cancer Screening Trainings

A number of projects trained community health workers and health assistants to conduct B&CC screenings. Kwajalein AHCB trained six female health assistants to perform B&CC screening, and participants demonstrated statistically significant increases in B&CC screening knowledge, skills and confidence.

Two projects conducted trainings on visual inspection with acetic acid (VIA) screenings, a low cost cervical screening method involving a visual inspection of the cervix using acetic acid. The Pohnpei Department of Health partnered with the Pohnpei WAC, trained 18 health assistants and four nurse practitioners from nine dispensaries, five on the outer islands and four on the main island. Yap CCC trained a total of 16 health assistants, certified birth attendants, community health workers, and future health providers in many aspects of primary health care and cancer prevention, including how to conduct VIA screenings.

Pre and post training scores from the VIA trainings in Pohnpei and Yap indicated that knowledge and skills improved significantly among all participants.

Preventive Health Behaviors

Other projects aimed to improve preventive health knowledge and behaviors. In the KKWCA's project in Pohnpei, 13 out of 32 youth participants reported that they quit using tobacco and alcohol while post test scores indicated improved knowledge of tobacco and alcohol use.

The Island Foods Community of Pohnpei changed nutritional practices through system changes when the College of Micronesia – FSM (COM-FSM) selected coconut juice and water at their graduation ceremony, instead of serving soft drinks.

Kapinga Village also reported using new recipes on banana flower and green papaya, further incorporating locally available foods.

Summary of Cancer Prevention and Health Communications Projects

Elements supporting positive changes in cancer prevention knowledge and behaviors, are: 1) partnerships, 2) collaboration, 3) participation, 4) volunteer interest, 5) cultural appropriateness and 6) resource sharing.

All of the projects identified strong collaborations between the respective CCC coalition and community partners, including churches, local non-government organizations, women's groups, and community colleges.

Committed individuals and community members were instrumental in mobilizing the project and partnerships. The partnerships often involved the ability to organize a network of community volunteers who were critical in helping implement these projects. The projects were also culturally tailored by involving community members in the planning and implementation and delivering the project in local languages.

Another important aspect of these projects is their ability to engage and address youth on culturally relevant best practices, which often require alternate approaches to those used with adults. Three of the projects were successful in obtaining youth interest and participation by working within channels of delivery where youth are more likely to hear health messages.

The Island Foods Community of Pohnpei worked in schools but also delivered messages via songs and through radio, television, and email. The Micronesian Community Network engaged youth interest when they developed Public Service Announcements for broadcast on local community television.

The KKWCA delivered their program through local churches in Pohnpei while maintaining links to home origins in Kosrae. These channels may serve as promising models to engage youth in health promotion programs on lifestyle behaviors including cancer prevention.

Policy and Advocacy Projects

Five Pacific CEED Projects focused on or influenced advocacy and policy changes toward breast and cervical cancer prevention and intervening factors (see table 1).

- *Formation of policy advocacy committee:*
  - The Micronesian Health Advisory Coalition's (MHAC) Micronesian Language Access Program organized advocacy efforts among Compact of Free Association

(COFA) migrants against the Basic Health Hawai'i Plan, which reduces health access to COFA migrants.

o The Republic of the Marshall Islands CCC program assembled an ad hoc committee of health experts, hospital nurses, and public health professionals to draft national screening standards for breast, cervical, and colorectal cancer to be endorsed by the Ministry of Health (MOH).

- *Creation of cancer screening policy:* The Republic of the Marshall Islands CCC Program's ad hoc committee created cancer screening standards and developed a community navigation program. The evidence and process utilized in RMI was informed by a similar process that took place in 2008 in the FSM for a Pacific CEED Local Project. National standards of practice for B&CC prevention, diagnosis, treatment, and palliative care were developed and made national policy in the FSM. The RMI proposed standards included minimum or core standards to be implemented throughout the jurisdiction, desirable standards to be implemented over the next two to three years, and expanded ideal standards given adequate resources.

- *Assessment of existing policies:*
  o FSM National CCC: The FSM National Tobacco Policy Summit Review completed an assessment of anti-tobacco policies in FSM and convened a summit of 34 participants to review the findings from the policy assessment according to the Framework Convention for Tobacco Control (FCTC).
  o Guam CCC Program: The Guam Breast and Cervical Cancer Early Detection Program administered a survey to assess the extent providers were implementing the new national B&CC screening guidelines approved by the CDC-funded Breast and Cervical Cancer Early Detection Program. Provider training needs including identifying ways to improve patient-provider interaction and patient satisfaction related to B&CC screening and care were assessed.

- *Formation and policy implementation*: Island Foods Community of Pohnpei: The Community Awareness on Diet and Lifestyle to help prevent cancer advocated healthy "Go Local" eating and resulted in local level policy change with a number of communities banning soft drinks at their community events.

Summary of Advocacy and Policy Projects

Partnerships and collaboration between the CCC Programs, community groups, national governments and other CDC funded programs, i.e., tobacco and diabetes, were critical to the success of these advocacy and policy projects. Neither Island Foods Community of Pohnpei nor the MHAC Language Access project originally proposed advocacy and policy objectives for their projects. However, as a result of implementing their original objectives and forming partnerships, the increased community awareness led to a desire to implement advocacy and policy changes. Both projects mobilized rapidly around key policy related issues as result of the extensive community partnerships.

Systems Changes

Two Pacific CEED projects, both in Palau, created changes in the cancer prevention and control system within the MOH, across other health-related sectors such as education, and in partnership with the community (Table 1). The NCD Strategy Workshop was conducted to collaborate, coordinate, and integrate the Palau CCC Program with relevant programs within the MOH and among major community groups and leaders. This project resulted in the creation of an NCD Strategic Implementation Plan. Partnership with organizations were also brought together including the NCD Community Coalition Ulekereuil a Klengar, the national CCC Coalition-Belau Cancer Coalition-Omellemel ma Ulekerreuil a Bedenged, legislators, other CDC funded programs, the World Health Organization and the Secretariat for the Pacific Communities.

The Republic of Palau Ministry of Health College of Health created the Palau College of Health as an institutional systems change to build human resource capacity and competencies within the current health workforce. Meetings were conducted with the Palau MOH Executive Committee to gain a better understanding of local problems in public health administration, planning, and implementation and to assess projects being developed and their progress. This project created new collaborations and initiated key community and regional partnerships while assessing educational and health services needs. These activities will support the continued development of the College of Health and ensure that its academic health programs address the academic and professional training needs of the workforce.

DISCUSSION

The Pacific CEED Promising Practices narrative reporting format was compatible with the Pacific CEED projects, contributing to the validity of the information reported, consistently revealing the general themes of promising practices, lessons learned, and project sustainability. This information in turn, allows a synthesis, summary, and recommendations to be made on the future directions of the Pacific CEED Legacy and Local Projects.

Community Partnerships and Collaborations

A recurrent feature and cornerstone of the Pacific CEED projects was their collaboration and coordination with diverse partners, engaging wide stakeholder participation in all phases of the projects while maintaining culturally compatible approaches. Community collaborations and partnerships are key to the development and implementation of community driven projects or initiatives (12). The Pacific CEED projects collaborated with existing networks and with new partners. The KKWCA attributes its project success to having committed partners prior to commencement of the project. The Palau MOH's project activities to establish a College of Health involved partnership building to assess health workforce education and training needs and to engage community and regional partners. The lesson learned is that before starting an initiative, either existing partnerships must be in place or the organization must have the ability to mobilize interested partners.

Shared or Leveraged Resources

Another lesson learned is that the Pacific CEED projects drew on existing assets and their collaborative partnerships to leverage resources and opportunities to plan, implement, and evaluate their projects. The accomplishments of the Legacy and Local Projects are noteworthy given their small funding awards between $15,000 to $24,000, limited human resources, and limited infrastructure. Legacy and Local Projects were resourceful drawing on their additional community resources ranging from engaging key decision makers and professionals to community members.

Community members were often engaged in implementing the community assessments due to their skills and experience working with the community. The formative assessments conducted in Kosrae and Yap employed community members who were leaders in their communities to facilitate focus groups. The MHAC was mobilized as a result of obtaining support from Hawai'i legislators, congressional delegates, and community lawyers on Micronesian health concerns in Hawai'i and most importantly because of the indigenous leadership among the MHAC board members and staff.

Project Sustainability

Whether a project or its activities and efforts continue after short term seed funding for local improvement needs to be considered (21). Legacy and Local projects conducted formally or informally, process evaluations which served to document promising practices on implementation processes toward project progress and completion. A recurrent theme that was revealed of processes that allowed for successful project implementation was community collaborations and resource sharing. Maintenance of these two key project processes may contribute to project sustainability subsequent to Pacific CEED project funding (21). Furthermore, a factor that contributes to sustainability of any initiative are structures that are in place in a community after the project ends (22). Among the structural factors that foster sustainability of short term projects are community partnerships and exchange of resources (22, 23).

Factors related to the sustainability of Pacific CEED projects include organizational partnerships, collaborative program development and design, resource sharing, and infrastructure development. The promising practices and lessons learned related to community collaborations and resource sharing provide a foundation to sustain their efforts and activities.

Pacific CEED projects seeking to create changes at the systems and policy levels can also help to ensure sustainability. Consistent with the Socio Ecological Model, systems and policies changes create structural changes to sustain and institutionalize initiatives (24, 25). The policy changes addressed by these projects have been adopted by decision-makers and/or institutions as official policy to be implemented.

Pacific CEED projects have documented their activities, accomplishments, and results through the Promising Practices and other field reports prepared by the Pacific CEED Technical Assistance team. Such documentation may enhance sustainability and provide information to secure future funding.

Recommendations for Promising Practices

Pacific CEED Legacy and Local Projects should continue to focus on planning innovative interventions; documenting their activities, results, and lessons learned; conducting process and outcome evaluation; and identifying promising practices contributing to project sustainability. While some projects may not have achieved their intended goals and objectives, some have achieved unintended results to impact B&CC prevention and control.

Pacific CEED will revisit all Legacy and Local funded projects to document subsequent progress, results, and sustainability of these projects as Pacific CEED completes its fifth and final year of its cooperative agreement. The extent that adopted policies changes are now being enforced will be examined. A follow up of subsequent project related activities and results will document the extent that Pacific CEED Legacy and Local Projects contribute to the sustainability of B&CC efforts in the Pacific.

The Promising Practices Report template developed by Pacific CEED (Figure 1) based on the success story format of evaluation reporting aims has been user-friendly and helpful (18, 19). In turn lessons learned and promising practices may continue to be disseminated through accessible avenues such as the Pacific Cancer Programs website (www.pacificcancer.org), program publications, and other regional dissemination resources.

CONCLUSION

Pacific CEED projects addressed B&CC prevention and its determinants by focusing on community assessments and formative data collection, designing and implementing health education and communication programs, or influencing policy and conducting advocacy. The Pacific CEED Legacy and Local Projects demonstrate how community level partnerships and expertise are key to implementing projects at the local level. Up until recently, little was known about 'what works' for successful implementation of community based cancer prevention and control projects in the USAPI jurisdictions. Along with initial Pacific CEED funding to jumpstart these projects, the Legacy and Local Projects now provide promising approaches, models, and practices toward cancer prevention and control among hard to reach, geographically isolated Pacific Islander communities with limited resources and infrastructure. This information supports that these culturally relevant breast and cervical cancer prevention and control pilot projects at the local level may be replicated, expanded, and sustained. Community level projects should continue to focus on documenting their efforts and activities, regardless of whether this is required by external programs, as this documentation enhances sustainability and helps secure future funding.

ACKNOWLEDGMENTS

This project was supported by a REACH U.S. grant with the US Centers for Disease Control and Prevention through Pacific Center of Excellence in the Elimination of Disparities cooperative agreement # 5U58DP000976, Neal Palafox, MD, MPH and Lee Buenconsejo-Lum, MD, Principal Investigators. We appreciate the technical assistance provided for the evaluation and reporting of the Pacific CEED Legacy and Local Projects by Hali Robinett, MPH and Jeannette Koijane, MPH and the coordinators of the Legacy and Local Projects.

None of the authors have any conflict of interest to report, nor any financial interests represented with any products discussed or implied.

REFERENCES

[1]   Patrick K, CK G, T B, C L, Waldron J, Vezina R, et al. Meeting the challenge of HIV clinical traning within 2.5 million square miles of the Pacific Ocean. Pacific Health Dialog 2007;14(1):110-3.

[2]   Goodman R, Speers M, McLeroy K, Fawcett S, Kegler M. Identifying and defining the dimensions of community capacity to provide a basis for measurement. Health EducBehav 1998;25:258-78.

[3]   Feasley J, Lawrence Re, editors. Pacific partnership for health, charting a course for th 21st Century. Washington DC: National Academy Press, 1998.

[4]   Levy N. Micronesia handbook, 5th ed. Emeryville, CA: Avalon Travel Publishing, 2000.

[5]   Yamada S. Cancer, reproductive abnormalities, and diabetes in Micronesia: the effect of nuclear testing. Pacific Health Dialog 2004;2:216-21.

[6]   Tang KC, Nutbeam D, Kong L, Wang R, Yan J. Building capacity for health promotionóa case study from China. Health Prom Int 2005;20(3):285.

[7]   Yach D, von Schirnding Y. Towards a higher priority for health on the development agenda. Public Health Rev 1994;22(3-4):339.

[8]   Lansang MA, Dennis R. Building capacity in health research in the developing world. Bull World Health Organ 2004;82(10):764-70.

[9]   Molina-Guzman G. Third World experiences in health planning. Int J Health Serv 1979;9(1):139-50.

[10]   Simmons R, Hall P, Dìaz J, Dìaz M, Fajans P, Satia J. The strategic approach to contraceptive introduction. Stud Family Plann 1997:79-94.

[11]   Stinson N. HHS Health care activities in the Pacific Island Territories. Accessed 2012 Jan 01. URL: http://www.hhs.gov/asl/testify/t040225a.html.

[12]   Israel BA, Schulz AJ, Parker EA, Becker AB. Review of community-based research: assessing partnership approaches to improve public health. Annu Rev Public Health 1998;19(1):173-202.

[13]   Minkler ME, Wallerstein NE. Community based participatory research for health. San Francisco, California: Jossey-Bass, 2003.

[14]   Tsark J, Cancer Council of the Pacific Islands, Braun K. Reducing cancer health disparities in the US-associated Pacific. J Public Health Manag Pract 2007;13:49-58.

[15]   Palafox N, Tsark J. Cancer in the US Associated Pacific Islands (USAPI): history and participatory development. Pacific Health Dialog 2004;11(2):8-12.

[16]   National Cancer Institute. Surveillance epidemiology and end results cancer statistics. Accessed 2012 Jan 01. URL: http://seer.cancer.gov/statistics/.

[17]   Centers for Disease Control and Prevention. Behavioral risk factors surveillance system. Accessed 2012 Jan 01. URL: http://www.cdc.gov/brfss/.

[18]   Centers for Disease Control and Prevention. Impact and value: Telling your program's story. Atlanta, GA: Centers Disease Control Prevention, National Center Chronic Disease Prevention Health Promotion, Division Oral Health, 2007. Accessed 2012 Jan 01. URL: http://www.cdc.gov/oralhealth/publications/library/pdf/success_story_workbook.pdf.

[19]   Centers for Disease Control and Prevention. How to develop a success story. Atlanta, GA: Centers Disease Control Prevention, National Center Chronic Disease Prevention and Health Promotion, 2008.

[20]   Springett J, Wallerstein NE. Issues in participatory evaluation. In: Minkler ME, Wallerstein NE, eds. Community based participatory research for health. San Francisco: Jossey-Bass, 2008.

[21]   Scheirer MA. Is sustainability possible? A review and commentary on empirical studies of program sustainability. Am J Evaluat 2005;26(3):320.

[22]   Altman DG. Sustaining interventions in community systems: On the relationship between researchers and communities. Health Psychol 1995;14(6):526.

[23]   Alexander JA, Weiner BJ, Metzger ME, Shortell SM, Bazzoli GJ, Hasnain-Wynia R, et al. Sustainability of collaborative capacity in community health partnerships. Med Care Res Rev 2003;60(4 suppl):130S.

[24]   McLeroy KR, Bibeau D, Steckler A, Glanz K. An ecological perspective on health promotion programs. Health EducBehav 1988;15(4):351.

[25]   Stokols D. Translating social ecological theory into guidelines for community health promotion. Am J Health Promot 1996;10:282-98.

Submitted: January 03, 2012.*Revised:* February 04, 2012.*Accepted:* February 10, 2012.

In: Public Health Yearbook 2013   ISBN: 978-1-63321-095-0
Editor: Joav Merrick   © 2014 Nova Science Publishers, Inc.

Chapter 10

SHARED GOVERNANCE IN BUILDING COMMUNITY CAPACITY: A CASE STUDY OF SLEEP APNEA

Euny C Lee, MS[*1]*, Ellen P Simon, DSW*[2]*, Jillian Nickerson, BA*[1]*,
Barbara Brenner, DrPH*[1]*, Sandra Talavera, LMSW*[3]*,
Crispin Goytia, BS*[4]*, Guedy Arniella, MS, LCSW*[5]*,
and Carol R Horowitz, MD, MPH*[1]

[1]Departments of Health Evidence and Policy and Preventive Medicine,
Mount Sinai School of Medicine, New York, United States of America
[2]Union Settlement Association, New York, United States of America
[3]East Harlem Partnership for Diabetes Prevention and Senior Health Partners,
New York, United States of America
[4]East Harlem Partnership for Diabetes Prevention and Centers for Community and
Academic Research Partnerships, Mount Sinai CONDUITS, New York,
United States of America
[5]Institute for Family Health, Family Health Center at North General,
New York, United States of America

ABSTRACT

East Harlem has the highest diabetes mortality rate in New York City, NY. Using Community Based Participatory Research principles, the East Harlem Partnership for Diabetes Prevention—a community- academic partnership—formed to build community capacity with a goal to address health disparities in East Harlem. As part of prevention efforts, community partners chose to study the prevalence of obstructive sleep apnea and its relationship to pre-diabetes and progression to diabetes. However, community partners insisted any study of sleep apnea go beyond simple assessment to ensure the largely uninsured, minority population enrolled also have access to state of the art diagnosis and

---

[*] Correspondence: Euny C Lee, MS, Project Manager, Department of Health Evidence and Policy, Mount Sinai School of Medicine, One Gustave L. Levy Place, Box 1077, New York, NY 10029. E-mail: euny.lee@mountsinai.org.

treatment. Through compromise and collaboration, the partnership developed a culturally appropriate and scientifically rigorous method to diagnose and treat sleep apnea as part of a novel research program.

Keywords: Obstructive sleep apnea, diabetes prevention, community capacity building, community-based participatory research, underserved communities, East Harlem

INTRODUCTION

Diabetes is a growing epidemic nationally and internationally (1,2). There are racial and ethnic differences in prevalence, morbidity and mortality from diabetes, with African Americans, Hispanic/Latino and South Asians, particularly impacted (3). East Harlem is a predominantly low-income, African American, Hispanic/Latino community in northeast New York City, with the highest diabetes mortality rate and the highest obesity prevalence in Manhattan. In addition, 29% of East Harlem adults do not have a primary care provider and over one third (27%) are currently uninsured or, were uninsured at some time in the past year (10%)(4). Based on this information, community and academic partners in East Harlem came together in 2005 to develop programs to improve local health.

Once funded, a Community Action Board (Board), comprised of 20 local leaders, residents and investigators conducted local assessments and chose to focus on diabetes prevention. Using Community Based Participatory Research principles, the Board developed a peer-led, community-based diabetes prevention intervention (5). The intervention, named HEED (Help Educate to Eliminate Diabetes) aimed to help overweight and obese adults with pre-diabetes change their diets, increase physical activity and lose weight to prevent or delay diabetes (6-8). To test the impact of the intervention, we implemented a randomized controlled trial of peer-led, community- based lifestyle education, which resulted in significant and sustained weight loss (9). In consultation with the study's Scientific Advisory Board, we decided to add a new focus to this study, namely obstructive sleep apnea.

Obstructive sleep apnea is a condition when an individual has episodes of paused breathing cessation (apneas) due to a collapse in the upper airway during sleep (10). Sleep apnea affects 4% of the population, of whom only 20% are diagnosed (11,12). Resulting fragmented sleep and low oxygen intake increase the risk of heart disease, negatively impact quality of life, and physical and emotional health. (13,14) Sleep apnea also leads to insulin resistance and glucose intolerance,(15,16) and, if untreated, increases the risk of developing type II diabetes (17).

Surprisingly, little research exists exploring whether sleep apnea is an independent risk factor for progression of pre-diabetes to diabetes, particularly in African Americans and Hispanics/Latinos, who have higher prevalence of pre-diabetes, diabetes, obesity and sleep apnea (18). Will the metabolic changes associated with sleep apnea accelerate progression of pre-diabetes to diabetes? Will the fatigue from sleep apnea make it harder for people to increase physical activity and improve their diets so they can prevent diabetes? To answer these questions, the Board needed to determine ways to assess prevalence of sleep apnea among pre-diabetics with limited access to care, limited English fluency and limited financial resources. Thus, we aimed to develop a culturally sensitive, yet scientifically rigorous approach to diagnose sleep apnea and study the prevalence of sleep apnea in adults with prediabetes.

METHODS

A subcommittee of the Board formed to guide the sleep apnea substudy, in which a cohort of adults with prediabetes who were enrolled in the original diabetes prevention study would be offered an opportunity to undergo screening for sleep apnea. Initially, we had considered simply including the Berlin Sleep Questionnaire, a survey screening tool to assess sleep apnea. However, this led to two problems. First, before allowing the additional questions to be added, the Board wanted to ensure that this was a scientifically rigorous method to diagnose, not just to assess risk for sleep apnea (19). Second, the Board would not agree to include any sleep apnea assessment unless we also provided state of the art treatment. The Board members felt strongly that asking screening questions without providing accurate diagnosis was unethical. Furthermore, determining the prevalence of sleep apnea without ensuring all those diagnosed would be treated was continuing a practice many were uncomfortable with, namely estimating prevalence of a disease for research purposes without providing any benefit to research subjects. The Board felt this type of research practice disproportionately and negatively impacted the vulnerable populations we aimed to serve, particularly uninsured and underinsured participants. Interestingly, this was a contentious issue, as some Board members thought any increased capacity to diagnose or treat people for sleep apnea would be of benefit. Ultimately, however, the Board decided not to proceed unless we could diagnose and treat all participants enrolled.

Once the Board rejected using questionnaires to assess risk for sleep apnea, we needed to identify a method to diagnose it and to treat it. Both were complicated in that nearly half of those with pre-diabetes eligible for this substudy were uninsured and many were assumed to be undocumented. How could the group find a way to provide free diagnosis and treatment to this group? Otherwise, the Board voted that we would not pursue this avenue of research. The Investigators had to identify pulmonologists who were sleep apnea experts to meet this challenge.

Together, we first explored the standard diagnostic method, an overnight sleep study. Challenges to this method included cost, the need for an overnight stay (considered particularly difficult for a population with low trust in the medical system and with limited support, i.e., women with small children with no overnight childcare available). Thus, we explored use of an emerging technology, an in-home sleep testing device which would allow us to objectively identify risk for obstructive sleep apnea. These have been shown to be as reliable as overnight testing in a majority of subjects (20). The Board and sleep apnea experts then explored potential treatments. Obstructive sleep apnea is treated with Continuous Positive Airway Pressure (CPAP) machines, which are costly and require training in their use. However, there are no alternative treatments for individuals with moderate or severe apnea.

The guiding principal for Board members was ensuring access to care for research participants; concern about inability to access treatment was a perspective researchers had not fully considered. Researchers did not imagine that they would be able to provide free diagnostic or therapeutic services to participants. However, the sleep apnea experts met with the Board, demonstrated both portable diagnostic machines and CPAP therapeutic machines. In addition, they explained they could obtain donations of equipment and offer it to those in need. The sleep apnea experts were committed to working with the Board and investigators to secure device donations and develop a scientifically rigorous study protocol to assess the prevalence of sleep apnea. A period of adjustment and establishing of trust took place as the Board and the new sleep apnea experts got to know each other.

As new concerns surfaced, negotiations between the Board and researchers continued. The team developed a diagnostic plan, mechanisms to improve chances the very costly diagnostic machines would be returned to the study team for future use, a treatment plan, educational materials and evaluation plan. The planning and development of this study, to meet both scientific rigor and the requirement for equal access to treatment, took a year to implement. Ultimately, in response to the subcommittee's recommendation, the Board voted unanimously to pursue this descriptive prevalence substudy of sleep apnea among people with prediabetes. We describe the procedures developed in the results.

RESULTS

Participants from the parent diabetes prevention study, Project Help Educate to Eliminate Diabetes, were asked at their 12-month follow up if they were interested in participating in a separate substudy about sleep apnea and administered informed consent. If interested, a study team member would provide all of the specifics of the substudy as well as an in-depth description of sleep apnea and how it can be detected using bilingual (English and Spanish), low literacy materials developed by 2 sleep apnea experts, Board members from the community, and experts in health education. All materials were piloted with community members before their use, and revisions were incorporated with their recommendations. Six subjects also piloted the overnight study, and with their feedback and that from representatives of the company donating the machines, we finalized the training and testing of the protocol. Upon consent, participants made appointments to meet with study personnel, so they could be trained in the use of the donated, sleep apnea diagnostic machines called ResMed Apnea Link Plus.

Participants were trained on using the machines and took the machines home overnight for the sleep study, with written and pictorial instructions on its use and instructions for troubleshooting issues that might arise. All instructions were given to participants in either English or Spanish and provided in-person by bilingual study personnel. Upon return of the detection device (and receipt of a gift card for its return), study personnel uploaded data and sent it through an electronic server to the sleep lab. Data interpreted by the sleep technician stratified participants' results into four categories: (1) equivocal results, triggering a repeat portable study and if this too was equivocal, a traditional in-lab overnight study to clarify findings; (2) No sleep apnea, in which case participants would be given results and reassured; (3) Mild sleep apnea, in which case participants would be given advice on lifestyle modification to treat this mild condition; and (4) Moderate or severe sleep apnea, for which participants would be offered treatment with a CPAP machine. Results would be delivered in-person and in English or Spanish to ensure comprehension and to arrange for any needed follow-up. Those requiring treatment with a CPAP machine would be given the machine, instructed in English or Spanish on its use and re-contacted in 1-week and 1-month to assess comfort with the treatment machine, adherence, and to address any barriers that may exist in using the machine. The subcommittee also developed a semi-structured interview to be administered when testing results were given and at the 1-week follow up for those given machines, to assess knowledge, attitudes and beliefs about sleep apnea, portable testing and treatment.

DISCUSSION

The Board, investigators, and sleep apnea experts collaborated to identify a scientifically rigorous, evidence-based, yet practical, feasible, community-sensitive way to diagnose and treat obstructive sleep apnea in a population of overweight and obese people with prediabetes. The group had to address and overcome cultural, social, economic barriers that were present in the East Harlem community. In addition, they had to carefully straddle CBP (community-based participation), ensuring the needs of the community were being met, and R (research that is rigorous and in an emerging field). First, the Board needed to assert their conviction that it would be insufficient to assess risk of sleep apnea without objectively testing for the disease. Second, the Board needed to ensure that no study would be conducted unless all individuals, including those undocumented and uninsured, found a convenient mechanism to diagnose sleep apnea and be given treatment for this disease, both of which are traditionally costly endeavors. Surprisingly to the researchers, who initially viewed these demands as overly protective of the community and logistically impossible to meet, we were able to partner with sleep apnea experts and meet these requirements. Through this process of negotiation, we developed a study and procedures that embody Community Based Participatory Research (CBPR)- rigorous, relevant, community-responsive and with true potential for tangible benefit.

In terms of identifying a convenient, feasible mechanism to diagnose sleep apnea, we discovered a technology in use, but not in East Harlem, or to our knowledge, with underserved populations, namely portable overnight studies. These devices have a sensitivity of 88-98% and a specificity of 67-99% when compared to the in-hospital polysomnography (21). We anticipate the results of our study will show how well this technology works in vulnerable populations and provide simple strategies to teach such populations how to use the machines, again marrying scientific rigor and community acceptability.

This study also demonstrates mechanisms that can be used to address cost barriers to diagnosis and treatment of sleep apnea. With a largely uninsured and underinsured population in communities disproportionately impacted by diabetes and sleep apnea, such as East Harlem, new methods must be considered to address issues of underdiagnosis and undertreatment of health conditions. Insurance copayments, out of pocket costs and income level have been shown to thwart the initiation of CPAP treatment upon patients receiving a diagnosis of sleep apnea (22).

To an uninsured individual, any out of pocket costs would be daunting and deter them from seeking the much needed care and treatment. The partnership found new, practical ways to get people tested and treated upon diagnosis of obstructive sleep apnea. It demonstrates the need to find simpler ways of conducting research to meet the needs of people who are most vulnerable and also bear the greatest burden.

With data suggesting sleep apnea as an independent risk factor of diabetes, we also believe this study and its results bring to light the importance of exploring sleep apnea among the one in four U.S. adults (and those world-wide) with pre-diabetes. The International Diabetes Federation has set forth clinical recommendations urging clinicians to test for sleep apnea in type II diabetes patients (22). Our findings may also help medical providers become aware of socioeconomic and cultural factors such as language barriers, cost and access to care which contribute to sleep apnea's underdiagnosis among vulnerable populations.

The final study was significantly different than what was initially proposed because of community Board's input and advocacy. All participants have access to free screening for sleep apnea and treatment if needed, regardless of their insurance status and ability to pay. This process highlights how CBPR principles can be employed to resolve differences between academic and community partners resulting in a stronger study that meets both the community's need for service and the researchers need for rigor. Without the principles of shared governance developed over the initial eight years of the HEED study, community Board members might not have been as assertive in their efforts to ensure universal access to treatment. The Board's prior exposure and participation in research efforts also sharpened their understanding of the need for research rigor. The years of collaborative work strengthened their commitment and understanding of their role as advocates for the community and helped them stand their ground effectively for a single path to diagnosis and treatment.

While evaluating a diabetes prevention program in East Harlem, Community Board members and academic partners of Project HEED identified an opportunity to explore the prevalence of sleep apnea and its effect on community members with pre-diabetes. With guidance from the Scientific Advisory Board (SAB) and sleep apnea experts, a culturally appropriate and scientifically rigorous method to provide at home screening and treatment of sleep apnea for consenting participants at risk for diabetes was devised. The process of designing and implementing the study illustrates the value of Community Based Participatory Research (CBPR). In this instance, the process, although long and at times tedious, produced a study that has scientific rigor, provides equitable treatment for all participants, and enjoys wide acceptance among both community and academic partners.

ACKNOWLEDGMENTS

The sleep apnea pilot study was funded by a grant from the National Center for Research Resources of the National Institutes of Health and the New York State Department of Health Diabetes Prevention and Control Program. We would like to thank all members of the Community Action Board of the East Harlem Partnership for Diabetes Prevention and the Sleep Apnea subcommittee; partnering community members and organizations; study participants; our project staff including: Michael Nedelman, Alexander Moreta, Carol Yanisa Pimentel, Kenya Townsend, Hope Weissler; Drs. Rashmi Nisha Aurora and Ana C. Krieger in developing study instruments and providing scientific oversight; our sleep technicians Dzmitry Fiadosau, Vladislav Boyarskiy, Tomoko Ikuine.

REFERENCES

[1]   US Department of Health and Human Services, Centers for Disease Control and Prevention. National diabetes fact sheet: national estimates and general information on diabetes and prediabetes in the United States, 2011. Accessed 2011 Nov 10. URL:http://www.cdc.gov/diabetes/pubs/pdf/ndfs_2011.pdf

[2]   Shaw J, Sicree R, Zimmet P. Global estimates of the prevalence of diabetes for 2010 and 2030. Diabetes Res Clin Pract 2010;87:4-14.

[3]   Kim M, Berger D, Matte T. Diabetes in New York City: Public Health Burden and Disparities. New York City Department of Health and Mental Hygiene 2006. Accessed 2011 Nov 04. URL: http://www.nyc.gov/html/doh/downloads/pdf/epi/diabetes_chart_book.pdf

[4]   Olson EC, Van Wye G, Kerker B, Thorpe L, Frieden TR. Take Care East Harlem. NYC Community Health Profiles 2006. Accessed 2011 Nov 04. URL:http://www.nyc.gov/html/doh/downloads/pdf/data/2006chp-303.pdf

[5]   Horowitz CR, Eckhardt S, Talavera S, Goytia C, Lorig K. Effectively translating diabetes prevention: a successful model in a historically underserved community. Transl Behav Med 2011;1:443–52.

[6]   Jemal A, Ward E, Hao Y, Thun M. Trends in leading causes of death in the United States, 1970–2002. JAMA 2005; 294:1255–9.

[7]   Knowler WC, Barrett-Connor E, Fowler SE, Hamman RF, Lachin JM, Walker EA, Nathan DM. Reduction in the incidence of type 2 diabetes with lifestyle intervention or metformin. N Engl J Med 2002;346:393-403.

[8]   Barr EL, Zimmet PZ, Welborn TA, Jolley D, Magliano DJ, Dunstan DW, Cameron AJ, Dwyer T, Taylor HR, Tonkin AM, Wong TY, McNeil J, Shaw JE. Risk of cardiovascular and all-cause mortality in individuals with diabetes mellitus, impaired fasting glucose, and impaired glucose tolerance: the Australian Diabetes, Obesity, and Lifestyle Study. Circulation 2007;116:151–7.

[9]   Parikh P, Simon EP, Fei K, Looker H, Goytia C, Horowitz CR. Results of a pilot diabetes prevention intervention in East Harlem, New York City: Project HEED. Am J Public Health 2010;100:S232-9.

[10]   Punjabi NM, Polotsky VY. Disorders of glucose metabolism in sleep apnea. J Appl Physiol 2005;99:1998-2007.

[11]   Young T, Evans L, Finn L, Palta M. Estimation of the clinically diagnosed proportion of sleep apnea syndrome in middle-aged men and women. Sleep 1997;20:705-6.

[12]   Kapur V, Strohl KP, Redline S, Iber C, O'Connor G, Nieto J. Underdiagnosis of sleep apnea syndrome in U.S. communities. Sleep Breath 2002;6:49-54.

[13]   D'Ambrosio C, Bowman T, Mohsenin V. Quality of life in patients with obstructive sleep apnea: effect of nasal continuous positive airway pressure--a prospective study. Chest 1999;115:123-9.

[14]   Sjösten N, Vahtera J, Salo P, Oksanen T, Saaresranta T, Virtanen M, Pentti J, Kivimäki M. Increased risk of lost workdays prior to the diagnosis of sleep apnea. Chest 2009;136:130-6.

[15]   Pamidi S, Aronsohn R, Tasali E. Obstructive Sleep Apnea: Role in the Risk and Severity of Diabetes. Best Pract Res Clin Endocrinol Metab 2010;24:703-15.

[16]   Lurie A. Metabolic disorders associated with obstructive sleep apnea in adults. Adv Cardiol 2011;46:67-138.

[17]   Botros N, Concato J, Mohsenin V, Selim B, Doctor K, Yaggi K. Obstructive sleep apnea as a risk factor for Type II Diabetes. Am J Med 2009;122:1122-7.

[18]   Mahmood K, Akhter N, Eldeirawi K, Onal E, Christman JW, Carley DW, Herdegen JJ. Prevalence of type 2 diabetes in patients with obstructive sleep apnea in a multi-ethnic sample. J Clin Sleep Med 2009;5:215-21.

[19]   Netzer NC, Stoohs RA, Netzer CM, Clark K, Strohl KP. Using the Berlin Questionnaire to identify patients at risk for the sleep apnea syndrome. Ann Intern Med 1999;131:485-91.

[20]   Oktay B, Rice TB, Atwood CW Jr, Passero M Jr, Gupta N, Givelber R, Drumheller OJ, Houck P, Gordon N, Strollo PJ Jr. Evaluation of a single-channel portable monitor for the diagnosis of obstructive sleep apnea. J Clin Sleep Med 2011;7:384-90.

[21]   Chen H, Lowe AA, Bai Y, Hamilton P, Fleetham JA, Almeida FR. Evaluation of a portable recording device (ApneaLink) for case selection of obstructive sleep apnea. Sleep Breath 2009 ;13:213-9.

[22]   Shaw JE, Punjabi NM, Wilding JP, Alberti KG, Zimmet PZ. Sleep-disordered breathing and type 2 diabetes: a report from the International Diabetes Federation Taskforce on Epidemiology and Prevention. Diabetes Res Clin Pract 2008;81:2-12.

Submitted: January 03, 2012. *Revised:* February 05, 2012. *Accepted:* February 11, 2012.

In: Public Health Yearbook 2013
Editor: Joav Merrick

ISBN: 978-1-63321-095-0
© 2014 Nova Science Publishers, Inc.

Chapter 11

CHARACTERISTICS OF A COMMUNITY-BASED SENTINEL SURVEILLANCE SYSTEM: LESSONS LEARNED FROM TOOLKIT DEVELOPMENT AND IMPLEMENTATION

Tenaya M Sunbury, PhD*, and David L Driscoll, PhD
Institute for Circumpolar Health Studies,
University of Alaska Anchorage, College of Health, Anchorage,
Alaska, United States of America

ABSTRACT

Following several reports of current and potential health impacts from climate change in Alaska, the Institute of Circumpolar Health Studies (ICHS) developed a community-based sentinel surveillance system to capture baseline human health and ecosystem data. The multidisciplinary nature of climate change, like other environmental health exposures, demands surveillance systems that measure environmental exposure(s) and health outcome(s). Because public health surveillance systems vary in methods, scope, purpose, and objectives, attributes that are important to one system might be less important than another. We describe the challenges and steps involved in developing a sentinel surveillance system and the information it provides for improving public-health decision making. The final surveillance survey includes five thematic parts and consists of community observations on local weather, hunting and harvesting, food and water safety, general health and air quality, and any additional community observations. An understanding of climate change impacts on population health through public health surveillance is fundamental to planning and evaluating policies and programs.

Keywords: Climate change, community-based, sentinel surveillance system, Alaska

---

* Correspondence: Tenaya M. Sunbury, PhD, Post-doctoral Research Fellow, Institute for Circumpolar Health Studies, University of Alaska Anchorage, College of Health, DPL 404, 3211 Providence Drive, Anchorage, AK 99517 United States. E-mail: afts2@uaa.alaska.edu.

INTRODUCTION

Climate change is one of the most pressing environmental and public health concerns of the 21st century due to disruptions to interdependent cycles of plants, animals, and microorganisms that are occurring at a larger and faster scale than ecosystems are capable of adapting (1). Because these ecosystems provide humans with food, clean water, and air any drastic changes will influence global socio-economic systems (2), however the beneficial or negative effect of climate change on human health will vary by time and place (3,4). Following several reports of current and potential health impacts from climate change in Alaska, the Institute of Circumpolar Health Studies (ICHS) developed the CARECC (Community Action for Recording Effects of Climate Change) pilot project, a community-based sentinel surveillance system to capture baseline human health and ecosystem data. As other health professionals may have limited resources to develop and implement this type of surveillance, our experience should encourage other states and countries to develop their own sentinel surveillance system. The program can serve as an excellent resource for replication in communities facing similar emergent health problems to monitor and thus mitigate human morbidity and mortality from climate change.

Arctic and northern peoples inhabit a variety of ecosystems that are distributed across Alaska, Canada, Russia Federation, and the Scandinavian countries. Definitions of Arctic vary, but most researchers agree that it "includes areas of high northern latitudes dominated by snow, ice, and permafrost"(5). Alaska is the only Arctic state within the United States, but like other circumpolar nations faces unique challenges from climate changes. While approximately 40% of the state's 710,231 residents live in the Anchorage metropolitan area, a vast number of communities are spread along coastlines and interior regions in isolated rural villages off the road system (6). The health of indigenous and rural people in Alaska and other circumpolar regions may be particularly affected by changes in temperature, food sources, and livelihoods (7-12).

Rising winter temperatures in Arctic regions are expected to reduce excess winter mortality and cold-related injuries (1). However, the traditional diet of circumpolar residents is likely to be impacted by melting snow and ice, affecting animal distributions and accessibility for hunting (13-15). Water-borne and vector-borne diseases are expected to have a wider seasonal and geographical distribution (16). Most importantly, changes in the physical environment will make traditional ways of life impossible, forcing changes of behavior and means of supporting livelihoods, with associated effects on mental health and community cohesion (17,18).

Given that climate changes, and the accompanying effects on human health, vary geographically as a function of environment, topography, and of the vulnerability of local populations, understanding local needs and developing effective adaptation strategies are of greatest importance. Local or community capacity building has been defined as "the characteristics of communities that affect their ability to identify, mobilize, and address social and public health problems" (19).

Key features of community capacity are that it is a process, dynamic, an outcome, and context specific. A landmark symposium convened by the Centers for Disease Control and Prevention (CDC) recognized that enhancing community capacity is associated with health benefits and identified 10 dimensions of community capacity: participation and leadership, skills, resources, social and inter-organizational networks, sense of community, understanding of community history, community power, community values, and critical reflection (19). With no standard tool, or approach, for collecting and integrating community data, this pilot project aimed to develop a robust population level survey tool to collect surveillance data on ecosystem and human health outcomes appropriate for use primarily in Alaska rural villages. The primary aim of this paper is to describe the development and implementation of a community-based sentinel surveillance system and the lessons learned as a result of building community capacity to address climate change and human health impacts among Alaska communities.

How does a community-based surveillance system strengthen community capacity?

A sentinel surveillance system increases community capacity by supporting climate change adaptation. Climate change adaptation is a process by which "strategies to moderate, cope with, and take advantage of the consequences of climate events are developed and implemented"(20). With the bio-complexity of Alaska and other global environments, these processes cannot be understood or addressed in isolation from other stressors. Climate change, along with other social stressors, such as economic changes are mediated through a set of vulnerabilities – financial, social, political – that communities face; vulnerabilities that in turn create constraints to adaptive capacity. Knowledge and information play a key role in overcoming such constraints and are pivotal for building and strengthening the capacity of multiple stakeholders involved in adaptation strategies at the micro, meso, and macro levels (21). Community-based sentinel surveillance systems provide an opportunity to improve the collection and exchange of relevant climate change and human health information and knowledge.

METHODS

The process of developing the community-based sentinel surveillance system began by integrating two frameworks. The first framework outlined a process and method for identifying important surveillance constructs and topic inclusion criteria (22), while the second framework specifically emphasized the scientific basis and relevance of climate change as an environmental exposure for our Alaska populations (23).

This section provides relevant details on the development of a community-based sentinel surveillance system around 1) involving and engaging community stakeholders in identifying priority topic areas 2) survey methodology used for the design, collection, and analysis and 3) formulating an evaluation of the health component of the sentinel surveillance system which will be conducted using the framework promulgated by the US Centers for Disease Control and Prevention (CDC) (24). More details are available from the author upon request.

Involving and engaging community stakeholders in identifying priority climate change topic areas

Involving and engaging community stakeholders in identifying priority climate change topic areas was conducted in three ways: 1) organizing a colloquium with health and environmental professionals, 2) collaborating with community organization groups that have experience successfully working within each of the 8 invited Alaskan communities, and 3) contacting village environmental coordinators or formal/informal leadership for input and mobilizing community interest. The primary goal of the colloquium was to identify priority climate change topic areas effecting human health in Alaska (and other circumpolar populations), suggest current environmental health indicators or existing survey items that could be adapted for the surveillance survey, and discuss essential community-participatory methodologies used in past research. Table 1 outlines the priority climate change topic areas identified at the colloquium.

Table 1. Priority climate change topic areas effecting human health based on Alaska observations

Seasonality	Surveillance Elements	Observations
Fall/Winter/ Spring/ Summer	Water	Changes (reductions) in sea ice Changes in precipitation (rain, snow) (quantity and quality) Storm-surges (loss of protection from sea ice) Changes in river and lake systems (flow, sediment, contaminants, temp) Changes in freeze-up timing (later) Changes in break-up timing (earlier) Changes in ocean acidification (increase acidification or lower pH)
	Atmosphere	Changes in weather extremes/variability (increase) Changes in weather predictability (increase) Changes in particulate matter (increase) from fires Changes in allergen concentration (increase) Changes in UV-B radiation (increase) Changes in temperature (increase)
	Land	Erosion (due to: retreating glaciers) Changes in built environment (road networks, sanitation infrastructure, wastewater and solid waste systems) Land uplift (due to: retreating glaciers) Coastal areas Decrease in permafrost active layer
	Biology/ Ecosystems	Invasive flora (i.e., plant) species Changes in priority flora species (numbers, trends, and distribution) Invasive fauna species Changes in priority fauna species (numbers, trends, and distribution)
	Social	Cultural issues (e.g., changes in human and industrial activity due to ice-free ocean passage, traditional food gathering, preparation, storage, and consumption) Acute and chronic mental health Public health workers and/or emergency responders Causes of morbidity and mortality

After the creation of the priority climate change topics areas, project investigators reviewed the available peer-reviewed and grey literature conducted in Alaska and/or Canada for existing surveillance items and were unable to find any that met criteria inclusion based on: their severity or public health consequences, potential for large outbreaks, limitations of traditional passive public health surveillance systems, and existing data on local disease epidemiology.

Survey methodology used for the design, collection, and analysis

In order to collect structured observations from community participants, investigators developed a standardized survey. For the purposes of the pilot project, a surveillance system was developed to resemble a repeated cross-sectional survey to be conducted monthly for 12 months involving a purposive sample of community participants. Groves, Fowler, Couper, Lepkowski, Singer, and Tourangeau (25) describe several critical decisions regarding design, collection, and analysis that researchers need to examine before implementation. This section describes what and how these decisions were made and an overview is provided in Table 2.

The United States CDC National Health and Nutrition Survey (NHANES) and Behavioral Risk Factor Surveillance Survey (BRFSS) were used as surveillance survey design templates (26, 27) – both are large-scale, repeated surveys asking interviewers to self-report on health phenomena. The initial surveillance survey began with the final evaluation in mind.

Table 2. Modifications to Sentinel Surveillance Survey

Surveillance survey characteristics	Initial Design	Final Design
Data collection	Quantitative data only using likert scales	Qualitative and quantitative data using open-ended text fields and likert scales
Data collection mode	Web only	Mail-in, toll-free telephone number, and web
Language options	English, Inupiaq, and Tlingit	English only
Example of survey items	Detailed list of hunted animals/fish categorized by animal size and list of harvestable plants	Reduced to two survey items asking residents to report on any changes to hunting/harvesting
Survey style	None	Thematic sections and likert-scales were highlighted and directions were provided at regular intervals
Toolkit materials	None	Waterproof and re-useable material and self-addressed stamped envelopes

Project investigators prepared a spreadsheet utilizing colloquium climate change topics and started with major headings of: research question number, research purpose, interview question (as primary data collection), secondary data source (for the evaluation of health and ecosystem data), and any additional comments for the interview question. Pre-testing was undertaken using a small convenience sample of longtime Alaska residents, other researchers from Canada, and environmental coordinators from several Alaska villages. While the initial surveillance survey had 31-items with multiple response options, feedback from pre-test suggested that the survey was too long and detailed, and based on the original wording, some residents would not be comfortable reporting on other community residents that they did not know (28). The final iteration of the sentinel surveillance survey contains five thematic parts with a total of 34-items (33 items that consist of a 4- or 2-point likert scale).

The first thematic section consists of community observations on local weather (12 items), the second thematic section asks respondents to report on community observations on hunting and harvesting (8 items), the third thematic section covers community observations on food and water safety (7 items), the fourth thematic section covers community observations on general health and air quality (6 items), and the last thematic section is an open-ended text section that allows respondents to report on any additional community observations. The length of the monthly survey was shortened to approximately 30 – 40 minutes in duration.

Open-ended text and moderating factors

Other research challenges in addition to the lack of long-term health data are accounting for community level moderating factors. Moderating factors are described as population-level characteristics and non-climate factors that do not have an association between climate change and human health, but affect climate-related health outcomes by varying the health risk/susceptibility of populations.

Community members may report non-climate factors (e.g., unemployment, poverty, inadequate public health infrastructure, or substance abuse) which do not have an association between climate change and human health, but should be included as non-climate factors.

Some moderating influences include population growth and demographic change (e.g., seasonal employment/tourism), level of economic and technological development, preexisting health status, the quality and availability of health care, and public health infrastructure (23, 29).

Data collection

Initially, a web survey and response options limited to likert scales was the primary mode of data collection based on U.S. Current Population Survey data reporting that Alaska has one of the highest rates of computer ownership and internet access than any other state except for Utah (30). After discussions with community organizers and key informants, two other data collection modes and open-ended text boxes for optional qualitative data were utilized to increase response rates (25). Community organizers recommended that telephone surveys would be optimal for residents who preferred to communicate via phone for a variety of reasons (e.g., oral cultural tradition, insecure in spelling/writing skills). Program investigators established a toll-free 1-855 telephone number that was made available to all participating communities and tested to ensure that it was operable. Mail-in options were offered by traditional paper and pencil surveys. Self-addressed stamped envelopes were printed and included in each participant's toolkit and toolkit envelopes were selected that were made from a waterproof and re-usable material. Gaining access to communities was accomplished through community organizers that advised program investigators when telephone calls or webinars were needed to introduce the project to local officials. Several conference calls and webinars occurred with our northwest communities to describe the general purpose of the study, its importance for community health and planning, the organizations collaborating together, and sponsored agency. Recruitment of potential community participants was first identified by community organizers. Community organizers were asked to develop a list of prospective participants who represented health aids, elders, and civic or tribal employees. In appreciation of participant time, an incentive was offered of $20 per completed monthly survey.

Implementation of the sentinel surveillance system

Implementation of the sentinel surveillance system consisted of conducting visits to community sites, enrolling potential community participants, provide training on utilizing the surveillance system, data collection monthly process. Study participants include residents of the city and village of Ketchikan and Angoon in the Southeast region of the state, the villages of Healy, Anderson, and Cantwell in Interior, and the villages of Point Hope, Kivalina, and Noatak in Northwestern, Alaska (Figure 1).

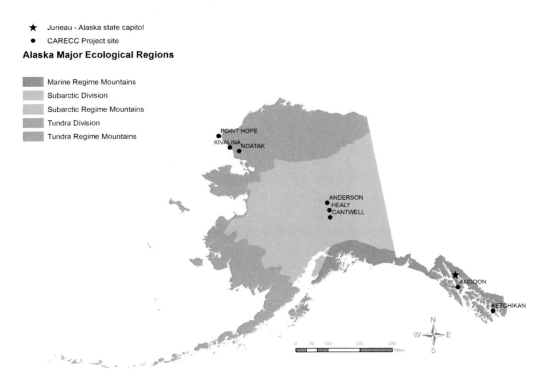

Figure 1. CARECC study sites in Alaska.

These population settlements provide a representative population cross-sample in three ecologically distinct regions of the state. Approximately 12 research participants per community site are involved in the study. This sample size takes into account the small size of each community site and anticipated attrition over the life of the study. Purposive sampling within communities was used to identify key informants that represent unique perspective differences (e.g., gender, race/ethnicity, and occupation) in climate change observations and human health impact literature (31). Because each community site differs demographically, inclusion criteria was also based on an individual ability to observe and communicate community environmental observations related to climate change events and other related processes that may take decades to occur. We excluded participants who did not possess the ability to observe and communicate climate change events from a historical perspective.

Exclusion criteria included: persons less than 18 years of age, residents who have lived in the community for less than 10 years, physically and mentally unable to read and understand a consent form and complete survey instruments, and persons who are not able to complete surveys in English.

To ensure that the CARECC surveillance survey collected relevant and timely data, we gathered extensive formative data regarding preferred communication methods from community organizers and residents to ensure that all program components were designed to address data collection challenges.

We identified convenient meeting times, locations, and methods of preferred information delivery. There are many physical and cultural barriers to conducting site visits in the Arctic due to low population density, weather conditions, and the associated difficulties such as transporting personnel, equipment, and samples to and from rural communities.

Cultural differences and prior negative experiences of indigenous people involved in past research studies can also be a barrier to participation. Even though travel is expensive in Alaska, visiting and staying overnight at each community was highly recommended by community organizers, especially in villages that do not have a hotel or an inn. Additionally, it is important for researchers to reflect on what Freudenberg referred to as 'determinants of community conditions' (21), otherwise known as fundamental determinants and other social/economic community characteristics that may seem banal and unnoteworthy to community participants, but researchers will recognize as potential moderating conditions to health outcomes.

Evaluation of the health component of the sentinel surveillance system

Evaluation of the health component of the sentinel surveillance system will be conducted in order to demonstrate the feasibility of community residents to collect community health and ecosystem data to detect the human health impacts from climate change. Using the framework promulgated by the US Centers for Disease Control and Prevention (2001) evaluation measures will include: 1) assessing the simplicity, flexibility, acceptability, timeliness, stability, validity, usefulness and representativeness of health data collected using this sentinel surveillance approach; 2) assessing the health data quality by examining 12 months of data collection; and 3) making recommendations to improve the system.

DISCUSSION

An understanding of climate change impacts on population health through public health surveillance is fundamental to planning and evaluating policies and programs. The multidisciplinary nature of climate change, like other environmental health exposures, demands surveillance systems that measure environmental exposure(s) and health outcome(s). The CARECC pilot project has completed the first year which included the development and implementation of a community-based sentinel surveillance system with 6-months of data collection, thus results are forthcoming. However, there are already several findings from this pilot project that are relevant for other rural and frontier regions, especially other circumpolar countries.

Based on the knowledge of the program investigator, this is the first community-based sentinel surveillance system developed to capture baseline ecosystem and human health data in Alaska. Similar projects to CARECC that have been conducted in the circumpolar north have been cross-sectional studies (32) that focused on one health outcome or were health impact assessments that were primarily conducted to determine probable health impacts from climate change instead of enabling communities to provide concurrent structured observations (33). There are many advantages of implementing a community-based sentinel surveillance system in Alaska, such as including communities and vulnerable population groups in the process of being a data resource and involvement in decision making. An advantage of implementing a sentinel surveillance system is the identification of outbreaks of public health importance earlier than passive (traditional) surveillance systems. However, there is currently limited evidence that sentinel surveillance systems add value to local public health disease surveillance (34).

Validity and reliability of the sentinel surveillance system has yet to be determined, yet preliminary results are promising. While potential sources of bias include the small sample, the generalizability is improved by selecting a purposive sample from each community of health aids, environmental coordinators, or civic/tribal employees. These women and men represent community residents who are able to report on community environmental and health conditions month-to-month.

Limitations of the project include observed ethical challenges in the field. The most difficult ethical challenge in the surveillance survey development was how to integrate traditional knowledge and western science. Traditional knowledge understands that knowledge is alive in the minds and hearts of indigenous peoples and resides within community elders, therefore great respect and care should be used in recording, storing, and analyzing traditional knowledge (35). While traditional Institutional Review Boards ensure the safety and security of data, the idea that 'living' knowledge could be captured in a structured survey format seems antithetical to the ideals of indigenous culture and will be further explored with our communities.

Other ethical questions discussed were how this pilot study could have been improved utilizing a community-based participatory research (CBPR) process (36).

While the colloquium attendees identified a broad set of human health indicators caused by climate change, there was little discussion on whether these indicators would be relevant to communities or establishing criteria that considered usefulness, objectivity, data quality, transparency, ability to show a meaningful trend, and relevance to climate change. Project investigators ultimately relied on peer-reviewed and grey literature to prioritize human health impacts from climate change, but considered what community priorities would have been identified utilizing CBPR methods.

CONCLUSION

The primary goal of public health surveillance is to guide the planning and evaluation of policy and programs, through the collection, analysis and interpretation of statistical information. The purpose of the sentinel surveillance system was to develop indicators that represent environmental and health conditions for Alaska communities for a specified period of time. These environmental and health indictors are important not only to the community, but to public health researchers, policy-makers, and others who use these indicators to track health trends over time.

Addressing the issue of human health effects from climate change in Alaska requires the interaction of public health researchers, state and federal environmental health workers who have experience in conducting climate change research in Alaska with experts who have experience working in Alaska (37-39).

Alaska is the only Arctic state within the United States, but like other circumpolar nations faces unique challenges in assessing the human health impacts from climate change. Conducting health research in the Arctic poses unique challenges given the rural and frontier areas and health research efforts offer a special challenge to investigators who aim to balance conducting culturally sensitive research with scientific rigor while providing a benefit to communities, disparities in research infrastructure and treatment delivery. Although recent health impact assessments provide new insights on what areas to focus research, they also build a strong case for including community participation in filling information gaps regarding the intricate causal mechanisms regarding climate change.

ACKNOWLEDGMENTS

The authors wish to acknowledge the input of the following community organizers: James Berner, MD, Michael Brubaker, and Jacob Bell from the Alaska Native Tribal Health Consortium, Jennifer Bell from Alaska Community Services, and Susan Renes, PhD from the University of Alaska Fairbanks. ICHS staff is acknowledged for their input and dedication to servicing Alaska communities.

Funding for the colloquium was provided by the Institute for Circumpolar Health Studies and Chancellor's office, University of Alaska Anchorage. Funding for the pilot project was provided by a cooperative agreement with the U.S. Centers for Disease Control and Prevention.

REFERENCES

[1]   Berner JE, Furgal C. Conclusions and recommendation on human health and climate change in the Arctic. New York: International Arctic Science Committee, Cambridge University Press, 2005:863-906.

[2]   O'Neill MS, Ebi KL. Climate Change. In: Galea S, editor. Macrosocial determinants of population health. New York: Springer, 2007:139-58.

[3]   Hess JJ, Malilay JN, Parkinson AJ. Climate change: the importance of place. Am J Prev Med 2008;35:468-78.

[4]   Campbell-Lendrum D, Woodruff R. Climate change: quantifying the health impact at national and local levels. Geneva: World Health Organization, 2007.

[5]   Serreze MC, Walsh JE, Chapin FS, Osterkamp T, Dyurgerov M, Romanovsky V, et al. Observational evidence of recent change in the northern high-latitude environment. Climatic Change 2000;46:159-207.

[6]   2010 U.S. Census Bureau. Table DP-1 Profile of General Population and Housing Characteristics. Accessed 2011 Sept 08.: 2010]. URL: http://factfinder2.census.gov/faces/tableservices/jsf/pages/productview.xhtml?pid=DEC_10_DP_DPDP1andprodType=table

[7]   Weatherhead E, Gearheard S, Barry RG. Changes in weather persistence: Insight from inuit knowledge. Global Environl Change Hum Policy Dimensions 2010;20:523-8.

[8]   Downing A, Cuerrier A. A synthesis of the impacts of climate change on the First Nations and Inuit of Canada. Indian J Traditional Knowledge 2011;10:57-70.

[9]   Green D, Raygorodetsky G. Indigenous knowledge of a changing climate. Climatic Change 2010; 100:239-42.

[10]   McNeeley SM, Shulski MD. Anatomy of a closing window: Vulnerability to changing seasonality in Interior Alaska. Global Environ Change Hum Policy Dimensions 2011;21:464-73.

[11]   Riseth JA, Tommervik H, Helander-Renvall E, Labba N, Johansson C, Malnes E, et al. Sami traditional ecological knowledge as a guide to science: snow, ice and reindeer pasture facing climate change. Polar Record 2011;47:202-17.

[12]   Wolf J, Moser SC. Individual understandings, perceptions, and engagement with climate change: insights from in-depth studies across the world. Climate Change 2011; 2:547-69.

[13]   George JC, Huntington HP, Brewster K, Eicken H, Norton DW, Glenn R. Observations on shorefast ice dynamics in arctic Alaska and the responses of the Inupiat hunting community. Arctic 2004;57:363-74.

[14]   Stieglitz M, Dery SJ, Romanovsky VE, Osterkamp TE. The role of snow cover in the warming of arctic permafrost. Geophysical Res Letters 2003;30.

[15]   Kellogg J, Wang JZ, Flint C, Ribnicky D, Kuhn P, De Mejia EG, et al. Alaskan wild berry resources and human health under the cloud of climate change. J Agricultural Food Chem 2010;58:3884-900.

[16]   Zhang Y, Bi P, Hiller JE. Climate change and the transmission of vector-borne diseases: A review. Asia-Pacific J Public Health 2008;20:64-76.

[17]   Lehti V, Niemela S, Hoven C, Mandell D, Sourander A. Mental health, substance use and suicidal behaviour among young indigenous people in the Arctic: A systematic review. Soc Sci Med 2009;69:1194-203.

[18]   Berry HL, Bowen K, Kjellstrom T. Climate change and mental health: a causal pathways framework. Int J Public Health 2010;55:123-32.

[19]   Goodman RM, Speers MA, McLeroy K, Fawcett S, Kegler M, Parker E, et al. Identifying and defining the dimensions of community capacity to provide a basis for measurement. Health Educ Behav 1998;25:258-78.

[20]   Houghton JT, Ding Y, Griggs M, Noguer PJ, van der Linden X, Dai K, Johnson CA. Climate Change 2001: The scientific basis. Contribution of working group I to the third assessment report of the Intergovernmental Panel on Climate Change. New York: Cambridge University Press, 2001.

[21]   Freudenberg N. Community capacity for environmental health promotion: Determinants and implications for practice. Health Educ Behav 2004;31:472-90.

[22]   Malecki KC, Resnick B, Burke TA. Effective environmental public health surveillance programs: A framework for identifying and evaluating data resources and indicators. J Public Health Manage Pract 2008;14:543-51.

[23]   Haines A, Patz JA. Health effects of climate change. JAMA 2004;291:99-103.

[24]   German RRL, Lisa M, Horan, JM, Milstein, RL, Pertowski, CA, Waller, MN. Updated guidelines for evaluating public health surveillance systems. MMWR, 2001:1-35.

[25]   Groves RMF, Floyd J, Couper, MP, Lepkowski, JM, Singer, E, Tourangeau, R. Survey methodology. Hoboken, NJ: John Wiley, 2004.

[26]   Centers for Disease Control and Prevention. Behavioral risk factor surveillance system user's guide. Centers for Disease Control and Prevention 2003. Accessed 2011 Sept 09. URL: http:// www.cdc.gov/brfss/

[27]   Centers for Disease Control and Prevention. National health and nutrition examination survey. Centers for Disease Control and Prevention 2003. Accessed 2011 Sept 09. URL: http://www. cdc.gov/nchs/nhanes/about_nhanes.htm

[28]   Tremblay M, Furgal C, Larrivee C, Annanack T, Tookalook P, Qiisik, M et al. Climate change in northern Quebec: Adaptation strategies from community-based research. Arctic 2008;61:27-34.

[29]   Portier CJ, Thigpen TK, Carter SR, Dilworth CH, Grambsch AE, Gohlke J, et al. A human health persepctive on climate change: A report outlining the research needs on the human health effects of climate change. Environmental Health Perspectives/National Institue of Environmental Health Sciences, Research Triangle Park, 2010.

[30]   Day JC, Janus A, David J. Computer and internet use in the United States: 2003. Washington, DC: US Census Bureau, 2005.

[31]   Furgal C, Martin D, Gosselin P. Climate change and health in Nunavik and Labrador: Lessons from Inuit knowledge. Fairbanks: Arctic Research Consortium United States, 2002.

[32]   Gessner BD, Middaugh JP. Paralytic shellfish poisoning in Alaska - a 20-year retrospective analysis. Am J Epidemiol 1995;141:766-70.

[33]   Brubaker M, Berner J, Warren J, Rolin A. Climate change in Point Hope, Alaska: Strategies for community health. Anchorage: Alaska Native Tribal Health Consortium, 2010.

[34]   Birkhead GS, Maylahn CM. State and local public health surveillance. In: Teutsch SM, Churchill RE. Principles and Practices of Public Health Surveillance. New York: Oxford University, 2000:253-86.

[35]   Alaska Native Science Commission. Traditional knowledge systems in the Arctic. Accessed 2010 Oct 03. URL: http://www.nativescience.org/communities/code.htm.

[36]   Israel BA, Schulz AJ, Parker EA, Becker AB. Review of community-based research: Assessing partnership approaches to improve public health. Annu Rev Public Health 1998;19:173-202.

[37]   Frumkin H, McMichael AJ. Climate change and public health thinking, communicating, acting. Am J Prev Med 2008;35:403-10.

[38]   Frumkin H, Hess J, Luber G, Malilay J, McGeehin M. Climate change: The public health response. Am J Public Health 2008;98:435-45.

[39]   Huang CR, Vaneckova P, Wang XM, FitzGerald G, Guo YM, Tong SL. Constraints and barriers to public health adaptation to climate change: A review of the literature. Am J Prev Med 2011;40:183-90.

Submitted: January 01, 2012. *Revised:* April 01, 2012. *Accepted:* April 21, 2012.

In: Public Health Yearbook 2013
Editor: Joav Merrick

ISBN: 978-1-63321-095-0
© 2014 Nova Science Publishers, Inc.

Chapter 12

CAPACITY BUILDING FOR LONG-TERM COMMUNITY-ACADEMIC HEALTH PARTNERSHIP OUTCOMES

M Kathryn Stewart, MD, MPH[1], Holly C Felix, PhD, MPA[,1], Naomi Cottoms, MA[2], Mary Olson, DDiv[2], Beatrice Shelby[3], Anna Huff[4], Dianne Colley, MPH[5], Carla Sparks[1] and Freeman McKindra[1]*

[1]Office of Community-Based Public Health, Fay W Boozman College of Public Health, University of Arkansas for Medical Sciences, Little Rock, AR, United States of America
[2]Tri County Rural Health Network, Helena-West Helena, AR, United States of America
[3]Boys Girls Adults Community Development Center, Marvell, AR, United States of America
[4]Mid-Delta Community Consortium, Helena-West Helena, AR, United States of America
[5]Seven Harvest Training Center, Forrest City, AR, United States of America

ABSTRACT

Too often, populations experiencing the greatest burden of disease and disparities in health outcomes are left out of or ineffectively involved in academic-led efforts to address issues that impact them the most. Community-based participatory research (CBPR) is an approach increasingly being used to address these issues, but the science of CBPR is still viewed by many as a nascent field. Important to the development of the science of CBPR is documentation of the partnership process, particularly capacity building activities important to establishing the CBPR research infrastructure. This paper uses a CBPR Logic Model as a structure for documenting partnership capacity building activities of a long-term community-academic partnership addressing public health issues in Arkansas, U.S. Illustrative activities, programs, and experiences are described for each of the model's four constructs: context, group dynamics, interventions, and outcomes. Lessons learned through this process were: capacity building is required by both academic and community partners; shared activities provide a common base of experiences and expectations; and creating a common language facilitates dialogue about

* Correspondence: Holly C Felix, PhD, MPA, Associate Professor of Health Policy, Fay W Boozman College of Public Health, University of Arkansas for Medical Sciences, 4301 West Markham Street, Slot 820, Little Rock, Arkansas, 72205 United States. E-mail: felixholly@uams.edu.

difficult issues. Development of community partnerships with one institutional unit promoted community engagement institution-wide, enhanced individual and partnership capacity, and increased opportunity to address priority issues.

Keywords: Community-based participatory research, partnerships, capacity building

INTRODUCTION

Too often, populations experiencing the greatest burden of disease and disparities in health outcomes are left out of or ineffectively involved in academic-led efforts to address the issues that impact them the most. This institutional or "expert"-driven approach, traditionally viewed as more efficient and easy to control, is often too narrowly construed and of limited impact when translated into practice. This "disconnect" has led to a movement of scholarship of engagement (1), which requires an alternative paradigm based on equity, collaboration, and transformative action on issues of importance to the community (2). Many communities have embraced deliberation as a mechanism for dialogue, identifying needs, and initiating action (3,4). Others have used a community-based participatory research (CBPR) approach to address these issues with outside researchers (5,6). Although now more widely accepted as critical to translating research into practice (7,8), the science of CBPR is still viewed by many as a nascent field (9).

Important to the development of the science of CBPR is documentation of the partnership process, particularly partnership capacity building activities important to establishing a community-based research infrastructure that can support CBPR. This paper uses Wallerstein and colleagues CBPR Logic Model (9) as a structure for documenting capacity building activities of long-term community-academic partnerships addressing public health issues in Arkansas, U.S. Wallerstein's model was produced using a systematic process including collection and analysis of primary data, synthesis of the literature, and input from a national advisory committee of CBPR experts. This model describes multiple constructs comprising the context of partnerships including structural inequities in socio-economic and environmental factors, and cultural influences over risk and protection; national and local policies and trends; community and university capacity and readiness, and perceived severity and salience of the health issue.

BACKGROUND

The Fay W. Boozman College of Public Health (COPH) at the University of Arkansas for Medical Sciences (UAMS) was founded in 2001, and immediately established the Office of Community-Based Public Health (OCBPH) based on the college's philosophy that "community lies at the heart of public health" (10,11). In the COPH's first year, two minority Arkansans with extensive community and organizational experience were hired to serve as community liaisons and to develop partnerships with community-based organizations (CBOs) in Phillips County (the focus of this paper) and Pulaski County. Boys Girls Adults Community Development Center (BGACDC), based in Arkansas' Mississippi River Delta region, was selected as an initial CBO partner. Also that year, network development funding from the Health Resources and Services Administration (HRSA) was secured to establish Mid-Delta Community Consortium (MDCC), a CBO providing technical assistance and funding to rural health networks for health program planning and implementation in the Delta region through its Arkansas Delta Rural Development Network (ADRDN) program. MDCC's director also serves as a COPH community liaison. The Tri-County Rural Health Network (TCRHN) formed in 2003, with ADRDN support, and became a COPH partner in 2004 (Figure 1).

These partnerships focus on improving the health and quality of life of individuals, families, and communities and on achieving health equity. Research is one among several mechanisms for achieving this goal. Indeed, partnership activities also include bidirectional technical assistance, program and resource development and sustainability, student service learning, community participation in classroom instruction, and community organizing.

UAMS and its COPH are located in Little Rock (the state capital), Pulaski County, Arkansas, U.S. UAMS is a major regional academic health center with five colleges and a graduate school, eight Area Health Education Centers, and six institutes of excellence (12). MDCC and TCRHN are located in Helena-West Helena, and BGACDC is in Marvell, all in Phillips County, 120 miles east of Pulaski County (Figure 1). Delta residents are primarily African American, have lower educational and employment levels, lower median household income, and a higher percentage living in poverty compared to those living in Little Rock or the state as a whole, although Little Rock and Arkansas lag behind the country on these same indicators. Phillips County has higher levels of mortality when compared to Pulaski County and Arkansas, U.S. as a whole, and racial health disparities are present. While access to quality healthcare is a factor in such disparities, structural determinants, such as political representation and control of major economic assets, also play an important role (Table 1).

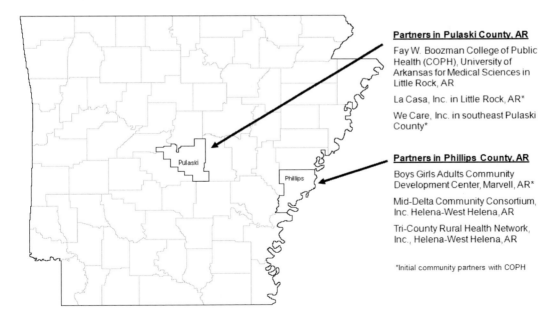

Partners in Pulaski County, AR

Fay W. Boozman College of Public Health (COPH), University of Arkansas for Medical Sciences in Little Rock, AR

La Casa, Inc. in Little Rock, AR*

We Care, Inc. in southeast Pulaski County*

Partners in Phillips County, AR

Boys Girls Adults Community Development Center, Marvell, AR*

Mid-Delta Community Consortium, Inc. Helena-West Helena, AR

Tri-County Rural Health Network, Inc., Helena-West Helena, AR

*Initial community partners with COPH

Figure 1. Partner Locations in Arkansas.

Table 1. Selected Demographic Characteristics and Mortality Rates of Partnership Communities

	Little Rock	Pulaski County	Helena	West Helena	Marvell	Phillips County	AR	US
Demographics								
Total population	191,130	381,907	6,323	8,689	1,395	20,921	2.9 mil	307 mil
Median age, years	36.2	37.0	31.7	30.0	37.6	35.7	37.1	36.7
Race								
White	52.1%	60.8%	30.6%	32.8%	40.4%	36.5%	80.6%	74.3%
Black/African American	41.6%	34.7%	67.9%	65.7%	58.1%	61.5%	15.8%	12.3%
Education								
High School grad or higher	89.6%	84.4%	62.3%	64.4%	64.6%	62.2%	75.3%	84.5%
College Degree or higher	39.0%	21.1%	17.4%	12.0%	13.9%	12.4%	16.7%	27.4%
In Labor Force	68.4%	67.8%	48.0%	55.1%	48.7%	56.6%	61.1%	65.2%
Income								
Median household income	$44,480	$45,215	$18,662	$21,130	$22,368	$26,436	$38,820	$52,175
Persons in poverty	12.2%	16.5%	38.4%	30.9%	22.6%	34.9%	17.3%	9.6%
Mortality Rates								
All Cause								
Total	na	930.2	na	na	na	1228.5	931.2	821.7
White	na	865.2	na	na	na	1091.1	905.1	806.3
Black/African American	na	1158.7	na	na	na	1369.2	1160.4	1051.2
Heart Disease								
Total	na	80.8	na	na	na	117.3	80.6	65.5
White	na	75.8	na	na	na	90.9	77.3	62.6
Black/African American	na	99.8	na	na	na	146.6	108.7	85.4

Mortality Rates

	Little Rock	Pulaski County	Helena	West Helena	Marvell	Phillips County	AR	US
All Cancer								
Total	na	211.4	na	na	na	270.4	210.9	194.1
White	na	200.5	na	na	na	259.8	206.4	192.6
Black/African American	na	257.5	na	na	na	279.8	256.5	236.9
Ischemic Stroke								
Total	na	38.8	na	na	na	68.7	43.4	31.2
White	na	38.3	na	na	na	54.1	41.9	30.3
Black/African American	na	41.1	na	na	na	86.0	57.8	42.9
Diabetes								
Total	na	26.6	na	na	na	64.1	26.6	24.5
White	na	18.7	na	na	na	30.3	22.9	22.3
Black/African American	na	58.5	na	na	na	99.7	57.8	47.6
Infant Mortality								
Total	na	7.9	na	na	na	na	7.8	6.7
White	na	na	na	na	na	na	6.4	5.7
Black/African American	na	11.6	na	na	na	na	7.8	13.3

General Notes: NA = not available; mil=million, Little Rock is located in Pulaski County; Marvell, Helena and West Helena are located in Phillips County. Helena and West Helena were individual cities until they consolidated in 2006.

Notes on Demographic Characteristics: Total population figures for all geographic regions are from 2009. Other demographic data for counties, AR and US are also from 2009. Data for Little Rock are from 2006-08. Data for Marvell, Helena and West Helena are from 2000 (39).

Notes on Mortality Rates: Infant mortality rate per 1000 live births, 2003-05. All other rates are age-adjusted rates per 100,000 persons. All mortality rates are for 2007. Heart Disease = ICD-10 I60-I78; All Cancer = ICD-10 C00-D48; Ischemic Stroke= ICD-10 I64-I64 (40).

Although disparities and other challenges exist, assets also abound. Delta-bred people are resilient and resourceful, often overcoming seemingly insurmountable odds.

The extended family structure and the small-church religious network support residents and local leadership development, and both unite local knowledge and experience that can be used to overcome barriers and survive a system not easily accessed by all. A perception by Delta-residents that no one is going to "do for us" has led to a sense of independence and determination that has prompted action. For example, when Marvell residents realized that they were lacking quality education and housing, they formed their own CBO, BGACDC, to address the issue. Recognizing gaps in healthcare access, Delta-based organizations formed MDCC to capture federal resources to support the development of rural health networks.

TCRHN was subsequently established to target access issues in ways consistent with the extended family culture and small-church social networks.

METHODS

Wallerstein's CBPR Logic Model (9) provides the structure for documenting partnership capacity building activities.

It focuses on CBPR processes and outcomes, and indicates how context and group dynamics affect interventions and consequently affect system, capacity and health-related outcomes, which can then circle back to affect context.

In this model, context refers to factors affecting partnership formation, and the nature of the partnership and its activities. Group dynamics refers to factors affecting interactions between partners.

Interventions are partnership activities undertaken to address identified problems. Finally, outcomes represent intermediate intervention results, including system and capacity changes, and improvements in health and health disparities (9) (Figure 2).

Procedures

An iterative process was used to obtain data from representatives of organizational partners for model constructs and to develop this paper. Each construct was discussed by partners to determine what illustrative experiences would be described. A qualitative group decision process was used to prioritize data using the criteria that each partner's participation would be represented, the breadth of activities and experiences would be reflected, and activities the group identified as being most crucial contributors to partnership outcomes would have higher priority for reporting. Each co-author wrote sections that were relevant to their experience, with the lead author incorporating sections and input from discussions into a final integrated piece.

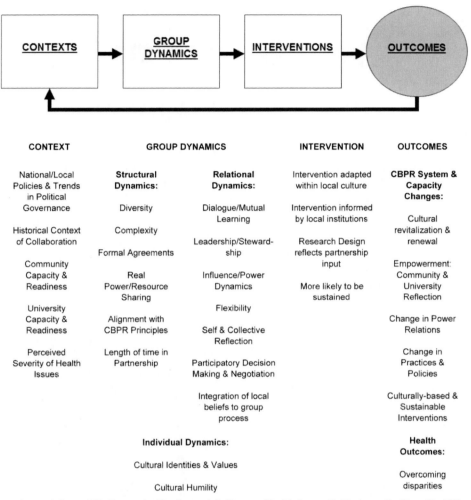

Source: Adapted from Wallerstein N, Oetzel J, Duran B, Tafoya G, Belone L, Rae R. What Predicts Outcomes in CBPR? In: Minkler M, Wallerstein N, editors. Community-Based Participatory Research for Health. 2nd ed. San Francisco: Jossey Bass; 2008. p. 371-388.

Figure 2. CBPR Logic Model.

RESULTS

National/local policies, trends, and political governance

Arkansas, U.S. used proceeds from the Tobacco Master Settlement Agreement to establish the COPH in 2001 (13). Early COPH leaders committed to community-based public health (CBPH) principles established the OCBPH to develop community partnerships; to provide resources for the COPH and community partners regarding CBPH theories and methods; to assist in developing new community-based educational, service, and research programs; and to support development and implementation of CBPR projects (11). This commitment was supported by the rapid development, nationally, of health-related CBPR in the 1990's and the increasing acceptance of, and funding for, this approach to research (14,15). The 2003 Institute of Medicine report on racial and ethnic disparities in healthcare (16) along with a growing body of research on social determinants of health (17,18) were also critical drivers and supports to these partnerships.

Historical context of collaboration

Community partners' perceptions of UAMS prior to partnering with the COPH centered around individuals' experiences with receiving healthcare at the University hospital and its clinics. These impressions varied. Some saw UAMS as a haven– a place for care for particularly serious problems. Others perceived UAMS as the "welfare hospital" where care might not be the best but where people went when they could not afford care elsewhere.

Strong and pre-existing relationships between COPH faculty and staff of two of the partnering CBOs provided a strong foundation for the partnerships between BGACDC, MDCC and the COPH. Other factors contributing to the early trust and understanding between partners include joint learning experiences and educational opportunities, and joint efforts to secure funding to support partner programs. For example, in 2001, a team of COPH and community partners visited the University of North Carolina Chapel Hill (UNC) and the University of Michigan (UM) to learn about their long-term efforts to integrate CBPH into their Public Health research, teaching, and practice. Partnership members also participated together in Undoing Racism Workshops (19,20), which created a common language for dialogue about issues of power, privilege, and institutionalized racism. These workshops, sponsored by the COPH and its institutional partners, were carried out by the People's Institute for Survival and Beyond with a focus on "understanding what racism is, where it comes from, how it functions, why it persists and how it can be undone..[using] a systemic approach that emphasizes learning from history, developing leadership, maintaining accountability to communities, creating networks, undoing internalized racial oppression and understanding the role of organizational gate keeping as a mechanism for perpetuating racism" (19). These shared activities, further described below, have established a common base of experience and expectations.

Community capacity and readiness

The community partners have strong roots and capacity for engagement within their communities, predating their partnership with the COPH. Their leaders have played significant community advocacy and organizing roles, such as serving on the local school board, chairing community development committees, and organizing local events.

BGACDC is a thirty-two year old CBO, serving residents of Marvell, Elaine and eight unincorporated communities, through its child and youth development, adult education, housing, health, and economic development programs. BGACDC emphasizes individual and organizational development and, as such, has sponsored staff and volunteers in training for leadership development, community and economic development, housing development, and organizational capacity-building. These efforts have succeeded in producing a number of high professional achievers, and in BGACDC becoming the county's leading producer of new and remodeled housing. BGACDC was recognized for its efforts through the receipt by its director, Mrs. Beatrice Shelby, of the Robert Wood Johnson Foundation (RWJF) Community Leadership Award, and of the Ford Foundation Leadership for a Changing World Award, and through invitations to partner with the WK Kellogg Foundation (WKKF) Rural People / Rural Policy Initiative and the Marvell Nutrition Intervention Research Initiative (NIRI), among others (21).

MDCC was established in 2001 to increase resources for, and understanding of, partnerships to enhance and promote community-driven health improvement initiatives. Through its HRSA-funded ADRDN program, MDCC provides technical assistance and funds to Delta-based multi-county networks to develop and implement health programs. MDCC also administers Arkansas, U.S.' only health-focused program and served as a community partner and community fiscal agent for the USDA Marvell NIRI (22).

TCRHN is a grassroots CBO whose mission is to improve access to healthcare. TCRHN's leadership, trained by the Kettering Foundation in the use of deliberative democracy forums, has used this approach to community engagement (CE) as an organizing tool. Its best-known program, the Community Connector Program (CCP), uses community health workers (CHW) to link residents to needed long-term care (LTC) services (23). The program was developed in response to community sentiment that, "we have great health resources in the Delta; but we don't access them," often because of lack of awareness or problems with trust in providers.

University capacity and readiness

In addition to having strong CBOs to partner with, the COPH has a number of internal structural supports for CBPR, including the OCBPH (described above) and its community liaisons, and the early opportunity to obtain education with partners about CBPH/CBPR through visits to UNC and UM. A combination of grants and core support to hire a part-time research assistant and to bring in academic and community consultants to assist with faculty development in CBPR and disparities also increased COPH partnering capacity. Other critical supporting structures have included monthly meetings between the OCBPH Director and the COPH Dean, a faculty committee designed to advise and connect the OCBPH with COPH departments, and core support for meetings focused on CBPH/CBPR and health disparities and for community partners to serve as co-instructors and guest lecturers in COPH courses. None of these assets would have been available had there not been strong leadership and support for the principles of CBPR from the COPH Dean and senior administrators.

OCBPH involvement in the Undoing Racism Workshops held at UAMS led to development of a workshop alumni group that met regularly to discuss potential opportunities and strategies for action and the need to organize those working on diversity issues at UAMS. The resulting cross-campus Racial and Ethnic Health Disparities Taskforce was influenced by several key publications (16,24,25) and subsequently identified three areas (quality of care, education, and faculty/student diversity) for UAMS to target to address racial and ethnic health and healthcare disparities in Arkansas, U.S.. In 2005, the Taskforce submitted a brief on its organization and purpose to the UAMS Chancellor, who subsequently asked the Taskforce to regularly report to him and to expand its membership to include representatives from all the Colleges and the Hospital. In addition, he charged the Taskforce with making recommendations for addressing language assistance services within UAMS clinical programs.

The Taskforce also served as a planning committee for a campus-wide retreat for addressing racial and ethnic health and healthcare disparities, which was sponsored by the COPH as a part of the WKKF's Engaged Institutions Initiative. The Taskforce recently completed a campus-wide survey of students on the racial and ethnic diversity attitudes and climate at UAMS, the findings of which will form part of an audit (described below).

Another COPH structural asset is a subset of faculty with interest and skills in CBPH/CBPR. The top-down/bottom-up emphasis on CBPH in the COPH has resulted in an environment in which CBPR has become more mainstream, facilitating involvement of more traditional researchers in CBPR. Outsiders can bring skills and resources when they enter the community and can use such assets to strengthen the community's power to serve their own needs (26). This kind of faculty capacity has played an important role in supporting community efforts (e.g., program evaluation and community research infrastructure development).

Perceived severity/salience of health issues

Health issues are of utmost concern to COPH community partners. Epidemiologic data indicate that citizens in the Arkansas Delta have the poorest health indicators and limited healthcare access. These statistics occur in a larger context of social determinants which create large racial and income disparities in health status (27). Against this background, COPH community partners have historically focused on addressing social determinants, disparities, and access to services.

Group dynamics

The group dynamics construct of Wallerstein's model's has three sub-dimensions: individual, structural, and relational dynamics of the partnerships.

Individual dynamics
Partnership activities have been extremely important in creating individual "cultural humility and critical self-reflection" (9). Undoing Racism Workshops, which have been attended jointly by COPH and community partners, focus on increasing awareness of white privilege and how it operates at both the conscious and unconscious level to perpetuate oppression. Incorporation of this content into courses co-taught by COPH and community partners has reinforced integration of these concepts and reflection on how these dynamics play out in the everyday context of these partnerships. The use of the privilege walk (28) and other individual and group reflection exercises provide tools and content for explicit discussion of these issues among community partners, faculty, and students, and serve to increase self-awareness and understanding of these social determinants of health.

Structural dynamics

Formal/informal agreements
While partnerships were not established with formal written agreements, a number of commitments were made by the COPH, such as support of community liaisons. In some cases, the COPH has entered into subcontracts with partners for specific activities or grant-funded projects. Students are also required to develop Memoranda of Agreement with community partners for course-related projects.

Agreement on values/expectations
OCBPH strategic planning conducted in 2004 with community partners identified a shared interest in social justice, health equity, and social determinants of health. The joint experience participating in Undoing Racism Workshops and conducting over 20 community screenings and facilitated discussions of the Unnatural Causes documentary series (29) helped to solidify mutual understanding of institutionalized and historical aspects of oppression that perpetuate disparities. This four-hour documentary series of seven episodes was produced by California Newsreel in collaboration with public health experts and organizational partners including the National Minority Consortium, the Joint Center Health Policy Institute and the National Association of County and City Health Officials. This series takes on the challenge of communicating the root causes of socio-economic and racial inequities in health status and seeks to broaden public understanding of the role of social structural factors in these outcomes.

Allocation and level of resources invested
The COPH has a long-term commitment to having community liaisons available to work with partners. Community liaisons help connect partners to resources and contacts, serve on boards, assist with planning, and provide trainings. One community partner serves as a paid co-instructor in required DrPH courses and other community partners have served as paid guest lecturers. The COPH has also helped partners to obtain grant funding (e.g., HRSA funds that supported MDCC's establishment and RWJF funds supporting the CCP).

Community partners have also invested significant time, effort, and resources to participate in COPH-initiated activities such as site visits by funders, training and planning sessions, presentations, conferences, web and face-to-face meetings, events, and classes. Sometimes their efforts have been supported by honoraria and/or travel reimbursement, but many times they have not been, reflecting their commitment.

Relational dynamics

Congruence of Core Values and Mutual Respect
While the structures supporting these partnerships have been essential to their success, their impact would be extremely limited if not for the personal relationships and shared core values that exist. These values include recognition of the mutual benefit of partners with different expertise; the significance of grassroots voices; the importance of CBPR principles; and the need to address the injustice of disparities.

Dialogue/mutual learning
Joint participation in Undoing Racism Workshops helped create a common language to discuss difficult issues related to racism; increased recognition of institutional racism; and enhanced faculty understanding of how structures can benefit them while oppressing others. For example, prior to this training, some of the faculty involved were not fully aware of the under-representation of racial minorities on high-level decision-making bodies at UAMS or the day-to-day discrimination experienced by minority colleagues and community partners. Likewise, community partners talked about aspects of their communities or personal experiences they felt reflected their internalized oppression.

Having community partners participate as co-instructors or guest lecturers has provided a significant learning opportunity for partners and faculty involved throughout course development, annual updating and modification, and during class discussions. Community partners have become more knowledgeable about CBPR principles, program design, and evaluation methods. COPH faculty and students have learned about community power dynamics, the importance of history, the community's mixed perceptions of academics and other outsiders trying to "help", and experiences that established and deepened these impressions.

Leadership and stewardship
Community partners have taken on significant local and national leadership roles over the course of the partnerships including serving on National Institutes of Health's Council of Public Representatives, serving as the Deputy Co-Director of the Arkansas Prevention Research Center (APRC), and two being recipients of the RWJF Community Leadership Award. COPH liaisons also serve on the Boards of several partnering organizations.

Influence and power dynamics
Clearly, there are many times when traditional dynamics play out with professional knowledge, skills, and expertise having a stronger influence on choices made, issues raised, and projects that get discussed; but, there have also been instances where community preferences have driven final decisions. It has been important for the COPH, as the institutional partner, to avoid pushing partners to take on projects with which they are uncomfortable. For example, when faculty approached BGACDC to partner on a study on agricultural-related factors in air and water quality (which they had previously identified as of concern), there was significant resistance from BGACDC staff. They felt such a project could have negative repercussions for their organization and others in their community whose livelihood was dependent on the agricultural economy. As a result, the partnership did not pursue that study.

Researchers' community involvement
COPH faculty and staff have participated in community events (e.g., MLK Day Marade, Arkansas Delta Green Expo); in locally-driven initiatives (e.g., ADRDN's regional conference, Unnatural Causes documentary screenings, and Delta Bridge's community development efforts (30)); in joint projects (e.g., Community Research Workshops and the CCP evaluation (both described below)); and in bringing visitors to the Delta to learn about the community and the community partners.

Participatory decision-making and negotiation
Community partners developed a code of ethics for researchers who want to conduct research in their communities. A COPH student worked with partners using multiple deliberative forums to engage communities in discussions about having agreements on goals, data ownership, and dissemination of information. The final code includes the key concepts of shared power; equitable inclusion; mutual benefit; equal opportunity for capacity building; respect and recognition; and ongoing communication.

Integration of community beliefs
Community partners focus on engaging residents in identifying community assets and needs, implementing solutions that incorporate community experience and perspectives, and building on identified resources. TCRHN's CCP was developed to respond to the need for trusted advocates with information about accessing existing services and builds on community interest in helping citizens access home and community-based LTC services and avoid unnecessary institutionalization (31, 32).

INTERVENTIONS

The "Interventions" construct considers whether interventions are designed, implemented, and researched to fit with community values and involve the community. A critical issue is sustainability.

Fits with community explanatory models
While community explanatory models have not been explicitly studied within these partnerships, a core set of beliefs and values of the partners' communities informs the approaches they use, including 1) trust is given to those who understand based on their own experience; 2) relationships should come first; and 3) priorities are based on need and on perceived relevance and possibility.

TCRHN's CCP and MDCC's Prescription Assistance Program (PAP) grew out of community-identified needs. These programs hire and train local individuals to meet those needs, in keeping with the critical role of community relationships and with their desire to build on existing assets. In the CCP, CHWs live in the community and share characteristics with those they serve. Key to their success is their ability to increase trust and provide valuable information about available services. They identify individuals in need through both formal methods (e.g., provider referrals) and through informal social networks.

Attends to bi-directional translation/ implementation/dissemination
Many of the partnership interventions were developed in an iterative manner. For example, after TCRHN developed and implemented the CCP pilot, COPH provided technical assistance on evaluation, sustainability, and the need for evidence of cost impact.

Community partners have also provided critical input into COPH activities as consistent participants in site visits by agencies or foundations funding or evaluating the COPH, co-presenters in conferences, and preceptors and educators of students and faculty.

Appropriate research design

The CCP is an example where a quasi-experimental design was selected because random assignment of participants to the CCP intervention or a control condition was not possible. COPH faculty evaluating the CCP used propensity score matching in which CCP participants in intervention counties were matched to Medicaid beneficiaries residing in non-intervention counties to strengthen the design (31, 32).

Outcomes

The outcomes construct has two sub-dimensions: 1) intermediate system and capacity changes, and 2) health and disparities outcomes.

Intermediate system and capacity changes

Partnership activities have led to several intermediate system and capacity changes. The increased financial stability and sustainability of these minority-controlled community organizations and their programs has increased their power within their communities and increased their ability to contribute to community empowerment and renewal. Their programs are aligned with the cultural values of those they serve and provide community models from which COPH students and faculty are learning. These relationships have also increased opportunities to fund infrastructure for community-based and translational research and have served as exemplars, speeding the pace of formation of other community partnerships (33).

An example of a system change resulting from these partnerships is the change in outreach methods used by Arkansas Medicaid to serve residents in need of LTC services. Prior to the CCP, residents in need of LTC primarily learned about LTC services by contacting service providers or state agencies. There was no direct LTC service outreach in the community. The COPH evaluated the TCRHN's CCP three-county demonstration which used CHWs to canvas communities, identify elderly and adults with disabilities in need of LTC services, and then link them to services, particularly those available in the home or community. The evaluation showed the CCP generated a $2.92 savings to the Medicaid program for every $1 invested by reducing the use of institutional care and increasing the use of home and community-based LTC (32,34). These findings led Arkansas Medicaid to expand the program into 15 counties.

The capacity of UAMS, the COPH and the community partners has been enhanced due to these partnerships. In 2009, UAMS received NIH funding to establish a Translational Research Institute (TRI). COPH faculty play important roles in the TRI core units, particularly, the Community Engagement Component. The OCBPH and community partners have helped identify community priorities, serving on the TRI's Community Advisory Board, and in obtaining additional NIH funding to build community capacity for CBPR by adapting the CCP model to increase minority participation in research. The COPH has also benefited from its community partnerships through CDC funding received in 2009 to establish the APRC, which focuses on using CBPR to reduce disparities in chronic disease. The COPH's underlying CBPH philosophy and experience with community partners guided the development of the ARPC's organizational structure, which is unique among PRCs across the US in having both community and academic Center Deputy Directors and community and academic Co-Directors for core units. Community Co-Directors are paid a stipend for carrying out their leadership roles. The APRC will be providing workshops to increase academic and community capacity to conduct CBPR. It also provides a rich community-based service learning environment for COPH doctoral students.

Community partners have increased their knowledge of CBPR and the research process through partnership with the COPH. Community and academic representatives involved in the USDA NIRI agreed that community members involved would benefit from knowing more about the research process and research ethics. The USDA retained the OCBPH to develop a workshop, which they did with input from community partners, who helped ensure the workshop content was appropriate and formatted in a way to be most accessible to community members (35). The evaluation of the workshop showed a positive trend in improvements in CBPR-related attitudes and behavior (36).

Students and partners have also increased their understanding of racial and ethnic health disparities through participation as Shepherd Poverty Center and UA Clinton School of Public Service interns, and through the Arkansas Health Disparities Service Learning Collaborative. This collaborative was developed as a result of participation in the Engaged Institutions Initiative (described above), which supported development and implementation of an interdisciplinary Masters-level service learning course on racial and ethnic health and healthcare disparities, with an emphasis on historical and social determinants and strategies for elimination, combined with community-based practice and reflection (37). In addition, community partners assisted in piloting a community-based workshop for individuals and CBOs to increase awareness about the social determinants of health and racial health disparities; to increase community action with respect to health disparities; and to increase community understanding and participation as service learning sites for students. This workshop prompted a Little Rock-based CBO, in partnership with residents of a low-income neighborhood, to establish a Healthy Communities initiative, which focuses on community gardening, healthy eating, energy efficient housing, the role of community ecosystems in sustainability, and environmental justice.

Health and Disparities Outcomes

Quantitative data are not available to determine whether these partnerships have led to improved health outcomes. However, several of the partnership programs are clearly affecting process measures associated with better outcomes such as improved access to home and community-based LTC services (TCRHN's CCP) and increased access to prescription medications (MDCC's PAP). MDCC's PAP has helped 9,228 Delta residents access free or low-cost prescription medications, saving them a total of $5 million in prescription medication costs for drugs needed largely to manage chronic diseases such as diabetes, high cholesterol, and hypertension. These programs are likely affecting racial and economic disparities in access as well, since those experiencing these disparities are targeted.

Table 2 summarizes partner involvement in various activities to illustrate the long-term, collaborative nature of the partnerships.

Changes in context

University capacity and readiness

Another important feature of the model is its allowance for outcomes to loop back around to affect context. The experiences of these partnerships has affected the capacity of both community and university partners to engage in research. This is exhibited by successes of these partnerships and by the role community partners are playing in building the capacity of newer COPH community partners.

The University context has also been affected as the COPH has increased its capacity and understanding of issues related to diversity and health disparities and played a key role in the UAMS Racial and Ethnic Health Disparities Taskforce.

The UAMS Center for Diversity Affairs (CDA) was recently re-organized with promotion of its director to Assistant Vice-Chancellor and giving it a cross-campus purview.

The University also has a new Chancellor who supports centralized coordination through the CDA of campus diversity efforts (including those of the Taskforce) and implementation of an audit to better define and create momentum to address these issues.

CONCLUSION

This partnership "story" illuminates several important lessons for the development and maintenance of academic-community partners.

First, both academic and community partners need capacity building to engage in CBPR work. Both "sides" of the partnership, particularly the academics, may perceive themselves as being adequately knowledgeable of pressing public health problems and methods to address them. However, the experience of these partnerships reveals that all participants benefited from shared experiences and learning opportunities that were important for establishing a common base of experience and expectations as well as establishing a common language for discussing difficult issues.

Second, the development of a small core group of academics and community partners interested in CBPR was important for expanding its adoption more widely, both in the academic institution and in the community.

Consistent with notions of Diffusion Theory (38), early adopters of CBPR were able to share their experience and knowledge which led to others at UAMS choosing to use this approach to research.

Finally, continuing to engage in individual and joint capacity building activities, even when there was no active CBPR project, enabled the partners to be poised to leverage past work and take advantage of emerging opportunities.

Many CBPR partnerships may come together around a specific study and disband when the study ends. However, by continuing a strong bi-directional relationship, even in the absence of a current CBPR study, these partners were able to rapidly respond to new challenges and funding announcements.

Table 2. Summary of Activities, Programs, and Centers, and Partners Involved

Activities, Programs, and Centers	Timeframe	UAMS[a]	COPH[b]	OCBPH	MDCC	BGACDC	TCRHN
				Partners Involved			
Trip to UNC and UM	2001		X		X	X	
MDCC Arkansas Delta Rural Development Network	2001-present	X	X	X	X	X	X
OCBPH established	2002		X	X	X	X	X
TCRHN Community Connector Program	2003- present		X	X	X	X	X
Undoing Racism Workshops	2003-2007	X	X	X	X	X	X
Deliberative Community Forums	2003-present		X	X	X	X	X
MDCC AmeriCorps/ Prescription Assistance Program	2004-present		X	X	X	X	X
UAMS Health Disparities Taskforce	2004-present	X	X	X	X	X	X
Co-Teaching	2005-present		X	X	X	X	X
Shepherd Poverty Center and UA Clinton School Interns	2005-present			X	X	X	X
USDA NIRI Community Research Workshops	2006-2008		X	X	X	X	X
WK Kellogg Engaged Institutions Initiative	2006-2007	X	X	X	X	X	X
WK Kellogg Rural People / Rural Policy Initiative	2006-2010			X		X	X
CNCS/CCPH AR Health Disparities Service Learning Collaborative	2007-2010		X	X	X	X	X
Unnatural Causes Screenings	2008-present	X	X	X	X	X	X
AR Prevention Research Center	2009-present		X	X	X		X
Translation Research Institute	2009-present	X	X	X	X	X	X
Arkansas Delta Green Expo	2010		X	X	X	X	X
Community Linked Research Infrastructure	2010-present	X	X	X		X	X

[a] UAMS is selected if entities other than the COPH have been involved.
[b] COPH is selected if other than OCBPH faculty/staff have been involved.

ACKNOWLEDGMENTS

Support was provided in part by the University of Arkansas for Medical Sciences Translational Research Institute (TRI) (National Center for Research Resources Award No. 1UL1RR029884) and TRI career development award (KL2RR029883).

The content is solely the responsibility of the authors and does not necessarily represent the official views of the National Center for Research Resources or the National Institutes of Health. Support for the Community Connector Program was provided by the Robert Wood Johnson Foundation, the Enterprise Corporation of the Delta, the Arkansas Department of Human Services, the Foundation for the Mid-South, and the MDCC. MDCC is supported by the Health Resources and Services Administration.

REFERENCES

[1]   Barker D. The Scholarship of Engagement: A Taxonomy of Five Emerging Practices. [J Higher Educ Outreach Engage] 2004;9(2):123-37.

[2]   Israel BA, Schulz AJ, Parker EA, Becker AB, Community-Campus Partnerships for Health. Community-based participatory research: policy recommendations for promoting a partnership approach in health research. [Educ Health] (Abingdon) 2001;14(2):182-97.

[3]   Scutchfield FD, Ireson C, Hall L. The voice of the public in public health policy and planning: the role of public judgment. [J Public Health Policy] 2004;25(2):197-205; discussion 206-10.

[4]   Downey LH, Anyaegbunam C, Scutchfield FD. Dialogue to deliberation: expanding the empowerment education model. [Am J Health Behav] 2009;33(1):26-36.

[5]   Farquhar SA, Wing S. Methodological and ethical considerations in community-driven environmental jJustice research: Two case studies from rural North Carolina. In: Minkler M, Wallerstein N, eds. Community-based participatory research for health, 2nd ed. San Francisco: Jossey Bass, 2008:263-83.

[6]   Tau Lee P, Krause N, Goetchius C, Agriesti JM, Baker R. Participatory action research with hotel room cleaners in San Francisco and Las Vegas: From collaborative study to the bargaining table. In: Minkler M, Wallerstein N, eds. Community-based participatory research for health, 2nd ed. San Francisco: Jossey Bass, 2008:335-53.

[7]   Wallerstein N, Duran B. Community-based participatory research contributions to intervention research: the intersection of science and practice to improve health equity. [Am J Public Health] 2010;100(Suppl 1):S40-6.

[8]   Ahmed SM, Palermo AG. Community engagement in research: frameworks for education and peer review. [Am J Public Health] 2010;100(8):1380-1387.

[9]   Wallerstein N, Oetzel J, Duran B, Tafoya G, Belone L, Rae R. What predicts outcomes in CBPR? In: Minkler M, Wallerstein N, eds. Community-based participatory research for health, 2nd ed. San Francisco: Jossey Bass, 2008:371-88.

[10]   Community-Based Public Health Caucus. CBPH Caucus Vision Statement. Available at: http://www.sph.umich.edu/cbphcaucus/vision.html#. Accessed 11/13, 2010.

[11]   Felix H, Stewart MK, Raczynski JM, Bruce TA. From the schools of public health. Building a college of public health: structuring policies to promote community-based public health. [Public Health Rep] 2004;119(2):225-227.

[12]   University of Arkansas for Medical Sciences. Website. Available at: http://www.uamshealth.com/why-uams/. Accessed 9/1, 2010.

[13]   Thompson JW, Boozman FW, Tyson S, Ryan KW, McCarthy S, Scott R, et al. Improving health with tobacco dollars from the MSA: the Arkansas experience. Health Aff (Millwood) 2004;23(1):177-85.

[14]   Bruce TA, McKane SU eds. Community-based public health: A partnership model. Washington DC: American Public Health Association, 2000.

[15]   Minkler M, Wallerstein N, eds. Community-based participatory research for health, 2nd ed. San Francisco: Jossey Bass, 2008.

[16]   Smedley BD, Stith AY, Nelson AR. Unequal treatment: Confronting racial and ethnic disparities in health care. Washington, DC: Natl Acad Press, 2003.

[17]   LaVeist TA, ed. Race, ethnicity, and health. A public health reader. San Francisco: Jossey-Bass, 2002.

[18]   Link BG, Phelan J. Social conditions as fundamental causes of disease. [J Health Soc Behav] 1995;Spec No:80-94.

[19]   The Peoples' Institute for Survival and Beyond. Undoing Racism Community Organizing Workshops. Available at: http://www.pisab.org/. Accessed 2/12/12.

[20]   Aronson RE, Yonas MA, Jones N, Coad NE, E. Undoing racism training as a foundation for team building in CBPR. In: Minkler M, Wallerstein N, eds. Community-based participatory research for health, 2nd ed. San Francisco: Jossey Bass, 2008:447-51.

[21]   Arkansas Citizens First Congress. Arkansas Citizens First Congress homepage. Available at: http://citizensfirst.org/about-us. Accessed 10/20, 2010.

[22]   United States Department of Agriculture, Agricultural Research Service. Delta Obesity Prevention Research Program. Available at: http://www.ars.usda.gov/research/projects/p rojects.htm? accn_no=413503. Accessed 11/13, 2010.

[23]   Felix HC, Stewart MK, Mays GP, Cottoms N, Olson MK, Sanderson H. Linking residents to long-term care services: first-year findings from the community connector program evaluation. [Prog Community Health Partnersh] 2007;1(4):311-9.

[24]   Nash C, Ochoa E. Arkansas racial and ethnic health disparity study report. Little Rock, AR: Arkansas Minority Health Commission, 2004.

[25]   The Sullivan Commission. Missing persons: Minorities in the health professions. A report of the Sullivan Commission on Diversity in the Healthcare Workforce. Sullivan Commission, 2004.

[26]   McKnight JL. Rationale for a community approach to health. In: Bruce TA, McKane US, eds. Improvement community-based public health: A partnership model. Washington, DC: American Public Health Association, 2000:13-8.

[27]   Hotez PJ. Neglected infections of poverty in the United States of America. [PLoS Negl Trop Dis] 2008;2(6):e256.

[28]   Privilege Walk, from Teaching for Diversity and Social Justice Available at: http://www. life.arizona.edu/residentassistants/programming/social_justice/PRIVILEGE_WALK.pdf.   Accessed 12/18, 2010.

[29]   California Newsreel I. California Newsreel, Inc. Unnatural Causes: Is Inequality Making us Sick? Available at: http://www.unnaturalcauses.org/. Accessed 12/18, 2010.

[30]   Delta Bridge Project. Available at: http://deltabridgeproject.com. Accessed 10/31, 2010.

[31]   Mays GP, Felix HC. Economic evaluation of the Arkansas Community Connector Program: Final report of findings from the Demonstration and Extension Periods. Little Rock, AR: Arkansas Department Human Services, 2009.

[32]   Felix HC, Mays GP, Stewart MK, Cottoms N, Olson M. Medicaid savings resulted when community health workers matched those with needs to home and community care. [Health Affairs] 2011;30(7):1366.

[33]   Clayton PH, Bringle RG, Senor B, Huq J, Morrison M. Differentiating and assessing relationships in service-learning and civic engagement: Exploitative, transactional, or transformational. [Michigan J Commun Serv Learning] 2010;16(2):5-22.

[34]   Using Community Health Workers to Target Home and Community-Based Long-Term Care: A Propensity Score Analysis of Economic Impact. Oral Presentation at the 2010 Annual Meeting of Academy Health, Boston, MA; 2010.

[35]   Stewart MK, Colley D, Huff A. Participatory Development and Implementation of a Community Research Workshop: Experiences from a community-based participatory research partnership. [Commun Health Partnerships] 2009;3(2):165-178.

[36]   Stewart MK, Colley D, Felix H, Huff A, Shelby B, Strickland E, et al. Evaluation of a workshop to improve community involvement in community-based participatory research efforts. [Educ Health] 2009;22(3).

[37]   Development and Early Experience with a Masters Level Public Health Service Learning Course on Racial and Ethnic Health Disparities. Oral Presentation at the 2010 Annual Conference of Community Campus Partnerships for Health, Portland, Oregon; 2010.

[38]   Rogers EM. Diffusion of innovation, 5th ed. New York: Free Press, 2003.

[39]   US Census. Available at: http://www.census.gov. Accessed 11/13, 2010.

[40]   Centers for Disease Control and Prevention. Available at: http://wonder.cdc.gov. Accessed 11/13, 2010.

Submitted: November 14, 2011. *Revised:* March 01, 2012. *Accepted:* April 21, 2012.

SECTION TWO - GLOBAL HEALTH ISSUES

In: Public Health Yearbook 2013
Editor: Joav Merrick

ISBN: 978-1-63321-095-0
© 2014 Nova Science Publishers, Inc.

Chapter 13

CHILDHOOD ASTHMA IN GEORGIA: COMPARISON AGAINST THE NATION

Hani M Samawi, PhD, James H Stephens, Gerald R Ledlow and Ren Chunfeng*

Karl E Peace Center for Biostatistics, Jiann-Ping Hsu College Public Health, Georgia Southern University, United States of America

ABSTRACT

This article investigates childhood asthma in Georgia compared with the combined data of the forty-nine states of the United States based on survey data from the National Survey of Children's Health (NSCH) (2003), provided by the Centers for Disease Control and Prevention in Hyattsville, Maryland. Several risk factors of asthma in Georgia are found to be statistically significant. The comparison with the factors between Georgia and all other states combined is performed to get insight about the problems of childhood asthma in Georgia. Preliminary logistic regression analysis revealed that race, poverty level, weight, and respiratory allergies are significant covariates for childhood asthma in Georgia. However, in the other states, besides those risk factors for Georgia, the analysis revealed that gender, medical preventive care, metropolitan statistical area location, and insurance status are also significant with regard to childhood asthma. Second-hand smoking is beyond the reach of statistical significance as a risk factor for childhood asthma in both Georgia and the combined states.

Keywords: Childhood Asthma, Logistic Regression, Pearson Chi-Square test, Mantel-Haensael Chi-Square Test Model Diagnostics, Lemeshow and Hosmer Goodness-of-fit

---

∗ Correspondence: Hani Samawi, PhD, Jiann-Ping Hsu College of Public Health, Georgia Southern University, P.O. Box 8015, Statesboro, GA 30460-8015 United States. E-mail: hsamawi@georgiasouthern.edu.

INTRODUCTION

Asthma has been defined by the National Heart, Lung and Blood Institute as a common chronic disorder of the airway. The disorder is complex and characterized by variable and recurring symptoms, airflow obstruction, bronchial hyper responsiveness (bronchospasm), and an underlying inflammation amid various acuity levels. Asthma is one of the leading causes of chronic illnesses among children and adolescents in the United States. Childhood asthma can be very disruptive, causing bothersome daily symptoms that interfere with play, sports, school and sleep. In some children, unmanaged asthma can cause serious or even life-threatening acute asthma attacks. Mayo Clinic Staff (1) stated common childhood asthma symptoms are:

- Coughing;
- A whistling or wheezing sound when exhaling;
- Shortness of breath; and
- Chest congestion or tightness.

Other signs and symptoms of asthma in children include:

- Trouble sleeping caused by shortness of breath, coughing or wheezing;
- Bouts of coughing or wheezing that get worse with a respiratory infection such as a cold or the flu;
- Delayed recovery or bronchitis after a respiratory infection; and
- Fatigue or trouble breathing during active play or exercise — signs of exercise-induced asthma.

Nationally, asthma prevalence, health service utilization, and mortality (2) have increased among children and adolescents since 1980. The CDC indicated that nationwide, asthma was the third leading cause of hospitalization among children 15 years and younger. The EPA reported that about 23 million people, including 6.8 million children, have asthma in USA. The national economic burden of asthma increased to $14.5 billion by the year 2000 (3). Similarly, a 2008 Georgia health report indicated that approximately 230,000 (10%) children in Georgia have asthma, with approximately 41,000 (11%) middle school students, and approximately 44,000 (10%) high school students. Hospitalization charges related to asthma totaled more than $124 million in 2006. More than 10,000 hospitalizations for asthma occurred in Georgia in 2006. On average, from 2001 to 2006 there were 116asthma deaths per year.

Thus, investigating factors and disparities in childhood asthma in Georgia is an important issue to public health and health care delivery organizations.

Current knowledge may not draw definitive conclusions about the causes of asthma onset. Better adherence to current recommendations for medical therapy and environmental management of asthma would decrease the burden of this disease. Although asthma is a potentially serious disease, with appropriate medical treatment and environmental measures, most asthma symptoms and associated morbidity can be prevented or managed if risk factors can be identified.

Actually, based on the literature, some possible risk factors can be associated with asthma such as metropolitan statistical area (4, 5), racial/ethnic minority populations (4, 6), gender (7), medical prevention (8, 9), insurance (10), family income (6, 11), weight (12, 13), household secondhand tobacco smoke (14, 15), respiratory allergy (4), and breastfeeding (16, 17). Besides the above variables, this project also incorporated age into the study since this variable is biologically important to the response variable.

METHODS

This study investigates childhood asthma risk factors in Georgia and compares these factors against the combined forty-nine states in the United States. The total population of Georgia in 2000 was about 8.2 million as indicated by US Department of Commerce (18) with about 2.2 million children age 17 or less (see table 1).

The National Survey of Children's Health (19), served as the database for the study. The description of the Georgia sample is provided in table 2. Table 2 shows that the majority of the sample is Caucasian/white; this may due to that fact that some of the participants did not provide information on their racial/ethnic background, and this subgroup is identified as "Unknown" in the table.

In this paper the focus is on the data that were obtained from the NSCH database, which contains information from all states. To handle and analyze the data, SAS Version 9.2 (20) was used. Several statistical techniques were used to achieve the purpose and the aims of our investigation.

Those statistical techniques, including the Pearson Chi-square test (21), was used to investigate proportional differences between Georgia (serving as the referent state) and the other states combined, involving participants who were diagnosed with asthma, versus those who were not diagnosed with asthma ($\alpha = 0.05$).

Also, odds ratios and 95% confidence limits were calculated to assess the magnitude of observed association by racial/ethnic group, age groups and the other risk factors. Finally, to control for the effect of other factors, two multivariate logistic models are used, one for Georgia and one for the other forty-nine states.

RESULTS

There were 12.84% of children in Georgia that have been advised that they had asthma by a doctor or a health professional. This is higher than 11.93% in the other combined states (see table 3). Thus, investigating the cases of asthma within the state of Georgia is important.

A cross-tabulation of childhood's asthma status by potential risk factors for Georgia and the combined other states is presented in Table 4.

Table 1. 2000 populations

State	Population-All Ages			Under 18 years			Race (Total Population)			
	Total	Male	Female	Total	Male	Female	White	Black	Hispanic	Other
Georgia	8,186,453	4,027,113	4,159340	2,169,234	1,111,589	1,057,645	5,327,281	2,349,542	435,227	74,403

Source: U.S Census Bureau 2000. Total percentage might be over 100% because some people reported more than one race or ethnicity.

Table 2. National Survey of Children's Health sample

	White		African American		Multi-Racial		Other		Unknown		TOTAL	
	♂	♀	♂	♀	♂	♀	♂	♀	♂	♀	♂	♀
GA	629	534	243	228	19	33	28	23	54	55	973	873

Legend: ♂ = Male; ♀ = Female.

The data contains mixed types of possible variables that arenominal, ordinal, and continuous. We grouped the continuous variables to transform them to categorical variables. Chi-square tests of association are first conducted to search for potential risk factors on childhood asthma in Georgia and in the other combined states (Table 4). At an alpha level of significance of 0.05, we found that age, respiratory allergy, weight level, race, and poverty level are significant factors affecting childhood asthma in Georgia. In the other states, all factors are found to be significant to asthma.

Table 4 indicates that age is a significant factor for childhood asthma without controlling for other factors. It seems that in Georgia and in the other states, the odds of getting asthma at an older age are less than for a child at a younger age.

MULTIVARIATE ANALYSIS

Multivariate analysis is used to study the effect of the significant factors found in Table 4 on childhood asthma controlling for other factors. The use of 0.25 as the criterion of screening for factors in the multivariate models is based on the work by (22) on linear regression and by (23on logistic regression.

Table 3. Frequency table for Georgia and the other states together

	Childhood Asthma		
States	No	Yes	Total
Georgia	1622 87.16%	239 12.84%	1861 100%
The other states together	88311 88.07%	11963 11.93%	100274 100%
Total	89933 88.05%	12202 11.95%	102135 100 %

Table 4. Cross-tabulation of childhood asthma with potential risk factors of Georgia and other states together

Covariates	Georgia				All States			
	DF	Chi-square test	P-value	Odds ratio	DF	Chi-square test	P-value	Odds ratio
Age group (0-5, 6-10, 11-17)	2	11.22	0.0037		2	936.08	<0.0001	
Gender (male, female)	1	2.44	0.1180	1.24	1	286.42	<0.0001	1.40
Household Smoking (Yes, No)	1	0.52	0.4717	1.12	1	69.87	<0.0001	1.20
Respiratory Allergy (Yes, No)	1	87.59	<0.0001	3.81	1	8235.50	<0.0001	5.88
Metropolitan area (Yes, No)	1	1.23	0.2682	0.85	1	4.21	0.0401	1.06
Weight groups (Overweight, Normal, underweight)	3	17.93	0.0005		3	170.48	<0.0001	
Race (White, black, Hispanic, multi-racial, other)	4	44.30	<0.0001		4	409.42	<0.0001	
Health care coverage (Yes, No)	1	0.68	0.4089	1.25	1	81.16	<0.0001	1.45
Preventive health care (Yes, No)	1	0.76	0.3829	1.26	1	12.97	0.0003	1.14
Breastfed (Yes, No)	1	2.41	0.1203	1.54	1	124.63	<0.0001	0.61
Poverty level (0-99%, 100-199%, 200-399%, 400+% FPT)	3	5.17	0.1596		3	121.90	<0.0001	

After fitting the multivariate model, the importance of each variable should be verified by first checking the individual Wald test, then log-likelihood ratio test and potential confounder checking. Variables not contributing to the model based on these criteria should be removed from the model and a new model fit. The new model should be compared to the old model using log-likelihood ratio test. This process of deleting, refitting, and verifying continues until all important variables are included in the model and the excluded variables are not either significant or biologically important to the model.

Model assumption checks of the final models are performed to check the validity of our final models (24). Before the logistic regression models for Georgia and the other states combined are used to describe the relationship between asthma and its predictors, the fit of the models should be assessed. The approach usually consists of five steps: multicollinearity diagnostics, interaction check, computation and evaluation of overall measures of fit; and graphical examination of the individual components of the summary statistics.

For Georgia data, all the interaction terms are not significant in the model. However, for the combined states data, there are 5 interaction terms significant to the model. When an explanatory variable is nearly a linear combination of other explanatory variables in the model, the estimates of the coefficients in the regression model are unstable and have high standard errors. This problem is called collinearity.

The Collinearity Diagnostics table is calculated using the Eigen structure of the X'X matrix. A collinearity problem exists when a component associated with a high condition index contributes strongly to the variance of two or more variables. Belsley, et al. (25) proposed that a condition index of 30 to 100 indicates moderate to strong collinearity. The highest condition number is 15.24 which appear not to support multicollinearity. However, for the other states together, the largest condition index is 57.02 (19.01 for the model without any interaction term), which seems high multicollinearity does exist. After we removed several interaction terms, the highest condition index was 22.29.

Hosmer-Lemeshow Tests are usually used to evaluate overall measures of fit. The value of Lemeshow and Hosmer about goodness-of-fit test statistic computed is 8.88 for Georgia data. The corresponding p-value is 0.3528, indicating the model seems to fit quite well for Georgia data.

Similarly, the value of Lemeshow and Hosmer about goodness-of-fit test statistic computed is 12.83 for the other states together data. The corresponding p-value is 0.1177, indicating the model seems to fit well for the other states together data.

The index plots are useful to identify extreme values. The index plots of the Pearson residuals and the deviance residuals for Georgia indicate that no cases are poorly accounted for by the model. The index plot of the diagonal elements of the hat matrix for Georgia indicates that there are some extreme cases in the data. After removing these observations, the largest coefficient rate change is 94.2%. Thus, from statistical analysis perspective, these observations cannot be removed from the model.

For the combined states, 3 cases are found to be extreme. However, after removing these observations, the largest coefficient rate change is less than 5%. Thus, we can conclude that there are no potential outliers in the other states together model.

CONCLUSION AND FINAL REMARKS

Using univariate analysis for Georgia data, we found that age, respiratory allergy, poverty level, weight level, and race were all factors affecting childhood asthma with 95% odds ratio confidence intervals (0.939, 0.988), (2.84, 5.12), (1.011,1.324), (1.154,1.560), (1.667,2.977) (White versus Black), (1.078, 3.883) (other versus Black), respectively. Similarly, for the combined states, we found that in addition to the five variables listed above, second-hand smoking, metropolitan statistical area location, medical preventive care, and insurance status are all significant factors associated with childhood asthma.

The final model for Georgia (table 5) revealed that when other independent variables are controlled, one year increase in age has no significant effect on childhood asthma. From one weight level to another weight level (underweight, normal weight, at risk for overweight, and overweight), the odds of children overweight are higher than the odds of lower weight children to develop an asthma. The odds for blacks to develop asthma is 2.41 (1.679, 3.457) times higher than for whites and 5.58 (1.69, 18.86) times more than other groups. There are no significant differences on asthma based on poverty level. Moreover, the odds of children with respiratory allergy are 4.413 (3.122, 6.229) times higher than children without respiratory allergies to develop asthma.

For the combined states (Table 6), controlling for the other variables in the model, a one year increase in age didn't result in a significant effect on asthma. Similar to the result of Georgia, from one weight level to another weight level (underweight, normal weight, at risk for overweight, and overweight), the odds of overweight children is higher than the odds of lower weight children to develop asthma. Moving from one poverty level to another (0-99% FPL,100-199% FPL, 200-399% FPL, and 400% FPL or greater), the odds of poorer children to acquire asthma is higher than those with better income. The odds for Blacks are 1.555 (1.432,1.687) times higher than Whites to develop asthma and 1.19 (1.05, 1.36) times higher than others to develop asthma. The odds for children living in metropolitan statistical areas are 1.161 (1.087,1.241) times higher than those not living in metropolitan statistical areas to develop asthma. Medical preventive care and insurance status are also statistically significant to childhood asthma, whose 95% confidence intervals of odds ratios (No versus Yes) were (0.718, 0.868) and (0.713, 0.932), respectively.

Gender and respiratory allergies were difficult to interpret since there is significant interaction terms expressed in the models. In short, when the other variables were controlled, age was not significantly associated with childhood asthma in both Georgia and the combined states.

In Georgia, race, weight, and respiratory allergies are risk factors for childhood asthma while poverty level is barely significant in the model. However, in the combined states, besides those risk factors, gender, metropolitan statistical area, and poverty level are also found to be risk factors for childhood asthma. Medical preventive care and insurance status were negatively associated with childhood asthma. Compared with the combined states, Georgia had less risk factors associated with childhood asthma; also, there are no significant differences for race.

Table 5. Final model for Georgia (after removing some observations)

Parameter	Estimate	Standard Error	Wald Chi-Square	Odds Ratio		Pr > ChiSq
				Point estimate	95% CI	
Age groups (0-5, 6-10, 11-17)	0.0197	0.0186	1.1162	1.020	(0.983,1.058)	0.4410
Weight level (Underweight, normal, at risk of overweight, overweight)	0.3083	0.0920	11.2168	1.361	(1.136,1.630)	0.0024
RACER (black vs other)	-1.7377	0.6164	7.9487	0.176	(0.053, 0.589)	0.0028
RACER (black vs white)	-0.8793	0.1843	22.7711	0.415	(0.289,0.596)	<.0001
Poverty level (0-99%, 100-199%, 200-399, 400+% FPT)	-0.1027	0.0867	1.4043	0.902	(0.761,1.069)	0.2375
Respiratory Allergy (Yes, No)	1.4845	0.1759	71.2233	4.413	(3.126,6.229)	<.0001

Table 6. Final model for the other states together

Factors	Estimate	Standard Error	Odds ratio Point Estimate*	95% CI
Age groups (0-5, 6-10, 11-17)	0.00840	0.0101	1.008	(0.989,1.029)
Gender	-0.6724	0.0751	1.234	(0.865,1.258)
(Male, female)			1.043	(0.992,1.097)
Respiratory allergy (Yes, no)	-1.9019	0.0751	0.905	(0.986,1.104)
			1.043	(0.992,1.097
Weight level (Underweight, normal, at risk of overweight, overweight)	0.1489	0.0163	1.121	(1.124,1.198)
Poverty level (0-99%, 100-199%, 200-399, 400+% FPT)	-0.1484	0.0157	0.862	(0.836,0.889)
Insurance (yes, no)	-0.2045	0.0685	0.815	(0.713,0.932)
RACER (black vs white)	0.4412	0.0418	1.555	(1.432,1.687)
Others vs white)	0.2631	0.0555	1.301	(1.167,1.451)
Preventative Medical Care (yes, no)	-0.2364	0.0481	0.789	(0.718,0.868)
Metropolitan Statistical Area	0.1497	0.0339	1.161	(1.087,1.241)
Interaction (age*respiratory allergy)	0.0336	0.00647		
Interaction (age*gender)	-0.0284	0.00653		

*The point estimate of odds ratio for each group of gender and respiratory allergy represents when age changes in 5 years and the other covariates are fixed.

The data in this project is a representative sample based on the National Children Health Survey (NCHS) 2003. Two logistic models were developed to draw meaningful conclusions and comparisons on the basis of purposeful logistic model selection. Insurance status and medical preventive care are negatively associated with asthma. Further analysis should be implemented based on the NCHS 2007 survey data to verify this result. If the response variable is "currently, does your child have asthma?" instead of "in the past 12 months, has your child ever been told they have asthma", different results may be found. However, this study agrees with prior findings in the literature.

ACKNOWLEDGMENTS

We are grateful to the Center for Child and Adolescent Health for providing us with the 2003 National Survey of Children's Health. Also, we would like to thank the referees and the associate editor for their valuable comments which improved the manuscript.

REFERENCES

[1] Mayo Clinic Staff. Childhood asthma. Accessed 2009May 5. URL:http://www.mayoclinic.com/health/childhood-asthma/DS00849/DSECTION=symptoms

[2]   Gergen PJ. The increasing problem of asthma in the United States. [Am Rev Respir Dis] 1992;146:823-4.

[3]   Jack E, Boss L, Millington WA. Speakers kit for public health professionals. Atlanta, GA: Centers Disease Control Prevention, 1999.

[4]   Noreen MC, Randall WB, Edith PL. Childhood asthma. [Environl Health Perspect] 1999;107:421-9.

[5]   Floyd JM, Sheryl AF. Environmental risk factors of childhood asthma in urban centers. [Environ Health Perspect] 1995;103(Suppl6):58-62.

[6]   Lauren AS, Juliet LH, Richard W, Robert SK. Rethinking race/ethnicity, income, and childhood asthma: Racial/ethnic disparities concentrated among the very poor. [Public Health Rep] 2005;120:109-20.

[7]   Bernard A, Carbonnelle S, Burbure CD. Chlorinated pool attendance, atopy, and the risk of asthma during childhood. [Environ Health Perspect] 2006;114(10):1567-73.

[8]   Shahani AK, Korve N, Jones KP, Paynton DJ. Towards an operational model for prevention and treatment of asthma attacks. [J Operation Res Soc] 1994;45(8):916-26.

[9]   Yates CE. Prevention and treatment of asthma. Dissertation. Southhampton: Faculty Math Stud, Univ Southampton, 1989.

[10]   Yu C, Martin JB. Helicobacter pylori colonization is inversely associated with childhood asthma. [J Infect Dis] 2008;198:553-60.

[11]   Miller JE. The effects of race/ethnicity and income on early childhood asthma prevalence and health care use. [Am J Public Health] 2000;90:428-30.

[12]   Schachtera LM, Salomea CM, Peatb JK. Obesity is a risk for asthma and wheeze but not airway hyper responsiveness. [Thorax]2001;56:4-8.

[13]   Tim JT, Sutherland JOC, Sarah Y. The association between obesity and asthma-interactions between systemic and airway inflammation. [Am J RespirCrit Care Med] 2008;178:469-75.

[14]   Gilliland FD, Li YF, Peters JM. Effects of maternal smoking during pregnancy and environmental tobacco smoke on asthma and wheezing in children. [Am J RespirCrit Care Med] 2001;163(2):429-36.

[15]   Sturm JJ, Yeatts K, Loomis D. Effects of tobacco smoke exposure on asthma prevalence and medical care use in North Carolina middle school children. [Am J Public Health] 2004;94(2):308-13.

[16]   Yousuke T, Yutaka S, Satoshi H. Relation between breastfeeding and the prevalence of asthma. [Am J Epidemiol] 2001;154(2):115-9.

[17]   Raisler J, Alexander C, O'Campo P. Breast-feeding and infant illness: A dose- response relationship? [Am J Public Health] 1999;89:25–30.

[18]   US Department of Commerce. United States Census: 2000 census of population and housing. Washington, DC: US Department of Commerce. Accessed 2009 Jul 09. URL: http://www.census.gov/prod/cen2000/index.html.

[19]   Child and Adolescent Health Measurement Initiative 2003. National survey of children with special health care needs: Indicator dataset 6. Data Resource Center for Child and Adoles-cent Health website. Accessed 2009 Jul 9. URL: www.childhealthdata.org.

[20]   SAS Institute. SAS/STAT Version 9.1. Cary, NC: SAS Institute, 2010.

[21]   Agresti A. Categorical data analysis. New York: John Wiley, 1990.

[22]   Bendel, RB, Afifi, AA. Comparison of stopping rules in forward regression. [J Am Statistical Assoc] 1977;72:46-53.

[23]   Mickey J, Greenland S. The impact of confounder selection criteria on effect estimation. [Am J Epidemiol] 1989;129:125-37.

[24]   Hosmer DW, Lemeshow S. Applied logistic regression. New York: John Wiley, 1989.

[25]   Belsley DA, Kuh E, Welsch RE. Regression diagnostics. New York: John Wiley, 1980.

Submitted: August 20, 2011.*Revised:* October 15, 2011.*Accepted:*October 24, 2011.

In: Public Health Yearbook 2013   ISBN: 978-1-63321-095-0
Editor: Joav Merrick   © 2014 Nova Science Publishers, Inc.

Chapter 14

FORCED SEX AMONG FEMALE ADULTS IN ZAMBIA: RESULTS FROM THE ZAMBIAN SEXUAL BEHAVIOURAL SURVEY, 2009

Seter Siziya, BA (Ed), MSc, PhD[1]*,
Adamson S Muula, MBBS, MPH, PhD[2],
Aseel Mansour, BSc, MSc[3],
Emmanuel Rudatsikira, MD, MPH, DrPH[3],
Selestine H Nzala, MBChB, MPH[4],
Cosmas Zyaambo, MBChB, MPhil[4],
Peter Songolo, MBChB, MPH[5]
and Olusegun Babaniyi, MBBS, MPH, MSc[5]

[1]Department of Clinical Sciences, Public Health Unit, The Copperbelt University, School of Medicine, Ndola, Zambia
[2]Department of Community Health, University of Malawi, College of Medicine, Blantyre, Malawi
[3]School of Community and Environmental Health, Old Dominion University, Virginia, United States
[4]Department of Community Medicine, School of Medicine, University of Zambia, Lusaka, Zambia
[5]World Health Organization Country Office, Lusaka, Zambia

ABSTRACT

There is growing interest in the study of prevalence and experience of forced sexual intercourse (forced sex), because it is human rights violation with severe physical and

---

* Correspondence: Professor Seter Siziya, BA (Ed), MSc, PhD, The Copperbelt University, School of Medicine, Department of Clinical Sciences, Public Health Unit, Box 71191, Ndola, Zambia. E-mail: ssiziya@gmail.com.

psychosocial consequences. The literature on forced sex in southern Africa suggests this could be an important driver of HIV infection in the region. The objectives of the study were to estimate the prevalence and correlates of self-reported history of forced sex among females aged 15-49 years participating in the Zambian Sexual Behavioural Survey of 2009. We used logistic regression to identify correlates of forced sex victimization. Of the 2270 study participants, the majority was from 15 to 35 years age group (56.3%), married (81.4%) and with primary level of education (60.2%). The prevalence of self-reported history of forced sex was 27.8%. Factors associated with history of forced sex were: alcohol use (AOR=1.58, 95%CI [1.06, 2.36]); being employed (AOR=1.43, 95%CI [1.03, 1.99]); younger age (AOR=3.12, 95%CI [1.49, 6.48] for 15-30 years and AOR=2.94, 95%CI [1.41, 6.15] for 31-45 years); sexual debut at less than 21 years old (AOR=1.96, 95%CI [1.33, 2.91]; number of sex partners (AOR=0.13, 95%CI [0.03, 0.57]; and age of sex partner at first sexual intercourse (AOR=0.49, 95%CI [0.29, 0.82]). History of forced sex among Zambian women was common. There is need for concerted effort to address this major public health problem.

Keywords: Sexual violence, prevalence, correlates, females, Zambia

INTRODUCTION

There is growing recognition of sexual violence (within or outside marriage) as a major public health problem as well as a serious human rights issue (1).

Sexual violence such as forced sexual intercourse (forced sex) is associated with multiple reproductive and sexual health risks (2-5) and other adverse effects such as suicidality (6). In a Nepalese study women described backache, headache, lower abdominal pain, vaginal bleeding and thoughts of suicide as negative physical and psychological health consequences following forced sex within marriage (7).

Other gynaecological and reproductive health problems associated with forced sex include transmission of HIV and other sexually transmitted infections (STIs), unwanted pregnancy, infection, decreased sexual desire, genital irritation, pain during sexual intercourse, chronic pelvic pain, and urinary tract infections (8-11).

In a study conducted at alcohol serving venues in South Africa, Sikkema et al., (12) reported that post-traumatic stress disorders and depression were associated with history of forced sex.

In Botswana, Tsai et al., (13) reported that the problem of heavy drinking was associated with forced sex victimization among women. Pettifor et al., (14) have reported the association between forced sex and non-use of condoms among young people in South Africa, thus potentially exposing the victims to sexually transmitted diseases and unwanted pregnancies. Chigbu et al., (15) reported that a culture of male dominance was responsible for forced sex in women.

Forced sex has been reported at sexual debut among unmarried adolescents in India (16).

In a qualitative study from Uganda, Hayer (17) reported that young women narrowly defined forced sex as only rape while excluding other forms of forced sex. It was also reported that overall, respondents were tolerant of sexual coercion, and, in some cases perceived that the occurrence was justified. Thus, an estimate for the true prevalence of forced sex may be an underestimate of the true magnitude of the problem.

The objective of this study was to contribute to the literature from a population-based survey on sexual behaviours and forced sex experiences in southern Africa, the 'epicentre' of HIV and AIDS. Data from Zambia were used to achieve this aim. First, we estimated the prevalence of self-reported history of forced sex among females. Second, we examined the variables that may be associated with history of self-reported forced sex.

METHODS

Data were obtained from the Zambian Sexual Behavioural Survey of 2009. This was a national survey which was designed to produce nationally representative estimates stratified by residence (urban/rural) and sex. The sample size was 2500 households from 100 clusters in which all females aged 15-49 years and males aged 15-59 years were eligible to participate in the survey. However, we only used data for females because no male reported having ever experienced forced sex. A Standard Enumeration Area (SEA) was considered a cluster.

DATA COLLECTION

This was a questionnaire survey study. The questionnaires were translated into the seven major languages spoken in Zambia: Bemba, Nyanja, Tonga, Lozi, Lunda, Luvale and Kaonde. Data were collected using a household and an individual questionnaire. The information that was sought included: age, marital status, education, employment, residence (rural/urban), religion, AIDS test, alcohol consumption, sexual behaviour, condom use and forced sex. The question on forced sex was: have you ever been forced by a man to have sexual intercourse with the following options for answers: 1 was considered yes and 0, otherwise.

DATA ANALYSIS

We conducted a descriptive analysis to understand the socio-demographic characteristics of the sample. Also, logistic regression analysis was done to evaluate the relationship between forced sex (outcome) and explanatory variables. Unadjusted odds ratios (OR) from bivariate analyses and adjusted odds ratios (AOR) from a multivariate analysis are reported together with their 95% confidence intervals (CI).

RESULTS

Altogether, 2270 females participated in the survey. The majority of the respondents were in the 15-35 years age group (56.3%), married (81.4%), of primary level of education (60.2%) and were not employed (61.8%). Further description of the sample is shown in Table 1.

About a quarter (27.8%) of the respondents reported having had forced sex. Table 2 shows factors associated with forced sex. Factors associated with forced sex at bivariate analyses were: age, alcohol use, age at first sexual intercourse, schooling, age of sex partner at first sexual intercourse and number of sex partners.

In multivariate analysis, all the factors that were significantly associated with forced sex at bivariate analyses remained significant, except for the factor "schooling" that was no longer significant in the multivariate analysis. The factor "working" became significant in the multivariate analysis, although it was not significant in a bivariate analysis. The factor "age when first married/lived with sex partner" was not associated with forced sex at both bivariate and multivariate analyses.

Table 1. Socio-demographic characteristics of female study participants in the Zambia Sexual Behavioral Survey 2009

Characteristic	Frequency* (%)
Age	
15 – 30	1277 (56.3)
31 – 45	706 (31.1)
>45	287 (12.6)
Marital Status	
Married	1392 (81.4)
Single	319 (18.6)
Education	
Primary	1214 (60.2)
Secondary	695 (34.5)
Higher	106 (5.3)
Working	
Yes	862 (38.2)
No	1393 (61.8)
Centrality	
Lusaka City	213 (9.4)
Ndola City	79 (3.5)
Kitwe City	121 (5.3)
50 km of Lusaka, Ndola, Kitwe	16 (0.7)
Provincial Capital	117 (5.2)
30 km southern to Copperbelt line of rail	39 (1.7)
30 km along northern line of rail	17 (0.7)
30 km of provincial Capitals	214 (9.4)
District centres	347 (15.3)
30 km of district centres	223 (9.8)
Remote areas	884 (38.9)
Resident	
Rural	1402 (61.8)
Urban	868 (38.2)
Religion	
Catholic	409 (18.2)
Protestant	1842 (81.8)
AIDS Test	
Yes	1249 (55.0)
No	1021 (45.0)

Frequencies* may not add up due to missing information.

Compared to respondents who were aged more than 45 years, respondents who were of age 45 years or younger were more likely to have forced sex (AOR=3.12, 95%CI [1.49, 6.48] for 15-30 years, and AOR=2.94, 95%CI [1.41, 6.15] for 31-45 years). Respondents who consumed alcohol were 58% (AOR=1.58, 95%CI [1.06, 2.36]) more likely to have forced sex. Compared to respondents who were aged more than 45 years, those who were aged less than 21 years at sexual debut were 96% (AOR=1.96, 95%CI [1.33, 2.91]) more likely to have forced sex. Respondents who were employed were 43% (AOR=1.43, 95%CI [1.03, 1.99]) more likely to have forced sex compared to those who were not employed. Compared to respondents who had sex partners aged more than 45 years at first sexual intercourse, those who had sex partners of age 21-45 years at first sexual intercourse were 51% (AOR=0.49, 95%CI [0.29, 0.82]) less likely to have forced sex.

DISCUSSION

In a nationally representative survey of female adults in Zambia, the prevalence of self-reported history of forced sex was 27.8%.

Previous studies have reported prevalence rates of forced sex among African women ranging from 13.8% in Nigeria (18) to 50.7% in Sierra Leone (19).

Table 2. Associations between explanatory variables and forced sex in bivariate and multivariate logistic regression analyses in Zambia, 2009

Characteristic	OR[1]	95% CI[2]		AOR[3]	95%CI	
Age (years)						
15–30	2.81	1.69	4.63	3.12	1.49	6.48
31–45	1.98	1.17	3.35	2.94	1.41	6.15
>45	1			1		
Alcohol consumption in last 4 weeks						
Yes	1.40	1.03	1.92	1.58	1.06	2.36
No	1			1		
Age (years) when first had sexual intercourse						
< 21	2.28	1.65	3.15	1.96	1.33	2.91
21–45	1.75	0.99	3.08	1.48	0.57	3.80
>45	1			1		
Attended school						
Yes	2.00	1.22	3.28	1.70	0.94	3.05
No	1			1		
Employed						
Yes	1.21	0.93	1.56	1.43	1.03	1.99
No	1			1		
Age (years) of sex partner at first sexual intercourse						
<21	0.94	0.63	1.41	0.66	0.39	1.09
21–45	0.53	0.35	0.78	0.49	0.29	0.82
>45	1			1		

Table 2. (Continued)

Characteristic	OR[1]	95% CI[2]		AOR[3]	95%CI	
Number of sex partners						
<2	0.10	0.02	0.29	0.13	0.03	0.57
2+	1			1		
Age (years) when had first married/lived with sex partner						
<21	1.41	0.96	2.06	1.33	0.85	2.08
21+	1			1		

OR[1] unadjusted odds ratio, CI[2] Confidence Interval, AOR[3] Adjusted odds ratio.

In this study, we found that attending school was not significantly associated with forced sex contrary to the findings reported in Nigeria (18) and Tanzania (20). In a study conducted in four tertiary institutions in Nigeria, Kullima et al., (18) found that 13.8% of the respondents were sexually assaulted as a student and 7.1% were assaulted by their lecturers and fellow students. In Tanzania, Matasha et al., (20) reported that nearly half of students in primary and secondary schools had forced sex with adults including teachers and relatives.

It was found that respondents who were employed were more likely to have forced sex than those who were not employed. Sexual harassment of women in a workplace has been reported in other countries such as South Africa (21), India (22), and Turkey (23). Jewkes and Abrahams (21) reported that, in South Africa, sexual coercion is common in the workplace. In our study, however, we did not assess the circumstances or setting of reported forced sex.

In this study, we found that having taken alcohol was associated with history of forced sex. While some of the women may have experienced forced sex before alcohol intake, it is reasonable to suggest that having taken alcohol should be taken as a marker of lifestyle and personal experiences. These findings are consistent with previous reports from India by Berg et al., (24) and United States (25). Berg et al., (24) reported that alcohol use was associated with forced sex against women in Mumbai, India. In a study of perceptions and barriers when reporting forced sex among African American College female students, Amar (25) found that factors associated with reporting forced sex included violence, if they were drinking at the time.

Other factors associated with forced sex in this study include younger age and earlier age at sexual debut. Kullima et al., (18) reported that younger age at sexual debut, history of forced sexual debut, marriage, sexual debut with relations and unknown persons, significantly influenced subsequent risks of sexual assault. They suggested improved security, having a designated person on campus to handle sexual assault, and the perception of how one would be treated, and stiffer penalties against perpetrators. Prevention strategies should include education that targets significant perceptions of resources and the elimination or minimization of barriers.

Limitations of the study

Among the strengths of the current study is that data were collected as a national sample; results may therefore be generalized to the wider population of Zambia. Despite the strengths, several limitations exist. Firstly, data were self-reported and to the extent that the respondents intentionally or inadvertently mis-reported, our results may be biased. Secondly, there may be some unmeasured confounders which were not controlled for in the analysis. This study was based on survey data (cross sectional), which means that the associations that we found should be understood in that context and not as causal.

CONCLUSION

Reported history of forced sex among females is common in Zambia. Not only is the practice a violation of individual human rights and dignity, it predisposes victims to infectious diseases such as HIV/AIDS and long-term psychological sequalae. We suggest the following: enhanced community awareness of forced sex; design and implementation of multisectoral programmes aimed at prevention and control of forced sex.

ACKNOWLEDGMENTS

We thank the Central Statistical Office (Zambia) for the data collection and the respondents for contributing their time and responding to the questions in the survey.

REFERENCES

[1]   World Health Organisation. World report on violence and health. Geneva: World Health Organization, 2002.

[2]   Caceres CF, Marin BV, Hudes ES. Sexual coercion among youth and young adults in Lima, Peru. [J Adolesc Health] 2000;27:361-7.

[3]   Kishor S, Johnson M. Profiling domestic violence: a Multi-country study. Calverton, MD, USA: Macro International, 2001.

[4]   Koenig MA, Zablotska I, Lutalo T, Nalugoda F, Wagman J, Gray R. Coercive first intercourse and reproductive health among adolescent women in Rakai, Uganda. [Int Fam Plan Perspect] 2004;30:156-63.

[5]   World Health Organisation. WHO Multi-country study on women's health and domestic violence against women. Geneva: World Health Organization, 2005.

[6]   Epstein JA, Spirito A. Risk factors for suicidality among a nationally representative sample of high school students. [Suicide Life Threat Behav] 2009;39:241-51.

[7]   Puri M, Tamang J, Shah I. Suffering in silence: consequences of sexual violence within marriage among young women in Nepal. [BMC Public Health] 2011;11:29.

[8]   Garcia-Moreno C, Watts C. Violence against women: its importance for HIV/AIDS prevention. [AIDS] 2000;14(Suppl 3):S253-65.

[9]   Maman S, Campbell J, Sweat MD, Gielen AC. The intersections of HIV and violence: directions for future research and interventions. [Soc Sci Med] 2000;50:459-78.

[10] Watts C, Mayhew S. Reproductive health Services and intimate partner violence; shaping a pragmatic response in Sub-Saharan Africa. [Int Fam Plan Perspect] 2004;30:207-13.

[11] Zierler S, Feingold L, Laufer D, Velentgas P, Kantrowitz-Gordon I, Mayer K. Adult survivors of childhood sexual abuse and subsequent risk of HIV infection. [Am J Public Health] 1991;81:572-5.

[12] Sikkema KJ, Watt MH, Meade CS, Ranby KW, Kalichman SC, Skinner D, et al. Mental health and HIV sexual risk behavior among patrons of alcohol serving venues in Cape Town, South Africa. [J Acquir Immune Defic Syndr] 2011;57:230-7.

[13] Tsai A, Leiter K, Wolfe W, Heisler M. Prevalence and correlates of forced sex perpetration and victimization in Botswana and Swaziland. [Am J Public Health] 2011;101:1068-74.

[14] Pettifor A, O'brien K, MacPhail C, Miller WC, Rees H. Early coital debut and associated HIV risk factors among young women and men in South Africa. [Int Perspect Sex Reproduct Health] 2009;35:82-90.

[15] Chigbu CO, Ekweazi KE, Chigbu CC, Iwuji SE. Sexual violations among married women in southeastern Nigeria. [Int J Gynaecol Obstet] 2010;110:141-7.

[16] Santhya KG, Acharya R, Jejeebhoy SJ, Ram U. Timing of first sex before marriage and its correlates: evidence from India. [Cult Health Sex] 2011;13:327-41.

[17] Hayer MK. Perceptions of sexual coercion among young women in Uganda. [J Health Organ Manag] 2010;24:498-504.

[18] Kullima AA, Kawuwa MB, Audu BM, Mairiga AG, Bukar M. Sexual assault against female Nigerian students. [Afr J Reprod Health] 2010;14:189-93.

[19] Coker AL, Richter DL. Violence against women in Sierra Leone: frequency and correlates of intimate partner violence and forced sexual intercourse. [Afr J Reprod Health] 1998;2:61-72.

[20] Matasha E, Ntembelea T, Mayaud P, Saidi W, Todd J, Mujaya B, Tengo-Wambua L. Sexual and reproductive health among primary and secondary school pupils in Mwanza, Tanzania: need for intervention. [AIDS Care] 1998;10:571-82.

[21] Jewkes R, Abrahams N. The epidemiology of rape and sexual coercion in South Africa: an overview. [Soc Sci Med] 2002;55:1231-44.

[22] Chaudhuri P. Experiences of sexual harassment of women health workers in four hospitals in Kolkata, India. [Reprod Health Matters] 2007;15:221-9.

[23] Celik Y, Celic SS. Sexual harassment against nurses in Turkey. [J Nurs Scholarsh] 2007;39:200-6.

[24] Berg MJ, Kremelberg D, Dwivedi P, Verma S, Schensul JJ, Gupta K, Chandran D, Singh SK. The effects of husband's alcohol consumption on married women in three low-income areas of Greater Mumbai. [AIDS Behav] 2010;14(Suppl 1):S126-35.

[25] Amar AF. African-American college women's perceptions of resources and barriers when reporting forced sex. [J Natl Black Nurses Assoc] 2008;19:35-41.

Submitted: January 18, 2012. *Revised:* April 02, 2012. *Accepted:* April 21, 2012.

In: Public Health Yearbook 2013
Editor: Joav Merrick

ISBN: 978-1-63321-095-0
© 2014 Nova Science Publishers, Inc.

Chapter 15

THE SOCIAL AND ECONOMIC PATTERNING OF SLEEPING PILL USE AMONG WORKING AGE CANADIANS: IDENTIFYING VULNERABLE SUBGROUPS

*William H Laverty[1], Ivan W Kelly[*2] and Bonnie L Janzen[3]*

[1]Department of Mathematics and Statistics, University of Saskatchewan, Saskatoon, Canada
[2]Department of Educational Psychology and Special Education, University of Saskatchewan, Saskatoon, Canada
[3]Department of Community Health and Epidemiology, University of Saskatchewan, Saskatoon, Canada

ABSTRACT

While previous research has indicated the prevalence of both sleep problems and sleeping pill usage increases with age, and that women use more sleeping medicines than men, this research has focused on single variable (main effect) analyses and ignored how various factors may interact together to influence sleeping medicine usage. Our results have uncovered subgroups of men (and women) that use sleep medicine in far greater proportions over what has been previously reported in research.

Keywords: Sleep, male, demographic variables, social variables

INTRODUCTION

The use of sleeping pills (hypnotics) is widespread in Western populations, with estimates of their use close to 10% overall, with larger percentages of usage in older populations. Most research on sleeping pill use has therefore focused on the elderly (1-3). This widespread

*Correspondence: Ivan Kelly, Department of Educational Psychology and Special Education, College of Education, University of Saskatchewan, 28 Campus Drive, Saskatoon, Saskatchewan, Canada, S7N 0X1. E-mail: ivan.kelly@usask.ca.

usage of sleeping pills has recently been of concern to health professionals with research indicating long-term health side-effects, including increased cancer rates and mortality in users (4-6).

Relatively little is known about sleeping pill use among working age Canadians, despite the growing literature pointing to sleep difficulties in this group and the economic and social impact of such difficulties. Thus, one aim of this study is to examine the prevalence and social patterning of sleeping pill use among 20-59 year old Canadians. While recent research has found sleeping pill use to be greater among women than men, less consistent findings across studies have tended to support higher sleeping pill use with lower income, higher use with lower educational attainment, and higher use among those divorced or widowed (7-9). However, such analyses have focused on main effects only (ie., comparisons between values of single variables such as between types of marital status or types of education-level groups). Main effects however can mask subgroup differences. Relatively little is known about how gender may interact with various indicators of social position (e.g., education and income) and family and work roles in relation to sleeping pill use.

This study aimed to correct the previous shortcomings of research in this area, and to examine the socio-demographic and economic patterning of sleeping pill use in a large representative sample of working age Canadians. Our central focus was on whether work, family and economic characteristics affect sleeping pill use and whether these variables interact to predict sleeping pill use. Which sub-groups of people report the greatest percentage of sleeping pill use? Are there population subgroups in which the proportion of sleeping pill use is greater among men than women (or no difference)?

METHODS

Our research was based on Cycle 1.2 of Statistics Canada's 2002 Canadian Community Health Survey (CCHS) on mental health and well-being (10), the most recent national survey that asked questions on prescription drug use among Canadians age fifteen years and older. A detailed methodological overview of the CCHS is available in other publications (11). In short, the response rate for the CCHS was 77%, and excluded residents in the northern Canadian territories, Indian reserves and institutions. Data was collected using a complex (multistage) sampling method and the majority of interviews (86%) were conducted in person. To address our research goals, the sample was restricted to 20, 974 participants between the ages of 20 and 59 years. Survey sample weights were used that accounted for the complex survey design of the CCHS (12).

MEASURES

The dependent variable was participants' response to the question "In the past 12 months, that is, from the date one year ago to yesterday, did you use any medication to help you sleep, such as Imovane, Nytol or Starnoc?" Thus, the question includes reference to either prescribed or over the counter sleep medication. The independent variables, all categorical in scale, were: gender (male/female); age (20-39, 40-59 years); educational attainment (less than high school, high school graduate, post-secondary graduate); income adequacy (low, middle/high); employment status (employed all year, not employed); partner status (married/living together, single/never married, and divorced/separated/widowed); and parent status (at least one child under the age of 25 years living in the household/none).

ANALYSIS

Preliminary analysis involved calculating the proportion of Canadians who reported use of sleeping medication according to each of our key study variables separately (ie., main effects). To achieve our primary objective, that is, to determine whether the independent variables interacted to produce effects on sleeping pill use, a linear logit model was fitted. The logit model contained main effects together with two-factor, three-factor, and higher order interactions. A backwards elimination method was used to determine the simplest model that adequately fit the data. The statistically significant interaction effects uncovered are displayed (together with lower-order interactions and main effects) in multi-way frequency tables.

RESULTS

Overall, 9.6 % (9.2%-10.0%) of respondents reported using medication to help sleep in the last year; 65.9% of sleeping pill users reported that the sleep medication was prescribed by a physician (data not shown).

Table 1 displays the frequency of sleeping pill use according to various demographic, social and economic factors. Sleeping pill use was greater among women (11%) compared to men (8.2%) and among older (11%) than younger respondents (8%). With regard to socioeconomic indicators, persons with low incomes (14.2%) had a significantly higher prevalence of sleeping pill use than middle/high income groups (9.2%), as did persons with less than high school (13.3%) compared to those with higher educational attainment (~9.3%), and those unemployed (12.0%) versus employed (8.4%). Regarding family role occupancies, parents (7.8%) reported lower usage of sleeping pills than non-parents (11.5%), as did partnered respondents (8.6%) compared to those who were divorced/separated/widowed (15.6%) or single/never married (10.9%).

Using backward selection, one statistically significant two-way interaction and five four-way interactions were uncovered. Table 2 displays the two-way interaction, showing the highest sleeping pill use amongst participants who are both divorced and unemployed (22.3%).

Greater complexity is introduced with the statistically significant four-way interaction between gender, income, age and parent status on sleeping pill use (Table 3).

What is noteworthy is that while 8% of men as an overall group (Table 1) reported taking sleeping pills, this usage jumps to 24% of men who are 40-59 years of age, non-parents, and living in low income circumstances; women with the same socio-demographic characteristics reported sleeping pill use almost identical to men (24.3%).

Table 1. Sleeping pill use by gender, work and family roles, and socioeconomic indicators

	Number	Percent (95% CI)
Gender		
Male	10314	8.2 (7.7-8.8)
Female	10659	11.0 (10.4-11.6)
Age		
20-39 yrs	9341	8.0 (12.7-15.8)
40-59 yrs	11632	11.0 (10.4-11.5)
Partner status		
Partnered	15836	8.6 (8.2-9.0)
Single/never married	2064	10.9 (9.8-12.0)
Divorced/separated/widowed	3073	15.6 (14.0 – 17.1)
Parent status		
One or more children (<25 years) living in home	10678	7.8 (7.3-8.3)
No children	10295	11.5 (10.9-12.1)
Income adequacy		
Low	1895	14.2 (12.7-15.8)
Middle/high	19078	9.2 (8.8-9.6)
Employment		
Employed all year	13742	8.4 (7.9-8.8)
Not employed	7231	12.0 (11.2-12.7)
Educational attainment		
Less than high school	1403	13.3 (11.5-15.1)
High school graduate	4240	9.2 (8.3-10.1)
Post-secondary graduate	15329	9.4 (8.9- 9.9)

Also interesting, among men, living in low income was not universally associated with higher use of sleeping pills; that is, among 20-39 year old fathers living in low income, only 3.5% reported using sleep medications in the last year. Also, mothers in the middle/high income group reported use of sleeping pills which was similar to the lower overall average (main effect) for men – approximately 8%.

Another statistically significant four way interaction emerged between gender and parent status combined this time with employment and educational attainment (Table 4).

Table 2. Percentage (95% CI) reporting sleeping pill use by employment and partner status

	Employed	Not employed
Partnered	7.8 (7.3-8.4)	10.1 (9.3-11.0)
Single/never married	11.5 (9.8-13.3)	22.3 (19.3-25.3)
Divorced/separated/widowed	9.3 (7.9-10.7)	13.3 (11.4-15.2)

Table 3. Percentage (95% CI) reporting sleeping pill use by gender, income, parent status and age

	Men			
	Low Income		Middle/high income	
	Parent	Non-parent	Parent	Non-parent
20-39 years	3.5 (0.2-6.8)	14.3 (9.6-19.0)	5.7(4.6-6.7)	6.7 (5.6-7.7)
40-59 years	10.8 (6.5-15.0)	24.0 (18.4-29.6)	7.8 (6.8-8.8)	10.1 (8.9-11.3)
	Women			
	Low Income		Middle/high income	
	Parent	Non-parent	Parent	Non-parent
20-39 years	9.9 (6.9-12.9)	12.0 (7.6-16.3)	8.2 (7.1-9.4)	10.0 (8.7-11.4)
40-59 years	11.1 (6.8-15.5)	24.3 (19.1-29.6)	8.4 (7.3-9.5)	15.5 (14.4-16.9)

Table 4. Percentage (95% CI) reporting sleeping pill use by gender, employment status, parent status and educational attainment

	Men			
	Employed		Not employed	
	Parent	Non-parent	Parent	Non-parent
Less than high school	0.9 (-0.8-2.7)	7.3 (3.9-10.7)	17.9 (8.3-27.4)	14.9 (10.4-19.4)
High school graduate	5.9 (4.2-7.6)	5.3 (3.7-7.0)	8.6 (4.7-12.5)	13.6 (10.2-17.0)
Post-secondary graduate	7.0 (6.1-7.9)	8.8 (7.7-9.9)	7.9 (6.0-9.8)	11.2 (9.3-13.2)
	Women			
	Employed		Not employed	
	Parent	Non-parent	Parent	Non-parent
Less than high school	10.3 (4.2-16.4)	22.2 (15.7-28.6)	8.7 (4.8-12.5)	21.3 (16.2-26.4)
High school graduate	7.2 (5.1-9.2)	11.3 (8.6-14.0)	10.3 (7.5-13.1)	16.7 (13.2-20.2)
Post-secondary graduate	7.9 (6.9-9.0)	11.1 (9.8-12.4)	9.3 (7.9-10.7)	15.4 (13.4-17.4)

Almost 18.0% of unemployed fathers with a less than high school educational attainment reported use of sleeping pills in the previous year. Women who were not mothers and had not graduated high school reported the highest sleeping pill use (~21.8%), which, in contrast to men, varied little by employment status.

Similar patterns for both men and women are illustrated in Table 5 where the combination of being non-parents, unemployed, and between the ages of 40 and 59 years, are associated with higher sleeping pill use (men: 15.9%; women: 20.1%). These socio-demographic subgroups utilize close to twice the proportion of sleeping pills used by men and women on average (Table 1).

Table 5. Percentage (95% CI) reporting sleeping pill use by gender, employment status, parent status and age group

	Men			
	Employed		Not employed	
	Parent	Non-parent	Parent	Non-parent
20-39 years	4.6 (3.5-5.7)	6.8 (5.6-8.0)	8.8 (6.1-11.5)	8.5 (6.6-10.4)
40-59 years	7.9 (6.8-8.9)	9.1 (7.7-10.4)	8.6 (6.4-10.8)	15.9 (13.5-18.4)
	Women			
	Low Income		Middle/high income	
	Parent	Non-parent	Parent	Non-parent
20-39 years	8.4 (6.9-9.8)	9.8 (8.2-11.4)	8.6 (7.0-10.2)	10.9 (8.7-13.1)
40-59 years	7.5 (6.2-8.7)	13.5 (11.8-15.2)	10.4 (8.6-12.1)	20.1 (17.8-22.3)

A significant 4-way interaction with gender by age by education by partner status (not shown) showed similar patterns of sleeping pill use, namely, the effects that age, along with being divorced have on both men's and women's use of these medications. What was also noteworthy is that education itself is not a guarantee that sleeping pill usage will be low, even though lower educational attainment by itself is associated with lower use (Table 1): especially with men, being single and middle aged can be overall associated with higher use even among those with a post-secondary degree (16.8%). Divorce also is a contributor to higher use with divorced middle aged men being higher sleeping pill users even with completed high school. In addition, sleeping pill use was exacerbated among the sub-group of divorced women who were older (40-59), and had a less than post-secondary degree.

DISCUSSION

This study utilized a large representative sample of working age Canadians to examine the relationships among sex, age, educational attainment, income adequacy, and employment status on sleeping medicine use. Our logit analysis has illustrated the importance of considering subgroups in studies (identified through examination of variable interactions). The advantage is that single variable (main effect) analyses will very often mask subgroups that are strongly affected by the variables under consideration but not uncovered in the results. Our analysis in this study has shown that work, family, and economic characteristics all predict sleeping medicine use in complicated ways. Looking at the overall relationship between sleeping medicine use and gender show that males, on average use less medicine to combat sleeping problems than women, but this statistic alone can lead us to overlook subgroups of men (and women) whose usage is far higher than what would be expected considering the male and female averages alone. For example, having low income, not being a parent, and being middle aged (40-59 years) is associated with three times the age usage across the overall working age (20-59 years). Again, while women overall take more sleep medicine than men, some sub-groups of men have higher usage of sleep medicine than the corresponding subgroup of women (e.g unemployed male parents with less than high school).

A post hoc examination of this subgroup of men with low income, who were also non-parents, and in middle age indicated 24% of this group used sleeping medicine during the previous year. This subgroup is further associated with a variety of mental and physical health issues, namely insomnia, mental disorder diagnoses, and chronic health conditions.

The limitations associated with this study are generally related to lack of further information in the survey. First, the data was restricted to self-reported use of sleep medicines over only one year. Second, the dependent variable (sleeping medicine usage) combined over the counter (OTC) and prescribed medicines (Rx). Third, the survey did not indicate the frequency of sleep medicines used in the previous year of participants. Fourth, role quality was not considered in this study.

This study provides several productive avenues for future research on sleeping pill usage in Canadians. Some further questions are: Does social and economic patterning vary by Rx vs OTC? Does the social and economic patterning of insomnia mirror the uncovered patterns of sleeping medicine usage? How does sleeping pill usage relate to the patterning of other psychotropic drugs? Does role quality (as opposed to just role occupancy) affect sleeping pill usage?

Although the higher usage of sleeping medicines in women has been well documented, our study highlights the importance of going beyond single factor (main effect) investigations, and the consideration of subgroups in analyses. Our exploratory study has uncovered a number of vulnerable sub-groups of both men and women whose high sleeping medicine usage has been hitherto masked in previous studies. By documenting such overlooked groups and identifying them, we are in a stronger position to alert health professionals about these vulnerable subgroups.

REFERENCES

[1]   Neutel C, Patten S. Sleep medication use in Canadian seniors. [Can J Clin Pharmacol] 2009;16:443-51.

[2]   Busto UE, Sproule BA, Knight K, Herrmann N. Use of prescription and nonprescription hypnotics in a Canadian elderly population. [Can J Clin Pharmacol] 2001;8:213-21.

[3]   Sproule BA, Busto UE, Buckle C, Herrmann N, Bowles S. The use of non-prescription sleep products in the elderly. [Int J Geriatr Psychiatry]. 1999;14:851-7.

[4]   Kojima M, Wakai K, Kawamura T, Tamakoshi A, Aoki R, Lin Y, et al. Sleep patterns and total morality: A 12-year follow-up study in Japan. [J Epidemiol] (Japan) 2000;10:87-93.

[5]   Kripke DF, Langer RD, Kline LE. Hypnotics' association with mortality or cancer: a matched cohort study. [BMJ Open] 2012;2:e000850.

[6]   Belleville G. Mortality hazard associated with anxiolytic and hypnotic drug use in the National Population Health Survey. [Can J Psychiatry] 2010;55: 558-67.

[7]   Kassam A, Patten S. Hypnotic use in a population-based sample of over thirty-five thousand Canadians. [Pop Health Metrics] 2006; 4:15.

[8]   Beck C, Williams J, Wang J, Kassam A, El-Guebaly N, Currie S, Patten, S. Psychotropic medication use in Canada. [Can J Psychiatr] 2005;50:605-13.

[9]   Graham K, Vidal-Zeballos D. Analysis of use of tranquilizers and sleeping pills across five surveys of the same population (1985-1991): The relationship with gender, age, and other use of substances. [Soc Sci Med] 1998; 46:381-95.

[10]   Statistics Canada. Canadian Community Health Survey, Mental Health and Well Being. Public Use Documentation. Tunney's Pasture, Ottawa: Statistics Canada, 2002.

[11]   Gravel R, Be´land Y. The Canadian community health survey: mental health and well-being. [Can J Psychiatr] 2005;50:573–9.

[12]   Rao JNK, Thomas DR. The analysis of cross-classified categorical data from complex sample surveys. [Sociol Methodol] 1988;18: 213-69.

Submitted: February 08, 2012. *Revised:* April 05, 2012. *Accepted:* April 24, 2012.

In: Public Health Yearbook 2013
Editor: Joav Merrick

ISBN: 978-1-63321-095-0
© 2014 Nova Science Publishers, Inc.

Chapter 16

NEEDS ASSESSMENT OF MEDICAL CARE FOR RURAL JAMAICANS THAT REQUIRE ASSISTANCE FROM SHORT-TERM MEDICAL MISSIONS

Marko Popovic*, Milos Prica, MBBS(C),
Milan Minic, MBBS LRCP&SI(C), Beatrice Steele, RN,
Edward Chow, MBBS and Jelena Popovic, MD
Short-term medical mission with Crystal Mission International,
Toronto, Ontario, Canada

ABSTRACT

Short-term medical missions (STMMs) are a well-established means of providing healthcare to the developing world. Jamaica is a nation that enjoys the benefits of a multitude of STMMs. The objective of this study was to offer a collection of statistics about the medical needs of a sample of patients seen at a Jamaican STMM. We participated in a STMM with Crystal Mission International to Jamaica from July 1st to July 8th, 2011. We devised a comprehensive medical profile of patients admitted to the STMM Over half of accrued patients (50.8%) reported their health as being either 'fair' or 'poor'. The most common observed conditions were: hypertension (26.0%), dermatitis (19.4%), asthma (8.2%), diabetes and hyperglycemia (6.6%), and arthritis (6.6%). Almost half of the sample (49.1%) reported that it took $\geq$ 60 minutes for them to get to their nearest doctor, indicating that temporal and financial implications may have been the primary obstacles barring rural Jamaicans from receiving regular medical care. To our knowledge, this is the largest study outlining the medical needs of the rural Jamaican population that require care from STMMs. With this study we hope to provide a comprehensive set of medical issues faced by members of this population, and we hope this study will be of great use to those travelling to Jamaica to take part in a STMM.

Keywords: Needs assessment, medical care, Jamaica, short-term medical missions

---

* Correspondence: Jelena Popovic MD, FRCPC, Department of Pediatrics, Toronto East General Hospital, Toronto, Ontario M4C 3E7 Canada. E-mail: jpopo@tegh.on.ca.

INTRODUCTION

Short Term Medical Missions (STMMs) are defined as "travel by a group of physicians to a foreign country for the purpose of making a special study or of undertaking a special study of a short-term duration" (1). This broad definition encompasses a wide range of services, ranging from surgical missions providing craniofacial reconstruction or cataract extraction (2,3) to medical and/or pediatric missions providing care for acute illness and chronic disease (4). STMMs have been hugely successful in delivering greatly needed medical care to much of the developing world. Annually, there are approximately 6000 STMMs sent out from the United States alone, totaling an annual expenditure of around $250 million (5). They appeal to physicians and other medical professionals due to their unique combination of philanthropy and direct approach to patient care (6). Missions differ widely in size (2 to 90 health care providers per mission) (7), budget (from a few hundred dollars to $39 million in annual expenses) (8), duration (from 2 days to several months in length) (9), and logistical detail.

Although STMMs have good intentions, there are sometimes issues that arise with the practical implementation of STMMs; these may include thepaucity of follow-up data, inadequate relations with the local health care system, and lack of sustainability (5). In order for these problems to be addressed more successfully, a collection of relevant literature concerning the medical needs of the typical population cared for by STMMs in the country of focus is needed. Without proper research beforehand, issues of efficacy, quality control, and impact assessment may be easily overlooked (5).

Jamaica is a nation of approximately 2.6 million people of which a sizeable minority (14.8%) lives in poverty (10).

The unemployment rate in Jamaica (12.9%) is relatively high, and the country has a considerable debt-to-GDP ratio of 120% (10). Jamaica has a public and free health care system. Even though each year the Government of Jamaica invests millions of dollars into health care, many rural Jamaicans may feel that they either don't have the funds or the time to travel to regional health centers, which are often a number of kilometers away. Thus, there is a great need for STMMs to help with overcoming the vast medical needs of the rural population. In order for STMMs to be efficient and focused in their execution, they must have a sound understanding of the medical needs of the rural population being cared for. Unfortunately, to date, there has been a lack of published information in this field. Prior to the creation of this study, a literature search using PubMed (1947 to 2010) and PubMed Central (1947 to 2010) was conducted. The search terms "Jamaica", "short term medical mission", and "needs assessment" were used to elicit relevant literature. Studies were deemed relevant if they tried to comprehensively outline the medical needs of the rural population in Jamaica. No relevant studies were found. Therefore, to date, this is the first study that aims to offer a collection of statistics concerning the medical needs of a sample of rural Jamaicans being cared for by a STMM.

METHODS

We participated in a STMM with Crystal Mission International (CMI) to Jamaica from July 1st-July 8th, 2011. CMI is a privately owned charitable organization based in Toronto, Canada that is funded exclusively by private donations. Our STMM team consisted of a variety of physicians, nurses, medical students, and volunteers.

The medications that were brought to Jamaica included the Physician Travel Pack as outlined by Health Partners International of Canada, as well as a charitable pharmaceutical donation from Teva Canada. The STMM was fully approved by the Jamaican Ministry of Health.

To the rural population, our mission was advertised towards a pediatric population; however, with the help of local health authorities, our scope of work was extended to adults as well. During the STMM, we visited three different parishes.

To collect our data, we created a comprehensive medical profile for all patients seen at our STMM. We extracted the following information: age, sex, district, parish, health care information, past medical history, family history, and social information. In addition, the physicians and/or nurses on our STMM were required to conduct a history enquiry, perform a physical examination, analyze the chief complaint, and finally offer a diagnosis and treatment, if applicable. An in-depth look at the medical profile that we used can be found in Appendix 1.

RESULTS

A total of 248 patients from 3 different parishes (Manchester, Clarendon, and Saint Ann) were accrued. Only 31.9% (79) of patients were male, while 68.1% (169) were female. Furthermore, 44.0% (109) of patients were over the age of 18, while 56.0% (139) were 18 or under (Range: 1 month to 89 years) (Table 1). Examined patients came from the following 11 parishes: Manchester, Saint Mary, Saint James, Saint Ann, Clarendon, Saint Andrew, Kingston, Saint Catherine, Trelawny, Saint Elizabeth, and Westmoreland. The variety of districts in each of these 11 parishes was considerable; we had patients from 24 different districts in total.

Prior health care findings

A total of 247 of 248 patients were able to respond to this portion of the medical profile. 48.2% (119/247) said that they had a regular doctor that they saw at least once a year. In addition, 35.2% (87/247) of patients told us that they were currently being treated for symptoms or conditions.

A total of 99.2% (246/248) of patients did not have a medical provider within walking distance, while 0.8% (2/248) said that they walked to their nearest physician. Of the entire sample, 60.1% of patients (149/248) reported that they went to see their doctor by taxi, 38.3% (95/248) said that they used their own car, and 0.8% (2/248) said that they used public transportation.

Patients were asked how long it took them to travel to their nearest physician. A total of 46.8% of patients reported that it took ≤ 30 minutes to travel to their nearest physician, while another 49.1% stated that it took ≥ 60 minutes for them to get to their nearest physician. On average, patients reported that it took them 59.8 minutes to travel to their nearest doctor (Table 2).

A total of 5.2% of patients (13/248) were unable to answer this section of the medical profile. When asked how often they went to see a doctor, either for a check-up or for a complaint, 10.6% of patients (25/235) said they saw their doctor less than once every 3 years, 17.0% of patients (40/235) said they saw a physician once every 2 to 3 years, 26.8% of patients (63/235) said that they regularly saw a doctor at least once a year, and a large percentage of patients, 45.5% (107/235), told us that they saw a doctor regularly every several months. Only 27.7% of patients (65/235) did not see a doctor at least once a year.

When asked about their present health, 10.9% (27/248) of patients stated that their present health was poor, 39.9% (99/248) stated that their present health was fair, 44.0% (109/248) stated that their present health was good, and 5.2% (13/248) of patients stated that their present health was excellent. Therefore, over half of the patients accrued to the study (50.8%) reported their health as being either 'fair' or 'poor'.

Past medical history findings

Of the 248 patients accrued to the study, 154 of them (62.1%) were willing and able to complete this section of the profile. Of these 154, 82 (53.2%) were adults and 72 (46.8%) were children. A small group of patients (13.0%, 20/154) reported that they have been either diagnosed with asthma or they have been frequently wheezing. Problems with either hearing or vision loss were reported by 13.6% of patients (21/154). Dermatologic conditions such as dermatitis were reported by 11.7% of patients (18/154). 14.9% of patients (23/154) previously had arthritis, while 21 patients reported headaches and/or sinus conditions (13.6%). Almost a third of patients (51/154, 33.1%) reported that they had problems with their blood pressure and cholesterol.

A large majority of patients, 78.6% (195/248), stated that they had never been hospitalized in the past while 21.4% (53/248) stated that they had been previously hospitalized. Of those that had been previously hospitalized, 24.5% of patients (13/53) were hospitalized due to asthma, while 9.4% (5/53) were hospitalized due to hypertension. An overwhelming amount of patients (81.0%, 201/248) stated that they did not regularly take any medications, while 19.0% of patients (47/248) stated that they did. Out of the 47 people who took medications, 53.1% (25/47) took antihypertensives, 19.1% (9/47) took medication for asthma, and 10.6% (5/47) took medication for diabetes.

Only 12.5% of patients (31/248) reported that they had at least one allergy, while 87.5% of patients (217/248) did not have any allergies or were unsure. 21 out of 27 (67.7%) had seasonal allergies, 2 out of 27 (6.4%) were allergic to certain medications, and 4 out of 27 (14.8%) had allergies, but were unsure of the exact etiology. 4 patients out of 248 (1.6%) were lactose intolerant.

When asked about their immunizations, 61.7% of patients (153/248) reported that they were fully immunized, 4.8% (12/248) reported that they were missing certain immunizations, and 33.5% (83/248) stated that they were unsure if they were fully immunized or not.

Table 1. Age distribution of patient sample

Age Group	Number of Patients (n=248)	Percentage of Total (%)
1 month-2 years	32	12.9
3 -9 years	70	28.2
10 -19 years	39	15.7
20 -29 years	11	4.4
30 - 39 years	20	8.1
40 -49 years	18	7.3
50 -59 years	18	7.3
60 -69 years	16	6.5
70 -79 years	18	7.3
80 -89 years	6	2.4

Table 2. Patient-reported times to nearest physician

Time (minutes)	Number of Patients (n=248)	Percentage of Total (%)
Less than 15	29	11.7
16-30	87	35.1
31-45	10	4.0
46-60	66	26.6
61-90	9	3.6
91-120	32	12.9
121-150	6	2.4
151-180	5	2.0
181-210	1	0.4
211-240	3	1.2

Family history findings

This section was answered by 84.3% of patients (209/248). Of these 209 patients, only 18.7% (39/209) reported that there was no pertinent history of any medical conditions in their family. 11.0% percent of patients (23/209) reported that there was a history of heart trouble in their family. The same number (11.0%, 23/209) of patients reported a family history of cancer. 13.9% of patients (29/209) reported stroke in the family, while 23.0% of patients (48/209) stated that there was a history of asthma in the family. More than a quarter of patients (54/209, 25.8%) explained that arthritis was present in their family history. A great number of patients (85/209, 40.7%) reported a family history of diabetes. We found that 57.9% of patients (121/209) reported at least one person in their family suffering from high blood pressure.

Social findings

All 248 patients accrued to our study answered this portion of the profile. 96.8% of patients (240/248) reported having electricity in their homes. However, only 35.9% of patients (89/248) reported that they had running water at home. Collection of rainwater into tanks was the most cited alternative for people that did not have running water at home, followed by the collection of water from nearby springs. 7.3% (18/248), 10.1% (25/248), and 1.2% (3/248) of patients reported that at least one person at homedrank alcohol, smoked, or did illicit drugs on a regular basis, respectively.

We asked the adult population (>18 years old) to provide us with a verbal record of their furthest education. We were able to extract the furthest education of all 109 adults. 61.5% (67/109) never started high school, 26.6% (29/109) previously started high school, 8.3% (9/109) finished high school, 2.8% (3/109) finished vocational college, and 0.9% (1/109) finished university.

Physical exam findings

A detailed view of the normal ranges we used for heart rates, blood pressures, and respiratory rates can be found on tables 3, 4, and 5, respectively. All measurements were taken when patients were at rest.

Most patients (88.7%, 220/248) were able and willing to receive a heart rate reading. Of these, 92.3% (203/220) were reported to have a normal heart rate. 6.8% of patients (15/220) were found to have bradycardia, and only 0.9% of patients (2/220) had tachycardia.

Only 106 accrued patients (42.7%, 106/248) had a respiratory rate measurement performed. Of these, 68.9% (73/106) had normal respiratory rates, 18.9% (20/106) had tachypnea, while 12.3% (13/106) had bradypnea.

We were able to perform blood pressure measurements on almost half of the sample (44.8%, 111/248). We did not take blood pressure readings for patients who were less than 13 years of age. Of those that had their blood pressure read, 41.4% (46/111) were normotensive, 7.2% (8/111) were hypotensive, and 51.4% (57/111) had hypertension. Malignant hypertension, defined as diastolic blood pressure above 130mmHg, was found in 3 out of 57 patients with hypertension, representing 5.3% of patients with hypertension.

Diagnosis and treatment findings

Only 11.3% (28/248) of all admitted patients came for a check-up; most of the patients that we cared for in our STMM had a chief complaint. Of the 248 patients in our sample, 52 (21.0%) were found to be health, or were not given a definite diagnosis. We referred 13.7% of our patients (34/248) elsewhere for further tests or surgeries; X-rays, ultrasounds, and various blood tests were cited as the most common reasons for further referral. 196 patients were diagnosed with a medical condition.

Again, the most significant diagnosis was that of hypertension. Hypertension was extremely common in our patient population; 26.0% of all diagnosed patients were diagnosed with hypertension (51/196). The next most common conditions were those of the skin;

dermatitis represented 19.4% of all diagnoses (38/196). Other common conditions included asthma (8.2%, 16/196), diabetes and hyperglycemia (6.6%, 13/196), arthritis (6.6%, 13/196), sinusitis or other conditions of the sinus (6.1%, 12/196), upper respiratory tract infection (6.1%, 12/196), and various hernias (5.6%, 11/196). Also, 4.6% (9/196) of patients had a fungal infection. None of our patients were found to have preventable conditions from immunizations such as tetanus, measles, or mumps.

The most significant areas of disease seen in our sample were, in increasing order: gastrointestinal disorders (10.7%, 21/196), otolaryngologic conditions (12.2%, 24/196), pulmonary disorders (12.8%, 25/196), infectious diseases (15.3%, 30/196), dermatologic disorders (19.4%, 38/196), and cardiovascular disorders (31.1%, 68/196). A comprehensive summary of the medications given to patients in the STMM can be found on Table 6. Of the entire patient sample (n=248), 20.1% (50/248) required no medication because they were deemed healthy by the attending physician. We did not have adequate medications for 15.1% (26/248) of patients; the most cited cases were creams for dermatitis, medications and blood glucose monitors for diabetics, medications for various species of worms, and shampoos for fungal infections.

Table 3. Normal heart rate ranges

Age (years)	Heart Rate (beats per minute)
< 1	110 - 160
1 - 2	100 - 150
2 - 5	95 - 140
5 - 12	80 - 120
> 12	60 - 100

Table 4. Normal blood pressure ranges

Ages (years)		Blood pressure (mmHg)		
From	To	Average	Minimum	Maximum
15	19	177/77	105/73	120/81
20	24	120/79	108/75	132/83
25	29	121/80	109/76	133/84
30	34	122/81	110/77	134/85
35	39	123/82	111/78	135/86
40	44	125/83	112/79	137/87
45	49	127/84	115/80	139/88
50	54	129/85	116/81	142/89
55	59	131/86	118/82	144/90
60	64	134/87	121/83	147/91

Table 5. Normal respiratory rate ranges

Age (years)	Breathing Rate (breaths per minute)
< 1	30 - 40
1 - 2	25 - 35
2 - 5	25 - 30
5 - 12	20 - 25
> 12	15 - 20

Table 6. Medications used in the STMM

Medication	Number of Patients (%) (n=248)
Multi-vitamins	70 (28.2%)
Acetaminophen	24 (9.7%)
Ibuprofen	19 (7.7%)
Amoxicillin	12 (4.8%)
Hydroxyzine	11 (4.4%)
Naproxen	10 (4.0%)
Ranitidine	8 (3.2%)
Clarithromycin	4 (1.6%)
Doxyciline	3 (1.2%)
Acyclovir	1 (0.4%)
Ciprofloxacin	1 (0.4%)
Cloxacillin	1 (0.4%)

DISCUSSION

In the rural areas of Jamaica, high levels of unemployment and poverty substantially decrease the access to appropriate medical care. In Jamaica, there is a need for STMMs to help with overcoming the vast medical needs of the population, especially in rural areas, which do not have easy access to regular health care providers. In order for STMMs to be efficient and focused in their execution, they must have relevant literature outlining the needs of the population they will be caring for. Unfortunately, to date, there has been a lack of published information on the medical needs of the rural population in Jamaica. We have developed a study which gives a collection of statistics on our rural patient sample, which we hope can be used to provide a clearer understanding of the medical needs of the rural areas of Jamaica.

At our STMM, we cared for a greater number of female patients than males. Out of the 248 accrued patients, 79 were male while 169 were female. This discrepancy surely raises a few questions. Are women in rural Jamaica a more underprivileged group that depend on STMMs? Are they, on average, more open to seek help from STTMs? Are they a group that naturally has more health problems in rural Jamaica? It is our hope that future studies analyzing STMMs to Jamaica will help answer these important questions.

A significant pattern was noted when patients were asked how long it took them to travel to their nearest physician. A considerable number of patients, 49.1%, reported that it took ≥ 60 minutes for them to get to their nearest physician. From the medical profile, length of travel and financial implications were cited as obstacles to seeing physicians regularly; in our sample, many Jamaicans felt that going to the doctor for check-ups was simply unnecessary and costly. In a country suffering from unemployment and poverty, it is no wonder why the demand for STMMs is so high; the rural population simply does not have the means, either financially or logistically, to regularly see physicians for check-ups or any health complaints that they may have. For approximately half of the rural population, doctors are found tens of kilometers away, and thus they are able to receive adequate medical care only through STMMs.

We observed intriguing results when asking the adults (>18) in our sample to provide a record of their furthest education. Of the 109 adults in our sample, only 12.0% of our patient sample had at least a high school education. Our sample therefore remains largely uneducated as many continue to work in professions in which they do not have a need for a high school education. This continues to be an issue for the rural Jamaican population; without proper education, many are at a predisposition to live in lower socioeconomic backgrounds and therefore neglect their health in order to cut costs.

A surprising statistic was found when patients were asked if they had running water or electricity at home. It was encouraging to find out that 96.8% of patients (240/248) reported having electricity in their homes. However, only 35.9% of patients (89/248) reported that they had running water at home. Thus, it is no wonder why we diagnosed 25 of our 248 patients (10.1%) as suffering from some form of gastrointestinal or parasitic disease, and why many more had past medical histories or family histories of gastrointestinal or parasitic diseases.

Our data shows strong indication for cases of hypertension, diabetes, dermatitis, asthma, arthritis, gastritis, viral upper respiratory tract infection, and sinusitis to be common in rural Jamaicans that are cared for by STMMs. This is in line with much of the major literature examining facets of the epidemiology of Jamaica (12-21).

The most pressing conditions that face many rural Jamaicans are hypertension and diabetes. The national prevalence rate of hypertension in the adult population of Jamaica, according to the Medical Association of Jamaica, is 20% for males and 29% for females (22). Our results, which focus solely on the rural population of Jamaica that need regular assistance from STMMs, found that these people have a higher prevalence rate of hypertension than their counterparts living in urban settings, as 46.8% (51/109) of our adult sample was diagnosed with either mild or malignant hypertension. Furthermore, we observed a large number of patients (40.9%) stating that they had a family history of diabetes of those that responded to the family history section of the medical profile. In the population of rural Jamaica, these prevalence rates may even be higher as much of the population does not possess the means to regularly assess their blood pressure and blood sugar.

Another common condition seen by our team was dermatitis. In Jamaica, the prevalence rate of dermatitis is unknown as criteria for the diagnosis of the condition is currently not universally accepted. Our sample of 248 people had 38 members (15.3%) that suffered from some form of dermatitis. Thus, future STMMs to Jamaica must prepare beforehand because this disorder will most likely be common.

A final common condition seen in our clinic was asthma. The worldwide prevalence of asthma is estimated at 7-10% (23); the nationwide prevalence of asthma in Jamaica is still unclear. 16 of our 248 patients were diagnosed with some form of asthma, representing 6.5% of our sample. Thus, we believe that members of the rural population in Jamaica may have comparable prevalence rates of asthma as those experienced worldwide.

Surprisingly, a relatively small percentage of our patient sample was found to have fungal infections (3.6%, 9/248) or parasitic conditions (1.6%, 4/248); however, the number of parasitic conditions may be underestimated because we were unable to check stool samples.

None of our patients had clinical symptoms of preventable conditions such as tetanus, diphtheria, poliomyelitis, measles, mumps, or rubella. Further, we cannot comment on the incidence rates of tuberculosis or sexually transmitted infections (STIs), such as HIV/AIDS, syphilis, and gonorrhoea because we did not have the means to test for these diseases.

Our study is not without limitations. A limitation exists in in that we did not have data from all 14 parishes of Jamaica. As such, our study cannot be comprehensive for the parishes of Hanover, Portland, and Saint Thomas. However, the combined population of these 3 parishes is only 9.2% of the total population of Jamaica (238 846/2 607 631), according to the Jamaican 2001 census. Therefore, we hope that this study will give an intriguing insight into various issues that the vast number of rural Jamaicans that are cared for by STMMs face.

To our knowledge, this is the largest population-based cohort study in the literature outlining the medical needs of the rural Jamaican population that require care from STMMs. With this work, we hope to stimulate scholarly awareness on the medical issues faced by the rural Jamaican population. The authors of this study encourage future investigators to begin similar work in other regions cared for by STMMs. Only then can the vast resources of time, money, and people that are continually poured into STMMs be used most effectively and efficiently.

ACKNOWLEDGMENTS

The authors would like to thank the invaluable volunteers, nurses, and physicians working for Crystal Mission International in Jamaica from July 1st to 8th, 2011 for their services and help in the data collection process. This study and publication was supported by Crystal Mission International. We thank Ms. Stacy Yuen and Ms. Michelle Zhou for secretarial assistance.

CONFLICTS OF INTEREST

The authors have no conflicts of interest to disclose.

APPENDIX 1. PATIENT MEDICAL PROFILE

Name: _____

Date: _____

Date of Birth: _____ Age: _____ Sex: _____

District: _____ Parish: _____

HEALTH CARE

Do you have a regular doctor?   Yes/No   Are you being treated by a doctor now?   Yes/No

Time to travel to the nearest doctor: _____   Mode of travel to see a doctor: _____

How often do you see a doctor?

<Once/3 years   Once/ 2- 3years   Once/Year   Several times/year

My present health is: excellent   good   fair   poor

PAST MEDICAL HISTORY

Have you ever had or do you still have any of the following conditions? If there is an asterisk (*) beside a condition, and you state that you do have it, please further specify the type of condition.

STD[1]*	Yes	No	NS[4]	Stroke	Yes	No	NS[4]	Tonsillitis	Yes	No	NS[4]	Migraines	Yes	No	NS[4]
Heart Disease				Asthma				Tuberculosis				Skin Diseases			
Cancer*				Bronchitis				H1N1				Hepatitis*			
Diabetes				Emphysema				Nut. Def.[6]				Tumours*			
Broken Bones				Pneumonia				Meningitis				Malaria			
High BP[2]				DC[5]*				Arthritis				Cystic Fibrosis			
IC[3]*				Depression				UC[7]*				Anemia			

- Sexually Transmitted Diseases (Includes HIV/AIDS)[1]; Blood Pressure[2]; Intestinal Conditions[3]; Not Sure[4]; Dental Conditions[5]; Nutritional Deficiencies[6]; Urinary Conditions[7].

Other Conditions/ Additional Specifications:

Hospitalizations: _____
Current medications: _____
Allergies: _____ Immunizations: _____

FAMILY HISTORY

Diabetes		Easy Bleeding		Obesity		Allergy
High Blood Pressure		Jaundice		Arthritis		High Blood Fats
Stroke		Alcoholism		Asthma		Cancer of:_____
Heart Trouble		Tuberculosis		Psychiatric Illness		Other:_____

SOCIAL

Furthest Education (if applicable): _____

Running water at home: Yes/No   Electricity at home: Yes/No

Alcohol use: Yes/No   Smoking: Yes/No Drug use: Yes/No

To Be Completed By a Physician

CHIEF COMPLAINT

PHYSICAL EXAM

Weight: _____ Height: _____

Heart Rate: _____ Respiratory Rate: _____ Blood Pressure: _____

Temperature: _____ AC: _____

GENERAL INFORMATION

Head and Neck: Musculoskeletal System:

Respiratory System: Neurological System:

Cardiovascular System: Overall Impression:

Abdominal/Genital:

Skin: Treatment/Additional Comments:

REFERENCES

[1] The National Library of Medicine. The United States National Library of Medicine. Accessed 2011 July 02. URL: http://www.nlm.nih.gov

[2] Yeow VK, Lee ST, Lambrecht TJ, et al. International Task Force on Volunteer Cleft Missions. [J Craniofac Surg] 2002;13(1):18-25.

[3] Mulliken JB. The changing faces of children with cleft lip and palate. [N Engl J Med] 2004;351(8):745-7.

[4] Mitka M. Advice for aspiring volunteer physicians. [JAMA] 1999;282(5):413

[5] White B, Qualls M, Maki J, et al. Health impact assessment and short-term medical missions: A methods study to evaluate quality of care. BMC Health Services Research 2008; 8 (1):121

[6] Vastag B. Volunteers see the world and help its people. [JAMA] 2002;288(5):559-65.

[7] Alabama Honduran Missions. Alabama Honduras Medical and Educational Network. Accessed 2011 July 16. URL: http://www.honduranmissions.com

[8] Operation Smile. Operation Smile Canada Foundation. Accessed 2011 July 16. URL: http://operationsmile.org

[9] Surgical Eye Expeditions International. Surgical Eye Expeditions International, Inc. Accessed 2011 July 16. URL: http://www.seeintl.org

[10] Jamaica Economy, 2011. Chief Intelligence Agency World Factbook. http://www.theodora.com/wfbcurrent/jamaica/jamaica_economy.html (Accessed July 11 2011)

[11] Berkow R, Fletcher AJ, Bondy PK, et al. The Merck manual, Sixteenth Edition. Whitehouse Station, NJ: Merck Research Laboratories, 1992.

[12] Morrison E. Diabetes and hypertension: Twin trouble. [Cajanus] 2000;33:61-63.

[13] Blake G, Hanchard B, Mitchell K, et al. Jamaica Cancer Mortality Statistics, 1999. [West Indian Med J] 2002;2:64-7.

[14] Gage TB. Population variation causes of death: Level, gender, and period effects. [Demography] 1994;31:271-96.

[15] World Health Organization. World health report 1999. Geneva: WHO; 1999.

[16] Bloom DE, Canning D. The health and poverty of nations: From theory to practice. [J Hum Dev] 2003;4:47-72.

[17] Muller O, Krawinkel M. Malnutrition and health in developing countries. [Can Med Assoc J] 2005;173:279-86.

[18] Forrester T, Cooper RS, Weatherall D. Emergence of Western diseases in the tropical world: the experience with chronic cardiovascular diseases. [Br Med Bull] 1998;54:463-73.

[19] Fraser HS. Hypertension: The Silent Killer and the Deadly Quartet. Editorials. [West Indian Med J] 1999;49:91-3.

[20] World Health Organization. Preventing Chronic Diseases a vital investment. Geneva: WHO; 2005.

[21] Bourne PA. Impact of poverty, not seeking medical care, unemployment, inflation, self-reported illness, and health insurance on mortality in Jamaica. [North Am J Med Sci] **2009; 99-109.**

[22] The Medical Association of Jamaica. Current Treatment Options in the Management of Hypertension. Accessed 2011 August 26. URL: http://www.medicalassnjamaica.com/hypertension.html

[23] Lazarus SC. Clinical practice. Emergency treatment of asthma. [N Engl J Med] 2010;363(8):755–64.

Submitted: April 15, 2012. *Revised:* May 29, 2012. *Accepted:* June 08, 2012.

In: Public Health Yearbook 2013
Editor: Joav Merrick

ISBN: 978-1-63321-095-0
© 2014 Nova Science Publishers, Inc.

Chapter 17

SPECTRUM OF HEMOGLOBINOPATHIES AND EVALUATION OF BETA-THALASSEMIA TRAIT IN TRIBAL LAND OF MIDDLE INDIA

Ranbir S Balgir, M Sc Hons, PhD[*]

Department of Biochemistry, Regional Medical Research Centre for Tribals (Indian Council of Medical Research), Jabalpur, Madhya Pradesh, Central India

ABSTRACT

It is fascinating that about half of the world's indigenous communities live in India. They constituted 8.2% of the total population as per 2001 census. Tribal communities are highly vulnerable to many hereditary hemolytic disorders that cause high degree of morbidity and mortality. Pattern of hemoglobin disorders in Central India is still unknown. Based on 1251 referral cases studied during March 2010 to March 2012 from a tertiary hospital, has shown the highest incidence of sickle cell trait (24.6%) and β-thalassemia trait (12.1%) in the general population of Central India. From the tribal land of Odisha, the highest frequency of β-thalassemia trait (12.7%) was noticed among Paraja Bhuyan tribe of Sundargarh district, followed by Paraja tribe (8.5%) of Koraput district, Dudh Kharia (8.1%) of Sundargarh district, Santhal (8.0%) of Mayurbhanj district, Paik Bhuyan (7.8%) of Sundargarh district. High frequency of β-thalassemia trait (10.4%) was recorded among Hill Korwa of Chhattisgarh. A very low frequency of β-thalassemia trait (range: 0.4-3.8%) was observed among other major scheduled tribes of Chhattisgarh. The prevalence of β-thalassemia trait (range being 0.2-3.6%) was found very low in Madhya Pradesh. However, the highest frequency of β-thalassemia trait (10.0%) was recorded among Gond tribe of Damoh district in Madhya Pradesh. The frequency of β-thalassemia trait was equally high among scheduled castes such as Jharia caste (10.0%) of Jabalpur district, and followed by Chaudhury (9.0%) of Damoh district, and other backward castes (8.6%) of the state. The frequency of β-thalassemia trait was recorded to be around 3%

---

[*]Correspondence to: Ranbir S Balgir, Scientist F/Deputy Director (Senior Grade) and Head, Department of Biochemistry, Regional Medical Research Centre for Tribals (Indian Council of Medical Research), Near NSCB Medical College & Hospital, P.O: Garha, Nagpur Road, Jabalpur-482 003, Madhya Pradesh, Central India. E-mail: balgirrs@yahoo.co.in.

among Bagata tribe of Andhra Pradesh. The frequency of β-thalassemia trait in primitive tribes of Gujarat (3.1-4.6%), Maharashtra (1.6-3.2%) and Tamil Nadu (0.9-2.3%) was also found very low. In view of the high prevalence of β-thalassemia trait among some tribal communities, emphasis was laid on intervention and prevention through antenatal carrier screening, genetic/marriage counseling and establishment of prenatal diagnostic facilities in localities of at risk tribes in India.

Keywords: Tribal land, tribal communities, hemoglobin disorders, β-thalassemia trait, intervention, prevention, Middle India

INTRODUCTION

It is fascinating that about half of the indigenous people of the world, i. e. 84,326,240 as per 2001 census live in India and they constitute 8.2% of the total population of the country. The common terminology used for these people is aborigenese, indigenous people, tribal communities, and tribals; the primitive tribes/communities being the most backward of all people. There are about 635 tribes and subtribes including 75 primitive communities registered in 2001 census. These communities are highly vulnerable to hereditary hemolytic disorders that cause high degree of morbidity, infant and maternal mortality in India.

The malady of hemoglobinopathies in India is an important public health problem. Of the erythrocytic disorders of hemoglobin (Hb), beta (β)-thalassemia is the most common among the general castes/ communities of India. In the North/North-western part of India, α- and β-thalassemia, and sickle cell and hemoglobin D significantly represents a public health problem. The β-thalassemia is an inherited disorder in which the body is unable to synthesize adequate amount of hemoglobin due to a genetic defect that leads to absence or reduced synthesis of one or more polypeptide globin chains of hemoglobin molecule. This causes a spectrum of anomalies among the vulnerable individuals/communities leading to ineffective erythropoiesis. It has a wide geographical spread throughout the country, the highest prevalence being in the North-western, followed by North-eastern, and the lowest being in Southern parts of India (1, 2). With a wide range of variation of its prevalence in different communities of India, it would be interesting to explore the prevalence of β-thalassemia among the under privileged indigenous people of India.

This research paper would considerably be of interest to the international scientific community to know that the indigenous communities that are endogamous in India were originally more or less completely free from hereditary β-thalassemia. However, with the advent of penetration of invaders and/or migration of local/nonlocal nontribal communities and/or invaders from other parts of the world, especially from Mediterranean/gulf and/or South East Asian regions, the β-thalassemia was introduced in them. In addition to knowing the pattern of hemoglobinopathies in a tertiary hospital in Central India, it would be fascinating to see geographical/regional or ethnic variations with respect to distribution of β-thalassemia trait in tribal land belt of India.

METHODS

This study is a part of a major ongoing research project undertaken on 'Reproductive Outcome in Carrier Couples of Hemoglobinopathies in a Tertiary Hospital in Central India.' Ethical approval was obtained from the Human Ethical Committee, Regional Medical Research Centre for Tribals (ICMR), Jabalpur, Madhya Pradesh, Central India. A total of 1251 subjects suspected to be suffering from anemia/hemoglobinopathies referred from a tertiary hospital, Netaji Subhash Chandra Bose Medical College & Hospital, Jabalpur in Central India were screened for β-thalassemia and other hemoglobinopathies during the period from March 2010 to March 2012.

About 2ml. of blood was taken intravenously under aseptical conditions using disposable syringes and needles with disodium salt of ethylene diamine tetra acetic acid (EDTA) as anticoagulant from each individual after taking informed/written consent and was free of blood transfusion for at least one month for screening of hemoglobinopathies and β-thalassemia syndrome. Blood so collected was transported to laboratory at RMRCT, Jabalpur under wet-cold conditions for analysis. All the adopted procedures and techniques standardized in the laboratory were followed for diagnosis as described elsewhere (3, 4). Hematological indices were measured using $MS_5$9 Hematological Analyzer (Melet and Schloesing Laboratories, Cergy-Pontoise Cedex, France). Laboratory investigations were carried out following standard procedures. All the blood samples were further subjected to confirmation by hemoglobin variant analysis (made for Bio-Rad Diagnostics Group, Hercules, California, USA). For quality control, results were cross-checked periodically. Family studies were carried out to confirm the diagnosis, wherever it was necessary.

RESULTS

Table 1 shows the pattern of hemoglobinopathies in a tertiary hospital in Central India. It is interesting to note that the sickle cell trait is the most common hemoglobinopathy (24.6%), followed by β-thalassemia trait (12.1%), sickle cell disease (7.7%), β-thalassemia major (2.4%), sickle cell-β-thalassemia (2.4%), sickle cell-E disease (0.2%), hemoglobin E trait (0.3%), and hemoglobin E-β-thalassemia (0.1%) in the decreasing order. Out 1251 blood samples screened, 50.2% were found normal, i.e., without any hemoglobinopathies. During this study, three typical families of β–thalassemia were encountered and their illustrated details are presented in tables 2-4, which are self-explanatory. In the state of Madhya Pradesh, we have encountered not only the $β^0$, $β^+$-thalassemia but also the $β^{++}$-thalassemia in some tribal as well as nontribal communities with mild clinical manifestations, thus indicating that $β^{++}$-thalassemia is not a rare disease entity in India (Table 2 to 4).

Ranbir S Balgir

Table 1. Spectrum of hemoglobinopathies in a tertiary hospital in Central India

Types of Hemoglobinopathies	Number	Percentage
Normal	628	50.2
Sickle cell trait	308	24.6
Sickle cell disease	96	7.7
Sickle cell-β-thalassemia	30	2.4
Sickle cell-E disease	2	0.2
Hemoglobin E trait	4	0.3
Hemoglobin E-β-thalassemia	1	0.1
β-thalassemia trait	152	12.1
Thalassemia Major	30	2.4
Total	1251	100.0

Table 2. A Gond family with Sickle cell-β^0-thalassemia belonging to scheduled tribe community from Jabalpur district of Madhya Pradesh, India

Parameters of study/ Hematological indices	Parents		Offsprings
	Sadaram Haveli (Father)	Saroj Bai (Mother)	Two stillbirths (Daughters) and one miscarriage of 5 months
Age in years	28	26	
Sex	Male	Female	
Hb (g/dl)	11.0	9.0	
RBC($\times 10^3$/μl)	4.8	4.2	
HCT (%)	35.9	30.3	
MCV (fl)	74.7	72.8	
MCH (pg)	22.8	21.6	
MCHC (g/dl)	30.6	29.7	
RDW (%)	11.6	11.6	
WBC ($\times 10^3$/μl)	8.8	8.1	
Sickling test	-ve	+ve	
Electrophoresis:			
Major bands	AA_2	SFA_2	
Hb A_2 (%)	6.2	5.3	
Hb F (%)	1.6	6.7	
Hb S (%)	-	88.0	
Hb A (%)	92.2	-	
Red Cell Morphology	Microcytosis, Hypochromia	Microcytosis, Hypochromia	
Clinical Symptoms	-	Pallor, Back Ache, Mild Jaundice, Splenomegaly (4 cm), H/o Hospitalization	

*Name of patient changed.

DISCUSSION

The thalassemias and related hemoglobinopathies are responsible for a large number of genetic disorders and hence are of great public health importance especially in Central India. A large number of hemoglobin variants prevalent among the populations of Central India (Table 1) indicate that hemoglobinopathies and also their related clinical complications are not uncommon at birth. The inherited disorders of hemoglobin synthesis are one of the important public health challenges in the region. The present scenario of hemoglobinopathies reflects the genetic heterogeneity of the population of the region. Historical accounts (5) reveal that several ethnic elements with varied genetic heritages have been absorbed into the mainstream, resulting in population diversity with the passage of time (6). The findings of high incidence of different hemoglobinopathies in the region are in agreement with the population admixture in Central India.

All the β-thalassemia major patients were transfusion dependent, whereas only 10% of the sickle cell disease cases needed blood transfusion. High levels of fetal hemoglobin ranging from 2 to 30% were observed among the sickle cell disease patients. It is interesting to note that splenomegaly was consistently observed in β-thalassemia trait, β-thalassemia major and in sickle cell disease cases in this population. *Plasmodium falciparum* malaria is rampant in this region, which may also be responsible for splenomegaly in subjects with either a normal hemoglobin profile or with sickle cell or β-thalassemia trait.

Due to the intriguing nature of the people, historical accounts (5) regarding the gene flow or migrations of different waves of people from different corners of Central India are still obscure.

Epidemiology and clinical profile of β-thalassemia in tribal land belt of India

Reporting of thalassemia major in the tribal communities in the rural India is either almost absent or very rare due to non-availability of reliable diagnostic and medical facilities or due to missed diagnosis because of untrained medical manpower. Thus, in the absence of a true picture of clinical manifestations, prognosis and management strategies for the prevention and control of β-thalassemia in the country, there is a demand for special attention to be given in vulnerable communities in rural areas especially to the indigenous people in India.

Inherited disorders of hemoglobin are the commonest monogenic disorders in the Indian subcontinent. They are frequently encountered in scheduled castes (SC) and scheduled (indigenous) tribes (ST), and in other backward castes (OBC) than in other endogamous communities residing in adjacent geographical regions of Central India. The tribal land belt in India constitutes the states of West Bengal, Jharkhand, Odisha, Northern Andhra Pradesh, Chhattisgarh, Madhya Pradesh, Maharashtra, Gujarat, Rajasthan, Uttar Pradesh, and some pockets of Kerala and Tamil Nadu in South India. The β-thalassemia syndrome and sickle cell (Hb S) disorders are the most predominant genetic and clinical disease burden in Central India (3, 7). These disorders present heterogeneity in their geographical distribution, scatter or spread in the vulnerable people. The undivided state of Madhya Pradesh (i.e., Madhya Pradesh and Chhattisgarh) harbors about one-fourth of the total tribal (aboriginal or indigenous people) population of India.

The sporadic surveys carried out by different medical/research institutes/centers either independently or in collaboration with medical colleges (hospital based data), research institutes/centers or nongovernmental organizations (NGOs) indicate the occurrence of β-thalassemia in the tribal land of India.

Therefore, the reports of published data pertaining to incidence/prevalence of β-thalassemia trait in some primitive tribe/scheduled tribal/nontribal communities in tribal land are available for a few states of India. However, the data pertaining to prevalence of β-thalassemia trait are still scanty. A summary of the prevalence data available from the published sources is presented here in table 5.

Out of a total of 12 primitive tribes in the state of Odisha, 9 were studied for β-thalassemia syndrome. The highest prevalence (β-thalassemia trait) of 10.8% among the Kutia Kondh primitive tribe of Kandhamal district in Odisha was reported (Table 5).

Table 3. A Yadav family with β^+-thalassemia belonging to other backward community from Narsinghpur district of Madhya Pradesh, India

Parameters of study/ Hematological indices	Parents		Offsprings	
	Komal Singh (Father)	Saroj Bai (Mother)	Vipin (Son)	Vineet (Son)
Age in years	35	30	8	5
Sex	Male	Female	Male	Male
Hb (g/dl)	13.8	9.6	11.3	8.4
RBC(x10^3/µl)	5.4	3.3	4.7	3.9
HCT (%)	45.9	28.0	34.3	27.3
MCV (fl)	85.1	86.1	72.8	70.6
MCH (pg)	25.6	27.6	24.1	21.6
MCHC (g/dl)	30.1	32.1	33.0	30.6
RDW (%)	11.7	12.4	12.8	15.4
WBC (x10^3/µl)	9.1	7.2	13.1	16.2
Sickling test	-ve	+ve	+ve	+ve
Major bands	AA$_2$	SF	AS	ASFA$_2$
Hb A$_2$ (%)	5.3	3.0	2.2	7.2
Hb F (%)	1.3	20.0	1.6	30.5
Hb S (%)	-	77.0	32.2	32.6 -
Hb A (%)	93.4	-	64.0	29.7
Red cell Morphology	Microcytemia Hypochromia	Microcytemia, Hypochromia	Leucocytosis, Microcytemia, Hypochromia	Leucocytosis, Microcytemia, Hypochromia
Clinical symptoms	-	Splenomegaly		Occasional joint and abdominal pains, Hepatosplenomegaly (3 cm)

*Name of patient changed.

Table 4. A Jharia family with β⁺⁺-thalassemia belonging to scheduled caste community from Jabalpur Town of Madhya Pradesh, India

Parameters of study/Hemato-logical indices	Parents		Offsprings		
	Pradeep (Father)	Sadhna (Mother)	Sunita (Daughter)	Shivani (Daughter)	Chaman (Son)
Age in years	35	31	13	11	10
Sex	Male	Female	Female	Female	Male
Hb (g/dl)	15.3	12.6	11.3	10.3	11.2
RBC (x10³/μl)	4.6	5.2	4.4	3.6	4.4
HCT (%)	47.8	42.3	37.4	33.6	37.9
MCV (fl)	103.1	80.7	84.2	93.3	86.2
MCH (pg)	33.1	24.1	25.5	28.5	25.5
MCHC (g/dl)	32.1	29.8	30.3	30.5	29.5
RDW (%)	10.2	11.9	12.9	12.9	11.8
WBC (x10³/μl)	10.2	6.6	14.2	6.9	5.4
Sickling test	+ve	+ve	+ve	-ve	+ve
Electrophoresis:					
Major bands	ASA₂	AS	AS	AA	ASA₂
Hb A₂ (%)	6.6	3.0	2.2	2.2	6.7
Hb F (%)	11.8	1.0	1.2	1.0	10.6
Hb S (%)	42.0	34.7	32.6	-	37.2
Hb A (%)	39.6	61.3	64.0	96.8	45.5
Red cell Morphology	Macro-cytemia	-	Leucocytosis, Normochromic anemia	Normochromic anemia	Normochromic anemia
Clinical symptoms	-	-	-	-	Occasional joint and abdominal pains

*Name of patient changed.

Table 5. Prevalence of βthalassemia trait in major primitive tribes, scheduled castes/tribes/other backward castes of Chhattisgarh, Gujarat, Madhya Pradesh, Maharashtra, Odisha, and Tamil Nadu states of India

State	Caste/Tribe	Group	N	β-Thalassemia Trait	
				n	%
Odisha[1]	Primitive Tribes	Bondo	165	4	2.4[2]
		Paudi Bhuyan	379	8	2.1
		Didayi	227	9	4.0[2]
		Juang	457	22	4.8[2]
		Kutia Kondh	65	7	10.8
		Kondh	375	16	4.3[2]
		Lodha	78	6	6.7
		Saora	177	11	6.2
		Lanjia Saora	74	2	2.7
		Sabar	102	6	5.9
	Scheduled Tribes	Bathudi	95	0	0.0
		Bhatra	166	11	6.6

Ranbir S Balgir

Table 5. (Continued)

State	Caste/Tribe	Group	N	β-Thalassemia Trait n	%
		Bhumiz	116	2	1.7
		Bhuyan	92	0	0.0
		Bhuyan	836	53	6.2
		Paik Bhuyan	244	19	7.8
		Paraja Bhuyan	213	27	12.7
		Gond	219	1	0.5
		Kharia	54	1	1.9
		Kharia	767	48	6.2
		Dudh Kharia	422	34	8.1
		Dhelki Kharia	345	14	4.1
		Kissan	130	2	1.5
		Kolha	102	2	2.0
		Kondh	254	16	6.3
		Munda	96	5	5.2
		Oraon	104	2	1.9
		Paraja	176	15	8.5
		Santhal	100	8	8.0
Chhattisgarh[3]	Primitive Tribes	Birhor	270	6	2.2
		Hill Korwa	744	62	8.4
		Hill Korwa	402	42	10.4
		Kamar	320	21	6.6
		Kawar	114	0	0.0
		Kawar	72	0	0.0
		Hill Maria	93	0	0.0
		Maria	94	0	0.0
		Maria	101	0	0.0
		Muria	101	0	0.0
	Scheduled Tribes	Bhatra	102	0	0.0
		Bhatra	99	0	0.0
		Dhurwa	81	0	0.0
		Gond	127	0	0.0
		Gond	157	0	0.0
		Halba	122	0	0.0
		Halba	99	0	0.0
		Halba	365	9	2.4
		Halba	95	0	0.0
		Kodaku	400	15	3.8
		Oraon	422	0	0.0
		Oraon	215	4	1.9
		Pando	458	2	0.4
		Patelia	166	0	0.0
Madhya Pradesh[3]	Primitive Tribes	Baiga	175	6	3.5
		Baiga	1566	3	0.2
		Baiga	990	28	3.6
		Baiga	219	4	1.6
		Bharia	183	0	0.0
		Bharia	102	0	0.0

State	Caste/Tribe	Group	N	β-Thalassemia Trait	
				n	%
	Scheduled Tribes	Barela	345	0	0.0
		Barela	316	4	1.3
		Bhil	904	0	0.0
		Bhil	433	0	0.0
		Bhil	316	3	1.0
		Bhilala	403	0	0.0
		Bhilala	370	5	1.3
		Gond	299	3	1.0
		Gond	321	32	10.0
		Gond	3224	281	8.7
		Gond	280	0	0.0
		Gond	158	0	0.0
		Gond	75	0	0.0
		Gond	83	0	0.0
		Gond	286	0	0.0
		Gond	252	12	4.6
		Gond	311	7	2.2
		Kol	290	17	5.9
		Korku	250	12	4.8
		Korku	301	7	2.3
		Korku	296	12	3.9
		Panika	210	3	1.4
		Pradhan	226	0	0.0
		Pradhan	990	28	3.6
		Raj Gond	321	10	3.1
	Scheduled Castes	Balai	276	7	2.5
		Basod	150	6	4.0
		Basod	123	0	0.0
		Chaudhary	339	31	9.0
		Chaudhary	195	7	3.6
		Jharia	637	15	2.3
		Jharia	409	41	10.0
		Katiya	181	2	1.1
		Mehra	352	1	0.3
		Mehra	114	6	5.2
		Mehra	216	3	1.4
		Mehra	219	0	0.0
	Other Backward Castes	Backward Castes	58	5	8.6
Gujarat[2]	Primitive Tribes	Kotvaida	285	13	4.6
		Kolcha	653	20	3.1
		Kathodi	124	4	3.2
		Total	1062	37	3.5
Maharashtra[2]	Primitive Tribes	Madia	602	18	3.0
		Kolam	595	19	3.2
		Katkari	879	14	1.6
		Total	2076	51	2.5

Table 5. (Continued)

State	Caste/Tribe	Group	N	β-Thalassemia Trait	
				n	%
Tamil Naidu[2]	Primitive Tribes	Irula	687	15	2.2
		Kurumba	384	6	1.6
		Moolu Kurumba	322	3	0.9
		Paniya	301	7	2.3
		Total	1694	31	1.8

[1]Data from reference 7.
[2]Data from reference 8.
[3]Data from reference 3.

Out of 62 major scheduled tribes in Odisha, 13 tribes were investigated for hemoglobin disorders and β-thalassemia. The highest frequency of β-thalassemia trait: 12.7% among the Paraja Bhuyan tribe of Sundargarh district, followed by Paraja tribe (8.5%) of Koraput district, Dudh Kharia (8.1%) of Sundargarh district, Santhal (8.0%) of Mayurbhanj district, Paik Bhuyan (7.8%) of Sundargarh district, and so on in the decreasing order was noticed in the state of Odisha (Table 5).

In a recently carved state of Chhattisgarh, out of four primitive tribes, all were studied for hemoglobinopathies and β-thalassemia. The highest frequency of β-thalassemia trait, i.e., 10.4% was recorded among the Hill Korwa of Korba district of Chhattisgarh. A very low frequency of β-thalassemia trait (ranging between 0.4-3.8 percent) was observed among other major scheduled tribes of the state (Table 5).

Of the three primitive tribes in the state of Madhya Pradesh, two tribes, namely, Baiga and Bharia were studied for hemoglobinopathies and β-thalassemia, but the prevalence of β-thalassemia trait (range being 0.2-3.6%) was found very low (Table 5). Out of 46 major scheduled tribes of Madhya Pradesh, 9 were studied for hemoglobinopathies and β-thalassemia. The highest frequency of β-thalassemia trait (10.0%) was observed among Gond tribe of Damoh district of Madhya Pradesh. However, in other tribes, the prevalence of β-thalassemia trait was found to be low (Table 5). Among the scheduled caste communities of Madhya Pradesh, the frequency of β-thalassemia trait was equally high among Jharia caste (10.0%) of Jabalpur district, and followed by Chaudhury (9.0%) of Damoh district, and other backward castes (8.6%) of the state.

The frequency of β-thalassemia trait in primitive tribes of Gujarat (3.1-4.6%), Maharashtra (1.6-3.2%) and Tamil Nadu (0.9-2.3%) was found very low (Table 5) by Mukherjee et al. (8). The frequency of β-thalassemia trait was recorded to be around 3% (6/202) among Bagata tribe of Andhra Pradesh (9).

These findings are thought provoking. In order to explain, interpret and synthesize the above prevalent scenario of β-thalassemia trait among the tribal communities of India, the following etiquettes, factual evidence, and vicissitudes must be kept in mind. Historical evidence shows the existence of at least three well established open corridors (passages) to penetrate India, i.e., Northwestern, Northeastern, and Southwestern (sea routes) part of the country (10-12). These corridors in the distant past had facilitated the invasions/migrations of the people for several reasons, i.e., looting, plundering, conquering/grabbing the wealth accumulated in India. A majority of them came to India as dacoits/soldiers without wives and some had taken away Indian people with them as slaves. Biological contact was not a hindrance for these people under the circumstances. Being subdued by the mighty invaders, the people of India might have assimilated the inherited genetic characters of the incomers and some of these invaders (e.g., Mughuls) did not go back to their home land and settled permanently in India. With the passage of times, the offspring of these people mingled with the main stream of the people of India (13, 14).

Apart from this, India has witnessed the inter-state, inter-community or inter-religion battles/feuds/wars for rivalry/capture of power, dominancy, etc. which has forcefully amalgamated the population of India (13, 14). Natural disasters such as earthquakes, draughts, floods, and epidemics in several parts of India from time to time have also contributed for the emigration (exodus) of the people from one place to another in search of food, better safety and security, and economic viability. In some cases due to poverty and indebtedness, daughters were sold (bride price) to rich landlords/wealthy people to pay the debt or sustain livelihood, etc. These people carried good as well as bad gene pools with them wherever they migrated to other places and some of them were seduced and had also mixed and merged with the local people. Under this population scenario, the occurrence of different frequencies of β-thalassemia is not unexpected and the tribal people of India are not exception to this vulnerable seductive situation. In fact, β-thalassemia trait frequency in the tribals represents the degree (multiplication) of penetration of foreign elements (β-thalassemia) and the inbreeding.

As regard the clinical manifestations, the sickle cell-β^+thalassemia is found to have milder course than the sickle cell-β^0 thalassemia (15). Sickle cell-β^+thalassemia produces Hb S, Hb F and Hb A_2 with variable amount of Hb A. The severe forms have low, i.e., <10% (16) and (3-15%) (17) Hb A level. Mild forms have higher, i.e., >10% (18) and (18-30%) (17, 19) levels of Hb A. On the contrary, clinically there was no significant difference between these genotypes (β^+ and β^{++}) indicating that the low levels of Hb A (3-5%) were insufficient to modify the clinical features (18, 20). However, in the latter study (18), the figures for total hemoglobin (Hb S, Hb F, Hb A_2) level were found exaggerated in some reported cases.

Since it (β^{++}thalassemia) has encountered in a few communities with low prevalence/frequency so far investigated, therefore, it is said to be of rare occurrence, but actually it is not of rare occurrence in India (21). Several communities have not yet been investigated due to mild clinical manifestations of β^{++}-thalassemia gene and it is likely to present in high frequency in India. It is equally important that in some studies only the variants of hemoglobin have been investigated depending upon the laboratory infrastructural facilities available and not the whole abnormal hemoglobin spectrum, with the result either the actual diagnosis is missed or misdiagnosed, accordingly the results were reported.

Several β–thalassemia mutations, namely, IVS 1-5 (G-C), IVS 1-1(G-T), CD 41-42, CD 30 (G-C), CD 15 (G-A), CD 8-9, 619bp deletion, nonsense codon 15, frame shift at codon 16, etc. are commonly known to occur in Asian Indians (16-18, 20, 22, 23). According to Nishank et al. (24), the tribal population possessed only the IVS 1-5 (G-C) mutation, whereas, nontribals had the IVS 1-1 (G-T), IVS 1-5 (G-C), FS 41/42 (-CTTT), FS 8/9 (+G), and CD 30 (G-C) β-thalassemia mutations in Odisha state. Similarly, Mukherjee et al. (18) encountered only CD 15 (G-A) mutation in tribals, and IVS 1-5 (G-C), CD 15 (G-A), CD 8/9 (+G), and CD 30 (G-C) mutations of β-thalassemia in nontribal populations of Western India.

Geographical distribution

The thalassemias are wide-spread with about 5% of the world population affected by it. It is most prevalent around the Mediterranean Sea i.e., countries like Greece, Italy, Turkey and Northern Africa. It is also seen in Saudi Arabia, Iran, Afghanistan, Pakistan, India and South East Asian countries like Thailand and Indonesia (25). The prevalence is the highest in Italy, Greece and Cyprus. Population migration and intermarriage between different ethnic groups have introduced thalassemia in almost every country of the world. In India, the prevalence of β-thalassemia is very high among certain linguistic communities like Punjabi, Sindhi, Gujarati, Bengali, Parsee, Lohana and certain scheduled tribes belonging to northern, western and eastern parts of India, while it is much less in the southern parts of India (2).

β-thalassemias are a group of hereditary blood disorders characterized by genetic anomaly in the synthesis of β-globin chain of hemoglobin resulting in variable phenotypes ranging from severe anemia to clinically asymptomatic individuals (15). In the homozygous state, β-thalassemia (i.e., thalassemia major) causes severe transfusion-dependent anemia. In the heterozygous state, the β-thalassemia trait (i.e., thalassemia minor) causes mild clinical manifestations with mild to moderate microcytic anemia. Beta-thalassemias are caused by point (genetic) mutations or, more rarely, deletions in the β-globin gene on chromosome 11, leading to reduced (β^+) or absence of synthesis (β^0) of the β-chains of hemoglobin, however, several additional (epigenetic) factors influence the clinical manifestations of the disease (15). That is, the same particular mutation may have different clinical manifestations in different patients. The following factors are known to influence the clinical phenotype in hemoglobin disorders: (i) Intra-cellular fetal hemoglobin (Hb F) concentrations: (a) Level of expression of Hb F (i.e., the expression of the β-globin gene) determines, in part, the severity of disease. (b) Patients with high Hb have milder disease. (ii) Co-inheritance of α-thalassemia: (a) Patients with co-inheritance of α-thalassemia have a milder clinical course because they have a less severe α–β chain imbalance. (b) The coexistence of sickle cell trait and β-thalassemia is a major symptomatic hemoglobin disorder with most of the symptoms and complications of the sickle cell disease.

Persons heterozygous for sickle Hb and β-thalassemia (Hb S/β-thal) also may experience sickle cell disease, although their symptoms tend to be less severe than those persons homozygous for sickle cell disease. The sickle cell-β–thalassemia varies in severity, depending on the inherited β-thalassemia mutation. There are two main varieties of β-thalassemia in different populations, β^0-thalassemia, in which no β-globin is produced, and β^+-thalassemia, in which some β-globin is produced, but less than normal. The diagnostic feature of β-thalassemia is an elevated level of Hb A_2 in heterozygotes, which is found in most forms of β^0 and β^+-thalassemia (15). The β^{++}-thalassemia, with more than 10% of adult hemoglobin (Hb A), also occurs having milder symptoms and less severe clinical manifestations.

Clinical Severity of β-thalassemia Major

Individuals with thalassemia major usually present symptoms within first two years of life with severe anemia, requiring regular red blood cell (RBC) transfusions. Findings in untreated or poorly transfused individuals with thalassemia major, as seen in some developing countries, are growth retardation, pallor, jaundice, poor musculature, hepatosplenomegaly, and development of masses from extramedullary hematopoiesis, and skeletal changes that result from expansion of the bone marrow (2, 26).

Regular transfusion therapy leads to iron overload-related complications including endocrine complication (growth retardation, failure of sexual maturation, diabetes mellitus, and insufficiency of the parathyroid, thyroid, pituitary, and less commonly, adrenal glands), dilated myocardiopathy, liver fibrosis and cirrhosis.

Patients with thalassemia intermedia present later in life with moderate anemia and do not require regular transfusions. Main clinical features in these patients are hypertrophy of erythroid marrow with medullary and extramedullary hematopoiesis and its complications (osteoporosis, masses of erythropoietic tissue that primarily affect the spleen, liver, lymph nodes, chest and spine, and bone deformities and typical facial changes), gallstones, painful leg ulcers and increased predisposition to thrombosis (2, 26).

Thalassemia minor (trait) is clinically asymptomatic but some subjects may have moderate anemia. These patients are either asymptomatic or have mild anemia and rarely moderate degree of anemia. Symptoms of β-thalassemia trait include: fatigue, irritability, jaundice, trouble in breathing, slow growth in child (2). Clinical examination is normal except for mild anemia. Usually subjects are given iron and vitamin supplements to which they do not respond.

The peripheral blood smear shows microcytosis, hypochromia, anisocytosis, poikilocytosis and target cells. Serum iron studies are normal, except in those who have coexisting iron deficiency - a condition not uncommon in India (2).

Diagnosis is made by hemoglobin electrophoresis which shows increase in Hb A_2 to more than 3.5%. Hb F is usually normal but may be elevated in some cases. When both parents are carriers, there is a 25% risk at each pregnancy of having children with homozygous thalassemia (27, 28).

Management and treatment therapy

The condition of β-thalassemia trait usually requires no treatment. Folic acid supplements may help to prevent relative folate deficiency which may occur as a result of increased cell turnover. Though red cells are hypochromic and microcytic, they do not need iron. Unfortunately, this fact is ignored by many doctors and results in injudicious prescription of hematinics containing iron to all those patients who look pale or have anemia. Not only this therapy is of no use but it could lead to iron overload and its complications (4, 26). Thus use of iron supplements is contraindicated unless there is coexisting iron deficiency. Iron supplements are required in pregnant women with β-thalassemia minor, but serum iron should be carefully monitored. These patients should be educated about thalassemia major if they do not have a child suffering from the disease in their family. They should be told about means of preventing the birth of a thalassemia major baby, i.e., by screening the spouse of the carrier parent and by prenatal diagnosis. Regular transfusion of red blood cells at the interval of a fortnight/month with timely chelation therapy is the optimal solution/treatment under Indian setting (2, 4).

Intervention and prevention

To tackle such a huge population suffering from β-thalassemia and other hemoglobinopathies, the following practical options are available in the Indian context:

1. Genetic counseling and prenatal diagnosis

Prevention of β-thalassemia is based on carrier identification, genetic counseling and prenatal diagnosis (29). Carrier detection and genetic counseling provide information for individuals or couples at high risk (i.e., both carriers) regarding the mode of inheritance, the genetic risk of having affected children and the natural history of the disease including the available treatment and therapies under investigation. Prenatal diagnosis for pregnancies at increased risk is possible by analysis of DNA extracted from fetal cells obtained by amniocentesis, usually performed at approximately 15-18 weeks' gestation or chorionic villi sampling at 11 weeks' gestation. Both disease-causing alleles must be identified before prenatal testing can be performed. Analysis of fetal cells in maternal blood (non-invasive technique) and analysis of fetal DNA in maternal plasma for the presence of the father's mutation are currently under investigations (30, 31). Pre-implantation genetic diagnosis may be available for families in which the disease-causing mutations have been identified (32).

2. Bone marrow and cord blood transplantation

Bone marrow transplantation (BMT) remains the only definitive cure currently available for patients with β-thalassemia. The outcome of BMT is related to the pretransplantation clinical conditions, specifically the presence of hepatomegaly, extent of liver fibrosis, history of regular chelation and hence severity of iron accumulation. In patients without the above risk factors, stem cell transplantation from an HLA identical sibling has a disease-free survival rate over 90% (33). The major limitation of allogenic BMT is the lack of an HLA-identical sibling donor for the majority of affected patients. In fact, approximately 25-30% of thalassemic patients could have a matched sibling donor. BMT from unrelated donors has been carried out on a limited number of individuals with β-thalassemia. Provided that selection of the donor is based on stringent criteria of HLA compatibility and that individuals have limited iron overload, results are comparable to those obtained when the donor is a compatible sib (34). However, because of the limited number of individuals enrolled, further studies are needed to confirm these preliminary findings. If BMT is successful, iron overload may be reduced by repeated phlebotomy, thus eliminating the need for iron chelation. Chronic graft-versus-host disease (GVHD) of variable severity may occur in 5-8% of individuals.

Cord blood transplantation from a related donor offers a good probability of a successful cure and is associated with a low risk of GVHD (35, 36). For couples who have already had a child with thalassemia and who undertake prenatal diagnosis in a subsequent pregnancy, prenatal identification of HLA compatibility between the affected child and an unaffected fetus allows collection of placental blood at delivery and the option of cord blood transplantation to cure the affected child (37). On the other hand, in cases with an affected fetus and a previous normal child, the couple may decide to continue the pregnancy and pursue BMT later, using the normal child as the donor.

Considering the Indian social and cultural pattern, highlighting the awareness programs and genetic counseling in high risk communities is the only powerful and economic tool to control thalassemia (2). This strategy imparts the information to the target population without creating undue fear and concern, and takes into consideration the social structure and taboos, religion and economic aspects. Major constrains are poverty and illiteracy in India. In conclusion, apart from the above mentioned available options, genetic/marriage counseling in the high risk communities is a useful strategy to control β-thalassemia disorder in India.

ACKNOWLEDGMENTS

Author is grateful to Dr. V. M. Katoch, Secretary, Department of Health Research, Government of India, and Director General, Indian Council of Medical Research, New Delhi for providing the necessary research facilities. My heart-felt thanks go to all those authors whose research works have directly or indirectly been quoted here.

CONFLICT OF INTEREST

The author declares that he has no conflict of interest.

REFERENCES

[1]   Madan N, Sharma S, Sood SK, Colah R, Bhatia HM. Frequency of β-thalassemia trait and other hemoglobinopathies in Northern and Western India. [Indian J Hum Genet] 2010;16:16-25.

[2]   Balgir RS. Community genetics and health approaches for bringing awareness in tribals for the prevention of beta-thalassemia in India. Thalassemia Reports 2011;1:4-7.

[3]   Balgir RS. Public health challenges of sickle cell disorders, β-thalassemia syndrome and G6PD deficiency in scheduled caste and scheduled tribe communities of Central India. [Int Public Health J] 2011;3:307-18.

[4]   Balgir RS (2011) Hematological profile of pregnant women with carrier status of hemoglobin disorders in coastal Odisha, India. [Int J Child Health Hum Develop] 2011;4: 325-32.

[5]   Russel RV, Lal H. Tribes and Castes of the Central Provinces of India. Four Volumes. London: Macmillan, 1916: 215–18.

[6]   Balgir RS, Dash BP, Murmu B. Blood groups, hemoglobinopathy and G6PD deficiency investigations among fifteen major scheduled tribes of Orissa, India. [Anthropologist] 2004; 6:69–75.

[7]   Balgir RS. Detrimental intrinsic factors contain population explosion for sustainable development in 18 indigenous communities of Orissa, India. In: Pati RN & Jain Atul Kumar (Eds) Biodiversity and Sustainable Development. 40th Chapter. New Delhi: Sarup Book Publishers Private Limited, 2010:507-16.

[8]   Mukherjee MB, Mohanty D, Colah RB, Wadia M, Ghosh K, Chhotray GP et al. β^S Gene diversity among fourteen primitive tribal groups of India. Paper presented in 4th International Congress on Sickle Cell Disease, 22-27th November 2010, Raipur, India.

[9]   Haritha P, Lakshmi V, Veerraju P, Sarkar BN, Rao VR. Prevalence of beta-thalassemia trait and Hb S among Bagatas of Visakhapatnum. Paper in 4[th]Int Congress on Sickle Cell Disease: Management and Prevention of Sickle Cell Disease in Developing Societies, 22-27 November 2010, Raipur, Chhattisgarh, India.

[10] Balgir RS. Blood groups, G6PD enzyme and hemoglobin studies among the three endogamous populations of Assam. [Indian J Hemat Blood Transfus] 1993;11:237-43.

[11] Balgir RS. Indigenous and independent origin of the β^S-mutation in ancient India: Is it a myth or reality? [Mankind Quart] 2001;42:99-116.

[12] Balgir RS. Scenario of hemoglobin variants in Central-East coast of India. [Curr Sci] 2006;90:1651-7.

[13] Balgir RS, Sharma JC. Genetic markers in the Hindu and Muslim Gujjars of North-western India. [Am J Phys Anthropol] 1988;75:391-403.

[14] Balgir RS. Epidemiology, population health genetics and phenotypic diversity of sickle cell disease in India. [Internet J Biol Anthropol] 2007;1:1-26.

[15] Weatherall DJ, Clegg JB. The thalassaemia syndromes. 4th edition. Oxford: Blackwell Science Limited. 2001:393-449.

[16] Balgir RS. Phenotypic diversity of sickle cell disorders with special emphasis on public health genetics in India. [Curr Sci] 2010;98:1096-1102.

[17] Ambekar SS, Phadke MA, Balpande DN, Mokashi GD, Khedkar VA, Bankar MP et al. The prevalence and heterogeneity of beta- thalassemia mutations in the Western Maharashtra population: a hospital based study. [Int J Hum Genet] 2001;1:219-223.

[18] Donaldson Alan, Fisher John Old, Serjeant Bryl E, Serjeant Graham R. Jamaican Sβ+thalassemia: mutations and hematology. [Br J Haemat] 2000;108:290-294.

[19] Kulozik AE, Bail S, Kar BC, Serjeant BE, Serjeant GE. Sickle cell β⁺thalassemia in Orissa state, [India. Br J Haemat] 1991;77:215-20.

[20] Mukherjee MB, Nadkarni AH, Gorakshakar AC, Ghosh K, Mohanty D, Colah RB. Clinical, hematologic and molecular variability of sickle cell β— thalassemia in western India. [Indian J Hum Genet] 2010;16:154-8.

[21] Balgir RS. The burden of hemoglobinopathies in India and the challenges ahead. [Curr Sci] 2000;79:1536-47.

[22] Kazanian HH, Orkin SH, Antonarakis SE, Serton JP, Boehm CD, Goff SC et al. Molecular characterization of seven beta thalassemia mutations in Asian Indians. [EMBO Journals] 1984;3:593-6.

[23] Varawalla NY, Old JM, Sarkar R, Venkatesan R, Weatherall DJ. The spectrum of beta-thalassemia mutations in the Indian subcontinent: the basis for prenatal diagnosis. [Br J Haemat] 1991;78:242-7.

[24] Nishank SS, Ranjit M, Kar SK, Chhotray GP. Molecular variants and clinical importance of β-thalassemia traits found in the state of Orissa, India. [Hematology] 2009;14:290-6.

[25] Weatherall DJ, Clegg JB. Inherited haemoglobin disorders: an increasing global health problem. [Bull] WHO 2001;79:1-15.

[26] Galanello R, Origa R. Beta-thalassemia. [Orphanet J Rare Dis] 2010;5:11.

[27] Balgir RS. Prevention of hereditary disorders in India: sickle cell disease, β-thalassemia and G6PD deficiency. Bhubaneswar: Division of Human Genetics, Regional Medical Research Centre (ICMR), 2001:1–12.

[28] Balgir RS. Challenges of imparting IEC for prevention of hereditary sickle cell disorders, β-thalassemia syndrome and G6PD deficiency in India. [Tribal Health Bull] 2007;13:14-22.

[29] Cao A, Galanello R, Rosatelli MC. Prenatal diagnosis and screening of the haemoglobinopathies. [Baillieres Clin Haematol] 1998;11:215-38.

[30] Lo YM. Recent advances in fetal nucleic acids in maternal plasma. [J Histochem Catechism] 2005;53:293-6.

[31] Mavrou A, Kouvidi E, Antsaklis A, Souka A, Kitsiou Tzeli S, Kolialexi A. Identification of nucleated red blood cells in maternal circulation: a second step in screening for fetal aneuploidies and pregnancy complications. [Prenat Diagn] 2007;27:150-3.

[32] Kullev A, Packalchuk T, Verlinsky O, Rechitsky S. Preimplantation diagnosis: efficient tool for human leukocyte antigen matched bone marrow transplantation for thalassemia. [Thalassemia Reports] 2011;1:1-3.

[33] Gaziev J, Lucarelli G. Stem cell transplantation for hemoglobinopathies. [Curr Opin Pediatr] 2003;15:24-31.

[34] La Nasa G, Argiolu F, Giardini C, Pession A, Fagioli F, Caocci G et al. Unrelated bone marrow transplantation for beta-thalassemia patients: The experience of the Italian Bone Marrow Transplant Group. [Ann NY Acad Sci] 2005;1054:186-95.

[35] Locatelli F, Rocha V, Reed W, Bernaudin F, Ertem M, Grafakos S et al. Related umbilical cord blood transplantation in patients with thalassemia and sickle cell disease. [Blood] 2003;101:2137-43.

[36] Pinto FO, Roberts I. Cord blood stem cell transplantation for haemoglobinopathies. [Br J Haematol] 2008;141:309-24.

[37] Orofino MG, Argiolu F, Sanna MA, Rosatelli MC, Tuveri T, Scalas MT et al. Fetal HLA typing in beta thalassemia: implications for haemopoietic stem-cell transplantation. [Lancet] 2003;362:41-2.

Submitted: May 08, 2012. *Revised:* June 08, 2012. *Accepted:* June 23, 2012.

In: Public Health Yearbook 2013
Editor: Joav Merrick

Chapter 18

RANKING COUNTRIES BY THEIR MAGNITUDE OF DISEASE: A RELIABILITY ANALYSIS

Tilahun Nigatu[*]

Department of Epidemiology and Preventive Medicine,
Monash University, Melbourne, Victoria, Australia

ABSTRACT

Number of cases, national prevalence and comparative prevalence of a disease are commonly used to rank countries by their magnitude of disease. However, the reliability of such rankings is usually challenged due to the nature of the measures used and the inherent demographic differences among populations. Objective: To analyze the reliability of three methods of ranking countries by their magnitude of disease. Methods: Three measures of disease magnitude were compared. Rank transformed country-level disease magnitude data were used for the purpose of the analysis. To measure the reliability of the prevalence measures the rank deviation and rank difference approaches were applied. Besides, correlation, kappa statistics, reliability model, and factor analysis were also used. Results: The reliabilities of number of cases in comparing disease magnitude across countries at a single point in time and at two points of time were -0.042 (P=0.54) and 0.211(P=0.002) respectively. The reliabilities of national prevalence in comparing disease magnitude at single point and at two points were 0.902(P=0.000) and 0.431(P=0.000) respectively. The reliability of Comparative prevalence measures in comparing disease magnitude across countries at two points in time was 0.498(P=0.000). Conclusion: Number of cases has lower reliability in comparing disease magnitude across countries as compared to national prevalence and comparative prevalence measures. Though better than others, comparative prevalence had lower reliability in comparing disease magnitude at two points of time.

Keywords: Prevalence, rank, reliability analysis

---

[*] Correspondence: Department of Epidemiology and Preventive Medicine, Monash University, The Alfred Centre, 99 Commercial Road, Melbourne, Victoria, Australia 3004. E-mail: tilahunigatu@gmail.com.

INTRODUCTION

Comparison of health and disease across countries has been an important aspect of public health in the last decades. Accordingly, several measures of comparison of disease magnitude and health status across countries were implemented. The earlier approaches include actual number of cases of a disease and prevalence of a disease at country levels (1).

The more recent approaches in the measurements disease are more standardized and needs the computation of time and event. Disability Adjusted Life year (DALY) which is the sum of Potential Years of Life lost (PYLL) and Prevalent Years Lived with Disability (PYLD) calculated at disease and country level is such a standardized measure to compare health and disease across countries (2).

However, these measures are not easy to calculate and simple to understand for most practitioners and community members. Besides, these methods measure disease burden in terms of health. While very useful at several levels, the utilization of these measures at many other levels seems low. This is partly due to the complexity of the measures and limited access of such data (3).

Disease magnitude data, such as number of cases and national prevalence, on the other hand are simple to compute and understand. These data are also regularly and continuously available for most countries and most disease conditions. The notion of having such data is to describe the disease status across countries at a specific point in time or at multiple points of time. Countries' relative status (i.e., ranks) with respect to a specific disease can also illustrated by those prevalence data sets (4).

However, there are several issues that need to be considered in making comparison of magnitude of a disease or diseases across countries. From the very beginning, countries differ in terms of their population size, density and age-sex structure. Secondly, what defines a case of disease varies from country to country based on the level of advancement of diagnostic facilities and health seeking behaviors. Thirdly, measurement issues and data qualities vary widely from one corner to another. With all these inherent differences related to the data, prevalence measures are still the most commonly used disease magnitude measures. These measures are also used to rank countries for their magnitude of specific disease (5).

Number of cases as a measure of disease magnitude has been used to rank countries with respect to a specific disease in several literatures. In most of those rankings, countries with higher population size tend to attain the highest ranks. India and china are best examples of this scenario for diabetes (6).

Ranking using the national prevalence on the other hand provides better picture by taking in to account the population size of the countries. However, countries have different population sizes. Hence, countries with the same number of cases of a disease could differ in their prevalence based on the size of their population. The one with the lower population size will have higher prevalence (7).

Countries also have differences in the age-sex structure of their population. The magnitude of most diseases is affected by these age-sex structures. Comparative prevalence using a standard population is thus used to compare disease prevalence among countries. This comparative prevalence was also used in many instances to rank countries for their magnitude of disease (8).

As to the author's knowledge of health metrics, there is no study conducted to establish the reliability of ranking of countries with respect to their disease magnitude using the different measures of disease magnitude as ranking factors. Besides, the reliability of changes in ranks of countries with respect to the magnitude of a disease at different points in time, using the different measures of disease magnitude as a ranking factor, is unknown. Therefore, this study was designed to analyze the reliability of different measures of disease magnitude in ranking disease magnitude across countries.

METHODS

Three types of measures of disease magnitude were compared in this study. It is clear that each measure conveys different information on its own at country level and at international level. Besides, each measure has its own advantage and disadvantage. In this study, the ability of these measures to make comparisons in relative magnitude of disease across countries both at a point in time and at different points of time was investigated. The three measures used are described as follows:

Number of cases of a disease: This prevalence measure is the number (count) of all cases of a disease in a country during a defined period. Similar measures under this category include number of cases in a country divided by constant figures like the global cases, and global population etc.

National prevalence: This measure is the number of persons with a disease in a country within a defined period divided by total population of the same country at the same period. It indicates the proportion of a population in that country with a disease at a certain point time.

Comparative prevalence: This prevalence measure is considered to be the number of people with a disease in a country at a defined period divided by a standard population of the same country as adjusted by the *WHO population* to account for variations in *age structure* of the population.

For the purpose of this analysis, two country-level prevalence data sets for Diabetes from international Diabetes Federation (IDF) were used. The two diabetes magnitude data sets used were country level estimates for 2011 and 2030. Diabetes data for both points of times were available for 216 countries/territories.

Rank transformation

Before the start of any analysis, the actual country-level prevalence values for the three prevalence measures were transformed in to ranks. Rank 1 was assigned to the smallest value in all cases. The *simple rank* ranking type was used in all cases. The *Mean rank* is assigned to ties. The national prevalence ranking and WHO standard ranking have 20 and 19 ties respectively.

After this transformation, the three prevalence measures are described as *ranking factors* as they are used to produce relative ranks of the countries. This rank transformation resulted in three rank variables. The resulting rank variables were termed as case ranks, national prevalence ranks and comparative prevalence ranks.

The Comparative prevalence (using world Population standard) was used as a ranking parameter to produce *reference ranks* against which each of the above three ranks were compared for reliability. This parameter is the number of people with a disease in a country at a defined period divided by a standard population adjusted to *World population* to account for variations in age structure of the population.

Rank deviation method

A *rank deviation* in this study refers to the difference between a country's reference rank and its rank in each of the three ranks: case ranks, national prevalence ranks and comparative prevalence ranks. A rank deviation for the case ranking, for instance, was case ranks minus the reference ranks. This process has resulted in three rank deviation variables: Rank deviation for case ranks, national prevalence ranks and comparative prevalence ranks.

The rank deviation variables were then described for each ranking factor using proportions, sum, mean, ranges and standard deviations. As the rank deviation variables had positive, negative and zero values, each of these types of rank deviations were described.

Rank reliability

To test the reliability of the ranks produced from the three ranking factors, three steps were applied. First, each of the ranks was correlated with the reference rank using the non-parametric correlation. Then all the rank variables were fitted in to the reliability analysis model to check for internal consistency among the ranks. Finally, factor analysis of all the ranks was conducted to check whether these ranks measure the same construct or not.

Rank difference method

A *rank difference* in this study refers to the difference between a country's rank in 2030 and 2011 (2030 ranks minus 2011 ranks) using the same ranking factor. This has resulted in three rank difference variables: Case rank difference, national prevalence rank differences and comparative prevalence rank differences.

Similar to the rank deviations, the rank differences were described using proportions, sum, ranges, means and standard deviations for each type of rank deviations in every rank difference variable.

Reliability of rank differences

In order to examine the reliability of the rank differences that have resulted from the three ranking factors, agreement statistics and non-parametric correlations among the rank difference variables were performed. Besides, *standard rank differences* were computed by *standardizing* the population.

This standardization was conducted by applying 2011 prevalence figures to 2030 population to calculate standard number of cases for 2011. The 2011 case numbers were also applied to 2030 population to calculate standard national prevalence for 2011.

Comparative prevalence for both 2011 and 2030 were applied to 2030 population to calculate standard number of cases for the comparative prevalence.

Each rank difference was then correlated with its standard rank difference to measure the reliability of comparison of disease magnitude at two points in time. The resulting values were presented as reliability of the measures in comparing disease magnitude across countries at two points in time.

RESULTS

The relative ranks of the countries in the three ranking factors were compared using agreement in the relative ranks to the reference ranks.

Ranks obtained from the three ranking factors were compared with this reference rank by subtracting the reference rank from each rank. This has resulted in rank deviations for each of the three ranking factors.

Case rank deviations

Comparison of case ranks and reference ranks has very low level of agreement. There were no absolute agreements (ties) between the case ranking and reference rank.

The rank deviations ranged from -208 to +164. The sum of the total deviations of the ranks from the reference rank was 16,473 indicating a mean (SD) deviation of 75.9 (49.2) units from the reference rank. When looking in to the direction of deviation of the ranks, the mean (SD) of 92 (42.4%) countries with negative deviations was -89.5 (57) while that of the 125 (57.6%) countries with positive deviations were +65.9 (39.8).

With regard to the distribution of the number of rank units that the case ranks deviate from the reference ranks, 90% were deviated by at least 15 rank units and 50% were deviated by at least 70 rank units from the respective reference ranks. About 30% deviated by at least 100 rank units from the respective reference ranks.

National prevalence rank deviations

The level of absolute agreement, ties, between the national prevalence ranks and reference rank was only 9 (4.1%). The rank deviations ranged from -82 to +72.5 rank units. Among all the countries, 114(52.5%) had a negative deviation with mean (SD) of -20 (17.5) units. The rest 94 (43.3%) countries had a positive deviation with mean (SD) of +24.4 (18.2) units. The sum of all deviations was 4,582 rank units.

Looking in to the distribution of the rank deviations, about 35% of the countries had a rank deviation of less than 10 units.

About half of the countries had rank deviations of less than 15 units. About 25% of the cases had rank deviations of more than 30 units. Less than 10% had rank deviations more than 50 units.

Comparative prevalence rank deviations

Both the comparative prevalence and the reference standard used in this study are forms of standardized prevalence measures but differ in the population structure used for the adjustment.

The absolute agreement between the ranks from these two ranking factors was 101 (45.9%). The rank deviations ranged from -6.5 to +5.

Fifty cases (23%) had negative deviation with mean (SD) of -1.86 (1.49) units. Sixty-six (30.4%) countries had a positive rank deviation, the mean (SD) of which was +1.4(0.86).

Table 1. Summary of the comparison of three ranks with the reference rank

Rank types	Absolute agreement	Positive deviations	Negative deviations
Number of cases	-	125(57.6%)	92(42.4%)
National prevalence	9(4.1%)	94(43.3%)	114(52.5%)
Comparative prevalence	101(45.9%)	66(30.4%)	50(23%)

Reliability analysis

The spearman's rank correlation between case ranks and reference ranks indicate a very low negative correlation (*spearman's rho*=-.042, p=0.54). The level of correlation between the national prevalence rank and the reference rank was high and statistically significant (*spearman's rho*=0.902, P=0.000). The correlation between comparative prevalence ranks and reference ranks shows singularity.

The chronbach's alpha which is based on the average inter-rank correlation was 0.768. The case rank has the lowest item-total correlation as compared to the other ranks. If this item is deleted, the internal consistency among the other three ranks will increase to 0.977. Analysis of the inter-rank correlation matrix also shows that the case rank has no statistically significant correlation with all the other three ranks.

To check whether these four ranks measure the same construct, factor analysis using the principal component extraction method was conducted. This analysis extracted one component suggesting that these four ranks measure the same construct. This component explained 71.8% of the variance. Here again, the rank that used number of cases had the lowest factor loading coefficient.

Comparison of rank differences

At this level, disease magnitude at two points of time were compared using the same ranking factor at a time. And then the results of these comparisons were contrasted. The purpose of this step is to analyze to what extent these ranks can effectively compare prevalence data of a single disease at different points in time. Country ranks for 2011 was subtracted from the 2030 rank to see the rank deviations, the change in the relative rank between 2011 and 2030.

Case rank differences

The difference between country ranks for 2030 and 2011 using the number of cases as a ranking factor shows that 82 (37.7%) countries had negative rank differences indicating that these countries will have lower rank on the spectrum in 2030 as compared to their rank in 2011. The mean (SD) rank difference for these countries was -7.3(5.5) and values ranged from -1 to -15. Based on this rank difference 28(12.9%) countries will maintain their current rank, had rank difference of zero. The rest 107 (49.3%) countries had positive rank differences ranging from +1 to +18 with mean (SD) of 5.6(4.2).

National prevalence rank differences

Analysis of the rank differences using the national prevalence as a ranking factor indicates that 118 (54.4%) countries have a negative rank difference that ranges from -0.5 to -22 with mean (SD) risk difference of -7.2(5.26). Based on this rank 14(6.4%) countries will maintain their current rank, zero rank difference. The rest 85 (39.2%) countries had positive risk difference with mean (SD) of +9.9(11.54) units.

Comparative prevalence rank differences

Using this ranking factor to compare country ranks in 2011 and 2030 indicates that 126 (58%) countries will have a negative rank difference indicating that they will have lower rank than their current status which indicates lower relative prevalence. The mean (SD) of these negative risk deviations was -3.6 (3.23) units. Based on this ranking factor, 18(8.3%) countries will maintain their 2011 rank of relative prevalence, zero rank difference. The rest 73 (33.7%) countries have positive risk difference with mean (SD) of +6.3(5.46) units. Comparison of rank differences in the three ranking factors is summarized in the following figure.

Reliability analysis of the rank differences

To examine the consistency of the three measures in comparing a country rank at two points in time, the rank differences from the three ranking factors were analyzed. After recoding of the negative, zero and positive rank differences in to -1, 0 and 1 respectively, the agreements in the rank differences between and among the three ranking factors were compared.

The level of agreement in the categories of rank difference between the case and comparative prevalence ranking factors was 114 (52.5%). The level of agreement in categories of rank differences between national prevalence and comparative prevalence ranking factors was 110 (50.7%). The level of agreement between Case and national prevalence was 116 (53.4%). The agreement among the three ranking factors was 72(33.2%).

The level of disagreement was described as *transcendence* when the ranking disagreement between two ranking factors crosses zero. That is when a positive rank difference in one factor is negative in the other factor.

Table 2. Agreement statistics of the rank differences from the ranking factors

Ranking factors	Agreement	Transcendence	Kappa
Cases vs comparative	114 (52.5%)	59 (27.2%)	0.214 (P=0.000)
National prev. vs comparative	110 (50.7%)	81 (37.3%)	0.099 (P=0.084)
Case vs. national prev.	116 (53.4%)	67 (30.8%)	0.215 (P=0.000)

The correlation among the rank differences from the three ranking factors indicates a statistically significant positive correlation. Similar to the kappa statistics the correlation between case rank differences versus comparative prevalence rank differences, and case rank differences versus national prevalence rank differences were 0.383 (P=0.000) and 0.345 (P=0.000) respectively. The correlation between comparative prevalence rank differences and national prevalence rank differences was relatively low with value of 0.153 (P=0.024).

Besides, analysis of the change in the overall magnitude of the disease between 2011 and 2030 indicates contradicting conclusions among the different measures. Based on the number of case and national prevalence measures, the change in the magnitude of the disease shows a dramatic increase between 2011 and 2030. But using the comparative prevalence method, there will be no statistically significant change in the magnitude of the disease between 2011 and 2030.

Final reliability analysis of each of the rank differences against their *standard rank* differences shows that the case rank difference, the national prevalence rank difference, and comparative prevalence rank difference have 0.211(P=0.002), 0.431(P=0.000) and 0.498(P=0.000) respectively.

DISCUSSION

Ranking countries for their disease magnitude using the number of cases as a ranking factor is less correlated to the reference rank and other rankings too. The other three ranks have higher level of correlation among them. Hence using number of cases and national prevalence would provide different ranks to countries with regard to the magnitude of disease. Therefore, it would be more informative if both measures are used to rank countries by their magnitude of disease at a point in time. Presenting ranks of countries from both parameters would help audiences understand a better picture of the status of the countries relative to each other.

There is generally low level consistency among the three measures in comparing changes in disease magnitude overtime. Even there is a difference in describing the overall change in magnitude of diabetes between the two periods. Comparison of 2011 and 2030 data using number of cases and national prevalence indicates a statistically significant increase in the magnitude of diabetes between the two periods. However, the comparison using the WHO standard prevalence doesn't show a statistically significant increase in the magnitude of diabetes between 2011 and 2030 based on the estimated figures.

The power of comparative prevalence in comparing disease magnitude across time needs to be revisited. Comparison using the number of cases and national prevalence figures to some extent should exhibit better correlation with comparisons using comparative prevalence if changes are going to be considered. Better measures changes in disease magnitude that can account for changes in population structure may be needed.

There are some limitations associated with this study. First, the data used were from a single disease. Reliability of the measures may vary based on the disease considered in the analysis. Second, only two points of time were used to measure the reliability of changes in disease magnitude among the different measures. More points in time would yield better picture of the reliability of measuring changes across time. Finally, an alternate measure was not used to compare the reliability of changes of disease magnitude at two points. Findings are based on internal consistency among the available measures.

In conclusion, this study has shown that national prevalence and comparative prevalence measures have high level of internal consistency in comparing disease magnitude across countries at a point in time. Even though the comparative prevalence had better reliability, all the three measures have lower reliability in comparing changes in disease magnitude across countries at two points in time.

ACKNOWLEDGMENT

I extend our acknowledgement to International Diabetes Federation (IDF) which owns the country level diabetes estimates for 2011 and 2030 that are used in this analysis.

Conflict of interest: none

Disclaimer: The views expressed in this article are solely that of the author and do not necessarily reflect that of IDF and Monash University. I also declare that the reliabilities analyzed in this study are exclusively the reliabilities the three measures in comparing disease magnitude across countries at a single point and two points in time. These are not, by any means, the reliabilities of the estimates of diabetes magnitude for 2011 and 2030.

REFERENCES

[1]   Rachel N. Chronic diseases in developing countries: Health and Economic burdens. Ann NY Acad Sci 2008;1136:70-9.

[2]   World Health Organization. Global burden of disease: Quantifying the burden of disease from mortality and morbidity. Accessed 2012 Jan 03. URL: http://www.who.int/healthinfo/global_burden_ disease/metrics_daly/en/

[3]   Sudhir A, Kara H. Disability adjusted life years: a critical review. J Economics 1997;16:685-702.

[4]   Central Intelligence agency. The world fact book: Country comparison for HIV prevalence rates. Accessed 2012 Jan 03. URL: https://www.cia.gov/library/publications/the-world-factbook/rankorder/ 2155rank.html

[5]   Rightdiagnosis.com. About prevalence and incidence statistics. Accessed 2012 Jan 03. URL: http://www.rightdiagnosis.com/admin/preval.htm

[6]   Sarah W. et al. Global prevalence of Diabetes: Estimates for the year 2000 and projections for 2030. Diabetes Care 2004;27(5):1047-53.

[7]   Countries of the world. Diabetes prevalence-country rankings 2010. Accessed 2012 Jan 03. URL: http://www.allcountries.org/ranks/diabetes_prevalence_country_ranks.html

[8]   Ahmad OB, et al. Age standardization of rates: A new WHO standard. Accessed 2012 Jan 03. URL: http://www.who.int/healthinfo/paper31.pdf

In: Public Health Yearbook 2013
Editor: Joav Merrick

ISBN: 978-1-63321-095-0
© 2014 Nova Science Publishers, Inc.

Chapter 19

INTEGRATION OF GRADUATES OF A HEALTHCARE MANAGEMENT PROGRAM IN PUBLIC AND PRIVATE HEALTHCARE SERVICES IN ISRAEL FROM AN INTERDISCIPLINARY PERSPECTIVE

*Nitza Davidovitch, PhD**

Ariel University Center of Samaria, Ariel, Israel

ABSTRACT

The Ariel University Center has a unique interdisciplinary program in healthcare management. Objective: In the current study we sought to investigate points of contact between the academic world and the professional field by following the professional integration of graduates of healthcare management at the Ariel University Center and their satisfaction with their training, job, and profession, from an interdisciplinary perspective. Study group: A survey was held among all 1,327 students who graduated from the Department of Healthcare Management in 2011. Methods: Data collection was performed through self-completed electronic questionnaires and personally distributed questionnaires, which included questions on graduates' current place of work and satisfaction with their degree. Results: The findings indicate that graduates are very satisfied with their interdisciplinary studies in the department. Students from the Arab sector, students who began their studies at an older age, and students who are more affluent, reported higher satisfaction with their studies. Most students intend to pursue an advanced degree in the profession. Conclusion: Significantly, graduates who worked in the field before beginning their studies at a relatively older age, when they already had families to support, were nonetheless very satisfied with the program, despite or maybe because of its interdisciplinary emphasis. Thus, this emphasis obviously plays a crucial part in the adequate training of healthcare professionals.

Keywords*: Graduates, health care management, interdisciplinary

---

* Correspondence: Nitza Davidovitch, PhD, Director of Academic Development and Assessment, Ariel University Center of Samaria, IL-40700 Ariel, Israel. E-mail: d.nitza@ariel.ac.il.

INTRODUCTION

Healthcare management studies train people for management positions in various levels of the healthcare system. Today, promotion within the public healthcare system in Israel requires an academic degree. Tools acquired at school allow healthcare personnel to apply for senior management positions and gain promotion. The Department of Healthcare Management at the Ariel University Center in Israel trains students for a Baccalaureate degree as part of the School of Health Sciences and aims to help train much-needed administrators for middle and high level management roles in the Israeli healthcare system. The Department of Healthcare Management boasts an innovative program, one of few in Israel. Studies combine classes in administration in different fields with specific professional knowledge related to the needs of the healthcare system. The program is based on the strong foundation provided at the Ariel University Center in the fields of teaching, research, and social sciences. The program imparts to students an extensive base in business management and behavioral sciences, together with a focus on components of the healthcare and medical systems. Based on these tools, students learn and practice how to apply management tools to unique problems in the Israeli healthcare system. The faculty hails from different medical and administrative fields and includes senior managers as well as heads of national health funds and hospital directors.

Once a year the department organizes a healthcare conference, held at the Israeli Knesset and focusing on healthcare issues on the public agenda. The conference is attended by senior representatives of the entire healthcare system, such as the chairman of the Knesset, the Minister of Health, Chairman of the Labor and Welfare Committee, directors of health funds and hospitals, Chairman of the Israel Medical Association, top medical officers, as well as Members of Knesset and ministers, and well-known public and academic figures. In addition, studies in diverse fields related to medical administration, health, and medicine, are conducted at the Department of Healthcare Management. Some of the subjects studied are public attitudes towards health promoting and risk behaviors, preparations within the healthcare system for applying the Dying Patient Act, healthcare systems around the world, topics in health education and public health, and topics in the field of policy planning. An annual national survey on core issues within the healthcare system is conducted as well. The department initiates collaborations with researchers of community- and hospital-based medicine and with the pharmaceutical industry.

In the field of healthcare management, graduates are required to demonstrate management and assessment skills, comprehension, interpersonal communication skills, an ethical approach to the moral standards of the profession, and the ability to work in a multidisciplinary team. Academization of the profession is relatively new. It has developed over the years together with the growing demand for evidence based practice (EBP) (1). Academization has led to enhancement through research, an extensive interdisciplinary system of instruction, and the high academic standards of the profession and its students.

Higher education systems in Israel and elsewhere are required to prove the effectiveness of their teaching programs. The authorities, as well as parents and students, wish to ensure that students receive the education promised them. Those in charge of accreditation require the various departments to operate measures for evaluation of outcomes in order to ensure that students have the opportunity to achieve the academic goals and to reach a high level of proficiency in their chosen field. In Israel, as in other western countries, the Council for

Higher Education (CHE) operates a quality control system of schools of higher education. However, in order to maintain constant control processes, the initiative for operating this system should come not only from government factors rather from within academic departments. An important component of the quality control process of study outcomes is graduate tracking. Tracking may be based on graduate surveys or on employer surveys, although for ethical reasons graduate surveys are more convenient. Richter and Ruebling (2) stated that surveys of healthcare management graduates should include three main components: 1) assessment of graduates' perceptions of the level of training they received at school, 2) gathering information on graduates' professional activities since graduation, 3) gathering demographic data on graduates, such as their workplace and field of work. Significantly, the purpose of the Department is to train graduates to work in a well-defined profession. Therefore, graduates' employment and job satisfaction are particularly important and reflect attainment of the major goal of the program.

In the current study we explore points of contact between the academic world and the professional field by tracking the professional integration of graduates of the Department of Healthcare Management at the Ariel University Center and their satisfaction with their training, job, and profession, from an interdisciplinary perspective.

CASE STUDY: THE HEALTHCARE MANAGEMENT PROGRAM

The Department of Healthcare Management at the Ariel Center was established in 1999, as part of the School of Health Sciences. Rationale for opening the department: The department was established to satisfy the need for skilled academic personnel in paramedical professions, in order to improve the standard of medical services in Israel. The School combines medical management studies with studies of the paramedical professions.

Program planners and faculty: The program was designed by academic faculty members from the department, senior healthcare managers from the field, senior physicians, and healthcare management personnel, as evident in several unique courses, as well as enrichment courses.

Structure of the program: The program includes the main areas that have a significant lack of personnel trained in modern healthcare management.

The program focuses on the academic field (training graduates to have independent learning and inquiry skills, professional interest, and a desire to learn about innovations in the profession, who recognize the importance of research as readers, research partners, and independent researchers), the ethical-behavioral field (training graduates in knowledge and awareness of patient rights, who maintain individual confidentiality, rules of professional ethics, legal aspects, and the needs of individuals and of the community; training graduates to be able to work in professional and multidisciplinary teams as required by modern medicine and to have the necessary skills and tools to conduct efficient and proper interpersonal communications), and in the professional field (training graduates in knowledge and skills in the field, imparting the necessary tools and skills to engage in healthcare management).

Faculty members who teach in the program come both from within the Ariel Center, academics engaged in teaching and research in the natural sciences and social sciences, as well as lecturers and expert teaching aides from the field.

In the current study we focused on the satisfaction of department graduates, both with their academic studies and with their work in the field, with the aim of examining the relationship between the academic world and the field as perceived by graduates, where our goal is to strengthen ties between academic studies and graduate achievements by the end of their studies, and between the labor market and work conditions that await them in the field.

HEALTH MANAGEMENT AS AN INTERDISCIPLINARY PROFESSION

The term "multidisciplinary" was introduced to the discourse of higher education in the mid-1990s, when a decision was made in Israel to recognize academic colleges as schools of higher education in addition to universities. Colleges were authorized to grant baccalaureate degrees in their own right, without the patronage of a university, degrees recognized by the Council for Higher Education (3). This development brought about a long-term change in the academic world, and significantly increased the popular demand for higher education. Opening the gates of higher education to colleges – both public and private – was part of the attempt to increase the accessibility of higher education. However for certain sectors of the population this was not enough. One result was the advent of "General BA" programs. These programs had been offered by universities even before the accessibility revolution, but the colleges were the first to give these programs a prominent place. The General BA degree, once considered less attractive, was recast and marketed under the title of a "multidisciplinary" degree. Programs offered a new approach to studies – learning a little in a variety of fields. What began as an attempt by colleges to attract potential consumers became a popular and trendy course of study. Moreover, universities too began marketing programs that had previously been played down, adopting the new refined title. At the same time, and with no real connection to "multidisciplinarity", a paradigmatic shift began to occur within the academic discourse, which edged closer to an "interdisciplinary" approach. The interdisciplinary approach involves transitions and the crossing of traditional disciplinary borders (4), creating new fields of collaboration between two or more disciplines. The terms "multidisciplinary" and "interdisciplinary" are often mistakenly used interchangeably.

MULTIDISCIPLINARY PROGRAMS

Multidisciplinary programs are higher studies that give students a broad academic foundation. Rather than specializing in a single subject, students study a variety of subjects to earn a degree. Studying in a multidisciplinary setting means avoiding the need to choose a predetermined list of subjects and disciplines that comprise a conventional basket of knowledge. Multidisciplinary studies enable presentation of topics not included in regular programs, without going through the formal process otherwise required for integrating disciplines in the curriculum. Some claim that initiation of multidisciplinary programs reflects the response of higher education to social changes and to its role as an agent of socialization (5), since multidisciplinary programs enable, among other things, flexibility in presenting contents and messages on construction of identity, adaptation to the oft-changing labor market, opportunities for closing gaps in society and for expanding equal opportunities.

Multidisciplinary programs began emerging throughout the world as early as four decades ago. At first they occupied a minor place, but they have since become a significant part of the academic world. For example, in the US, graduates of such programs numbered 7,000 in 1973, but by 2005 they numbered 30,000 a year (6).

Even programs not considered essentially multidisciplinary incorporate multidisciplinary courses. A survey held among US schools of higher education shows that 40% of all faculties offer at least one multidisciplinary course (7).

At the same time, there is also a contrasting trend in the US, whereby multidisciplinary programs are gradually being discontinued. For example, Arizona International, the multidisciplinary school at Miami University, and the multidisciplinary department at Wayne State University have been closed, despite reasonable and even high demand. Other multidisciplinary programs have suffered cutbacks, for example the Department of Multidisciplinary Studies at the Appalachian State University and at the George Mason University. Some claim that the cutbacks or closure of these institutions stems from the hegemony of the traditional disciplinary approach over the multidisciplinary approach (8).

In Israel multidisciplinary programs were first initiated with the establishment of academic colleges, which opened multidisciplinary programs for their students. However they were stigmatized as programs intended for students incapable of specializing in a specific discipline. They began as "general studies", a title later changed to overcome their negative connotations. Multidisciplinary programs first emerged in the social sciences and the humanities, but they are currently offered in many other fields as well. Multidisciplinary programs are characterized by a great deal of flexibility and they include a specialty in one or two fields, as well as study courses and units in diverse areas. The multidisciplinary track, once chosen by default, has become fairly popular in Israel. Multidisciplinary programs at the Bar Ilan University and its satellite colleges (Ashkelon, Western Galilee, Jordan Valley, Safed) alone encompassed 14,870 students from 2001 to 2007. This trend, which began in the colleges, has spread to all academic institutions, and a wide range of multidisciplinary programs are available. For example, Tel Aviv University has a variety of multidisciplinary programs in subjects such as the arts, religious studies, computational linguistics, etc. Ben Gurion University offers combinations of programs in the humanities and the natural sciences, management and safety engineering, as well as a multidisciplinary degree combining social sciences, natural sciences, and the humanities. The Hebrew University offers a multidisciplinary degree in social sciences and the humanities, the arts, psychology and education, etc. Similar programs can be found at other schools which seem to have joined the multidisciplinary trend. Despite the significant role of multidisciplinary programs in academia, the academic concept and the multidisciplinary concept are based on essentially different foundations.

ACADEMIC DISCIPLINES AND MULTIDISCIPLINARITY – ARE THEY COMPATIBLE?

The multidisciplinary approach is at odds with the academic concept that requires students to go into precise detail on specific subjects, cite sources and scholarly opinions, and present "strictly scientific" facts with no uplifting "deviations". The multidisciplinary approach may be perceived as a realistic necessity stemming from the circumstances – but the challenge posed by this approach is also evident, the need to combine diverse subjects and many aspects requiring generalization, knowledge, and scholarship. We have no choice but to admit that scholars, in their role as erudite intellectuals, are in decline. However the parallel courses of the multidisciplinary approach and academia fill different but interrelated needs, with the former approach mostly seeking to fill thirsty students' desire in subjects that interest them (9).

Academia and multidisciplinarity are to a great degree opposites. While multidisciplinary programs combine a wide range of disciplines, academia focuses by nature on narrow fields of expertise, and this trend increases in time. In order to reach academic achievements, which are translated into recognized status, research budgets and innovations, promotion, prestige, and publications, one has almost no choice but to specialize in a specific narrow field, i.e., "know more about less and less", as a result of the expansion of knowledge and the gargantuan databases currently available.

Universities are engaged in an accelerated process of professionalization and specialization in narrow fields, and innovations are limited to these fields. This is the basis for understanding the reserved attitude of the academic world to multidisciplinary programs, which include a variety of subjects in diverse fields, in contrast to academia, which prefers narrow expertise (9).

Today the west in general and the US in particular, place colleges at the base of the academic pyramid, together with undergraduate studies in very general programs such as "liberal arts" or "sciences". The goal is to provide a tertiary education that offers an introduction to the basic concepts of scientific disciplines, practice in reading scientific material, albeit at a basic level, and in writing papers based on data gathered from authorized sources (with proper references), as well as initial experience with structured summaries incorporating students' personal conclusions.

At this stage, students learn academic reading and written comprehension. At this stage and the next (specialized studies), academic schools are interested in imparting to students two additional skills: learning the "rules of the game" and the research methods of a defined discipline and the critical ability to ask well-defined and logical research questions (not necessarily limited to that discipline).

In the third stage, the school must train students for independent research, i.e., develop the ability to ask questions, formulate a structured plan for finding the answer, and develop tools for exploring the quality and validity of results. These abilities may form in a narrowing field, as students advance in their training and study the subject more intensively. But this is not imperative and certainly not exclusory. Recently, more and more academic settings of a distinct "multidisciplinary" nature are being established in the western world and in Israel as well.

This trend is arousing criticism and sometimes even hostility, derision, and malicious contempt on the part of long-time academic personnel and those who see themselves as keepers of the traditions of "serious" scientific research. However, the CHE has gradually been approving more and more programs of this type.

Today the western academic world is arriving at a recognition of the urgent need to train scientific personnel on a high academic level in the entire man-environment complex. There is an increasing need for graduates of schools of higher education with broad knowledge and judgment beyond their defined professional specialty.

The instinctive response of many academics is that this trend will necessarily lead to "amateurism" and "superficiality" – but is this indeed true? Does "understanding" necessarily rerequire specialization?

BETWEEN THE MULTIDISCIPLINARY AND THE INTERDISCIPLINARY

While the multidisciplinary approach refers to the non-integrative mixing of fields, albeit maintaining the methodology and premises of each discipline, the interdisciplinary approach refers to the crossing of traditional disciplinary borders to create a new collaboration between two or more disciplines. The purpose of interdisciplinarity is to create a cognitive advantage that would probably not have been possible by means of the disciplinary approach (10).

The academic split into disciplines has existed at modern and western universities since the late nineteenth century (11), when universities underwent secularization (12). Over the years, the accepted conception was that professionalization and scientization occur within disciplines – namely, focus and focusing are the only way of generating professional scientific knowledge (13).

Nonetheless, despite the hegemony of the disciplinary approach to knowledge, a paradigmatic shift towards the interdisciplinary approach to knowledge may be currently identified in Israel (14) and elsewhere (15), and some claim that its popularity is unprecedented (16). The adoption of a new approach to knowledge, research, and teaching, reflects social and cultural processes that occurred in western society and that have affected the system of higher education as well, creating an intellectual change reflecting the changes in how people think about how they think (17).

Today more than ever, schools of higher education are required to generate and produce interdisciplinary knowledge (18). Proof of this can be found in the significant attention and generous funding showered on interdisciplinary fields of research, such as nanotechnology, molecular biology, AIDS, and gender studies (6). This demand requires higher education to offer interdisciplinary programs, embrace an innovative approach, and be proactive in modifying former modes of operation.

There is a built-in conflict between the traditional academic concept and changes occurring in the world of knowledge (19). Researchers involved in interdisciplinary activities must come to terms with the possibility that this course of action will alienate them from the traditional disciplinary community to which they are professionally connected. In addition, they might endanger their professional prestige and legitimacy –strong forces that affect the professional life of faculty members. Thus, it seems that faculty members who identify with academia and strive to advance within it might find themselves between a rock and a hard place when required to act according to organizational norms of academia while recognizing that research within the discipline might limit their range of motion.

The reason for this has to do with the fact that success in contemporary academia depends on researchers' ability to advance within their discipline. This success determines various elements related to their academic position: tenure, promotion, and research budgets. Professional legitimacy in academia is entirely within the disciplinary specialty, and researchers are required to develop skills in a certain specific domain (20).

In contrast to academia, which has not reached a decisive view of interdisciplinarity, interdisciplinarity is considered extremely desirable in industry and scientific associations (21). The differences between the demands of academia and of the world at large have created a paradoxical state in which only academic institutions still require bispecialization (22). This matter creates certain problems, as faculty members who wish to engage in interdisciplinary activities cannot do so in a void, rather they need a supportive, sharing, and resourceful academic environment (23) to encourage interdisciplinary activities and allocate resources.

Some of those who tried and managed to conduct interdisciplinary research despite the built-in challenges reached interesting achievements and successes. For example Tucker (24) sought to explore the nature of interdisciplinary doctoral studies versus disciplinary studies in social work and social sciences. He sampled interdisciplinary data and compared them to disciplinary studies in social work and social sciences. Based on data from a period of 13 years, he found that students of interdisciplinary doctoral programs eventually gained a stronger research orientation and greater research productivity. Some claim that in order to assimilate the interdisciplinary approach both in research and in study programs, there is need for change not only in the distribution of work within schools of higher education, rather a more extensive transformation of the organizational culture of academia (15). In this context, one of the difficulties with assimilating the interdisciplinary approach in academia is the vagueness that surrounds the desire and capacity to change what is perceived as fundamental organizing principle – the disciplinary division of knowledge (25).

In conclusion, the interdisciplinary approach relies on sources from different fields and strives to integrate them. Many of these fields are part of a wider cultural whole, from which they are separated in a fairly arbitrary manner in order to create the complex of "multidisciplinarity". The multidisciplinary approach often lacks a clear research direction and scientific discipline. This is at odds with the academic orientation, sometimes radically so. For obvious reasons, university institutions striving for excellence find it difficult to resolve this tension. At two major Israeli universities, the Hebrew University and Tel Aviv University, no multidisciplinary tracks have been established, rather only multidisciplinary programs. One reason may be the concern that dealing with a wide variety of subjects with no option of intensive study might have a detrimental effect on excellence and result in superficiality.

The multidisciplinary tracks, worthy of all encouragement and appreciation, are problematic also for their lack of a defined goal; most graduates do not end up working in their field. Their academic status is unclear and options of employment and promotion are limited, both in the academic world and elsewhere. Interestingly, the multidisciplinary tracks are nurtured and encouraged by academic schools in Israel as they tend to attract many students, among other things from the security forces and people who are already part of the work force and have knowledge in some field. Studies in these tracks are considered relatively easy, due to their eclectic nature.

Obviously, students studying in multidisciplinary programs cannot be expected to demonstrate proficiency in all the fields they study. But in contrast to students who focus on a narrow topic within their field of specialty, they should theoretically demonstrate greater proficiency in several domains, even if it is not possible to study these fields intensively while at school. Studying multiple subjects from a multidisciplinary perspective requires integration of the various subjects from a broad, balanced outlook, while taking care to discern between the important and the less important, while avoiding deep inquiries or excessive detail in any specific field.

A primary conception of multidisciplinary studies, maybe even the most significant, is the ability to generalize and to avoid details. A multidisciplinary perspective means dealing with the fundamentals of the topic and forming a general view. The second most important concept is to convey a message and impart values, as much as possible. The third is to focus on the essence and the roots of the topic and its fundamentals from a general multidisciplinary angle that arouses public interest, including connections to current affairs. Multidisciplinary studies, in contrast to disciplinary studies, must be attractive and fascinating, since they appeal to a target population who mostly view them as a personal and challenging window of opportunity to the world, one that they could not otherwise access.

Despite the large number of multidisciplinary programs, they should be distinguished from interdisciplinary research. There is still a long way before the interdisciplinary approach can be adopted as a research approach. In order to enable such significant research in a wide setting, it will be necessary to enlist the academic consensus as well as to change the organizational structure and norms of schools of higher education. To a certain degree, in order for such a change to take place, the academic world must leave the "ivory tower" and recognize the changes that are occurring under its very nose. Today it is clear that interdisciplinarity is the world of tomorrow. We can either recognize this trend and join it or be left behind. However multidisciplinarity requires students, as well as researchers, to begin with disciplinarity. Moreover, disciplinarity is not inconsistent with multidisciplinarity and it is possible to strive for both at the same time, with fields of expertise forming the basic level, and then the sky is the limit.

The Ariel University Center opened a unique program for training high-class academic health management personnel in 1999, an essentially interdisciplinary program for managing healthcare systems. The program aims to facilitate improvements in the quality of service through superior management and it includes disciplinary fields such as management, economics, sociology, psychology, statistics, and health. The current study is unique for its attempt to explore points of contact between the academic and the professional field by tracking the professional integration of graduates of the Department of Healthcare Management at the Ariel University Center and their satisfaction with their training, jobs, and profession, from an interdisciplinary perspective.

METHOD

For this study a survey was conducted among all graduates of the Department of Healthcare Management who graduated between 2002 and 2011, forming a total of nine classes and 1,327 graduates.

Data collection was performed using two main methods: first, through self-completed electronic questionnaires, and secondly, by questionnaires distributed personally to graduates. Program graduates were asked to answer questions regarding their current employment, satisfaction with their degree, how they found their current job, etc., with the aim of identifying trends graduates' integration in the workplace, from an applied professional, personal, and academic perspective.

The research questionnaire –consisted of questions on job features (workplace, position); aspirations for further studies; general satisfaction with the job, the profession, and academic studies; satisfaction with job features, and the degree to which their academic studies trained them for different parts of their work in the field.

RESULTS

As shown in Table 1, most graduates are women and one quarter are men. Some two thirds are Israeli born and about one third were born elsewhere, mostly in the CIS. About two thirds are married with families of their own.

As shown in Table 2, most of the graduates are Jews and one quarter are Arabs. Some 70% reside in Tel Aviv and central Israel. The financial circumstances of most are fair to good.

Table 1. Personal-demographic characteristics (N=83)

Gender		Country of birth			Marital status			Number of children		
M	F	Israel	Eastern Europe and Russia	Other	Married	Single	Divorced	No children	1-2 children	3-5 children
25%	75%	64%	29%	7%	68%	24%	9%	30%	40%	30%

Table 2. Socio-demographic characteristics

Sector		Place of residence			Size of family			Assessment of financial circumstances		
Jews	Arabs	Judea and Samaria	T.A. and central Israel	Remote areas	Small	Medium	Large	Good	Fair	Very bad
75%	25%	13%	71%	16%	43%	32%	25%	52%	44%	4%

Table 3. Employment and studies

State of employment		First year of academic studies			Number of years studied at Ariel			Age upon beginning studies at Ariel			
Employed	Unemployed	2000-2007	2008	2009	3 years	4 years	5 years	25 or younger	26-30	31-40	41+
96%	4%	36%	32%	42%	26%	68%	6%	19%	21%	39%	21%

As shown in Table 3, almost all graduates are employed and the large majority (96%) were employed while studying for their degree. Their work places include: hospitals (49%, of them 40% nurses), health clinics (27%), private medical institutions (9%), Magen David Adom (the Israeli equivalent of the Red Cross) (6%), the Ministry of Health (1%). Only about one quarter completed their degree in the standard period (three years). About three quarters prolonged their studies by one year. Sixty percent were aged 31 or older upon beginning their studies.

Interestingly, 65% reported that they did not plan to change their place of work after graduating. Thirty five percent reported that they planned to change their place of work after graduation, and are even considering a change of career.

As shown in Table 4, over three quarters of graduates did not have a psychometric score when beginning their studies. Most had a matriculation certificate. Most had some experience in the following fields: nursing (54%), paramedics (20%), medical secretary (13%), practical engineer (13%), medical technology (7%), paramedical (3%), and dental assistant (2%). Notably, most of the graduates (80%) reported that a degree in healthcare management was their first choice for academic studies.

Evaluation of the program

As shown in Table 5, most of the graduates (57%) chose to study at the Department of Healthcare
Management because the field is close to their present occupation and will afford opportunities for promotion. About one third chose to study health management at the Ariel Center because the terms of admission were lenient, and about one fifth followed the recommendations of friends or other graduates.

Satisfaction with the baccalaureate program

Eighty percent of graduates were satisfied or very satisfied with their studies. Twenty percent were moderately satisfied None of the graduates were dissatisfied.

Graduates were asked: With what were you most satisfied? Fifty one percent cited the curriculum, 37% the faculty, and 13% the personal attitude, atmosphere, and program flexibility. Graduates were also asked: With what were you not satisfied? Thirty four percent cited the bureaucracy, 23% the inflexible or inconvenient curriculum. Twenty three percent cited repetitions in the curriculum. Thirty six percent stated that they felt the curriculum should have had more courses in management (risks, nursing homes, human resources). At the same time, 22% stated that the mathematics course was irrelevant for them and 18% stated that the courses in accounting, economics, and labor laws were unnecessary.

Recommending the Ariel Center to friends

Ninety one percent of graduates stated that they would recommend the Ariel Center to their friends, and 80% stated that they keep in touch with other graduates. Seventy nine percent would like the Ariel Center to keep in touch with them, and 89% expressed a wish to attend a reunion.

Image of the Department as perceived by graduates

The Department enjoys a good or moderate image, both in absolute terms and in comparison to similar departments in other academic institutions, as perceived by 80%-90% of graduates (see Table 6).

Average grade

The prevalent final grade ranges from 80 to 87. One third graduated with an average grade of 88 or higher. One third of students graduated with an average grade between 70 and 79. None of the students had an average final grade lower than 70 (see table 7).

Level of studies and level of difficulty of the baccalaureate program

Three quarters of the graduates (75%) perceived the level of the baccalaureate program as high or very high. Thirty percent of graduates reported that they found the studies difficult. Sixty nine percent reported that the level of difficulty was reasonable and only one percent reported that the studies were very difficult.

Attitude towards studies

No differences were found between men and women in their satisfaction with studies – which was high among both genders, although women reported having had more difficulty with their studies. Female graduates have a poorer image of the department than male graduates. Women more than men perceive the baccalaureate program as being on a high level (79% versus 62%). However, more women report that the Department has a poor image (see table 8).

Average grades upon graduation – by gender

Only small differences were found between men and women in their average grades upon graduation (see table 9).

Attitude towards studies at the Ariel Center by sector

Attitudes of graduates from the Arab sector were much more positive than those of their peers from the Jewish sector: Almost all Arab graduates (93%) were satisfied with their studies and perceive the baccalaureate program as being on a high level. Eighty percent think that the department has a very good image. Only 13% reported that their studies were difficult (compared to 35% in the Jewish sector).

Table 4. Circumstances and status at admission

Had a psychometric score			Had a matriculation certificate			Study track in high school					
No	Yes	Average score	No	Yes	Average score	Vocational	Technological	Social	Nursing	Literature	Scientific
71%	29%	526	13%	87%	88	5%	6%	19%	21%	39%	21%

Table 5. Reasons for choosing to study health management at the Ariel Center

Reason for choosing	Percentage of graduates
The field is close to my occupation and affords opportunities for promotion	57%
Easy terms of admission	35%
Recommended by graduates	22%
Recommended by friends	21%
The field that most interests me	17%
Geographical convenience	15%
Recommended by workplace	12%

Table 6. Image of the department as perceived by graduates

Image perceived	Percentage of graduates
High – very high	56%
Moderate	42%
Poor	3%

Table 7. Average final grade

Average final grade	Percentage of graduates
94 and higher	7%
88 – 93	26%
80 – 87	46%
70 – 79	21%

Average grade upon graduation by sector

The average grades of Jewish graduates upon graduation are higher than those of their peers from the Arab sector: 38% of graduates from the Jewish sector reported grades of 88 and higher versus only 14% of graduates from the Arab sector (see figure 1).

Attitude towards studies at the Ariel Center – by age upon beginning studies

Graduates who began their studies at a relatively advanced age are more satisfied with the degree, perceive it as being on a higher level, and believe that the department has a better image.

Table 8. Summary of attitudes towards studies at Ariel by gender

Gender	High satisfaction with baccalaureate degree	Good image of the department	Good image compared to other departments	High level of baccalaureate studies	High level of difficulty of studies
Male	81%	70%	68%	62%	15%
Female	78%	51%	53%	79%	37%

Table 9. Average grades upon graduation – by gender

Average final grade	Male	Female
94 and higher	10%	7%
88 - 93	24%	26%
80 - 87	43%	48%
70 - 79	24%	20%

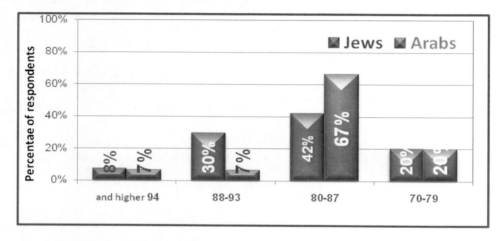

Figure 1. Average grade upon graduation by sector.

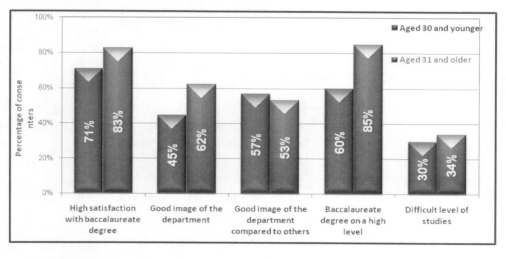

Figure 2. Attitude towards studies at the Ariel Center – by age upon beginning studies.

The difficulties experienced by graduates who began their studies at an older age are slightly higher than those of graduates who began their studies at a younger age (see Figure 2).

Average grade upon graduation – by age upon beginning studies

Older graduates achieved higher grades: 39% received a final grade of 88 or higher versus 26% of younger graduates, and only 15% received low grades versus 29% of younger graduates (see figure 3).

Attitude towards studies at the Ariel Center – by financial circumstances

Well-off graduates reported more positive attitudes than less affluent graduates: they are more satisfied with the program and its level and they perceive the department as having a better image. More affluent graduates reported that their studies were harder (see figure 4).

Average grade upon graduation – by financial circumstances

There are small differences in the average grade upon graduation by financial circumstances as reported by graduates (see Figure 5).

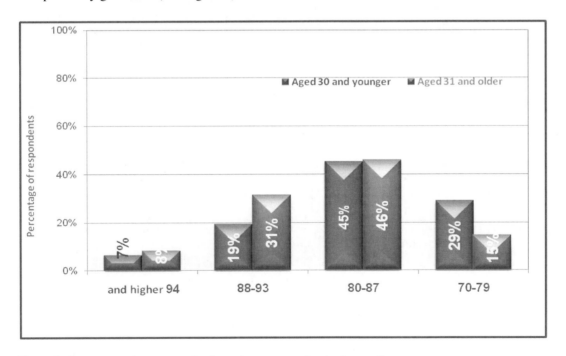

Figure 3. Average grade upon graduation – by age upon beginning studies.

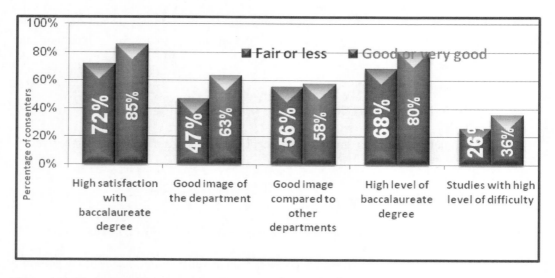

Figure 4. Attitude towards studies at the Ariel Center – by financial circumstances.

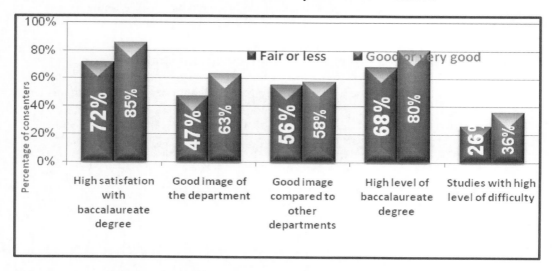

Figure 5. Average grade upon graduation – by financial circumstances.

Table 10. Summary of attitudes towards studies at the Ariel Center by sector

Sector	High satisfaction with baccalaureate degree	Good image of the department	Good image compared to other departments	High level of baccalaureate studies	High level of difficulty of studies
Jews	74%	48%	49%	69%	35%
Arabs	93%	79%	79%	93%	13%

Further studies

Eighty seven percent of graduates stated that they intend to continue their studies. Of these, 75% wish to continue studying at the Ariel Center and 71% wish to study for a Master's degree in healthcare management in the thesis track. Thirty nine percent further stated that they wish to continue to doctoral studies, and 28% said that they would like to join the faculty of an academic institution in the future.

DISCUSSION

In the current study we sought to explore points of contact between academia and the professional field by tracking the professional integration of graduates of the Department of Healthcare Management at the Ariel University Center, and their satisfaction with their training, job, and profession, from an interdisciplinary perspective. The findings of the case study indicate graduates' high satisfaction with the profession and its interdisciplinary approach.

Adopting a multidisciplinary approach, the healthcare management program derives its sources from various fields and strives to integrate them. Despite the concern that a multidisciplinary approach sometimes lacks a clear research focus and a single scientific discipline, often creating a conflict with the academic approach, the Department is currently developing graduate studies in this field, with has become popular around the world. Multidisciplinary tracks are nurtured and encouraged by academic institutions, as they tend to attract a large number of students, including people who are already employed and have a general idea of the field. Studies in these tracks are considered relatively easy due to their eclectic nature. Studies at the Department of Healthcare Management, as indicated by this case study, are selected by students for whom this challenging course of study constituted a significant choice, and the following characteristics were found: 75% of graduates are female, 68% are married, 75% are from the Jewish sector, most graduates live in central Israel, about half are financially well-off, and 60% began their studies at age 31 or older. Regarding their terms of admission: 87% have a matriculation certificate with an average grade of 88; only 29% had a psychometric score when beginning their studies and their average score was 526; 80% stated that healthcare management was their first choice of studies. Regarding employment: 96% are currently employed and a similar proportion were employed during their studies; 75% work at hospitals and clinics; 35% of graduates are thinking of changing their workplace following their studies and 32% are considering a change of career.

When evaluating the program in its multidisciplinary format, graduates referred to their reasons for choosing to study healthcare management at the Ariel Center: Most of the graduates chose to study at the Department of Healthcare Management since the field was close to their field of employment at the time and would afford opportunities for promotion, and one third chose healthcare management at Ariel due to the lenient terms of admission. Regarding satisfaction with the baccalaureate program in its interdisciplinary format: 80% of graduates are satisfied or very satisfied with the program; none of the graduates expressed dissatisfaction; 91% would recommend Ariel to their friends. Graduates' image of the department, both in absolute terms and compared to similar departments at other academic institutions, 80%-90% of graduates perceive the department as having a good or moderate image.

Average grade upon graduation: The prevalent grade ranges from 80 to 87, while one third graduated with a grade of 88 or higher. The standard of studies and their level of difficulty were perceived by three quarters of graduates as being high or very high; 30% of graduates reported that they found the studies difficult.

Attitudes towards the program

By gender: There are no differences between men and women in their satisfaction with the program – which was high among both genders; women had more difficulty with their studies; women more than men believe that baccalaureate studies are on a high level (79% versus 62%).

By sector: Attitudes of graduates from the Arab sector are much more positive than those of their peers from the Jewish sector: almost all (93%) are satisfied with the program and believe that the baccalaureate program is on a high level; 80% believe that the department has a good image; the grades of Jewish graduates upon graduation are higher than those of their peers from the Arab sector.

By age upon beginning studies: Graduates who began their studies at a relatively older age are more satisfied with their degree, believe that it is on a higher level and that the department has a better image; older graduates achieved higher grades.

By financial circumstances: More affluent graduates reported more positive attitudes than less affluent gradiates: they are more satisfied with the program and its standard, and perceive the department as having a better image; more affluent graduates reported that studies were very difficult; there are small differences between the average grade upon graduation by graduates' self-reported financial circumstances.

Plans for further studies: Most graduates had already taken part in advanced courses at the time of survey, possibly attesting to their professional interest and motivation to advance in the profession. Eighty seven percent intend to continue studying for a master's degree. Seventy five percent wish to continue studying for a master's degree at the Ariel University Center. Seventy one percent would like to study for a master's degree at the Department of Healthcare Management. About one half are interested in a change of career to other healthcare fields, particularly nursing. Some 40% are considering a doctoral degree. Nearly 80% are interested in continued contact with the Ariel University Center. Nearly 90% would come to a reunion.

The findings of the quantitative study show that most people studying in the healthcare management program were previously employed in a related field have families to support, and are relatively older. Therefore, their satisfaction with a program that is multidisciplinary by nature and includes elements that are not part of their daily practice is unique, interesting, and challenging, particularly when considering their desire to continue their studies beyond their current job requirements.

Research limitations

In the absence of data on similar surveys in other healthcare management tracks in Israel, the research results could only be compared to surveys conducted in other countries. There is further need for comparative surveys among graduates of departments of healthcare management in Israel.

ACKNOWLEDGMENTS

The author wishes to thank Yair Shapira and Yossi Weiss for the assistance in the preparation of this manuscript.

REFERENCES

[1]   Bridges PH, Bierema LL, Valentine T. The propensity to adopt evidence-based practice among physical therapists. BMC Health Serv Res 2007;7(1):103.

[2]   Richter RR, Ruebling I. Model for development of outcome assessment surveys for allied health educational programs. J Allied Health 2003;3:179-84.

[3]   Council for Higher Education Act [Amendment 10] [Colleges], section 8, 1995. [Hebrew]

[4]   Klein JT. Interdisciplinarity: history, theory, and practice. Detroit: Wayne State University, 1990.

[5]   Rubinstein Y. Disciplinarity, multidisciplinarity, and the education in their midst. In: Karniel T, Bartana O. Hachinuch Usvivato (College Annual). Seminar Hakibbutzim 2001;23:73-90. [Hebrew]

[6]   Levitan D. Interdisciplinary studies: Only a title or content as well? Study day in memory of the late Prof. Ozer Shield, Ariel University Center, 1 February 2011. [Hebrew]

[7]   Lindholm JA, Astin AW, Sax LJ, Korn WS. The American college teacher: National norms for the 2001-2002 HERI Faculty Survey. Los Angeles: UCLA Higher Education Research Institute, 2002.

[8]   Henry S. Disciplinary hegemony meets interdisciplinary ascendancy: Can interdisciplinary/integrative studies survive, and, if so, how. Issues Integr Stud 2005;23:1-37.

[9]   Shiller. Academia and knowledge of Israel – two parallels that will never meet. Ariel 2006;174:85-103.

[10]   BoixMansilla V, Duraising E. Targeted assessment of students' interdisciplinary work: An empirically grounded framework. J Higher Educ 2007;78:218–37.

[11]   Stein MB. Major factors in the emergence of political science as a discipline in Western democracies: A comparative analysis of the United States, Britain, France, and Germany. In: Easton JG, Gunnell L, Graziano D. The development of political science: A comparative survey. London: Routledge, 1991.

[12]   Bracken LJ, Oughton EA. What do you mean? The importance of language in developing interdisciplinary research. Trans Inst Br Geogr 2006;31:371-82.

[13]   Manicas PT. The social sciences since World War II: The rise and fall of scientism. In: Outhwaite W, Turner SP. The SAGE handbook of social science methodology. London: Sage, 2007.

[14]   Shenhar A. The challenge of education in the postmodern era. Makom Lemahshava Basha'ar, bulletins by the Academic Community for Society in Israel. Tel Aviv, December 1999:12. [Hebrew]

[15]   Holley KA. Interdisciplinary strategies as transformative change in higher education. Innovat Higher Educ 2009;34:331-44.

[16]   Catney P, Lerner D. Managing multidisciplinarity: lessons from SUBR:IM. InterdiscipSci Rev 2009;34:290-308.

[17]   Geertz C. The way we think now: Toward an ethnography of modern thought. Bull Am Acad Arts Sci 1982;35:14-34.

[18]   Pfirman S, Collins J, Lowes S, Michaels A. Collaborative efforts: Promoting interdisciplinary scholars. Chron High Educ 2005:B15–B16.

[19]   Lattuca LR. Creating interdisciplinarity: Interdisciplinary research and teaching among college and university faculty. Nashville, TN: Vanderbilt University Press, 2011.

[20]   Interdisciplinarity and Practice of Research. ASHE Higher Educ Rep 2009;35(2):59-74.

[21]   Rhoten D. Interdisciplinary research: Trend or transition. Items Issues 2004;5:6–11.

[22]   Caruso D, Rhoten D. Lead, follow, get out of the way: Sidestepping the barriers to effective practice of interdisciplinarity. A new mechanism for knowledge production and re-integration in the age of information. Hybrid Vigor White Paper, 2001. Accessed 2012 May 20. URL:www.hybridvigor.net/interdis/pubs/hv_pub_interdis-2001.04.30.pdf.

[23]   National Academy of Sciences. Facilitating interdisciplinary research. Washington, DC: National Academies, 2004.

[24]   Tucker DJ. Interdisciplinary in doctoral social work education: does it make a difference?. J Soc Work Educ 2008;44:115-38.

[25]   Chen S, Hsu IC, Wu C. Evaluation of undergraduate curriculum reform for interdisciplinary learning. Teaching Higher Educ 2009;14:161-73.

In: Public Health Yearbook 2013
Editor: Joav Merrick

ISBN: 978-1-63321-095-0
© 2014 Nova Science Publishers, Inc.

Chapter 20

HALTING AND REVERSING THE SPREAD OF HIV/AIDS BY 2015: THE CASE IN ETHIOPIA

*Mulu Abraha, MPH**

John Hopkins University, TSEHAI Project, Addis Ababa, Ethiopia

ABSTRACT

The Millennium Development Goal (MDG) 6 seeks to halt and reverse the spread of HIV by 2015. Objectives: The aim of this study is to predict the status of HIV/AIDS epidemic in Ethiopia by 2015 based on the progresses made so far and taking in to account the constant assumption for prediction. Methods: National level HIV/AIDS prevalence and incidence data were analyzed from different sources. Five levels of analysis were used for five major HIV/AIDS indicators. The analysis included description of trends of prevalence and incidence indicators, development of best-fit models and prediction for future points for the national HIV/AIDS indicators. Findings were presented using numerical and graphic summaries. Results: The prevalence of HIV at PMTCT (prevention of mother-to-child transmission) settings has decreased from 8% in 2006 to 2% in 2010 and is predicted to be 0.3% in 2015. The prevalence of HIV among HCT beneficiaries has decreased from 13.7 % in 2006 to 1.5% in 2010 and is predicted to be 0.3% in 2015. The prevalence of HIV from ANC surveillance sites has decreased from 6.6% in 2001 to 2.3% in 2009 and is predicted to be 0.2% in 2015. HIV prevalence among 15-24 years age group has decreased from 12.4% in 2000 to 2.6% in 2009 and is predicted to be close to zero in 2015. Conclusion: The magnitude of HIV has shown an exponentially decreasing trend during the last decade. Maintaining such rate of decline could possibly lead to the effective attainment of the MDG 6.

Keywords: HIV, AIDS, prevalence, trends, Ethiopia

---

* Correspondence: Mulu Abraha, John Hopkins University, TSEHAI Project, POBox 5605, Addis Ababa, Ethiopia.E-mail: muluabraha@gmail.com.

INTRODUCTION

According to the 2010 Global AIDS report, there were more than 33 million people living with HIV and more than 5 million people are now receiving HIV treatment. The HIV epidemic is getting close to zero in most Asia and pacific regions. However, the Sub-Saharan Africa still bears an inordinate share of the global HIV burden (1). An estimated 22.5 million people are living with HIV in the region - around two thirds of the global total. In 2009 around 1.3 million people died from AIDS in sub-Saharan Africa and 1.8 million people became infected with HIV. Since the beginning of the epidemic 14.8 million children have lost one or both parents to HIV/AIDS (2).

In 2010, about 68% of all people living with HIV resided in sub-Saharan Africa, a region with only 12% of the global population. Sub-Saharan Africa also accounted for 70% of new HIV infections in 2010, although there was a notable decline in the regional rate of new infections. The epidemic continues to be most severe in southern Africa, with South Africa having more people living with HIV (an estimated 5.6 million) than any other country in the world (3).

The current global HIV/AIDS strategy aims to advance global progress in achieving country set targets for universal access to HIV prevention, treatment, care and support and to halt and reverse the spread of HIV and contribute to the achievement of the Millennium Development goals (MDG) by 2015 (3).

With an estimated 1.1 million people living with HIV, Ethiopia has one of the largest populations of HIV infected people in the world. However, HIV prevalence among the adult population is lower than many sub-Saharan African countries. Adult HIV prevalence in 2009 is currently estimated to be between 1.4% and 2.8% (4).

Towards universal access, Ethiopia made significant progresses during the last decade. The number of Health Facilities providing HIV counselling and testing services, prevention and mother to child transmission services and HIV care and treatment services has increased dramatically. Subsequently, the number of people using these services has increased exponentially (5-8).

With these achievements, some suggest that the country can easily meet the stated MDG goals for HIV/AIDS. However, whether these achievements in access and utilization of services will lead to the achievement of MDG 6 for HIV is not systematically answered using a scientific method. Therefore, this study is designed to predict whether Ethiopia can halt and reverse the spread of HIV/AIDS by 2015 based on the progresses made so far and taking in to account the constant indicator assumption for prediction.

METHODS

National level HIV/AIDS prevalence and incidence data were analysed from different publicly available sources. The major data sources used in this study were:

- ANC (Antenatalcare) sentinel surveillance reports,
- Demographic and health survey reports,

- Annual HIV/AIDS monitoring and evaluation reports, and
- Health and health related indicator documents.

Indicators

Indicators addressing HIV prevalence (HIV positivity rate) among target groups were selected. The data sources were then reviewed to retrieve the prevalence data. The indicators retrieved from these documents were:

- National HIV prevalence projected from ANC sentinel surveillance reports,
- HIV positivity rate among HIV counselling and testing (HCT) clients,
- HIV positivity rate among prevention of mother to child transmission (PMTCT) service clients, and
- HIV positivity rate among blood donors, and HIV prevalence among young people 15-24 years of age.

Data compilation

The HIV indicator data with their respective year of measurement were aggregated on MS excel. Consistency of the data among different sources was checked. The data spread sheet was then made ready for analysis.

Data analysis and interpretation

Five levels of analysis were used for the major HIV/AIDS indicators considered in this study. These analyses included:

Description of prevalence values at critical points in time: As part of the first level of description, the HIV prevalence values were examined at different critical points in time. This level of analysis focused on description of the actual prevalence values. The major issues addressed were the total change during the analysis period, average annual change, and the time when the change was higher or lower.

Description of trends of HIV prevalence overtime: Trends of HIV prevalence from the different data sources were depicted in line graphs and bar graphs and the direction of the progress were described using technical terms. For easy look at actual indicator values used, data tables were included in every graph. For all graphs time in years was displayed in X-axis and magnitude of HIV in Y-axis.

Development of best-fit models for HIV prevalence: Best fit models for each trend data from the different data sources were selected and fitted using the R-squared values. Before the best fit model is selected, all possible trend-line equations and their respective R-square are evaluated. Exponential, logarithmic and linear models are found to fit best for the data used in this study.

Prediction for future points for the national HIV/AIDS indicators: Future values of the indicators used in this study for 2015 were predicted using the best-fit models. The number of forward points from the last indicator data was used as x-value to predict the outcome in 2015, the y-value. This prediction has the stringent assumption of similar trends in the magnitude of the indicators during the prediction period.

Comparison of trends among prevalence data of different sources: This level is a comparison of the trends depicted in the above step. The nature of the trends, rate of decrements, and the predicted values for 2015 were compared. The inherent differences in the measurement of the indicators were discussed.

All the findings were then presented using numerical and graphic summaries of prevalence, trends and trend-line equations with their R-squared. Limitations of the study and precautions that could be taken while using the findings were detailed in the discussions.

RESULTS

HIV prevalence projected from ANC surveillance

Based on the Ante-natal care site sentinel surveillance reports the prevalence of HIV in 1999 was about 7.4%. This prevalence has come down to 2.3% in 2009. This decrease implies an overall decrease of 5.1% in a decade, which is equivalent to an average of 0.5% per year.

Further look in to the pattern of decrement indicated that higher level of decrease was achieved in the early 2000's. The prevalence of HIV from ANC surveillance sites in Ethiopia across different years is shown in figure 1.

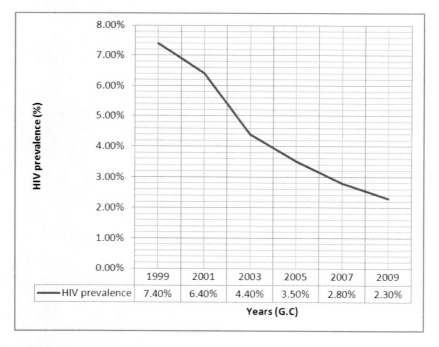

	1999	2001	2003	2005	2007	2009
HIV prevalence	7.40%	6.40%	4.40%	3.50%	2.80%	2.30%

Years (G.C)

Figure 1. Trends of HIV prevalence in Ethiopia from ANC sentinel surveillance: 1999-2009.

The best-fit trend-line equation for the trend of HIV prevalence from ANC sentinel surveillance was found to be the exponential equation, $Y=0.0962-0.244X(R2=.988)$. If the decrement pattern of HIV follows the same trend in the next six years, the projected prevalence of HIV from ANC sentinel surveillance sites will be about 0.2% in 2015.

HIV prevalence among HCT testers

The HIV prevalence among HCT users has decreased from 12.5% in 2005 to 1.5% in 2010. This is a very large decrease in prevalence of HIV by about 11% within five years, equivalent to an average of 2% decrease every year. There was an initial increase between 2005 and 2006 before a maximum annual decline was attained between 2006 and 2007. The patterns of decease in HIV prevalence among HIV testers is shown in figure 2.

The best-fit trend-line equation for the trends of HIV prevalence among HCT testers is again the exponential function, $Y=0.2556-0.454X$ ($R2=.942$). If the trend of HIV prevalence among HCT testers follows the same decrement pattern in the next five years, the predicted prevalence of HIV among HCT testers in 2015 will be about 0.3%.

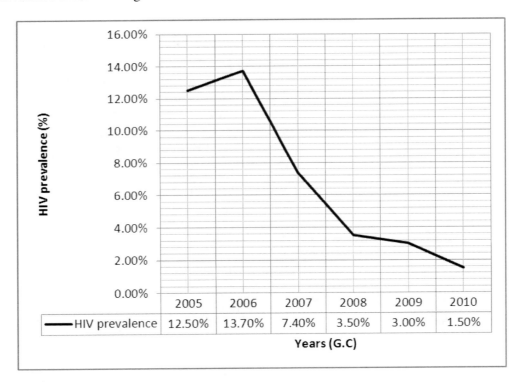

	2005	2006	2007	2008	2009	2010
HIV prevalence	12.50%	13.70%	7.40%	3.50%	3.00%	1.50%

Figure 2. Trends of HIV prevalence among HCT testers in Ethiopia: 2005-2010.

HIV prevalence among PMTCT testers

The HIV prevalence among PMTCT testers has decreased from 7.96% in 2006 to 2.03% in 2020. This is about a 5% decrease in five years period, equivalent to 1% decrease per year among PMTCT testers. Similar to the pattern of decrement of other HIV prevalence in this study, the decrement of HIV prevalence among PMTCT testers was higher at the first years of this analysis. The patterns of HIV prevalence among PMTCT testers is shown in figure 3. Unlike the previous trends, the best fit model for trends of HIV prevalence among PMTCT testers is the logarithmic function, $Y=-0.038\ln(x) + 0.0798$, R2=.995. If the HIV prevalence among PMTCT testers is assumed to follow the same decrement trend in the next five years, the predicted prevalence of HIV among PMTCT testers in 2015 will be about 0.3%.

HIV prevalence among blood donors

The prevalence of HIV among Ethiopian blood donors has decreased from 6.1% in 2002 to 2.2% in 2010. This shows an overall decrease of 4% in prevalence over 8 years. This pattern of decrease is similar to that of the decrease at ANC surveillance sites. This is another dramatic change in the prevalence of HIV in the country.

HIV prevalence among 15-24 years of age

The HIV prevalence among the 15-24 years of age population group has decreased from 12.4% in 2000 to 3.5% in 2007. This shows about an overall decrease of about 9% in seven years. As true for other prevalence rates, the decrement of this prevalence was higher between 2001 and 2003. The pattern of HIV prevalence among 15-24 years of age group is shown in figure 4. The best-fit model for the trends of the prevalence of HIV among the 15-24 years of age group was the linear function, $Y=-0.0232x+0.1518$, R2=.988. If the decrease in HIV prevalence among 15-24 years of age is assumed to follow the same trend in the subsequent eight years, the predicted prevalence of HIV in those age groups will come down to zero before 2015.

Comparison of the different sources

The comparison of the trends in the decrement of HIV prevalence shows a consistent pattern. All the best-fit models indicate that the HIV prevalence has decreased dramatically during the last decade. As shown above the highest predicted prevalence rate for 2015 is 0.3% which is among HCT and PMTCT testers. The prediction for the general prevalence from based on ANC sentinel surveillance data indicated a lower figure of 0.2%. A more impressing figure is that the predicted prevalence of HIV among 15-24 years of age which is close to zero.

DISCUSSION

The dramatic decrease in the prevalence of HIV during the past decade possibly shows the effectiveness of the commitment of the Ethiopian government in implementing the multi-sectoral approach of HIV/AIDS response (9). It also reflected the effectiveness of the support of external donors in funding the HIV/AIDS programs. It should be noted that the predicted values HIV prevalence among different groups for 2015 are under a stringent assumption of 'if things follow similar trend.'

This assumption carries a strong implication of continuing the existing commitment and efforts in mitigating the HIV epidemic in the country. The predicted figures would happen only when similar patterns of efforts and thus trends of HIV prevalence can be maintained. Of course the decrement patterns may not be constant as further decrease from a lower level is more difficult than further decrease from a higher level.

The HIV prevalence rates used in this analysis mostly imply the new HIV positives detected at different population groups. Most of these can be considered as HIV positivity rate than HIV prevalence rates except the ANC surveillance based figures. This indicates the figures may not fully take in to account those already identified people living with HIV. Hence the overall HIV prevalence might be higher than the predicted figures as the former takes in to account the number of PLHIV on ART.

It should also be noted that a lower HIV prevalence in highly populous countries like Ethiopia indicates a large number of people infected with HIV. This is due to both the population factors and better survival of people living with HIV as a result of higher level coverage of ART services. Therefore, both the actual number of HIV infected individuals and the HIV prevalence rates should be considered in planning and resource allocation decisions.

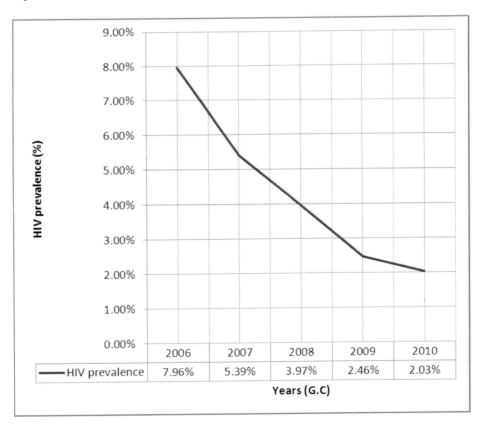

Figure 3. Trends of HIV prevalence among PMTCT testers in Ethiopia: 2006-2010.

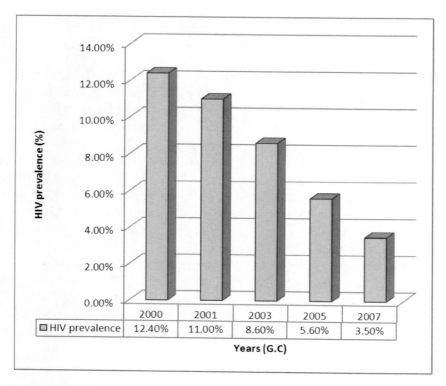

Figure 4. Trends of HIV prevalence among 15-24 years of age group: 2000-2007.

On the other perspective, there was an improvement both in the methods used to measure HIV figures and in the number of people seeking HCT and PMTCT services across time in the last decade along with the already known population increase. This study considered prevalence and HIV positivity rate figures from already published resources. These could have their own effect in the HIV prevalence figures. This study hasn't adjusted for these factors. Hence the interpretation and use of the findings should also consider this limitation of the study.

Though empirically it looks that the immense commitment and investment has resulted in the decrease in the prevalence of HIV, further studies are needed to deeply investigate the relative contribution of the various efforts. This will be particularly used in the era of emergence of non-communicable diseases whose mitigation can learn a lot from the experiences and the best practices of the HIV prevention and control efforts in the past.

CONCLUSION

The prevalence of HIV has shown exponentially and linearly decreasing trends during the last decade. Maintaining such rate of decline could possibly lead to the effective attainment of the MDG 6.

ACKNOWLEDGMENTS

I would like to extend my acknowledgement to the Ethiopian Federal Ministry of Health and the Federal HIV/AIDS Prevention and Control Office of Ethiopia for their published resources that were used as major sources of data. I also thank Tilahun Nigatu for his continious support in conducting this study. The views expressed in this study are solely the views of the author and do not necessarily reflect the views of the Federal Ministry of Health and the Federal HIV/AIDS Prevention and Control Office.

Conflict of interest: None declared.

REFERENCES

[1]   UNAIDS. Global Report: UNAIDS report on the Global AIDS Epidemic. Geneva: UNAIDS, 2010.

[2]   UNAIDS. Chronic care of HIV and non-communicable diseases: How to leverage the HIV Experience. Geneva: UNAIDS, 2011.

[3]   UNAIDS. How to get zero: Faster, smarter, better. World AIDS day report. Geneva: UNAIDS, 2011.

[4]   World Health Organization. Towards universal access progress. Accessed 2012 May 20. URL: http://www.who.int/hiv/pub/2009progressreport/en/

[5]   Federal HIV/AIDS Prevention and Control Office. Multi-sectoral HIV/AIDS response annual monitoring and evaluation report 2001 EFY, 4th ed. Addis Ababa: Federal HIV/AIDS Office, 2009.

[6]   Federal Ministry of Health. Health and health-related indicators report for EFY 2001. Addis Ababa: Federal Ministry Helth, 2009.

[7]   Federal Ministry of Health and National HIV/AIDS Prevention and Control Office. AIDS in Ethiopia, 6th ed. Addis Ababa: Federal Ministry Health, 2006.

[8]   Federal Ministry of Health. Ethiopia health sector development program. III annual performance report for EFY 2002. Addis Ababa: Federal Ministry Health,2010.

[9]   Federal HIV/AIDS Prevention and Control Office. Multi-sectoral HIV/AIDS response annual monitoring and evaluation report 2002 EFY. Addis Ababa: Federal HIV/AIDS Office, 2009.

In: Public Health Yearbook 2013
Editor: Joav Merrick

ISBN: 978-1-63321-095-0
© 2014 Nova Science Publishers, Inc.

Chapter 21

A RARE FAMILY AFFLICTED WITH MULTIPLE HEMOGLOBIN DISORDERS FROM REWA DISTRICT OF MADHYA PRADESH IN CENTRAL INDIA

*Ranbir S Balgir, M Sc Hons, PhD**

Department of Biochemistry, Regional Medical Research Centre for Tribals (Indian Council of Medical Research), Jabalpur, Madhya Pradesh, Central India

ABSTRACT

Hemoglobin disorders are genetically inherited hematological anomalies commonly encountered in the Central region of India. They cause a public health concern due to the high degree of morbidity, mortality, and fetal wastage in the vulnerable and underprivileged people. A rare family afflicted with multiple hemoglobinopathies from Rewa district of Madhya Pradesh in India was encountered during screening for cause of anemia. About 2-3ml intravenous blood samples were collected from all members of this referred family after obtaining the informed consent. Background data were recorded like age, sex, caste, place of origin, reproductive history, consanguinity, etc. Detailed hematological, biochemical, and genetical investigations were carried out following the standard procedures and technology for this family. This study highlights the rare and compound occurrence of abnormal hemoglobins, i.e., Hb E and Hb S interacting with β-thalassemia that is reported for the first time from the state of Madhya Pradesh. It was noticed that the cases with Hb E-β-thalassemia and sickle cell-β-thalassemia manifest variable clinical and hematological profile. High levels of fetal hemoglobin reduce the severity of clinical symptoms in patients. Apart from occurrence of SE disease in one parent, asymptomatic hemoglobin AS and AE carrier siblings were also detected in the family. This family provides for the first time a comprehensive database on the occurrence of double heterozygosity, testifying either ethnic admixture and/or genetic diversity in the state of Madhya Pradesh, India.

---

*Correspondence: Ranbir S Balgir, Scientist F/Deputy Director (Senior Grade) & Head, Department of Biochemistry, Regional Medical Research Centre for Tribals (Indian Council of Medical Research), Near NSCB Medical College & Hospital, P.O: Garha, Nagpur Road, Jabalpur-482 003, Madhya Pradesh, Central India. E-mail: balgirrs@yahoo.co.in.

Keywords: Hemoglobin disorders, compound heterozygosity, sickle cell-β-thalassemia, hemoglobin E-β-thalassemia, sickle cell trait, hemoglobin E trait, β-thalassemia trait, Central India

INTRODUCTION

Of the several hemoglobin variants so far identified and found predominantly prevalent, only three variants – sickle cell (Hb S), hemoglobin E (Hb E) and hemoglobin D (Hb D) are very common in the Indian population (1). The average allele frequency of sickle cell gene has been estimated to be 4.3% in India and that of hemoglobin E being 10.9% in North Eastern region of India (2). With a wide prevalence range of 3-17% and an average being 4.2%, the β-thalassemia commonly encounters throughout India with a wide range of geographical variations (1). The sickle cell disease is wide spread in tribal as well as nontribal communities especially belonging to Central-Eastern part of India (3).

No genetic disease could be as simple as the sickle cell disease. It is a simple disease but there is no cure. In the absence of any cure, the majority of the sickle cell patients have a miserable and short life span (4). Instances of sudden death in such cases have also been reported. This genetic disease is responsible for considerable morbidity and mortality (5). The majority of cases need first blood transfusion between one to three years of age reflecting a high morbidity especially in the preschool age. At this age, cross infection is more common, which could precipitate a sickle cell crisis (4, 6, 7). The anemia in sickle cell trait (AS) is mild and infrequent and one must look for other causes of anemia in them like iron deficiency, parasitic infestations, malaria, etc. The sickle cell disease affects the ability of red blood corpuscles (RBCs) to carry oxygen to various parts of the body by acquiring the shape of a sickle. In the absence of oxygen, the distortion in shape and size of cells leads to increased blood viscosity and blocking of the small vessels, resulting in devastating pain. The pain originates virtually at any time in any organ of the body in joints or bones. The disease carries the risk of debilitating fatigue, blindness, organ damage, and cardiac stroke within a life span of just about 20-30 years (4, 7). The symptoms of the disease include anemia, hand-foot syndrome and infection. The clinical course of these patients is punctuated by episodes of "crisis" and increased susceptibility to serious infections because of functional asplenia. The usual complications are vaso-occlusive crises (severe pain in almost all parts of the body), hemolytic crises (yellow eyes, jaundice or hepatic infection), aplastic crises (diminished production of RBCs) and the deadliest of complications, the sequestration crises (blood suddenly goes to spleen) (4, 7).

Double heterozygosis for hemoglobin disorders is a rare entity. Due to the paucity of adequate literature available on the occurrence of heterosis for hemoglobinopathies in India and the hemoglobinopathies being a major genetic and public health problem in the state of Madhya Pradesh, the present family was investigated in details for double heterozygosity of sickle cell and hemoglobin E interacting with β-thalassemia. This study will not only add to prognostic understanding of the heterosis phenomenon for hemoglobinopathies in the state but also be useful for genetic counseling, prenatal diagnosis and future molecular studies on the subject in India.

METHODS

The index case was referred to us as a suspected case of hemolytic anemia and hemoglobinopathy from Pediatric Out-patient Department, Netaji Subhash Chander Bose Medical College and Hospital, Jabalpur for detailed investigations. Subsequently, the other members of the family were also investigated after taking informed/written consent and a family pedigree was drawn.

About 2-3 ml. intravenous blood samples were collected using ethylene diamine tetra acetic acid (EDTA) as anticoagulant by disposable syringes and needles from each individual after obtaining the informed consent. All the signs and symptoms related to hemoglobinopathy after clinical examination were recorded. Laboratory investigations were carried out following the standard procedures after cross checking for quality control from time to time. Hematological parameters were studied by using an automated Blood Cell Counter (Model-MS$_5$9, Melet Schloesing Laboratories, Cergy-Pontoise Cedex, France).

The sickling test was performed by using freshly prepared sodium metabisulphite solution as reducing agent for the presence or absence of sickle cell hemoglobin (8). The routine hemoglobin lysate electrophoresis was carried out on cellulose acetate membrane (CAM) in Tris-EDTA-Borate buffer at pH 8.9 and quantification of A$_2$ fraction of adult hemoglobin was done by elution method (9). The value more than 3.5% of A$_2$ fraction of adult hemoglobin was taken as cut off point for determining the β-thalassemia trait. Those individuals having the very high hemoglobin A$_2$ value, i.e., more than 10% were suspected to have Hb A$_2$ plus Hb E, which was confirmed by the investigation of other family members. Estimation of fetal hemoglobin was done as described by Weatherall (9).

The diagnosis of sickle cell-β-thalassemia was based on the findings of hemoglobin (Hb) A, F, S and A$_2$ on electrophoresis under alkaline pH, elevated HbA$_2$ levels (>3.5%). All the blood samples were further subjected to hemoglobin variant analysis for detecting any discrepancy (made for Bio-Rad Diagnostics, Hercules California, USA).

RESULTS

The clinical, hematological and genetical findings of cases of sickle cell-β-thalassemia and cases of hemoglobin E-β-thalassemia and their family members have been summarized in table 1.

A 13 year old female child (index case; Daughter-2) with severe anemia, recurrent fever, icterus and retarded growth and development who has become transfusion dependent was referred to us for complete hematological investigations. She had enlarged spleen (4-5cm) with palpable hepatomegaly. Her sickling test was found negative. Almost all the red cell indices were below normal range, i.e., hemoglobin level (2.7g/dl), RBC counts (0.9.10^3/μl), HCT (8.8%), MCV (65.2fl), MCH (17.5pg), MCHC (15.6g/dl), RDW (27.7%), and normal WBC and Platelet counts (Table 1). Red cell morphology showed hypochromatosis, microcytosis, and target cells. After alkaline (pH 8.9) electrophoresis, it was known that she had raised A$_2$/E hemoglobin (54.6%), fetal hemoglobin 14.5%, and only 30.9% normal adult hemoglobin (AA band).

The 45 year old thin and lean father of this child had complaints of irritability, dysponea, chest pains, upper respiratory tract infection (URTI), splenomegaly (5-6cm) with palpable liver. His sickling test was found positive. His red cell indices picture was like this: hemoglobin level (9.9g/dl), RBC counts ($3.8.10^3/\mu l$), HCT (31.7%), MCV (84.6fl), MCH (26.4pg), MCHC (31.2g/dl), RDW (14.6%), WBC ($5.9.10^3/\mu l$) and Thrombocytopenia ($88.10^3/\mu l$). Red cell morphology showed hypochromia and microcytemia. The alkaline electrophoresis showed only two major bands at the position of A_2/E (26.5%) and a thick band (65.9%) at sickle position with a minor band at fetal hemoglobin band level. No normal adult hemoglobin (AA) band was observed.

Table 1. A typical family belonging to Oilman Caste (Teli) with Multiple hemoglobinopathies from Rewa District of Madhya Pradesh, India

Parameters of Study/ Hematological Indices	Parents		Offsprings			
	Father	Mother	Daughter-1	Daughter-2	Daughter-3	Son
Sex	Male	Female	Female	Female	Female	Male
Age in years	45	39	15	13	10	8
Hb (g/dl)	9.9	10.0	6.2	2.7	9.9	11.1
RBC ($x10^3/\mu l$)	3.8	3.1	2.8	0.9	4.5	5.2
HCT (%)	31.7	32.0	18.6	8.8	29.0	34.5
MCV (fl)	84.6	102.8	70.6	65.2	71.3	70.3
MCH (pg)	26.4	32.0	21.3	17.5	21.8	21.3
MCHC (g/dl)	31.2	31.2	27.6	15.6	27.6	29.1
RDW (%)	14.6	14.5	13.2	27.7	11.5	12.7
WBC ($x10^3/\mu l$)	5.9	6.8	5.4	9.7	8.1	7.6
PLT ($x10^3/\mu l$)	88	250	102	280	10	268
Sickling Test	+ve	-ve	-ve	-ve	+ve	+ve
Electrophoresis:						
Major bands	SE	AA_2	AE	AEF	ASA_2	AS
Hb A_2 (%)	26.5	5.2	26.3	54.6	7.7	2.1
Hb F (%)	7.6	1.2	1.0	14.5	15.0	1.2
Hb S (%)	65.9	-	-	-	43.2	30.5
Hb A (%)	-	93.6	72.7	30.9	34.1	66.2
Red cell Morphology	Hypochromia, Microcytemia, Thrombocytopenia	Microcytosis, Hypochromia	Hypochromatosis, Thrombocytopenia	Hypochromatosis, Microcytosis, Target cells	Hypochromatosis	Normochromia
Clinical symptoms	Irritability, Dysponea, Chest pains, URTI, Palpable liver, Splenomegaly	No complaints	No compalints	Pallor, Severe anemia, Recurrent fever, Jaundice, Splenomegaly, Retarded growth & development	Joint & abdominal pains, Pallor, Dysponea, Spleno-megaly	No complaints

The 39 year old healthy mother of the index case had no clinical complaints. However, her periphery red cell smear showed hypochromia and microcytosis. The sickling test was found negative. Her hemogram showed: hemoglobin level (10.0g/dl), RBC counts ($3.1.10^3/\mu l$), HCT (32.0%), MCV (102.8fl), MCH (32.0pg), MCHC (31.2g/dl), RDW (14.5%), and normal WBC and platelet counts (Table 1). The alkaline electrophoresis showed only two major bands: one at the position of A_2/E (5.2%) and the other thick band (93.6%) at the position level of adult hemoglobin (AA).

Thus the index case (Daughter-2) was diagnosed as hemoglobin E-β^{++}thalassemia. Patient was given whole blood transfusion and showed the signs of improvement. The siblings of this index case were also studied and their findings are presented in table 1.

The 15 year old sibling sister (Daughter-1) of this index case with severe anemia had no clinical complaints, but the red cell morphology showed hypochromia and microcytosis. The sickling test was found negative. The red cell indices were like this: hemoglobin level (6.2g/dl), RBC counts ($2.8.10^3/\mu l$), HCT (18.6%), MCV (70.6fl), MCH (21.3pg), MCHC (27.6g/dl), RDW (13.2%), and normal WBC and Thrombocytopenia (Table 1).

The alkaline electrophoresis showed only two major bands: one at the position of A_2/E (26.3%) and the other thick band at hemoglobin AA (72.7%) position, with the normal fetal hemoglobin (Table 1). Thus, this sibling was diagnosed as hemoglobin E trait (AE).

Another 10 year old female sibling (Daughter-3) of the index case had pallor, dysponea, joint and abdominal pains, and splenomegaly (3-4cm) with hypochromatosis. Her sickling test was found positive. The hemogram of this case showed: hemoglobin level (9.9g/dl), RBC counts ($4.5.10^3/\mu l$), HCT (29.0%), MCV (71.3fl), MCH (21.8pg), MCHC (27.6g/dl), RDW (11.5%), and normal WBC and platelet counts (Table 1). The alkaline electrophoresis showed four prominent bands, i.e., one at the position of A_2/E (7.7%), the other three at sickle (43.2%), fetal (15.0%) and AA (34.1%) positions, respectively. This sibling was diagnosed as sickle cell-β^{++} thalassemia case.

An eight year old brother of the index case had no clinical complaints. His red cell smear showed only normochromic cells. However, the sickling test was positive. His red cell indices presented the following picture: hemoglobin level (11.1g/dl), RBC counts ($5.2.10^3/\mu l$), HCT (34.50%), MCV (70.3fl), MCH (21.3pg), MCHC (29.1g/dl), RDW (12.7%), and normal WBC and platelet counts (Table 1). Electrophoresis showed only two thick bands at the position of sickle (30.5%) and AA hemoglobin (66.2%) level. Both hemoglobin A_2 and fetal were in the normal range (Table 1). This case was diagnosed as sickle cell trait (AS).

DISCUSSION

The genetic heterogeneity, double heterozygosity, or compound cases of hemoglobin disorders are not uncommon in the backward and under-privileged communities especially in the Central region. Heterosis, also called hybrid vigor or boost in performance, is the increase in growth, size, fecundity, function, yield, or other characters in hybrids over those of the parents. In other words, heterosis is increased strength of different characteristics in hybrids, the possibility to obtain a "better" individual by combining the virtues of its parents. Aberrant heterosis is antagonistic to heterosis, i.e., combination of ill effects or abnormal qualities in an individual. Therefore, it is not always true that the heterosis increases the strength of different characteristics in hybrid. Aberrant heterosis may occur with severer ill effects, abnormal qualities, or even lethal for the survival of an individual.

All the cases in the family under study had a large range of variation in hemoglobin levels (2.7-11.1%), but the majority had moderate to severe anemia. Patients of hemoglobin E-β-thalassemia and sickle cell-β-thalassemia disease manifest heterogeneity in clinical manifestations, prognosis, hematological picture, and management profile in India (10). The patients with early onset and severe anemia have the disease course similar to homozygous β-thalassemia in the former and that of sickle cell disease in the latter case, while those patients with late onset and mild anemia manage with occasional blood transfusions or remain completely asymptomatic without any hemolytic crisis in life. Similar observations were made for Hb E-β-thalassemia in Sri Lanka (11), Thailand (4), and for sickle cell-β-thalassemia in India (10, 12-14).

The phenotypic severity is dependent on the type of β-thalassemia mutation, levels of HbE and HbF, and the number of β-globin genes, which tend to reduce the severity of the disease (12, 13). The interaction of hemoglobin E with β-thalassemia results in a wide spectrum of clinical conditions, in some cases indistinguishable from β-thalassemia major, whereas, in others it has a milder course without dependent on transfusion. These findings get further support from the earlier studies (15-18). The Hb E is a mild structural variant of β-globin chain, being asymptomatic in homozygous state (19). The clinical and hematological profile of the index case of Hb E-β-thalassemia in the present study was identical with those of β-thalassemia major patient. This clinical picture is compatible with the studies reported from other parts especially from the North-Eastern region of India where its frequency is reported to be very high (6, 20, 21, 22). The index case had marked anemia, jaundice, bossy maxillary bones and prominent hepatosplenomegaly. The peripheral blood smear examination revealed a hypochromic and microcytic picture with predominance of target cells. Patients with hemoglobin E-β-thalassemia in Central-Eastern Indian belt, generally, are transfusion dependent from the age of one year onward and need multiple blood transfusions, varying from 1 to 25 units (10). This family is the 1st in series for Hb E-β-thalassemia from Madhya Pradesh. In the present study, apart from hemoglobinopathies, some other factors like iron/folic acid deficiency, nutritional deficiency disorders, parasitic infestations, malarial or viral infections, etc. which are very common in the state of Madhya Pradesh, may be responsible for mild or severe course of the disease.

It is apparent from table 1 that the sickle cell-β-thalassemia case before blood transfusion showed reduced values of red cell indices like HCT, MCV, MCH and MCHC manifesting hematological aberrations. The red cell morphology also showed hypochromia and microcytosis in this family. The complete blood cell count (CBC) values were either reduced or normal in carriers of Hb AS, Hb AE or β-thalassemia trait in the family.

The present study highlights the co-inheritance of β-thalassemia and hemoglobin E or sickle cell gene, which is wide spread in Eastern, Northern, Southern and Western Madhya Pradesh (7, 23). To conclude, it may be summarized that this family provides for the first time a comprehensive database on the occurrence of double heterozygosity, testifying either ethnic admixture and/or genetic diversity in the state of Madhya Pradesh, India. Further, it is a pity that a large number of such double heterozygosity cases remain mostly undiagnosed or misdiagnosed, wrongly interpreted and mismanaged leading to premature death without proper treatment in the state of Madhya Pradesh (24). For bringing awareness, motivation for carrier detection to reduce the genetic burden, and intervention in affected families and communities need to be launched vigorously in Central India.

ACKNOWLEDGMENTS

Author is grateful to Dr. V. M. Katoch, Secretary, Department of Health Research, Government of India, and Director General, Indian Council of Medical Research, New Delhi for providing the necessary research facilities. Technical support of Mr. V. K. Kachhi and Mr. P. Patel, Laboratory Technicians is thankfully acknowledged.

Conflict of interest: Author declares no conflict of interest.

REFERENCES

[1]   Balgir RS. The burden of hemoglobinopathies in India and the challenges ahead. Curr Sci 2000;79:1536-47.

[2]   Balgir RS. Genetic epidemiology of the three predominant abnormal hemoglobins in India. J Assoc Phys India 1996;44:25-8.

[3]   Balgir RS. Public health challenges of sickle cell disorders, □-thalassemia syndrome and G6PD deficiency in scheduled caste and scheduled tribe communities of Central India. Int Public Health J 2011;3:307-18.

[4]   Fucharoen S, Winichagoon P. Hemoglobinopathies in Southeast Asia: molecular biology and clinical medicine. Hemoglobin 1997;21:299-319.

[5]   Balgir RS. Infant mortality and reproductive wastage associated with different genotypes of haemoglobinopathies in Orissa, India. Ann Hum Biol 2007;34:16-25.

[6]   Chatterjea JB. Some aspects of Hb E and its genetic interaction with thalassemia. Indian J Med Res 1965;53:377-83.

[7]   Balgir RS. Clinical genetics and hematological profile of sickle cell cases in twenty families of Orissa. Indian J Hemat Blood Transfus 2006;22:45-52.

[8]   Dacie JV, Lewis SM. Practical Hematology. 7thEdn. Edinburgh: Churchill Livingstone1991:227-58.

[9]   Weatherall DJ. The Thalassemias. In: Methods in Hematology. Vol. 6. New York: Churchill Livingstone, 1983:1-53.

[10]   Balgir RS. Aberrant heterosis in hemoglobinopathies with special reference to β-thalassemia and structurally abnormal hemoglobins E and S in Orissa, India. J Clin Diagn Res 2007;1:122-30.

[11]   Premawardhene A, Fisher CA, Olivieri NF, de Silva S, Arambepola M, Perera W, O'Donnell A, Peto TEA, Viprakasit V, Merson L, Muraca G, Weatherall DJ. Haemoglobin E β–thalassaemia in Sri Lanka. Lancet 2005;366:1467-70.

[12]   Serjeant GR, Serjeant BE. Sickle cell disease. 3rdEdn. New York: Oxford University Press, 2001.

[13]   Weatherall DJ, Clegg JB. Inherited hemoglobin disorders: an increasing global health problem. Bull World Health Organization 2001;79:704-12.

[14]   Kulozik AE, Bail S, Kar BC, Serjeant BE, Serjeant GE. Sickle cell-β⁺thalassemia in Orissa state, India. Br J Hemat 1991;77:215-20.

[15]   Agarwal S, Gulati R, Singh K. Hemoglobin E-beta-thalassemia in Uttar Pradesh. Indian Pediatr 1997;34:287-92.

[16]   Balgir RS. Double heterozygosity for abnormal hemoglobins in six families of Orissa. Curr Med Trends 1998;2:378-85.

[17]   Chhotray GP, Dash BP, Ranjit MR, Colha, RB, Mohanty D. Hemoglobin E/β-thalassemia – an experience in the Eastern Indian state of Orissa. Acta Hemat 2003; 109:214-16.

[18]   Balgir RS, Mishra RK, Murmu B. Clinical and hematological profile of hemoglobinopathies in two tribal communities of Sundargarh district in Orissa, India. Int J Hum Genet 2003;3:209-16.

[19]   Balgir RS. Fertility and clinical profile of hemoglobin-E afflicted mothers in North Eastern India. Med Surg 1993;10:57-9.

[20]   De M, Das SK, Bhattarcharya DK, Talukder G. The occurrence of β-thalassemia mutation and its interaction with hemoglobin E in the Eastern India. Int J Hemat 1997;66:31-4.

[21]   Balgir RS. Prevalence of abnormal hemoglobin E gene in the Dhelki Kharia tribal population. Curr Sci 2003;85:1604-8.

[22]   Balgir RS. Emerging trends in genetic epidemiology of hemoglobinopathy in seven sister states of North Eastern India. In: North East India in Perspectives: Biology, Social Formation and Contemporary Problems. Das, Rajat Kumar, Basu, Debashish. Eds. New Delhi: Akansha Publishing House, 2005:17-37.

[23]   Balgir RS, Dash BP, Murmu B. Blood groups, hemoglobinopathy and G6PD deficiency investigations among fifteen major scheduled tribes of Orissa, India. Anthropologist 2004;6:69-75.

[24]   Balgir RS. Genetic epidemiology of the sickle cell anemia in India. Indian Practr 2001; 54:771-6.

SECTION THREE - CASE STUDIES TO BUILD COMMUNITY CAPACITIES

In: Public Health Yearbook 2013
Editor: Joav Merrick

ISBN: 978-1-63321-095-0
© 2014 Nova Science Publishers, Inc.

Chapter 22

MODEL COMMUNITIES AS A STRATEGY FOR ACHIEVING POLICY, SYSTEMS AND ENVIRONMENTAL CHANGE FOR OBESITY CONTROL AND REDUCTION

Rachael D Dombrowski, MPH[*,1], *Maryann Mason, PhD*[2,3,4,5],
Sarah B Welch, MPH[2], *Christina Welter, DrPH*[6],
Gina Massuda Barnett, MPH[6] *and Adlin Cedeño*[2]

[1]Public Health Institute of Metropolitan Chicago
[2]Consortium to Lower Obesity in Chicago Children/Ann and
J. Milburn Smith Child Health Research Program, Children's Memorial Research Center
[3]Feinberg School of Medicine, Northwestern University, Department of Pediatrics
[4]Feinberg School of Medicine, Northwestern University,
Department of Preventive Medicine
[5]Northwestern University Clinical and Translational Sciences Institute, Community
Engagement Research Center, Alliance for Research in Chicagoland Communities
[6]Cook County Department of Public Health, Illinois, United States of America

ABSTRACT

Suburban Cook County, Illinois is a large, geopolitically complex region in the Midwestern United States. To meet the unique needs of this jurisdiction, the Cook County Department of Public Health (CCDPH) in partnership with the Public Health Institute of Metropolitan Chicago (PHIMC) utilized funding from the US Department of Health and Human Services to initiate the Model Communities (MC) grant program as a component of their broad-based efforts to change policies and environments to promote healthy eating and active living, and prevent obesity. The MC strategy aims to build organizational and community capacity by providing local governments, school districts, and community-based institutions with resources and tools to address obesity through

* Correspondence: Rachael D Dombrowski, MPH, Assistant Program Director, Suburban Cook County Communities Putting Prevention to Work (CPPW), Public Health Institute of Metropolitan Chicago, 1010 Lake Street Suite 430, Oak Park, Illinois, United States. E-mail: rjankows@gmail.com.

implementation of policy, systems and environmental change (PSE). PSE changes are an effective strategy in addressing complex public health issues by prompting and reinforcing health behaviors at the population level. Through alliance strengthening, capacity building and health communications the MC strategy has already shown initial success among the 38 funded entities. At the midpoint of the grant cycle, five local governments have passed ordinances related to community design for active living; nine local governments and community-based institutions have increased healthy food access for residents; 83 schools have improved their school food environments and 59 schools have increased opportunities for physical activity among students and school staff. This program is likely to offer insights to other areas with similar complex environments and is a model that can be applied to other complex public health issues.

Keywords: Community, intervention, policy, obesity

INTRODUCTION

Obesity has reached epidemic proportions in the United States. In 2007-2008, 34% of US adults and 18.1% of adolescents 12 to19 years old were obese (1, 2). Nationally, obesity has hit a plateau with no significant increase for adults since 2003-2004 and among children from 2008-2010. In 2011, 27.7% of Illinois adults and 20.7% of Illinois children between the ages of 10 and 17 were obese (3,4). Obesity disproportionally affects minority and low-income individuals; including 39.5% of African Americans, 31.5% of Latinos and 33.8% of adults with an annual household income less than $15,000 in Illinois (3). While national obesity rates are stabilizing, Illinois continues to experience increases in the prevalence of obesity among adults and children with a disproportionate burden falling on minority populations and those living in poverty.

Obesity is associated with chronic diseases and conditions such as cardiovascular disease, diabetes mellitus II, arthritis, depression, certain cancers, hypertension and impaired mobility (4, 5). Chronic disease is a major cause of death and disability in the US with six out of ten causes of death attributed to chronic disease (6). Treatment of chronic disease is costly and is a major contributor to soaring medical expenses in the United States (4, 7). Obesity and its associated co-morbidities are influenced by lifestyle behaviors such as physical activity and diet and many chronic diseases and conditions can be prevented and managed through healthy behaviors (8).

Changes to policies, systems and the environment (PSE) are an effective strategy in addressing complex public health issues by prompting and reinforcing health behaviors at the population level. For example, the levying of "vice" taxes on tobacco and alcohol products has been shown to decrease use of these products (9-11). PSE changes can occur at the national (e.g., nutritional standards for the National School Breakfast and Lunch meal program; state (e.g., excise tax on sugar-loaded beverages) and local (e.g., sales tax, zoning and facility siting) levels. In addition to addressing complex public health issues, PSE approaches are effective means to address health disparities. Healthy behaviors exist within the conditions in which people work, live, and play, and broad PSE changes can affect underserved communities by creating sustainable changes that will promote healthy behaviors.

To prevent and reduce the epidemic obesity rates, the US Centers for Disease Control and Prevention (CDC) developed the Communities Putting Prevention to Work (CPPW) initiative, a large scale obesity and tobacco prevention and control effort focused on PSE change funded by the American Recovery and Reinvestment Act of 2009 and the Patient Protection and Affordable Care Act of 2010. In March 2010, the Cook County Department of Public Health (CCDPH) in collaboration with the Public Health Institute of Metropolitan Chicago (PHIMC), one of 55 community sites across the nation, was awarded nearly $16 million to increase access to healthy foods; decrease availability of unhealthy foods; and create more safe and convenient places to walk, bike and be physically active throughout suburban Cook County (SCC), Illinois.

CCDPH's vision to address chronic disease is to catalyze a culture shift that promotes healthy living and health equity across SCC, resulting in change that is far reaching and sustainable. Given the geopolitical complexity and disparity in SCC, CCDPH, along with partnering organizations, has employed a comprehensive approach that integrates systems thinking and community organizing principles within a socio-ecological framework and PSE change initiatives at the *state*, *county*, and *local* levels across multiple sectors.

To meet the unique needs of the jurisdiction, sustain efforts at the local level, and assure linkage with county, state and national initiatives, the Model Communities (MC) grant program remains a key health promotion and organizing strategy within the overall CPPW approach. It aims to build organizational and community capacity by providing local government, school districts, and community-based institutions with resources and tools to address obesity. Since this program is likely to offer insights to other areas with similar complex environments and is a model that can be applied to other complex public health issues, this paper describes the program; provides a theoretical background; and shares process and early outcome evaluation findings.

DESCRIPTION OF MODEL COMMUNITIES GRANT PROGRAM

Suburban Cook County covers a total of 700 square miles; encompasses 125 municipalities organized as cities, towns or villages with 2,233,179 people; and is home to 21 acute care hospitals, 18,000 licensed physicians, 143 school districts, and 650 licensed daycare centers (12). The intervention area for the CPPW initiative includes communities which fall within the jurisdiction of the CCDPH; excluding Evanston, Skokie, Oak Park, and Stickney Township.

Demographics in SCC are changing similar to the national trend, with increasing suburbanization of low income and minority populations (12, 13). The number of people living at or below 200% of the federal poverty level (FPL) increased 41% from 2000 to 2009 in SCC compared to a 4% increase in Chicago. In addition, the African American population increased 20% and the Hispanic population increased 44% in SCC (12, 14, 15).

Chronic diseases have a disparate impact on minority populations. The African American coronary heart disease rate (152.8 per 100,000) is 17% higher than the rate for Whites and is 52% higher than the Healthy People 2020 goal of 100.8 per 100,000. The diabetes any cause mortality rate for African Americans (93.5 per 100,000) in SCC is 85% higher than the rates for Whites. The pattern of disparity is repeated for African Americans and the South District region for many other chronic diseases, including stroke and cancer (15).

In SCC, chronic disease disparities are reflected in the region's economic disparities, the extent of which are highlighted by some of the nation's poorest and wealthiest communities in the country located in SCC. As a result, local capacity and delivery of human services to address growing needs is uneven across the jurisdiction (16). While various initiatives, programs, and services exist throughout the jurisdiction to meet increased need, disparities cannot be effectively addressed because the region lacks the infrastructure and coordination between the many systems that are already in place.

As part of CPPW, the Model Communities grant program was organized to support local level change while building a movement across the region. The program focuses on implementing PSE change in communities and schools to promote healthy eating and active living. The program places emphasis on reducing health inequities by focusing efforts in under resourced areas of SCC, and creating sustainable coalitions and partnerships to maximize the project's impact beyond the timeline of the grant.

Up to $4 million was awarded in Model Communities grant funds to 38 local governments (local gov't), school districts and community organizations throughout SCC. These projects focus on:

- Promoting breastfeeding,
- Making healthy foods more available and unhealthy foods less available,
- Creating convenient, safe places for walking, biking and other physical activities,
- Increasing opportunities for physical activity in schools,
- Supporting children in walking and biking to/from school, or
- Increasing access to services for adults at-risk or with chronic conditions.

THEORETICAL BACKGROUND

Grounded in the literature, the theoretical underpinning of the MC grant program encompasses three primary elements: (1) building constituency support; (2) enhancing organizational and community capacity; and (3) implementing health communications strategies.

Health communications

Using health communications and social marketing strategies to help influence perception and garner support toward policy change are key elements to any advocacy-based campaign (17, 18). The CPPW Initiative, in coordination with CDC and national experts, developed a media advocacy approach to influence public opinion and garner support for several of its major policy initiatives (18). The media products are intended to provide messaging to support local organizing initiatives.

Capacity-building

Capacity building is central to the program in order to cultivate leadership and sustainability, and is a core method in building a base of support for policy change (19, 20). The MC program promotes organizational and community capacity building through trainings, technical assistance and resource sharing.

Alliance strengthening

Building support for PSE change is crucial for success. Use of cooperative, inter-organizational networks has become a key strategy to help augment connectivity among partners, build legitimacy, and leverage and optimize resources (21). As part of the MC grant program, grant recipients are required to:

- coordinate among multiple sectors (e.g., school districts, local governments, community organizations and businesses) within a single community; among partners from the same sector (e.g., school districts) across multiple communities; or both. They were also encouraged to partner with grassroots organizations, community residents or youth, where possible; and
- participate in the Alliance for Healthy and Active Communities (AHAC), a collaborative that addresses chronic disease prevention and has representatives from several organizations and sectors supporting chronic disease prevention.

Additionally, several representatives from the countywide alliance participate in a statewide alliance to prevent obesity. This overall structure allows for connectivity between local, county and state chronic disease prevention efforts.

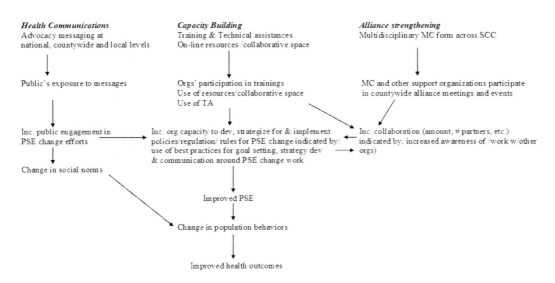

Figure 1. Theory of change for SCC CPPW Model Communities.

As demonstrated in the Theory of Change (Figure 1), the combination of the three primary elements described above aim to increase organizational capacity, allowing organizations to use best practices for goal setting, strategy development and communication to effectively advance PSE change. The changes in PSE are thought to support change in population behaviors and ultimately health outcomes.

METHODS

Outreach to garner interest in model communities grant program

Community-based outreach and capacity building opportunities were extremely important to the success of the MC grant program. A multi-faceted outreach strategy was integral for sharing the Request for Proposal (RFP) opportunity with over 1,000 eligible entities. In addition to posting information on the CCDPH website and mailing or e-mailing out the opportunity, targeted outreach was conducted by CPPW staff to reach eligible entities in areas of SCC with high need (less than 200% FPL or over 50% students registered for free and reduced lunch) and/or high population (populations were ranked from highest to lowest by region and prioritized). This approach was aligned with the CDC's emphasis on using CPPW funding to advance PSE changes with broad reach or impact and achievement towards health equity. To ensure applicants, including those from under resourced SCC communities, had the knowledge and capacity to submit competitive proposals we provided capacity building opportunities through a Grant Writing 101 and RFP Informational Session. The MC RFPs were due December 10, 2010 and funding decisions were announced January 24, 2011. The project period runs from February 1, 2011 to February 28, 2012.

Selection of model communities grant recipients

The MC grant program allowed eligible applicants to select strategies from a broad menu of PSE changes to account for factors like community assets and priorities, individual and unique political structures, and current partnerships already in place or needed. The menu of options was comprised of 16 PSE strategies organized around the three primary goals: increasing availability, accessibility and demand for nutritional options, decreasing opportunities for excess caloric intake, and increasing availability and/or utilization of safe places to be physically active. A list of the PSE strategy options is provided in Table 1.

Eligible applicants for the MC grant program included local and regional governments, not-for-profit community organizations, healthcare institutions, day care centers/providers, senior citizen centers and school districts serving SCC communities. Applicants were encouraged to work on multiple strategies, provide evidence of a strong collaboration and emphasize efforts towards health equity through their proposed PSE strategies.

Table 1. Model communities menu of options: PSE change strategies

Strategy		Description and examples (where possible)	Eligible applicant
1	Comprehensive plans	Develop or update local comprehensive plans with chapters on non-motorized transportation and sustainable food systems.	Local gov'ts
		Develop a non-motorized transportation chapter with strategies to improve the walking and biking environment in local communities.	Local gov'ts
2	Complete streets policy	Commit to accommodating pedestrian and bicycle traffic in all new transportation projects whenever appropriate. Examples: Build sidewalks, stripe bike lanes, and design streets for safer, slower vehicle speeds.	Local gov'ts
3	Zoning, development, and land use regulations	Require new developments to be more accessible by foot, by bike and by transit. Examples: Install pedestrian routes through parking lots and improve bike parking facilities.	Local gov'ts
4	Safe park zones (similar to safe school zones)	Set higher fines for speeding and disobeying traffic signals when children are present in parks. Revenue from fines can fund pedestrian safety projects at the local park district.	Local gov'ts
5	Bicycle route signs	Make streets more inviting to new cyclists by establishing a local network of way-finding signs. These signs are a guide to local destinations on streets preferred for cycling.	Local gov'ts
6	Sustainable food systems	Support small format grocery stores; farmers markets; co-ops; local buying clubs for corner stores.	Local gov'ts; Community organizations
7	Healthy food and beverage options	Change policies, nutritional standards, procurement practices or contracts to increase availability of healthy foods and beverages and decrease availability of unhealthy foods and beverages. Example: Revise nutritional standards for vending machines and change policies and procurement practices to enforce the standards.	Local gov'ts; Community organization; School districts
8	Chronic disease self-management program (CDSMP)	Implement systems supporting evidence-based CDSMP to increase accessibility of resources for residents in suburban Cook County who have a chronic disease or may be at-risk.	Local gov'ts; Community organizations; School districts
9	Breastfeeding-friendly environments	Develop and implement a plan to integrate some or all of ten steps to become a Baby Friendly Hospital and ensure babies get a healthy start to life.	Community organizations (hospitals)
		Develop policies and environments that promote breastfeeding at workplaces and locations throughout the community.	Local gov'ts; Community organizations; School districts
10	Worksite wellness	Develop or update policies to improve work settings that promote healthy living. Examples under this RFP include: increasing healthy food and beverage options (option #7); institutionalizing and setting aside resources to implement the chronic disease self-management program (option #8); creating a breastfeeding-friendly environment for employees (option #9); provision of maps for safe and convenient walking outside the office as part of an overall plan to promote physical activity; and securing and promoting free or markedly reduced access to exercise clubs.	Local gov'ts; Community organizations; School districts
11	Adopt a healthy schools program	*School Wellness Policies:* Require schools to develop quality wellness promoting infrastructures. The district will promote Healthy Schools Program six step process in order to build sustainable wellness promoting environments at the school level. Example: Revise wellness policies to promote healthy, active transportation, acknowledging and promoting walking and biking as a way to increase physical activity and improve students' overall health.	School Districts
		School Improvement Plan Enhancement: Incorporate wellness goals into their School Improvement Plan requirements. The district will require schools to include goals aligned with PSE change strategies in annual improvement plans, will monitor progress toward meeting goals, and will report on progress annually.	School districts

Table 1. (Continued)

Strategy		Description and examples (where possible)	Eligible applicant
		Before and After School Environment: Adopt policies relating to increasing physical activity and improving nutrition in their before and after school environments. Schools will collaborate with before and after school providing organizations to enhance programming and assess environments to maximize physical activity and access to healthy foods and beverages and decrease access to unhealthy foods and beverages.	School districts
		School Competitive Foods: Improve competitive food policies and policy implementation to increase access to healthy foods and decrease access to unhealthy foods and beverages.	School districts
		School Meals Program: Enhance or improve school lunch, school breakfast, or after school food programs to increase access to and consumption of healthy foods and decrease access to unhealthy foods.	School districts
		Physical Education (PE): Offer quality physical education for all grade levels. Physical education will be based on a written and sequential curriculum that is aligned to the national/state standards for physical education. The district will reduce or eliminates waiver policies for students in all grade levels and increase participation in quality PE.	School districts
		Physical Activity (PA): Adopt comprehensive physical activity policy grounded in quality Physical Education and inclusive of quality activity opportunities before, during, and after the school day. The comprehensive environment will include but is not limited to institutionalized physical activity breaks, quality recess development, and before and after school programming.	School districts
12	School siting policies	School districts and municipalities ensure that new schools are centrally located within the communities they serve, and are therefore more accessible on foot or by bike.	Local gov'ts; School districts; Community organizations
13	Land/cash ordinances	Land cash ordinances are impact fees paid by developers, related to the burden that new development places on municipalities. Instead of paying cash, developers may donate land intended for building new schools. By ordinance, school districts and municipalities ensure that new school lands contributed by developers meet healthy school siting standards.	Local gov'ts; School districts; Community organizations
14	School travel plans (safe routes to school [SRTS])	Schools adopt plans to address students' mode of travel to and from school, including strategies to improve infrastructure and safety programming. Any school applying for federal Safe Routes to School funding is required to complete a school travel plan approved by their school district and their local municipality.	School districts
15	School transportation department reform	Establish school policies that encourage walking and biking to school. Expand the scope of school transportation directors' roles to address the needs of students walking and biking to school, as well as those riding school buses.	School districts
16	Joint use agreement	Create formal agreements between school districts and non-school organizations to share use of facilities. Example: allowing a school gym to be used for a park district class in exchange for using a park district athletic field for school baseball games. This promotes value of the school as a community center and can reduce needed school site acreage, increasing walkability & preventing school sprawl.	Local gov'ts; School districts; Community organizations

An external review team informed the selection of Model Communities grant recipients. The review team of 74 Cook County professionals from various fields scored applications to favor those with the readiness and capacity to carry out PSE changes to reduce health disparities through strong collaborations, coalitions and partnerships. Leadership from

CCDPH and PHIMC made final funding decisions to align with the CPPW goals of broad reach and achievement of health equity.

Grant recipient technical assistance and training

As mentioned above, a multi-pronged training and technical assistance strategy was initiated with MC grant recipients to assist in their PSE change efforts. This included:

Training: The MC grant recipients began their work with enrollment in a year-long leadership institute, the Change Institute. This Institute includes five interactive opportunities, including three in-person conferences and two on-line training opportunities. The Change Institute provides a venue for all Model Communities grant recipients to share common barriers and successes as well as gain advanced training from locally and nationally-renowned experts in healthy eating and active living PSE change. The in-person conferences were planned with three themes in mind: 1) Kick off and workplan development; 2) Sustainability for PSE change and 3) Celebration and continuation. On-line training opportunities were selected from grant recipient assessments on training needs. In addition, over 10 additional training opportunities were offered to both MC grant recipients and non-funded agencies serving SCC on advancing policy change for obesity prevention.

Technical assistance: Ongoing technical assistance has been and will continue to be available to MC grant recipients throughout the project period in order to provide grant recipients with tailored one-on-one training and specialized sessions on advancing their specific PSE changes. The technical assistance team meets monthly to assess Model Communities grant recipient progress and identify common barriers and successes across the 38 grant recipients.

Resource sharing: MC grant recipients share best practices and success strategies through an online community called Cook County Connects. Cook County Connects provides grant recipients with an opportunity and venue to share resources, success stories, barriers to implementation and provide each other with support and problem solving suggestions. This online system encourages collaborations among Model Communities in geographically distant areas to communicate regularly, thereby sharing strategies and helping one another. This support network facilitates the work of Model Communities as well as strengthenes the network of organizations collaborating on activities to make healthier SCC schools and communities.

County-wide alliance

The Alliance for Healthy and Active Communities is a group of health advocacy organizations and individuals working under the leadership of the Cook County Department of Public Health to create healthier environments in SCC. AHAC provides members with networking opportunities, best practices and assistance with resource development for health promotion and is available to all SCC localities and organizations. Many Model Communities are active members in AHAC and are working to develop a far reaching policy agenda to guide the work of AHAC in 2012. AHAC provides an opportunity to leverage the work of Model Communities grant recipients and link them to other organizations and localities working on obesity PSE efforts, creating a sustainable alliance to support this work beyond the CPPW funding period.

Health communications

In addition to the work done on the local level with communities, specific media or communications activities have focused on the following five themes: decreasing consumption of sugar loaded beverages, increasing the availability of healthy foods in low access communities, increasing community opportunities for physical activity, promoting healthy schools and encouraging hospitals to support breastfeeding through passage of Baby-Friendly policies. A paid media campaign focused exclusively on decreasing sugar loaded beverage consumption. The campaign titled, "Rethink Your Drink," included media messages which were placed on television, print media, and billboards throughout SCC and sought to inform residents about the health impact of consumption of unhealthy beverages. The other priority areas utilized collateral materials and events (to generate earned media) to promote health messages informing residents about the importance of creating environments that are conducive to health and the critical role community, school and hospital leadership play in ensuring residents of Cook County have healthy places to live, work, learn and play.

RESULTS

Of 120 applications received, Model Communities grants were awarded to 41 local or regional governments (Local gov't; Regional gov't), hospitals, community-based organizations (CBO) and school districts in February 2010. Three selected entities declined the award. The PSE strategies of the 38 grant recipients have the potential to impact 71 communities and 127 schools (1.7 million residents). Table 2 provides a description of these grant recipients, the region they encompass in SCC (North [N], South [S], West [W] or Southwest [SW]) and their proposed PSE strategies and population impact.

Preliminary successes

Community design for active living: Five local governments in suburban Cook County achieved PSE strategies to incorporate active living into community design including Complete Streets ordinances, which require streets to be designed with all users (pedestrian, bikes, public transport and cars) in mind; Safe Park Zones ordinances, which require signage and speed limits around parks much like what is present around schools; bike signage installation and comprehensive community plan updates for active transportation development. Alone, the implementation of these policies and practices will impact up to 124,212 SCC residents. By the end of the project we expect to have at least six additional communities complete passages of this nature.

Table 2. Model communities grantee description and PSE strategies

Organization	MC grantee type	SCC region	Proposed PSE changes	PSE impact	Population
Arlington Heights School District 25	School District	N	Establish wellness councils and adopt health and wellness policy change; increase opportunities for PA/PE for staff and students; improve school food environment	5,117	Students and staff
Asian Health Coalition of Illinois	CBO	N	Institutionalize the Chronic Diseases Self-Management Program (CDSMP)	500	Residents
Broadview Park District	Local Gov't	W	Implementation of community gardens and a farmers market; passage of worksite wellness policy for healthy eating and active living	7,623	Residents and students
Brookwood School District 167	School District	S	Establish wellness councils and adopt health and wellness policy change; increase opportunities for PA/PE for staff and students; improve school food environment	1,269	Students and staff
Chicago Hispanic Health Coalition	CBO	W	Institutionalize CDSMP	600	Residents
Chicago Ridge School District 127 ½	School District	SW	Establish wellness councils and adopt health and wellness policy change; increase opportunities for PA/PE for staff and students; improve school food environment and integrate school gardens into curriculum	1,355	Students and staff
Cicero Elementary School District 99	School District	W	Establish wellness councils and adopt health and wellness policy change; increase opportunities for PA/PE for staff and students; passage of Safe Routes to School (SRTS); improve school food environment and integrate school gardens into curriculum	13,680	Students and staff
City of Berwyn	Local Gov't	W	Passage of active transportation plan, Complete Streets and Safe Park Zones ordinances; install bike signage; passage of SRTS in Berwyn school districts.	56,414	Residents and students
City of Blue Island	Local Gov't	SW	Passage of active transportation and food systems plans and Complete Streets ordinance; implementation of a community garden; institutionalization of Baby Friendly Steps at Metro South Hospital; passage of breastfeeding friendly worksite wellness	23,500	Residents and new moms
City of Countryside	Local Gov't	W	Passage of active transportation plan	5,784	Residents
City of Des Plaines	Local Gov't	N	Passage of active transportation plan and Complete Streets ordinance; installation of bike signage; passage of SRTS in Des Plaines school districts; passage of worksite wellness policy to increase opportunities for PA; passage of nutritional standards for concessions	63,459	Residents and students
Community High School District 218	School District	SW	Establish wellness councils and adopt health and wellness policy change; increase opportunities for PA/PE for staff and students; improve school food environment and institutionalize CDSMP	6,235	Students and staff
Council of Islamic Organizations of Greater Chicago	CBO	SW	Establish wellness councils and adopt health and wellness policy change; increase opportunities for PA/PE for staff and students; passage of SRTS and joint use agreements; improve school food environment; institutionalize CDSMP	1,430	Students and staff
Crossroads Coalition	CBO	S	Institutionalize CDSM	112,394	Residents
District 63 Education Foundation- TLC	School District	N	Establish wellness councils and adopt health and wellness policy change; increase opportunities for PA/PE for staff and students; improve school food environment; passage of SRTS; and integrate school garden into curriculum	3,914	Students and staff
Fourth Episcopal District AME Church	CBO	S	Implement 3 community gardens; establish nutritional standards; passage of 3 joint use agreements to improve physical activity opportunities	1,592	Congregation members and staff
Harvey School District 152	School District	S	Establish wellness councils and adopt health and wellness policy change; increase opportunities for PA/PE for staff and students; improve school food environment	2,600	Students and staff

Table 2. (Continued)

Organization	MC grantee type	SCC region	Proposed PSE changes	PSE impact	Population
Illinois Action For Children	CBO	W	Incorporating childcare facilities meal nutrition standards; standardizing nutrition and physical activity within the provider/family training curriculum; grassroots organizing to influence statewide health policies for early childhood education (working with faith communities)	5,000	Children in day care settings
J. Sterling Morton High School District 201	School District	W	Establish wellness councils and adopt health and wellness policy change; increase opportunities for PA/PE for staff and students; installation of bike racks	9,006	Students and staff
Little Company of Mary Hospital	Hospital	SW	Implementation of Baby Friendly USA steps	1,200	Maternity ward patients
Matteson School District 162	School District	S	Establish wellness councils and adopt health and wellness policy change; increase opportunities for PA/PE for staff and students; improve school food environment	3,384	Students and staff
Maywood/ Melrose Park/ Broadview District 89	School District	W	Establish wellness councils and adopt health and wellness policy change; increase opportunities for PA/PE for staff and students; improve school food environment; passage of joint use agreement	5,544	Students and staff
Northwest Community Hospital Foundation	Hospital	N	Implementation of Baby Friendly USA steps and community referral system for breastfeeding support	3,250	Maternity ward patients
Northwest Municipal Council	Regional Gov't	N	Installation of regional bike routes signage and bicycle facility planning	319,315	Residents
Oak Lawn Community High School District 229	School District	SW	Establish wellness councils and adopt health and wellness policy change; increase opportunities for PA/PE for staff and students; improve school food environment; passage of intergovernmental agreement; integration of school garden into curriculum	2,164	Students and staff
Prevention Partnership, Inc.	CBO	S	Passage of active transportation plan and safe park zones ordinance; installation of bike route signage; increase opportunities for PA/PE for school staff and students; improve school food environment; integration of school garden curriculum	35,283	Residents, students and staff
South Suburban Mayors and Managers Association	Regional Gov't	S	Establishment of 8 South Suburban transit oriented development sites (TOD sites)	144,340	Residents
Thornton Fractional Township High School District 215	School District	S	Establish wellness councils and adopt health and wellness policy change; increase opportunities for PA/PE for staff and students; improve school food environment; integrate school gardens into curriculum	3,606	Students and staff
Village of Forest Park	Local Gov't	W	Establish wellness councils and adopt health and wellness policy change; passage of SRTS; integration of school garden into curriculum; passage of active transportation plan and Complete Streets ordinance; installation of bike route signage; passage of worksite wellness policy for healthy eating and active living	16,035	Residents, students and staff
Village of Hoffman Estates	Local Gov't	N	Passage of Complete Streets ordinance; zoning code updates; installation of bike route signage	54,393	Residents
Village of Lemont	Local Gov't	SW	Passage of active transportation plan, Complete Streets and Safe Park Zones ordinances; installation of bike route signage	16,625	Residents
Village of Midlothian	Local Gov't	S	Passage of active transportation plan, Complete Streets, Zoning and Safe Park Zones ordinances; installation of bike route signage; passage of joint use agreement; nutritional standard for employee vending	20,122	Residents
Village of Oak Park	Local Gov't	W	Passage of Complete Streets and worksite wellness policy to promote biking to work	53,103	Residents
Village of Palos Park	Local Gov't	SW	Installation of bicycle route signage	4,689	Residents

Organization	MC grantee type	SCC region	Proposed PSE changes	PSE impact	Population
Village of Riverdale	Local Gov't	S	Passage of active transportation plan, Complete Streets and Safe Park Zones ordinances, implementation of community garden	13,549	Residents
Village of Schaumburg	Local Gov't	N	Passage of active transportation plan and zoning ordinances; installation of bike route signage; implementation of community garden	70,698	Residents
Village of Skokie	Local Gov't	N	Installation of bicycle route signage	64,784	Residents
Village of Tinley Park	Local Gov't	S	Passage of active transportation plan, establishment of wellness councils and adopt health and wellness policy change; passage of worksite wellness policy for healthy eating and active living	59,063	Residents and students

Increasing healthy food access: Eight local governments and one faith-based organization have improved community access to healthy foods through implementation of 8 community gardens and a farmers market. In addition, nutritional standards were passed to improve worksite food offerings in two localities. Alone, these changes will impact up to 168,741 SCC residents. At the completion of this project we expect to have at least three additional communities complete PSE changes which improve healthy food access for residents and employees.

Driving sustainable school wellness: Forty-five schools in nine school districts (with a total of 45,255 students) institutionalized wellness councils. Thirteen of those schools initiated action plans to implement changes in school food environments and opportunities for physical activity in and outside of school. Seven schools integrated wellness policies into their school improvement plans. It is our aim to implement action plans with active wellness councils in at least 12 additional schools, as these plans are integral to guide the work of the wellness councils and future school improvements in health and wellness.

Improving school food environments: The MC grant recipients have had greatest success in improving school food environments with 83 schools in 17 districts (with a total of 60,441 staff and students) making significant changes to encourage healthy eating among students and staff. Seven schools instituted a vending nutritional standard or provided healthier options in vending machines with competitive pricing to promote the healthier offerings. Forty-eight schools have made changes in their school meals programs, including school breakfast and lunch, to ensure that healthy options are available and are promoted to the students. Sixteen schools have implemented school gardens, and all are in the process of ensuring gardening is integrated into the school curriculum. Finally, 12 schools have made policy changes to ensure that competitive foods (foods other than the school lunch or breakfast served in schools) meet a nutritional standard.

Increasing opportunities for physical activity: Schools also had great success with implementing inside or outside of school policies and environmental change to increase opportunities for students and staff to be physically active. Out of a total of 59 schools, (impacting 47,099 staff and students) 23 have increased after-school opportunities through programs and classes for staff and students and 36 have improved physical activity during the school day. These schools will continue to work towards institutionalizing these changes through revisions of current administrative policies and updating their district wellness plans. In addition, 14 schools have completed bike rack siting plans and are well on their way to completing a Safe Routes to School policy to increase the number of students who bike and walk to/from school.

Collaboration and network building: Each of the 38 Model Communities grantees has coalitions at the local level with at least 2-3 unique partner organizations and at least a 5-10 member team. Alliance strengthening has occurred in several ways that help to build momentum and linkages between local level and county level change. AHAC membership increased by 70 member organizations throughout the time of the initiative, which includes but is not limited to Model Community grantees. More than 300 individuals working across organizational sectors belong to Cook County Connects. In addition, a strong faith-based collaborative has been built to include discussions with over 400 faith leaders and members across SCC on the connections between place (where you live, work and play) and health. Finally, the initiative successfully worked to develop a school-based health oriented network. Entitled the School Nurse Advisory Committee, school nurses representing each region of SCC participate in efforts to improve school health in SCC schools, including planning for an annual school health conference.

DISCUSSION

This paper presents a detailed description and early process outcomes of the MC grant program in SCC, Illinois. This strategy was specifically developed by public health practitioners and community-based leaders to support PSE change for obesity prevention and control in a geo-politically complex county.

Evaluating PSE change work can be challenging in part because strategies for achieving these types of changes are built incrementally, typically evolve over time and are initiated in response to many contextual factors which are often unpredictable. In this sense, evaluating PSE change work is a bit like shooting at a moving target. Further, because the impact of these change efforts often goes beyond the immediate PSE change itself, there can be multiple outcomes to assess – for example an organization's ability to sustain influence beyond immediate milestones or extend to a broader framework (e.g., local to county, county to state, state to national). In recognition of the multiple ways in which achievement can be characterized in PSE change work, the evaluation team in consultation with TA providers, stakeholders and CPPW program staff and upon review of relevant literature on evaluation of PSE change efforts, has identified a range of outcome areas for the local CPPW evaluation.

Strengthening the capacity of local communities to undertake obesity prevention PSE change work is supported by two approaches working in tandem. One approach is to work with "grass tops" (leadership). Another approach is to work with "grass roots" (community). Grass tops efforts concentrate on providing connections and linkages among leaders in PSE change for obesity prevention and control and operated largely through two main vehicles: the countywide Alliance for Active and Healthy Communities (a group of health advocates focused on reducing health disparities and improving the health of community members) and Cook County Connects (an online resource for sharing and collaboration around PSE change). Grass roots efforts concentrated on providing funding to local entities for staff time, raising community awareness, obtaining necessary equipment and supplies, and providing technical assistance and training in public health skills for achieving obesity-related PSE change at the local community level. Leadership and competency training and technical assistance were provided to organizations receiving MC grants both in generalized public health best practices and in specific and tailored tactics related to PSE change for obesity prevention.

The evaluation of the MC strategy is on-going. At the time of this writing, grant recipients are mid-way through their respective implementation period. While it is too soon to tell how successful this strategy was in supporting PSE change in funded communities, several lessons have been learned.

Data are needed early and often to drive the development and adjustment of supports and collaboration opportunities that meet communities where they are. While a "one size fits all" approach was never intended, based on early competency assessments during the earliest phases of the project, we learned that more upfront information on the specifics of community situations would be needed to best meet community needs.

Undertaking collaboration and capacity building simultaneously is necessary but challenging for most Model Communities. Based on participation and utilization of resources provided, we found communities engaged in more capacity building vs. collaboration activities, at least in the early phases of the project.

Many grant recipients were challenged with identifying the right staff person(s) to carry out their activities and there was a significant amount of change in assigned staff persons from the baseline to mid-point assessment time periods.

Sustainability of the capacity developed through the MC strategy will be one measure against which this approach will be judged. To date, communities with less capacity and infrastructure continue to struggle, even with provided training and technical assistance. It will be important to continue to assess this strategy for longer term outcomes and leverage.

One tactic within the MC strategy, building community partnerships, has been richly debated in the community health literature. This approach has been found to be difficult to evaluate and evaluations conducted have produced mixed results (22). Evaluation findings will further inform this rich debate.

Strategies used to increase MC grant recipient collaboration, such as our online collaborative tool, require intensive management to assure engagement of membership. While the tool has shown promise for facilitation and encouragement of collaborative relationship building, such systems should be weighed against the amount of staff time and resources in order to assess their appropriateness for a given project.

CONCLUSION

The MC strategy of providing capacity development and collaboration support in multiple formats was designed specifically to address issues in a complex region marked by fragmented government, diverse populations with diverse needs and growing health disparities. The program provides opportunities for collaborating across boundaries while also allowing for customized approaches for working with individual communities based on the particulars of their needs and settings. This is a long term developmental strategy, requiring long term follow up to tracking organizational outcomes relative to capacity and collaboration for obesity prevention.

Early process outcomes have been used to adjust program implementation. Baseline capacity and collaboration assessments have been used to refine technical assistance and training opportunities provided to Model Communities grant recipients.

Early PSE achievement outcomes indicate that school environments are among the first to accomplish PSE changes, however more work needs to be done to understand the reasons for this. While promising in the number of SCC residents touched by MC PSE work, it remains to be seen how these achievements will impact health behaviors of SCC residents. An outcomes evaluation examining these issues is underway. Other complex regions may benefit from this account of the SCC, Illinois experience both in identifying strategy components and in shaping outcome expectations.

REFERENCES

[1]   Ogden CL, Carroll MD. Prevalence of overweight, obesity, and extreme obesity among adults: United States, trends 1960–1962 through 2007–2008. [Internet]. [Place unknown]. National Center for Health Statistics; c2010. Health E-Stats; June 2010 [cited 2011 Nov 8]. Available from: http://www. cdc. gov/NCHS/ data/hestat/obesity_adult_07_08/obesity_adult_07_08.pdf

[2]   Ogden CL, Carroll MD. Prevalence of obesity among children and adolescents: United States, trends 1963–1965 through 2007–2008. [Internet]. [Place unknown]. National Center for Health Statistics; c2010. Health E-Stats; June 2010 [cited 2011 Nov 8]. Available from http://www.cdc.gov/nchs/data/ hestat/obesity_child_07_08/obesity_child_07_08.pdf

[3]   Robert Wood Johnson Foundation, Trust for America's Health[Internet]. [Place unknown]. F as in fat: how obesity threatens America's future 2011. 2011 July [cited Nov 14 2011]; p.12, 18-20, 22. Available from: http://www.rwjf.org/files/research/fasinfat2011.pdf

[4]   National Conference of State Legislatures [Internet]. Denver and Washington: National Conference of State Legislatures; c2011 [updated 2011 August; cited 2011 Nov 8]. Obesity statistics in the United States. Available from: http://www.ncsl.org/default.aspx?tabid=14367

[5]   Centers for Disease Control and Prevention [Internet]. Atlanta, GA: Centers for Disease Control and Prevention; [updated 2011 Nov 14; cited 2011 Nov 14]. Health consequences. Available from: http://www.cdc.gov/obesity/causes/health.html

[6]   Kochanek KD, Xu J, Murphy SL, Miniño AM. Deaths: Preliminary Data for 2009. NVSS [Internet]. 2011 March [cited 2011 Nov 8]; 59(4). Available from: http://www.cdc.gov/nchs/data/nvsr/nvsr59 /nvsr59_04.pdf

[7]   Centers for Disease Control and Prevention [Internet]. Atlanta, GA: Centers for Disease Control and Prevention; [updated 2011 March 28; cited 2011 Nov 14]. Economic consequences. Available from: http://www.cdc.gov/obesity/causes/economics.html

[8]   Chaloupka FJ, Powell LM. Price, availability, and youth obesity: evidence from Bridging the Gap. Prev Chronic Dis. 2009 July [cited 2011 Nov 8]; 6(3):A93. Available from: http://www.cdc.gov/ pcd/issues/2009/jul/08_0261.htm

[9]   Mercer SL, Green LW, Rosenthal AC, Husten CG, Kettel Khan L, Dietz WH. Possible lessons from the tobacco experience for obesity control. Am J Clin Nutr. 2003 April [cited 2011 Nov 14]; 77(4): 1073S-1082S. Available from: http://www.ajcn.org/content/77/4/1073S.full.pdf+html

[10]   Chaloupka FJ, Tauras J, Grossman M. Public policy and youth smokeless tobacco use. Southern Economic Journal. 1997; 64(2):503-16.

[11]   Centers for Disease Control and Prevention. Responses to cigarette prices by race/ethnicity, income, and age groups – United States 1976-1993. MMWR. 1998 Jul; [cited 2011 Nov 8]; 47(29):605-609. Available from: http://www.cdc.gov/mmwr/preview/mmwrhtml/00054047.htm

[12]   U.S. Census Bureau. State and county quickfacts: Cook County, Illinois. c2011 [cited 2011 Nov 8]. Available from: http://quickfacts.census.gov/qfd/states/17/17031.html

[13] Berube A, Kneebone E. Two steps back: city and suburban poverty trends 1999-2005. Brookings. 2006 Dec [cited 2011 Nov 8]. Available from: http://www.brookings.edu/reports/2006/12poverty_ berube.aspx

[14] U.S. Census Bureau. Census 2000 Summary File: Cook County, IL. c2000 [cited 2011 Nov 14]. Available from: http://factfinder.census.gov/servlet/QTTable?_bm=n&_lang=en&qr_name=DEC_ 2000_SF1_U_DP1&ds_name=DEC_2000_SF1_U&geo_id=05000US17031

[15] Cook County Department of Public Health [Internet]. Oak Forest, IL. WePLAN 2015, suburban Cook County community health assessment and plan. 2011 [cited 2011 Nov 8]. Available from: http://www.cookcountypublichealth.org/files/pdf/weplan-2015.pdf

[16] Hendrick R, Mossberger K. Uneven capacity and delivery of human services in Chicago suburbs: the role of townships and municipalities. Chicago, IL; University of Illinois Chicago and Chicago Community Trust. 2009. [cited 2011 Nov 14] Available from: http://www.uic.edu/cuppa/gci/news/ Hendrick-Mossberger_CCT_report_3-24-09.pdf

[17] Mibach E, Duyn M, Bloodgood B. A marketing perspective on disseminating evidence-based approaches to disease prevention and health promotions. Prev Chronic Dis [Internet]. 2006 July [cited 2011 Nov 8]; 3(3): A97. Available from: www.cdc.gov/pcd/issues/2006/jul/05_0154.htm

[18] Louie J, Guthrie K. Strategies for assessing policy change efforts: A prospective approach. Evaluat Exchange 2007;13(1):5.

[19] Glanz K, Rimer BK, Lewis FM, eds. Health behavior and health education, 3rd Ed. San Francisco, CA: Jossey-Bass, 2002.

[20] Goldsmith S, Eggers W, Richardson K, Gregory W, Midgley G. System thinking and complexity science: insights for action. Proceedings of the 11th ANZSYS/Managing the Complex V Conference. Mansfield, MA: ISCE Publishing, 2006.

[21] Best A, Clark P, Leischow SJ, Trochim WMK, editors. Greater than the sum: systems thinking in tobacco control [Internet]. Bethesda, MD: U.S. Department of Health and Human Services, National Institutes of Health, National Cancer Institute; 2007 [cited 2011 Nov 8]. Available from: http://cancercontrol.cancer.gov/tcrb/monographs/18/

[22] Shortell SM, Zukoski AP, Alexander JA, Bazzoli GJ, Conrad DA, Hasnain-Wynia R, et al. Evaluating partnerships for community health improvement: tracking the footprints. J Health Polit Policy Law 2002; 27(1):49–91.

In: Public Health Yearbook 2013
Editor: Joav Merrick

ISBN: 978-1-63321-095-0
© 2014 Nova Science Publishers, Inc.

Chapter 23

BREAKING THE CODE OF SILENCE: LESSONS LEARNED IN BUILDING COMMUNITY CAPACITY TO ADDRESS INTIMATE PARTNER VIOLENCE

Mary Frances Oneha, PhD, MN, BS[*1],*
Jan Shoultz, DrPh, MPH, MS, BS[2], Cindy Spencer, BA[3],
Joy Lacanienta, MA[4], Melissa Mamasig, BS[5],
Lois Magnussen, EdD, MS, BS[2] and Nanci Kreidman, MA[3]

[1]Waianae Coast Comprehensive Health Center
[2]University of Hawaii School of Nursing and Dental Hygiene
[3]Domestic Violence Action Center
[4]JL Community Consulting
[5]Department of Health Public Health Nursing Branch Leeward Oahu Section, Hawaii, United States of America

ABSTRACT

Violence between intimate partners results in significant health consequences that impact individuals within households and across communities. The purpose of this paper is to describe the lessons learned as a result of working to build community capacity to address the persistent public health issue of intimate partner violence (IPV). The Consortium for Health Safety and Support (CHSS) convened to strengthen responsive support for women suffering the presence of abuse in their families and intimate relationships in the Native Hawaiian and Pilipino communities along the Leeward coast of Oahu in the State of Hawaii. Methods used by consortium members to increase community capacity to address IPV from a culturally appropriate, community participatory, and gender focused public health approach included: a) research to

* Correspondence: Mary Frances Oneha, PhD, MN, BS, Waimanalo Health Center, 41-1347 Kalanianaole Hwy, Waimanalo, HI 96795 United States. E-mail: moneha@waimanalohealth.org.

understand IPV among specific cultural groups; b) a community health needs assessment to identify primary focus areas; c) participation in community events to increase awareness related to IPV and recruitment of natural allies; and d) identification of other coalitions with similar interests to create a safe and supportive community. Lessons learned over the past year fall into the following broad categories of sustaining partnerships, respecting cultural differences, recognizing the importance of family and friends, and collective leadership. Cultivating a community of sustainability, particularly in the areas of partnerships, leadership, and community driven solutions to address IPV, and celebrating unique cultural and place differences through collective leadership are important next steps for the consortium.

Keywords: Intimate partner violence, community, culture

INTRODUCTION

The mission of the Consortium for Health Safety and Support is to:

- Work together to reach a day when girls, women and their families are free of violence, when communities have influence to end domestic violence, and when everyone takes responsibility for being part of the solution.
- We envision a healthy future for girls and women.
- We envision safe communities, where support is community driven, culturally appropriate and accessible to all.

The purpose of this paper is to describe the lessons learned as a result of working to build community capacity to address the persistent public health issue of intimate partner violence (IPV). Efforts of a community based participatory research team to understand this issue from a community and cultural perspective has informed a community based consortium's endeavor to develop community driven solutions to addressing IPV.

Intimate partner violence

Violence between intimate partners results in significant health consequences that impact individuals within households and across communities. IPV includes patterns of ill-health that are physical, psychological, social, and economic. The overwhelming burden of IPV occurs in women at the hands of men (1). The General Assembly of the United Nations (1948) adopted the Universal Declaration of Human Rights reaffirming their faith in fundamental human rights. Further, Article 5 emphasizes, "No one shall be subjected to torture or to cruel, inhuman or degrading treatment or punishment (2)." IPV impacts not only women who are abused but also their children, families and others in the community.

Victimization by an intimate partner was associated with higher odds of women being injured than men (3). In the State of Hawaii, 12% of the general population report experiencing IPV at some point in their lives (4); 1 in 16 women experience IPV around the time of their most recent pregnancy; 90% of sexual assault victims are women, average of 18 years old, and Hawaiian/part-Hawaiian (5). Between 2000 and 2009 there were 58 murders of women resulting from IPV and greater than 70% were Pilipino or Native Hawaiian women (6). While the population of women who are affected is not homogenous, intervention strategies have commonly been based on Western notions of family life, and do not thoroughly take into account the unique perspectives, values and belief systems of different cultures.

METHODS

Funding for IPV has focused on tertiary services from legal and social service professionals working with women who have been victimized. Victims do not necessarily seek assistance from the mainstream agencies, including the criminal justice system. It is well understood that new strategies must be employed to assist those in our communities who have not been served well, or will not pursue support from others outside their own community. Research has validated that victims of IPV go first and foremost to their family members or friends for assistance and only access professional services if family and friends cannot help (7-8). Communities have also identified faith-based groups or cultural civic clubs as sources of support. Current options that depend primarily and sometimes exclusively on the criminal justice system severely limit the resources for those relationships, families and communities who are unable or unwilling to use these services.

The Consortium for Health, Safety and Support (CHSS) in 2010 advanced the work begun by the Oahu Domestic Violence Task Force including its commitment to work in the community, motivate system engagement, and strengthen responsive support for women suffering the presence of abuse in their families and intimate relationships. The Oahu Domestic Violence Task Force was an initiative born out of a statewide Strategic Plan commissioned by Hawaii's Department of Health, Maternal and Child Health Branch. The Domestic Violence Action Center (DVAC) assumed the role for coordinating the body, to facilitate examination, discussion and relationships among community entities involved with IPV. The Task Force began the process of inviting people to the table who were not normally invited and began to empower the community members to own the issue of IPV. Moving this agenda forward, the work of the CHSS focused on the leeward coast of Oahu, serving a high concentration of Native Hawaiian and Pilipino individuals. Eleven organizations and individuals representing a health department, medical organization, community-based organizations, wellness organization, an academic institution, and other natural community allies committed to addressing this issue. Significant contributions were received from a 16-member advisory group, representing community based organizations, a community college, state government, and members of the ethnic groups in the geographic area.

The task of community engagement is one that requires a deliberate and long term approach and commitment. The end result however is an increase in capacity building within families, neighborhoods, faith based organizations and other community entities created by engaging natural helpers or advocates within these specific communities. Methods used by consortium members to increase community capacity to address IPV from a culturally appropriate, community participatory, and gender focused public health systems approach have included: a) research to understand the documented incidence and cultural perceptions, responses, and needs of IPV among specific cultural groups; b) completion of a community health needs assessment, gender analysis, and strategic action plan to identify primary focus areas for the CHSS; c) participation in community events to increase awareness related to IPV, share information on the consortium and recruit natural allies; and d) identification of other coalitions interested in building the capacity of their members to create a safe and supportive community for women and girls.

Research: Understanding IPV from a cultural perspective

The context for IPV is a belief system about relationships of power, societal structure and the resulting conditions in society. Dominant voices hold power over more underrepresented voices. Such dominance creates both privilege and marginalization. Sources of such dominance tend to be connected to the privileges accorded by gender, race and class. Critical social theory (CST) served as the theoretical framework that guided the course of the identified research studies. The intent of this theory is to "challenge conventional assumptions and social arrangements and to move beyond the 'what is' to the 'what could be' (9)." Such knowledge is proposed to be emancipatory. As a community defines its own stories and creates solutions, the community members are recognizing and reclaiming their own power.

A community based participatory research (CBPR) team came together in 2003 to address the issue of IPV, a priority within the community. The CBPR team consisted of members of the Consortium, including DVAC, Waianae Coast Comprehensive Health Center, and the University of Hawaii School of Nursing and Dental Hygiene. Three other community health centers in urban Oahu also participated on the team. Several research studies were conducted and articles published by this team. The first study (10) relevant to this paper was a retrospective review of documented reports of IPV in 337 medical records across four community health centers on the island of Oahu. In that study, IPV was found in 9% of the total records reviewed. Within the records of the Native Hawaiian subgroup, 32.3% were found to have documentation of IPV (higher than any other ethnic group), but represented 19% of the sample population reviewed. Sixteen percent (16%) Pilipina women reported IPV, but represented 23.7% of the total sample population, and women ages 40-49 reported IPV at a higher level than any other age group.

The second research project (7-8, 11) was to understand how IPV and culture come together for selected cultural groups (Native Hawaiians, Pilipina (Tagalog speaking), and Chuukese) served by each community health center. The research question was, "What are the cultural perceptions, responses, and needs of selected individuals and groups served through a variety of programs that are affiliated with three participating community health centers regarding IPV?" Both qualitative and quantitative data were collected. Individual interviews with women who experienced IPV and focus groups with women who may not have experienced IPV were conducted with each cultural group. A "Perceptions of the Acceptability of Violence" (12) tool was administered to individual interview participants. The importance of the perceptions, responses and needs of participants from each cultural group became clearer and can be used as a basis for intervention and policy development. Unique cultural aspects emerged; however, common themes identified across the cultural groups included: Living within a Collective; Cultural Protective Factors; Cultural Barriers to Helpseeking; Gender Specific Roles; and Belonging to a Place (13).

Currently, the CHSS is embarking on a five year community based and developed intervention to engage Native Hawaiians and Pilipinos on the Leeward coast of Oahu in the State of Hawaii regarding the gender based crime of IPV. The intervention will assist in determining if community owned, community led "talk story" group sessions lead to increased awareness of IPV, gender role expectations, and increased community engagement and leadership to achieve social change. The quasi-experimental intervention is based on findings from a community health needs assessment completed by the CHSS.

The proposed evidence-based intervention will use the Community Engagement Model (CEM) (14) that includes community outreach, education, mobilization, organizing and accountability, with two culturally specific communities to prevent and address IPV within community groups, ranging from families/friends, businesses, health/social service organizations, to cultural/social groups. This model sets out a culturally appropriate approach to IPV prevention and intervention.

Community health needs assessment

The CHSS convened monthly and set up a structure to complete a community health needs assessment (CHNA) in order to understand the context of IPV within the targeted geographic (Waipahu to Waianae) and cultural communities (Native Hawaiians and Pilipinos) and developed a strategic action plan. Focused questions for the CHNA were identified by the CHSS. Information gleaned through a literature review or already available or known to CHSS members was identified first. A process was conducted with CHSS members to identify the information gaps. Key areas for examination and questions were identified. Focus groups and surveys were conducted by the CHSS and/or Community Advisory members with identified groups and at community events representing the targeted populations. Consultation was sought from Community Advisory members on the process and the summary findings of the focus groups and surveys. A subcommittee was formed with members of the Consortium to conduct the analysis.

As derived from the community health needs assessment, the following goals became the focus of the strategic action plan: 1) Build on relationships developed in both the Native Hawaiian and Pilipino focus groups and the community to advance community engagement and leadership development to create safe and supportive communities for women and girls through community owned talk story groups; 2) Strengthen linkages to build capacity with other coalitions or organizations within the targeted community to further identify natural helpers; 3) Identify the need for specialized services as identified by the talk story groups to support women and girls; and 4) Identify strategic best practices by service providers responding to IPV. The CHSS is currently moving forward with the goals of the strategic action plan.

Participation in community events to raise awareness

In an effort to raise awareness of IPV, engage the community, and recruit new members to the CHSS, Consortium members participated in various community events. The events presented an opportunity to share information and initiate conversation through a random selection of questions related to IPV. Participants at the event that stopped by the Consortium information booth were asked to take part in a game. In the game, they were asked to select a question card; the Consortium member would ask the question on the card and wait for a response. Examples of yes/no questions included: 1) "Healthy relationships allow for each person in the relationship to have friends with people of the opposite sex;" and 2) "A man's home is his castle and he gets to make all the rules and if those rules are not obeyed by his wife and children then he has the right to punish them for breaking the rules." Multiple choice questions were also asked such as: 1) "Why do people stay in an abusive relationship?" Multiple Choice Answers to this question included: A) "Because they want the family to stay together," B) "Because they do not have financial resources to leave," C) "Because they are afraid of their partner," D) "Because they love their partner," or E) "All of the above." Depending on the response, a conversation or discussion may follow with the participant and/or their family members or friends present. CHSS information was also shared and participants were given the opportunity to sign up to be on a mailing list or become a member of the CHSS.

These events presented learning opportunities for CHSS members as participant responses (to the question) provided baseline information on how the targeted community perceives or understands IPV. This knowledge helps to inform the various activities of the CHSS.

Collaboration with other coalitions

An outcome of the CHSS is to build the capacity of participating community organizations to create a safe and supportive environment for women and girls. This is also consistent with Healthy People 2020 Educational and Community-Based Programs, (ECBP-10.2), community-based primary prevention services objective to increase the number of community-based organizations providing population-based primary prevention services in the area of violence.

Several requests have come before the CHSS to join efforts in addressing related issues of child abuse and sexual violence. In an effort to decrease the burden on community members (due to multiple requests to participate on various community groups), increase Consortium participation, and meet the needs expressed in the community, the CHSS invites key coalitions/community members to join as contributing partners. The CHSS has agreed to join forces with the Sexual Violence Prevention Coalition, Consuelo Foundation (addressing child abuse and neglect), and the Hawaii State Coalition against Domestic Violence to identify common interests/activities and consolidate efforts.

RESULTS

The ground rules for Consortium members set the tone for our work together:

- We will come together with the commitment to agree for our common purpose.
- We will begin with the awareness that we are involved in a process of universal healing.
- We will have respect for one another as part of the collective passion that guides our work. Given our relative roles and skills, we are moving forward from a place of equality.
- We will impart wisdom to bind our conscience until we meet again.

Over the past year that Consortium members have been together, and eight years for the CBPR team, there have been many lessons learned. The lessons can be grouped into the following broad categories of sustaining partnerships, respecting cultural differences, recognizing the importance of family and friends, and collective leadership.

Sustaining partnerships

The DVAC has served as the facilitator and administrator of the CHSS. In year one, the DVAC entered into cooperative agreements with relevant partners from the original members of the task force and with new community partnerships. Consisting of 11 members, the Consortium has gone through periods of low participation. Gaps in the Consortium representation have reflected the impact of the state's dire budget deficits. Some Consortium members have had to change employment or have had additional job responsibilities added to their work schedule which has impacted their ability to be active participants in the Consortium. In an effort to increase and sustain partnerships, Consortium members, shifted the criteria for membership from merely community organizations and institutions to individual community members who may have experienced IPV themselves or indirectly within their family or community, conducted outreach through community events, joined forces with other coalitions working on similar interests, and will initiate Consortium meetings in the morning and evening and in two different locations to allow for maximum participation and cultural representation.

The CHSS honors and respects the time and effort interested individuals have within their capacity to give. We also anticipate that natural helpers will emerge from the talk story groups which will lead to increased Consortium and Advisory group membership. In order to sustain the work of the CHSS, it was essential to explicitly state expectations of members and collectively enjoy the benefits of this unique partnership. Renewed agreements in year two with comparable compensation included attendance at one meeting per quarter, participation in training about domestic violence, assisting at community presentations and events twice a year (i.e., staffing booths), and assisting with evaluation, by participating in interviews, completing surveys, and collecting data.

Respecting cultural differences

The Consortium's efforts to address two distinct cultural groups, representing an indigenous and immigrant populations have indeed provided invaluable lessons. Both groups contribute different ways of knowing and engaging community members and understanding IPV and the associated needs to addressing IPV. Consistent cultural representation on the Consortium and Advisory group is vital to better understanding the cultural context within which individuals, families, and communities who experience IPV have responded. Ensuring that distinct needs of each cultural group are represented throughout the activities of the CHSS is paramount.

Cultural beliefs, practices and norms can function as protective or contributing factors to IPV. One cultural belief that might be a source of conflict between partners revolves around the role of the women – "In the US, changes involving greater female empowerment or independence may disrupt a previously established balance of power within a family and precipitate forms of emotional, psychological or physical abuse" (15). Adequate cultural representation throughout consortium activities provides for clarification, education, and understanding towards enhancing cultural assets and dispelling common cultural myths. In the Philippine value system

- Kapwa is at the very foundation of human values. This core value then determines not only the person's personality but more so his/her personhood or Pagkatao. Without Kapwa, one ceases to be a Pilipino. One also ceases to be human.
- Pakikiramdam (feeling for another) is the pivotal value of shared inner perception. It refers to a heightened awareness and sensitivity. Pakikiramdam is an active process involving great care and deliberation…

Using Pakikiramdam, a person seeks to clarify an ambiguous and therefore critical situation to arrive at an appropriate response. It is a legitimate move leading to Pakikiisa (being one with others); later, to being able to identify with another's being; and ultimately, to being able to share complete trust" (16).

Recognizing the importance of family and friends

Funding for IPV has focused on tertiary services from legal and social service professionals working with women who have been victimized. The CHSS recognized from earlier studies that women and their children do not rely on traditional victim services or health care providers until injury has occurred (7-8). Family preservation in some cultures has been seen as a priority rather than safety (15). The opportunity to engage community members from Native Hawaiian and Pilipino communities during the planning phase of this program has clearly underscored the idea that women seek support and safety from their families, friends and other community members (neighbors, businesses) to prevent and intervene early when relationships are difficult. It is well understood that new strategies must be employed to assist those in our communities who have not been served well, or will not pursue support from others outside their own community group. Current options that depend primarily and sometimes exclusively on the criminal justice system severely limit the options for those relationships, families and communities who are unable or unwilling to use these options. Many people will not use the conventional IPV resources due to language or cultural barriers and basic fear of the police, jails and the legal and immigrations systems. For example, within Hawaii's Pilipino community, IPV is currently perceived more as a "social taboo." The cultural concept of bringing Hiya (shame) to one's self and family often prevents the survivors/victims from disclosing the nature of their abusive relationship. This cultural barrier also extends to the survivor's support network, economic and social independence. As a community, it is imperative to create awareness about IPV as an urgent Pilipino community health issue.

IPV is more than a criminal justice or legal system issue and more than a health care system issue. IPV is a public health epidemic and a human rights issue that requires communities – neighbors, friends, families, and nontraditional community allies to generate new approaches to preventing IPV. These efforts include creating equality between the genders, and changing social norms to begin physical, psychological and spiritual healing in order to rebuild family and community support networks.

Collective leadership

Five principles to collective leadership have been described in order to affect sustained change within communities (17). Lessons learned by the CHSS will be described within each principle. First, collective leadership is place-based, honoring historical context, local cultures, and their environments. The CHSS is place-based, convening, recruiting members, and implementing activities within the communities of focus. Native Hawaiians and Pilipinos have encountered unique historical experiences that have influenced their way of life and the environments in which they reside. Consortium members representing not only the cultural group, but the places of focus, provide a rich context to developing effective intervention strategies. Understanding unique community patterns, infrastructure, access, resources, social structure, and politics contribute to the decision making process of the consortium, while being respectful of cultural norms and practices.

Second, leadership capacity building occurs at three levels: individual, collective, and the organization. At the start of the CHSS, shared meaning around the topic of IPV needed to occur. How it is understood in the literature versus how it is articulated in the community presented some differences and continues to be an evolving process.

Webinars sponsored by the Department of Health and Human Services Office of Women's Health related to community engagement, gender analysis, and economic evaluation have been invaluable in creating a shared vision and building leadership capacity. Local and national workshops or activities, attended by consortium members, have also provided an opportunity to increase our knowledge related to developing community based interventions to prevent IPV. While team participation in these activities has been useful, balancing personal learning and team-building skills among consortium members is a vital and continuous process.

Collectively, the CHSS has developed a formative evaluation plan to examine the collective and organizational processes identified to achieve the goals of the strategic action plan. Individual interviews with key consortium members and intervention participants will be conducted at defined time points along with a continuous review of the proposed work plan timeline. Recommendations will be incorporated into the CHSS work plan. An evaluation to measure the economic impact of the proposed intervention will also be completed.

The third principle of collective leadership is learning, understanding and enacting democratic principles that lead to a just community. The ground rules developed by the CHSS reflect this principle. Renewed agreements and comparable compensation with consortium partners describe the level of participation required to affect the work of the CHSS. Facilitation skills focused on shared-decision making, strategic planning, conflict management and community organizing.

Fourth, effective relationships are built and sustained with a network of partners and alliances that support and sustain the collective mission of the group and its work. As described previously, the CHSS has joined forces with other coalitions in order to move this issue forward through an expanded network of people and organizations. Finally, the fifth principle, collective leadership is supported by an organizational infrastructure that ensures sustainability. As the CHSS enters its second year, sustainability is critical and collective leadership is necessary to move the consortium in this direction. Potential strategies to ensure sustainability and build on the work of the consortium include dissemination (presentation, publications, translation to practice, institutional policies) of work products and research findings, development of future related projects at the consortium or organizational levels, and maturation of the CHSS to possibly its own non-profit entity.

CONCLUSION

As the work of the consortium continues, there will be more valued lessons learned. A significant next step, based on the lessons learned, includes cultivating a community of sustainability, particularly in the areas of partnerships, leadership, and community driven solutions to address IPV. This requires ensuring that the appropriate voices are identified, developed, heard, and supported within the consortium. Celebrating and respecting unique cultural and place differences through collective leadership will provide a rich context to the work of the CHSS.

ACKNOWLEDGMENT

We would like to acknowledge members of the CHSS and advisory group and those organizations who have provided funding for this important work: National Institute of Nursing Research 1 R15 NR009424-01A2 and Department of Health and Human Services, Office of Women's Health 1CCEWH101006-01-00 and 1CCEWH111025-01-00.

REFERENCES

[1]   Heise L, Garcia-Moreno C. Intimate partner violence. In: Krug EG, Dahlberg LL, Mercy JA, Zwi AB, Lozano R, eds. World Report on Violence and Health. Geneva: World Health Organization, 2002.

[2]   United Nations. The Universal Declaration of Human Rights. Accessed 2011 May 12. URL: http://www.un.org/en/documents/udhr/

[3]   Warner TD. Violent acts and injurious consequences: An examination of competing hypotheses about intimate partner violence using agency-based data. J Fam Violence 2009;25:183-93.

[4]   Shor R, Hayes D, Roberson E, Fuddy L. Violence between intimate partners in Hawaii. Data from BFRSS, PRAMS, YRBS 2010. Honolulu, HI: Hawaii Department Health, Family Health Services Division, 2010.

[5]   Davidson J, Perrone P, Haro F, Yanagida E, Choi-Misailidis S. Sexual Assault Victims in Honolulu, A Statistical Profile 2004. State of Hawaii, Department of the Attorney General. Accessed 2010 Aug 8. URL: http://hawaii.gov/ag/cpja/main/rs/sp_reports_0306/SATC.pdf.

[6]   IPV Coalition. Deaths attributed to IPV in Hawaii 1996–present 2009. Unpublished report, 2009.

[7]   Oneha MF, Magnussen L, Shoultz J. The voices of Native Hawaiian women: Perceptions, responses and needs regarding intimate partner violence. Calif J Health Promotion 2010;8(1):72-81.

[8]   Shoultz J, Magnussen L, Manzano H, Arias C, Spencer C. Listening to Filipina women: Perceptions, responses and needs regarding intimate partner violence. Issues Ment Health Nurs 2010;31(1):54-61.

[9]   Mohammed S. (Re)Examining health disparities: critical social theory in pediatric nursing. J Spec Pediatr Nurs 2006;11(1): 68-71.

[10]   Magnussen L., Shoultz J, Oneha M, Hla M, Brees-Saunders Z, Akamine M, Talisayan B, Wong E. Intimate partner violence: A retrospective chart review. J Am Acad Nurse Pract 2004;16(11):502-12.

[11]   Shoultz J, Magnussen L, Hansen K, Brees-Saunders Z, Selifis S, Ifenuk M. Intimate partner violence: Perceptions of Chuukese women. Hawaii Med J 2007;66(10):268-71.

[12]   Torres S, Campbell J, Campbell D, Ryan C, Price P, Stallings R, et al. Abuse during and before pregnancy: Prevalence and cultural correlates. Violence Vict 2000;15(3):303-21.

[13]   Magnussen L, Shoultz J, Richardson K, Oneha M. Campbell J, Matsunaga D, Selifis S, Sapolu M, Samifua M, Manzano H, Spencer C, Arias C. Responding to the needs of culturally diverse women who experience Intimate Partner Violence. Hawaii Med J 2011;70(1):9-15.

[14]   Kim M. The community engagement continuum: outreach, mobilization, organizing and accountability to address violence against women in Asian and Pacific Islander communities 2005. Accessed 2011 Jun 22. URL: http://www.apiidv.org/files/Community.Engagement.Continuum-Report-2005(Rev.2010).pdf.

[15]   Uehling G, Bouroncle A, Roeber C, Tashima N, Crain C. Preventing partner violence in refugee and immigrant communities. Forced Migration Rev 2011;38: 50-1.

[16]   Enriquez V. From colonial to liberation psychology. Manila, Phillippines: Dela Salle Press, 1994.

[17]   Ah Nee-Benham MKP, Militello M, Ruder K. Learing and living-into collective leadership. Kellogg Leadership for Community Change: Crossing boundaries, strengthening communities. Battle Creek, MI: WK Kellogg Foundation, 2002.

In: Public Health Yearbook 2013
Editor: Joav Merrick

ISBN: 978-1-63321-095-0
© 2014 Nova Science Publishers, Inc.

Chapter 24

THE ROAD TO OZANAM:
A PLACE TO TEACH, LEARN AND HEAL

Casey M Rebholz, PhD, MPH[1,2], Taimur H Khan[2] and Marcia H Glass, MD[2]

[1]Department of Epidemiology, Tulane University School of Public Health and Tropical Medicine, New Orleans, Louisiana, US
[2]Department of Medicine, Tulane University School of Medicine, New Orleans, Louisiana, US

ABSTRACT

Homeless persons experience a greater burden of illness and barriers to accessing care. Furthermore, Hurricane Katrina had devastating and persisting effects on the healthcare system and health status of the New Orleans population. As a result, Ozanam Inn Weekend Clinic was founded in January 2010 by medical students to serve the homeless in post-Katrina New Orleans and has since expanded to involve public-health and social-work volunteers. The objective of this paper is to describe the community-based approach of this student-run clinic in addressing the health needs of the homeless in New Orleans. We retrospectively reviewed medical records for all 241 patients seen between January 1, 2010 and September 30, 2011. Medical teams conducted physical examinations, measured vital signs, provided blood pressure and glucose checks, wrote prescriptions, tested for tuberculosis, administered vaccines, and counseled on health promotion and disease prevention. Social-work and public-health teams provided case-based and group-based assistance, including health education and psycho-social counseling and referrals to medical care, community programs, and case-management services. The most common reasons for seeking care were musculoskeletal pain, cold symptoms, blood pressure and glucose checks, skin and foot problems, medication refills, and oral-health issues. The most common referrals were for primary care, dental care, psychiatric treatment, substance-abuse treatment, and orthopedics. The synchronized medical, social work, and public-health resources and community-academic partnership

* Correspondence: Marcia H Glass, MD, Clinical Assistant Professor of Medicine, Tulane University Health Sciences Center, Section of General Internal Medicine and Geriatrics, 1430 Tulane Avenue, SL-16, New Orleans, Louisiana, United States. E-mail: mglass@tulane.edu.

demonstrated by this clinic model could be emulated by other organizations to meet the varied needs of underserved populations.

Keywords: Homeless persons, students, health services, delivery of health care, community medicine, uncompensated care

INTRODUCTION

Homelessness is a significant public-health problem due to its associated increased risk for poor health status. In particular, various indicators of housing instability are related to chronic conditions (e.g., hypertension, diabetes, and asthma), acute conditions (e.g., infections and injuries), communicable diseases (e.g., tuberculosis, sexually transmitted infections), and premature mortality (1-4). In addition to physical ailments, there is an increased rate of substance abuse, mental health disorders, and social instability among the homeless compared to the general population, providing additional challenges to effective healthcare delivery (5, 6). Homeless persons experience increased barriers to accessing healthcare and managing their health conditions (7, 8).

In New Orleans, Louisiana, Hurricane Katrina and subsequent disasters, including Hurricane Rita and the BP oil spill, had devastating and persisting consequences for the healthcare infrastructure, particularly for underserved individuals (9, 10). The hurricane exacerbated existing health disparities in New Orleans, with both immediate and sustained adverse effects on disease management, mental health, and mortality (11-14). In addition, homelessness has increased 70% since Hurricane Katrina, with current estimates of over 9,000 individuals meeting the U.S. Department of Housing and Urban Development definition of being homeless (15). As a result, a greater burden of responsibility for providing care for the underserved has shifted onto community-based health and social-service organizations.

Ozanam Inn is one of the few shelters for men in the Greater New Orleans area that, in addition to housing, provides extensive social and occupation-development services. The student-run weekend clinic in Ozanam Inn homeless shelter was reopened in January 2010 after being closed since Hurricane Katrina in August 2005. Student leaders of the longstanding, weekday tuberculosis testing program at Ozanam Inn restarted the clinic after recognizing that access to and knowledge about affordable health and social services was limited in this population and in the overall New Orleans region. Patients and shelter administrators requested additional medical and social services beyond the capacity of the existing tuberculosis-testing program.

Through continuous feedback, evaluation, and communication, the clinic leadership strives to meet the evolving health and social needs of the patient population in collaboration with the shelter administration. The stated mission of the Ozanam Inn Weekend Clinic is to "expand access to primary care and promote wellness to the homeless community of New Orleans, while also providing a flexible and dynamic atmosphere for students to develop professional skills through a multidisciplinary approach to healthcare." The purpose of this paper is to describe the community-based approach of this clinic in addressing the healthcare needs of the homeless in New Orleans.

METHODS

Program design and patient selection

The student-run clinic takes place on Sunday afternoons throughout the calendar year. The clinic is held in administrative offices and designated healthcare offices in a homeless shelter. Patients are recruited by posting fliers around the shelter and by making an announcement over a loudspeaker system both inside and outside the shelter before lunch service. Additional outreach and promotion strategies for patient recruitment include posting clinic flyers in public locations throughout the city, posting updated clinic information on our own and other publically accessible websites, periodically volunteering to serve the homeless population in other capacities, and participating in community-based health outreach events. All services at the clinic are provided free-of-charge. All patients that seek care within the scheduled hours are seen on a walk-in basis, regardless of ability to pay, housing status, age, gender, or any other socioeconomic or demographic factors. The patient population consists primarily of those seeking a free meal at the shelter, those staying overnight at the shelter, and longer-term shelter residents participating in an occupational transitional-assistance program, volunteer corps-assistance program, or medical transitional-assistance program. The clinic is equipped almost completely through donated medical and office supplies. Several small grants, private donations, and a fundraiser have been the source of financial support for additional necessary items.

Program staff

The clinic is staffed entirely by volunteers. Preclinical medical student volunteers receive service-learning hours as academic credit. Clinical medical students participate in the clinic as part of the ambulatory medicine clerkship. Medical teams conduct physical examinations, measure vital signs, provide blood pressure and glucose checks, write prescriptions, test for tuberculosis, administer vaccines, and counsel on health promotion and disease prevention. Social work and public-health teams provide case-based and group-based assistance, including health education and psycho-social counseling and referrals to medical care, community programs, and case-management services. A Spanish language interpreter is on-call for all clinic dates. A board-certified volunteer physician and licensed clinical social worker are on-site during clinic to supervise students. A network of student leaders and an advisory board consisting of community site representatives, faculty, and medical, public-health, and social-work students oversee operations and management of the clinic and affiliated programs (i.e., tuberculosis testing and vaccine programs).

Data collection and analysis

Student leaders retrieved The Baltimore Health Care for the Homeless history and physical form from the National Health Care for the Homeless website and adapted it to use at the student-run clinic for recording patient information, medical student and physician assessment, and services rendered. Student leaders also designed an intake form for the student-run clinic to document patient self-reported reasons for seeking care and race/ethnicity. From the paper medical records for all patients seen since the clinic's inception (January 1, 2010-September 30, 2011), we abstracted date of visit, age, gender, race/ethnicity, number of visits, reason for seeking care, topics of health education and counseling, prescriptions given, referrals given, and administration of vaccines and tuberculosis skin test, and entered this information into a Microsoft Access 2010 database. We performed logical quality-assurance checks periodically and upon completion of data entry and then gave feedback to data-entry personnel to correct errors we detected.

We also ran basic descriptive statistics, including frequencies, proportions, means, and standard deviations. We analyzed data with SAS statistical software, version 9.2 (SAS Institute, Inc., Cary, NC).

We followed procedures in accordance with the ethical standards of Tulane University's institutional review board and the Helsinki Declaration. The Tulane University institutional review board has approved the study protocol with a waiver of written informed consent.

RESULTS

We have summarized characteristics of the patient population in table 1. Between January 1, 2010 and September 30, 2011, 40 total weekend clinics were held, ranging from one to three clinic dates per month. The number of patients seen during each clinic ranged from 1 to 14, with a median of 7 patient visits. During this 21 month period, there were 241 patients and 284 patient visits. Most patients were seen at the clinic only once. Of the 241 patients seen, most were middle-aged, with a mean of 46.5 years and a standard deviation of 11.2 years, ranging from 19 to 77 years. Nearly all patients were male, and a majority of the patient population was African-American.

Table 1. Characteristics of Clinic Patient Population, January 2010-September 2011

Number of visits per patient	Frequency (n (%))
One	241 (84.9%)
Two	33 (11.6%)
Three	10 (3.5%)
Age, years	
<25	6 (2.5%)
25-44	88 (36.8%)
45-64	134 (56.1%)
>64	11 (4.6%)
Male gender	231 (95.9%)
Race/ethnicity	
African-American	129 (56.1%)
Caucasian	93 (40.4%)
Hispanic/Latino	3 (1.3%)
Other	5 (2.2%)

We describe the patient visits in Table 2. The most common reasons for seeking care were musculoskeletal pain, cold symptoms, blood pressure and glucose checks, skin and foot problems (blisters, dermatitis, abscesses, and fungal infections), medication refills, and oral-health issues. Clinic personnel provided counseling and health education most frequently for smoking-cessation and upper-respiratory symptom management. Clinic physicians prescribed non-steroidal anti-inflammatory drugs, anti-hypertensive medications, and topical antibacterial or antifungal ointment typically. The most common referrals given were for primary care, dental care, psychiatric treatment, substance-abuse treatment, and orthopedics, respectively. Seventeen patients were sent directly to the emergency department.

Table 2. Description of Patient Visits, January 2010-September 2011

Reason for seeking care	Frequency (n (%))
Musculoskeletal pain	52 (18.4%)
Cold symptoms	49 (17.3%)
Blood pressure check	30 (10.6%)
Skin problems	28 (9.9%)
Foot problems	16 (5.7%)
Oral-health issues	16 (5.7%)
Medication refill	15 (5.3%)
Vaccine	13 (4.6%)
Abdominal pain	10 (3.5%)
Tuberculosis test/treatment	9 (3.2%)
Glucose check	7 (2.5%)
Other	38 (13.4%)
Counseling and health education topics	
Smoking-cessation	29 (10.2%)
Upper-respiratory symptom management	23 (8.1%)
Hypertension management	13 (4.6%)
Diabetes management	6 (2.1%)
Other	7 (2.5%)
Referrals	
Primary care	89 (31.3%)
Dental care	26 (9.2%)
Psychiatric treatment	22 (7.8%)
Emergency department	17 (6.0%)
Substance-abuse treatment	10 (3.5%)
Social work	8 (2.8%)
Orthopedics	6 (2.1%)
HIV testing/treatment	5 (1.8%)
Tuberculosis clinic	5 (1.8%)
Gastroenterology clinic	5 (1.8%)
Hepatitis C clinic	5 (1.8%)
Sexually transmitted infections clinic	4 (1.4%)
Other	14 (4.9%)
Prescriptions	
Non-steroidal anti-inflammatory drugs / aspirin	62 (21.8%)
Anti-bacterial or anti-fungal ointment	40 (14.1%)
Anti-hypertensive medications	31 (10.9%)
Other	86 (30.3%)
Hepatitis A & B vaccine	19 (7.0%)
Influenza vaccine	17 (6.3%)
Tuberculosis test	13 (4.8%)

DISCUSSION

In post-Katrina New Orleans, the overall health care system and Tulane University have slightly shifted focus from a central hospital to community health centers, especially for the underserved population (16, 17). Community-based health and social service organizations have the advantage of being easier for patients to access and better tailored to the local community's needs. Ozanam Inn Weekend Clinic is part of this expanding network of neighborhood-based healthcare sites. This shelter-based, free, student-run clinic has effectively delivered services that address both the presenting acute medical conditions and underlying social determinants of health for a high-risk, hard-to-reach, and vulnerable population.

It has been well-documented that homeless adults have multiple unmet health needs, including physical and mental illness, and experience barriers to accessing care (4, 7, 8). There are some promising reports of improved health for individuals that are engaged in a homeless-shelter system, and for models of care that address behavioral factors and vulnerability indicators (4, 6, 18). This evidence lends support to our shelter-based clinic model with a multidisciplinary team of volunteer staff to address various dimensions of illness. The observation that most patients are seen at our clinic on only one occasion highlights the importance of meeting as many of the patient's health and social needs as possible during the first visit, which we have been able to achieve with the use of targeted referrals and maintaining an inventory of clinical supplies that mirrors recent demands.

When access to primary care is limited and health insurance coverage rates are low, as is the case in post-Katrina New Orleans and among the homeless population, one concern is inappropriate and costly utilization of the emergency department (8, 19, 20).

In our patient population, on a nearly monthly basis, we encounter a patient that requires urgent medical attention and we refer directly to the emergency department in such a situation. However, the vast majority of patient-reported chief complaints are relatively benign medical conditions, which we are able to address on-site or for which we refer to primary care. These findings demonstrate the effectiveness of our clinic in triaging by disease severity, directing urgent cases to better-equipped healthcare sites and diverting non-urgent cases away from inefficient healthcare use.

There are many strengths of this clinic. For the patients, this is a level of care and access to resources that is convenient and free. With the added dimension of social workers, translators, and community health professionals to the medical team, this program has evolved into a synchronized healthcare-delivery team, providing more holistic care for patients. For students, it provides early and necessary exposure to the local patient population and many common medical and social issues, along with insight into the culture and environment of the community. This service-learning experience is invaluable training for future health professionals. Student volunteers benefit from small-group teaching from faculty, focused mainly on practicing basic skills in talking to and examining patients. Students also benefit from peer teaching through interactive case presentations and multidisciplinary, team-based approaches to patients.

There are also some limitations to this program. Ozanam Inn Weekend Clinic is still in its formative years since it reopened in January 2010. Scarce funds, space, and personnel continue to present challenges to the clinic leadership and jeopardize the clinic's sustainability, with physician volunteers being the principal limiting factor. Nonetheless, the clinic has grown remarkably in a short period of time to become recognized as a mutually beneficial partnership for members of the homeless, the shelter, and the academic communities alike. The clinic operations have been possible on a limited budget due to the generosity of donors and participation of volunteers. The use of existing office space in the shelter during periods of non-use is an economical alternative to creating designated clinic space and is a familiar and non-threatening environment for patients.

Our future goal for the clinic is to build a stronger foundation and to improve the likelihood of its long-term sustainability, as well as to ensure that it continues to be community-relevant. The clinic will further collaborate with allied health disciplines, such as pharmacy, to develop a basic dispensary and otherwise meet medicinal needs of patients based on the most frequently dispensed over-the-counter medications and most frequency prescribed medications. The most common patient counseling topics will be revisited in a health-fair format facilitated by the public-health team in order to reach a broader audience. Several strategies will be employed to facilitate an effective referral process, such as supporting a continuity-of-care specialist to follow-up with agencies and patients about appointments during the week. Appropriateness of the program components in meeting the local homeless community's needs will be assessed through patient-satisfaction surveys, communication with shelter administrators, review of volunteer reflections, and monthly meetings with student leaders.

Given that the homeless population is inadequately represented in research and few student-run clinics have been reported in the published literature, further methodologically rigorous and culturally appropriate research is warranted. In particular, an epidemiologic study utilizing respondent-driven sampling methods to identify a representative sample of this hard-to-reach population would be useful for understanding prevalent diseases and risk factors among the homeless. Qualitative studies would aid in the determination of barriers to accessing care and program strategies to address these barriers since existing quantitative tools have not been validated in homeless populations. Due to a recent surge in development of student-run clinics, updated multi-site and national surveys are warranted to describe the role of these programs in caring for underserved populations and in providing educational experiences.

This description of the early development and implementation of a student-run, shelter-based, free clinic provides a model that could be emulated by other organizations in New Orleans or in other regions of the U.S. and the world. Community-academic partnerships that synchronize medical, social and public-health resources at preexisting shelters to deliver services directly to a largely neglected patient population would be of great value to the patients, the students, and the overall community.

ACKNOWLEDGMENTS

The authors would like to acknowledge the contribution of several people. Deacon Biaggio DiGiovanni, Executive Director of Ozanam Inn homeless shelter, reviewed the manuscript and has provided support for all student-run programs at Ozanam Inn. Many student leaders, student volunteers, and faculty members have been involved in various aspects of the clinic's operations. We are grateful for the continued support of the Ozanam Inn homeless shelter administration, staff, and Executive Board. We are most thankful for and indebted to our patients for attending our clinic, trusting us to care for them, and teaching us about medicine and culture.

There was no funding provided for this study. The authors declare no conflicts of interest. This study was approved by the Tulane University Institutional Review Board, project #217649. A portion of these data were included in a poster presentation entitled "Implementation of a Free, Student-Run, Weekend Clinic in a Homeless Shelter" at the Society of Student-Run Free Clinics Conference in conjunction with the Society of Teachers of Family Medicine Conference on Medical Student Education in Houston, Texas in January 2011.

REFERENCES

[1]   Haddad MB, Wilson TW, Ijaz K, Marks SM, Moore M. Tuberculosis and homelessness in the United States, 1994-2003. JAMA 2005;293(22):2762-6.

[2]   Jones CA, Perera A, Chow M, Ho I, Nguyen J, Davachi S. Cardiovascular disease risk among the poor and homeless - what we know so far. Curr Cardiol Rev 2009;5(1):69-77.

[3]   Morrison DS. Homelessness as an independent risk factor for mortality: Results from a retrospective cohort study. Int J Epidemiol 2009;38(3):877-83.

[4]   Schanzer B, Dominguez B, Shrout PE, Caton CL. Homelessness, health status, and health care use. Am J Public Health 2007;97(3):464-9.

[5]   Brickner PW, McAdam JM, Torres RA, Vicic WJ, Conanan BA, Detrano T, et al. Providing health services for the homeless: A stitch in time. Bull N Y Acad Med 1993;70(3):146-70.

[6]   Gelberg L, Andersen RM, Leake BD. The behavioral model for vulnerable populations: Application to medical care use and outcomes for homeless people. Health Serv Res 2000;34(6):1273-302.

[7]   Baggett TP, O'Connell JJ, Singer DE, Rigotti NA. The unmet health care needs of homeless adults: A national study. Am J Public Health 2010;100(7):1326-33.

[8]   Kushel MB, Vittinghoff E, Haas JS. Factors associated with the health care utilization of homeless persons. JAMA 2001;285(2):200-6.

[9]   Berggren RE, Curiel TJ. After the storm--health care infrastructure in post-Katrina New Orleans. N Engl J Med. 2006;354(15):1549-52.

[10]   Rudowitz R, Rowland D, Shartzer A. Health care in New Orleans before and after Hurricane Katrina. Health Aff 2006;25(5):393-406.

[11]   Stephens KUS, Grew D, Chin K, Kadetz P, Greenough PG, Burkle FM Jr, et al. Excess mortality in the aftermath of Hurricane Katrina: A preliminary report. Disaster Med Public Health Prep 2007;1(1):15-20.

[12]   Fonseca VA, Smith H, Kuhadiya N, Leger SM, Yau CL, Reynolds K, et al. Impact of a natural disaster on diabetes: Exacerbation of disparities and long-term consequences. Diabetes Care 2009;32(9):1632-8.

[13]   Islam T, Muntner P, Webber LS, Morisky DE, Krousel-Wood MA. Cohort study of medication adherence in older adults (CoSMO): Extended effects of Hurricane Katrina on medication adherence among older adults. Am J Med Sci 2008;336(2):105-10.

[14]   Kessler RC, Galea S, Gruber MJ, Sampson NA, Ursano RJ, Wessely S. Trends in mental illness and suicidality after Hurricane Katrina. Mol Psychiatry 2008;13(4):374-84.

[15]   UNITY of Greater New Orleans. Homelessness in Greater New Orleans: A report on progress toward ending homelessness in the years after the nation's largest housing disaster. 2011.

[16]   DeSalvo KB, Muntner P, Fox CE. Community-based health care for "the city that care forgot." J Urban Health 2005;82(4):520-3.

[17]   DeSalvo KB, Sachs BP, Hamm LL. Health care infrastructure in post-Katrina New Orleans: a status report. Am J Med Sci 2008;336(2):197-200.

[18]   Hwang SW, Tolomiczenko G, Kouyoumdjian FG, Garner RE. Interventions to improve the health of the homeless: a systematic review. Am J Prev Med 2005;29(5):311-9.

[19]   Ku BS, Scott KC, Kertesz SG, Pitts SR. Factors associated with use of urban emergency departments by the U.S. homeless population. Public Health Rep 2010;125(3):398-405.

[20]   Mendelberg JH, Kuhn RE, Kohn MA. Epidemiologic analysis of an urban, public emergency department's frequent users. Acad Emerg Med 2000;7(6):637-46.

In: Public Health Yearbook 2013
Editor: Joav Merrick

ISBN: 978-1-63321-095-0
© 2014 Nova Science Publishers, Inc.

Chapter 25

IMPLEMENTING AND DISSEMINATING A FALL PREVENTION PROGRAM IN AT-RISK OLDER ADULTS LIVING IN A NATURALLY OCCURRING RETIREMENT COMMUNITY-SUPPORTIVE SERVICES PROGRAM

Dale Chaikin, RN, MS*[1], Renee Pekmezaris, PhD[1],
Rajni Walia, MA[1], Corinne Kyriacou, PhD[2],
Fredda Vladeck, LCSW[3] and Gayle Kolidas, LCSW[1]

[1]North Shore-LIJ Health System, Community Health and Public Policy, Great Neck
[2]Hofstra University, Health Professions and Kinesiology, Hempstead, NY, US
[3]United Hospital Fund, Director, Aging in Place Initiative, New York, US

ABSTRACT

The overarching goal of this study is to test the impact of the implementation and dissemination of a fall prevention program in at-risk older adults living in a Naturally Occurring Retirement Community-Supportive Services Program (NORC-SSP). The literature cites that the most effective interventions in targeting persons at risk to fall, include both a multi-factorial fall risk assessment and management program conducted by a team of health professionals. After NORC-SSP staff conducted a risk assessment utilizing a modified version of the Hartford Fall Risk Assessment (HFRA) tool, a multi-factorial intervention was implemented, utilizing a single group pre-post design. The process included communication of those risk scores to the residents' physicians, along with recommendations for follow-up interventions. NORC-SSP staff then facilitated the process by which those interventions could be accomplished. Post-intervention assessments showed a significant decrease in the mean composite fall risk score for residents (N=93) from 32.9 to 23.9, Wilcoxon signed rank, $p = 0.001$. It was our belief that the communication of those assessment results to the primary physician, and follow-up intervention by a health professional well known to the older adult, would decrease

---

*Correspondence: Dale Chaikin, RN, MS, Director of Community Health Nursing, North Shore-LIJ Health System, Community Health and Public Policy, 175 Community Drive, Second Floor, Great Neck, NY 11021 United States. E-mail: dchaikin@nshs.edu.

risk factors to fall. Future research initiatives should focus on evaluating the NORC-SSP setting as a dissemination vehicle for best practice chronic disease management.

Keywords: Older adult, falls prevention, naturally occurring retirement community

INTRODUCTION

Annually, nearly 30% of Americans over the age of 65 (one in three) fall and subsequently require medical treatment. In the population over the age of 80, the rate of falling increases to 50% (1). In 2005, of 433,000 older adults admitted to the hospital, about 16,000 died due to falls. Falls have become the leading cause of injury-related visits to emergency departments in the United States and the sixth leading cause of death (2). Furthermore, falls are the most common reason given by family members who seek nursing home placement for older adults, and have significant effects on the quality of life (2, 3).

According to 2008 census estimates, the population over the age of 65 accounted for roughly 36 million or 12% of the population (4). The population over the age of 65 years, in the United States, is expected to be 71 million in the year 2030, accounting for approximately 20% of the US population (5). Hence, the number of elderly individuals requiring services to meet their changing needs will increase dramatically. Frail older adults often do not qualify for government subsidized long term care but cannot afford private pay assisted living. In addition, a 2008 American Association of Retired Persons (AARP) survey indicates that 89 % of older Americans want to remain at home and in their community for as long as possible (6). Many, however, have not planned for management in their homes as their health deteriorates. Over the past two decades a new model of care has emerged that has the potential to revolutionize services for older adults living in the community. This new paradigm recognizes the considerable strengths of the older adult, as well as their inevitably changing needs. It also recognizes older adult's overwhelming preference to remain in the home and in the neighborhoods they have lived in for years and it acknowledges the importance of community for successful aging. This new model is Supportive Service Programs (SSPs) based in Naturally Occurring Retirement Communities (NORC). A NORC-SSP is a partnership that unites housing entities, health and social service providers, government and philanthropic organizations to locate a range of coordinated health care, social services and group activities, on site, that promote independence and healthy aging. One of the primary features of a NORC-SSP is the multidisciplinary approach to providing care, wherein nursing and social work staff provide the resident with a reliable source of information, referral, and chronic care management. Given the infrastructure of the NORC-SSP, as well as the trusting relationship that develops between the NORC resident and the nursing and social work staff, the United Hospital Fund (UHF), in collaboration with the New York Community Trust (NYCT), established the Deepdale CARES (Community Action Reach out to Elder Service) NORC Health Care Linkage Project. The goal of this project was to develop and strengthen effective linkages between NORC-SSPs and key healthcare providers serving their communities. An analysis of North Shore-Long Island Jewish Health System (NSLIJ) emergency room admissions of older adults from the previous year within this community revealed that 80% were due to trauma as a result of falls. In the quest to promote healthy aging and independence in older adults, a falls prevention program, in collaboration with physicians and community healthcare providers would be implemented and disseminated to at-risk seniors.

Despite the growing literature documenting prevention and best practices that have proven successful in well-controlled research, few of these interventions are consistently implemented in applied settings and as such, these gaps have been documented (2, 7-9). A systematic review and meta-analysis was performed to assess the relative effectiveness of various interventions to prevent falls in older adults. These interventions consisted of exercise programs, environmental modifications, as well as educational presentations (10). The most effective intervention was found to be a multi-factorial fall risk assessment and subsequent management program. Strong evidence exists demonstrating that multi-factorial interventions conducted by health professionals can prevent falls, particularly if they are targeting persons at-risk and include several intervention approaches (11-13). Successful fall prevention programs have demonstrated a significant reduction in fall risk (14).

There is, therefore, a clear need for translation of best practices to "real life" settings in order for them to be effective. Li et al. recently evaluated a Tai Chi fall prevention program for community-based use in six community centers (15). The program was found to have a 100% adoption rate and an 87% reach into the targeted older adult population. Baker et al. demonstrated that members of senior centers responded positively to one-on-one counseling delivered by credible senior center-based health care providers (16).

The NORC model/infrastructure

The growth of NORC-SSPs is likely to continue, and therefore, warrants considerable attention as a "real life" setting for disseminating best practices amongst community dwelling elders. Presently, NSLIJ provides nursing services to older adults in six Queens and Nassau, NY communities through the NORC-SSP model. Older adults who live in demographically similar non-NORC communities do not have the organized infrastructure of preventive, social and health programs which promote healthy aging. Another benefit is that NORC-SSP's forge partnerships with public and private sectors to maximize scarce financial resources that fund them (e.g., NORC-SSP staff ensure resident access to medical transportation programs, delivered meals, and medical insurance programs for which the typical senior does not have knowledge/access). The average NORC-SSP program budget is $150,000 per year and services approximately 650 older adults. The NORC-SSP program nurse plays a central role as a primary health resource and advisor to the residents. Since the NORC resident is essentially never "discharged," the NORC nurse and the resident become a team. The goal of the NORC nurse is to assist residents to function at optimal physical and mental capacity, while establishing and maintaining communication and accountability between the health care and social service team.

The specific aims of this study were to 1) utilize a fall assessment tool and then communicate the results of the assessment to the at-risk older adults, their physicians, and the relevant community-based agencies; 2) implement a multi-factorial intervention and; 3) determine whether these interventions impacted upon fall risk scores. Our hypothesis is that the implementation of a multi-factorial fall assessment and prevention intervention which disseminates the results to older adults, their physicians, and community-based agencies will result in a decrease in fall risk factors.

METHODS

The NORC-SSP targeted for intervention, Deepdale CARES, is a garden apartment cooperative in Northeast Queens, New York, and is home to approximately 1,000 older adults. Deepdale CARES was established as a NORC-SSP in 1999 under the auspices of the Samuel Field Bay Terrace Young Men's (YM) and Young Women's Hebrew Association (YWHA), in partnership with the NSLIJ and the Deepdale Gardens Housing Complex. Staffed by nurses and social workers, this program was ideally situated to develop a comprehensive fall prevention program. The NORC program nurse utilized a modified HFRA tool to screen residents for fall risk and to establish baseline measures. At the time the study was conducted, this fall assessment tool was utilized because it included both individual and environmental factors that contribute to falls. Although no specific reliability and validity reports of this tool were found in the literature, this tool allowed for assessment of fall risk to seniors in the community and subsequent prevention practices. For this study, 110 NORC residents deemed high-risk for falls by NORC-SSP staff were targeted. A resident was classified as being high-risk if they had scored 15 or greater on the HFRA tool, or if they expressed a fear of falling. An inclusion criterion for this study was being over the age of 60 and demonstrating the cognitive capacity to sign informed consent. Cognitive capacity was determined by the ability to score a 3 on the Mini-Cog exam. Ninety-six out of the 110 NORC residents agreed and consented to participate in this program. Of the 96 residents, 3 died prior to completion of the intervention and/or follow-up assessment.

Study design

This study utilized a single group pre-post design. A parallel group randomized trial was not feasible and, moreover, the objective was to perform a pilot investigation of whether a fall prevention program held any potential for benefit to this community. Due to the exploratory nature of this study, consent from the Institutional Review Board was not needed. Ninety-three NORC residents received a multi-component nursing intervention including: an assessment of prior fall history, a sensory assessment, a mobility assessment, a cognitive assessment, review of medications, orthostatic blood pressure check, incontinence/urgency assessment, and a home environment (internal and external) safety check.

In response to this assessment, the resident was advised to change factors in the home environment that were unsafe, and were assisted in obtaining aids to improve home safety (i.e., grab bars). Residents requiring any type of modification were asked to purchase the device or hardware. Once the purchase was made, the management company of the co-op accommodated the residents by offering installation free of charge, which had been previously negotiated by the NORC director. This type of arrangement lessened financial burden.

With consent from the resident, the primary care physician was consulted regarding the need for medication review and subsequent medication changes were made. In addition, orders were obtained for physical therapy and home care, as well as for assistive devices. The social work staff worked with the residents to decrease anxiety and lessen emotional liability by visiting regularly to provide counseling. Six months after initial assessment, the 93 residents were re-assessed with the modified HFRA tool.

In this study, fourteen risk factors identified on the HFRA tool were coded as present or absent pre- and post- intervention. These risk factors are listed in Table 1.

Table 1. HFRA tool risk factors

- History of falls
- Age (over 65)
- Confusion
- Impaired judgment
- Sensory deficit
- Unable to ambulate independently
- Decreased level of cooperation
- Increased anxiety/emotional liability
- Medications affecting blood pressure or level of consciousness
- Cardiovascular/respiratory disease affecting perfusion and oxygenation
- Incontinence/urgency
- Postural hypotension with dizziness
- Unsafe internal home environment
- Unsafe external home environment

Statistical analysis

The total number of risk factors present ("composite fall risk score") was the sum of the present component factors and was computed for pre- and post- intervention. For any component risk factor, McNemar's test for paired binary data was used to compare the prevalence rates pre- versus post-intervention. Additionally, the Wilcoxon signed rank test was used to compare the composite risk score pre- versus post-intervention.

RESULTS

The study population consisted of 24% males and 76% females (see Table 2). One-hundred percent of the population was of Caucasian descent. The multi-factorial intervention decreased at least one (or more) risks to fall in 65% of the residents. Overall, there was a significant decrease in the mean composite fall risk score for residents participating in the study (from 32.9 to 23.9, Wilcoxon signed rank, $p = 0.001$). Specifically, significant decreases in prevalence post-intervention, via McNemar's tests, in: 1) poor levels of cooperation, from 20 % to 12%, $p = 0.05$); 2) anxiety/emotional liability (55% to 29%, $p = 0.001$); 3) incontinence urgency scores (from 27 % to 13%, $p = 0.001$; 4) postural hypertension (from (36 % to 21%, $p = 0.001$), unsafe internal environment (from 74 % to 29%, $p = 0.001$), and unsafe external environment (from 49 % to 8%, $p = 0.001$) were seen. This study shows that a multi-factorial intervention can be successfully implemented and evaluated in a NORC setting. Our hypothesis that implementation of a multi-factorial fall prevention program which included enhanced communication between at risk older adults, their physicians and community-based agencies would result in decreased fall risk factors was confirmed.

Table 2. Subject demographics

Demographic	N	Percent of Total
Gender		
Male	22	24%
Female	71	76%
Age Distribution		
75-79	16	17%
80-84	52	56%
>85	25	27%

DISCUSSION

Fall risk has always been a part of successful health assessment. Given the magnitude of the problem, the involvement of medical and community-based staff is key in identifying and preventing fall risk. This enhanced involvement and communication system leads to increased engagement of frontline healthcare professionals. The use of NORC-SSPs as a dissemination and implementation vehicle is a novel idea which, to the best of our knowledge, has not been reported in the literature to date. A Department of Health and Human Services white paper cites the need to study dissemination in NORC-SSPs, particularly as it relates to older adults' trust of information sources (17). While our study only specifically addresses falls best practice, it demonstrates the potential of NORCs as a vehicle for best practice dissemination.

A barrier to implementation of this study was that the assessment tool utilized was not supported by clear evidence of validity and reliability within our study population. Perhaps a tool that is specific to older adult residents residing within the community should be developed and tested for its psychometric properties. A second limitation was that our study design did not consist of a control group. The study team felt that it would be unadvisable to withhold the intervention from those who are at high-risk to fall. A third limitation was that the study setting has not been extensively reported within the literature. This poses as both a limitation and strength of this study. As with any unexplored territory, the nuances that affect study design and implementation first need to be unveiled or discovered.

This project was initiated as a response to the high percentage of emergency room admissions related to falls in the client population of Deepdale CARES NORC-SSP and the belief that these falls would lead to subsequent decline in functional status. Many community-based fall prevention programs focus on reducing environmental risk factors, leaving the medical community to identify and address contributing health conditions. Our hypothesis that disseminating and implementing a multi-factorial fall prevention program in a community with the existing infrastructure of a NORC-SSP and utilizing a better system of communication between clients/patients, community physicians and community based agencies was confirmed by this intervention. This collaboration was found to have a positive effect on fall risk factor reduction in the older adult population.

The NORC-SSP is an existing public health infrastructure in many U.S. communities. Given the trusting relationship that develops between NORC staff and the resident, and the potential reach of the NORC-SSP model, the NORC-SSP may be a cost-effective, important new resource for the management of various chronic conditions and risks for community-dwelling older adults. Further study of this model and its role in the dissemination of best practice programs that enhance the management of chronic disease is warranted.

ACKNOWLEDGMENTS

The authors would like to acknowledge the United Hospital Fund, as well as the New York Community Trust for funding and guiding this initiative. The authors would also like to acknowledge the Samuel Field Y for lending support of their social work staff, as well as their administrative support. Lastly, the authors would like to thank the Biostatistics Unit at North Shore-LIJ Health System for providing their technical assistance.

REFERENCES

[1]   Improving the Lives of Older America. NCOA 2009. Accessed 2011 Sept 22. URL: http://www.ncoa.org/improving-health/falls-prevention/falls-prevention-issue-brief.html

[2]   MacCulloch PA, Gardner T, Bonner A. Comprehensive fall prevention programs across settings: a review of the literature. Geriatr Nurs 2007; 28:306-11.

[3]   Nevitt MC. Falls in the elderly: Risk factors and prevention. In: Masdeu JC, Sudarsky L, Wolfson L, eds. Gait disorders of aging: Falls and therapeutic strategies. Philadelphia: Lippincott-Raven, 1997: 13-36.

[4]   Age data of the United States. U.S. Census Bureau population division 2010. Accessed 2011 Sept 22. URL: http://www.census.gov/population/www/socdemo/age/general-age.html#older

[5]   Centers for Disease Control and Prevention. Public health and aging: trends in aging – United States and worldwide. JAMA 2003;289:1371-3.

[6]   The AARP Home Fit Guide. AARP 2008. Accessed 2011 Sept 22. URL: http://aota.org/DocumentVault/Documents/41878.aspx?FT=.pdf

[7]   Briss PA, Zaza S, Papaioanou M, Fielding J, Wright-De Agüero L, Truman BI, et al. Developing an evidence-based guide to community preventive service - Methods. Am J Prev Med 2000;18:35–43.

[8]   Hendriks MR, Bleijlevens MH, van Haastregt JC, Crebolder HF, Diederiks JP, Evers SM, et al. Lack of effectiveness of a multidisciplinary fall-prevention program in elderly people at risk: a randomized, controlled trial. J Am Geriatr Soc 2008;56:1390-7.

[9]   Whitlock EP, Orleans TC, Pender N, Allan J. Evaluating primary care behavioral counseling interventions: an evidence-based approach. Am J Prev Med 2002;22:267–84.

[10]   Chang JT, Morton SC, Rubenstein LZ, Mojica WA, Maglione M, Suttorp MJ, et al. Interventions for the prevention of falls in older adults: systematic review and meta-analysis of randomized clinical trials. BMJ 2004;328:680-7.

[11]   Rosen CJ. Postmenopausal Osteoporosis. N Engl J Med 2005;353: 595-603.

[12]   Gabriel SE, Tosteson AN, Leibson CL, Crowson CS, Pond GR, Hammond CS et al. Direct medical costs attributable to osteoporotic fractures. Osteoporos Int 2002;13:323-30.

[13]   Banez C, Tully S, Amaral L, Kwan D, Kung A, Mak K, et al. Development, implementation, and evaluation of an interprofessional falls prevention program for older adults. J Am Geriatr Soc 2008;56: 1549-55.

[14]   Campbell AJ, Robertson MC, Gardner, MM, Norton RN, Buchner DM. Falls prevention over 2 years: a randomized controlled trial in women 80 years and older. Age Ageing 1999;28:513-8.

[15]   Li F, Harmer P, Glasgow R, Mack KA, Sleet D, Fisher KJ, et al. Translation of an effective Tai Chi intervention into a community-based falls-prevention program. Am J Public Health 2008;98:1195-8.

[16]   Baker DI, Gottschalk M, Biance LM. Step by step: Integrating evidence-based fall-risk management into senior centers. Gerontologist 2007;47:548-54.

[17]   Ormond BA, Black KJ, Tilly J, Thomas S. Supportive services programs in naturally occurring retirement communities 2004. Accessed 2011 Sep 22. URL: http://aspe.hhs.gov/daltcp/reports/ NORCsspes.htm.

In: Public Health Yearbook 2013
Editor: Joav Merrick

ISBN: 978-1-63321-095-0
© 2014 Nova Science Publishers, Inc.

Chapter 26

YOU KNOW A TREE BY ITS FRUIT: GROWING A FELLOWSHIP PROGRAM FOR COMMUNITY PARTNERED MENTAL HEALTH DISPARITIES RESEARCH IN AN ACADEMIC MEDICAL CENTER

Ann Marie White, EdD[*][1], Kathryn Castle, PhD[1],
Silvia Sörensen, PhD[1], Sheila Briody, DMin[2], LMHC/LMFT,
Herman Dailey[3], Deborah King, PhD[1], Colleen Fogarty, MD[4]
and Paul Duberstein, PhD[1]

[1]Department of Psychiatry, University of Rochester Medical Center,
Rochester, New York, US
[2]Counseling/Community Works, St. Joseph's Neighborhood Center,
Rochester, New York, US
[3]Outreach Community Center, Rochester, New York, US
[4]Department of Family Medicine, University of Rochester Medical Center,
Rochester, New York, US

ABSTRACT

Pressing community needs to improve mental and physical health, decrease health disparities and lower health care cost burdens are increasing demand for mental health related research and practice collaborations across community sectors and health disciplines. Academic medical centers can develop and implement novel educational models that enable faculty and trainees to partner with community agencies to address specific community-identified needs in these areas while also advancing science. This

[*] Correspondence: Ann Marie White, EdD, Department of Psychiatry, University of Rochester Medical Center, 300 Crittenden Blvd, Box PSYCH, Rochester, New York 14642-8409, United States. E-mail: Annmarie_White@urmc.rochester.edu.

manuscript presents the design and results of a clinical research fellowship program that integrates research trainees with preceptors in community-based agencies. The Rochester Program of Research and Innovation in Disparities Education (PRIDE) brought the University of Rochester Medical Center's (URMC) Clinical Psychology training and research faculty leaders together with community-based, including faith-based, health and human service agency leaders in Rochester, NY. This article details how research institutions can, with modest grant resources, align pre-existing psychology training structures to learn from community partners and to advance community-based research opportunities in the context of mental health and medical education. We discuss implications and challenges of developing health professional training programs with foci on mental and medical health disparities as well as community engaged research in health promotion, illness prevention and effective community-based treatment options.

Keywords: Community-based research, fellowship, mental health disparities

INTRODUCTION

Despite increasing attention to developing community research partnerships to improve health and reduce health disparities, competencies supporting these aims remain underemphasized in health professional education programs. Many medical researchers continue to believe that collaboration interferes with science's pace as training paradigms emphasize autonomy of the scientist's judgment and vision (1). Academic medical centers can move these norms to more effectively address community health concerns and create ethnically and racially diverse research institutions (2). This paper describes the integration of educational goals within an academic health system's clinical psychology program to promote community research collaborations. Implications as the Program of Research and Innovation in Disparities Education (PRIDE) expanded recruiting to medical students and family medicine residents within the University of Rochester Medical Center (URMC) are discussed.

EMERGING NATIONAL PRIORITIES

It is one thing to know that eating healthy and exercising regularly in tandem promotes weight loss, but what if there are neither grocery stores selling produce nor safe streets where you live and obesity and diabetes rates continue to rise in your community? In 2006, the National Institutes of Health's (NIH) Clinical and Translational Science Awards program (CTSA), a premiere mechanism supporting medical centers' clinical research enterprises, responded to community needs. It mandated that core resources promote community engagement in research and translational research to facilitate the application of basic science advances (3). The CTSA program defines community engagement broadly as, *"...the intersection of the complementary efforts of members of the lay community, community non-profit organizations, health practitioners and medical and public health researchers to improve health...founded on mutual understanding and trust, between communities and local academic institutions.* (p. 4)" (4) Community engagement often occurs as coordination or collaboration among academic-community partnerships or coalitions so that research can fuel changes in practices, programs and policies (5). The NIH Director's Council of Public

Representatives (COPR) describes the community engagement process as one that, "*...supports mutual respect of values, strategies, and actions for authentic partnership of people affiliated with or self-identified by geographic proximity, special interest, or similar situations to address issues affecting the well-being of the community of focus....It requires academic members to become part of the community and community members to become part of the research team, thereby creating a unique working and learning environment before, during, and after the research. (p. 1)*" (5) COPR emphasizes ideals such as ensuring processes exist so that community members remain on the teams driving every step of these research projects. Expertise in developing and maintaining these unique science contexts is needed.

Relevance for health disparities education and research in mental health topics

Disparities in mental health exist around inadequate access to needed healthcare. Health disparities research focuses on health conditions that are persistently more prevalent in groups such as racial and ethnic minorities, low income or medically underserved communities (6). Blacks and to a lesser extent, Latinos, are less likely than Whites to seek and receive adequate mental health treatment in current treatment systems (7). Despite health promotion programs that build on traditional public health models, minority and low-income communities' disparities continue (8). Community-based research, another venue of community health improvement, often occurs with academics leading research. In many cases communities aren't involved in decisions about planning or implementing research projects situated in daily contexts; they have little input into intervention studies designed to "help" them (9, 10). Such research practices can arguably reinforce structural factors that contribute to health disparities, and work contrary to norms where community members inform the development of services.

Community engagement, when it includes community members as equal members of research teams as in community-based participatory research (CBPR) traditions, is a community-level health disparities intervention (11-12). CBPR is thought to accelerate implementation of new knowledge (and promote health outcomes) by increasing local capacity in leading health improvement initiatives and investments around community-defined priorities (13). PRIDE also emerges from Psychiatry's engagement with local clergy and goals to foster greater racial and ethnic diversity of medical and mental health professionals in Rochester. By 1945, two decades after the start of its medical school, URMC graduated its first black medical student ending an era of no admission to African-Americans (14). By 2007, only 60 U.S.-born black males had graduated from its medical school, and one of the few black psychologists who served Rochester's youth was a faculty member of PRIDE faculty (15).

Current state of workforce development in meeting new demands

In response to community engagement not being well incorporated into training, the CTSA consortium planned to promulgate a common framework of core competencies and learning objectives in community engaged research (e-mail from, Noelle Andrus, Assistant Professor of Clinical Nursing, University of Rochester, March 24, 2011). However, few examples of practical training in community-engaged research now exist in medical education. There remains a lack of research on how to conduct scientist training responsive to 21st century demands. Online curricula, discrete training opportunities like summer institutes and didactic CBPR coursework via conference workshops are steps in the right direction but tend to reach only faculty.

Developing awareness that community contexts matter to health, and synthesizing clinical practice with public health (e.g., by drawing on community assets in health action initiatives) are central aims of some education programs (16). Medical and other health professional education also expanded over the past two decades to include training in competent communication and fieldwork in cultural and community contexts (17-20). Recent health care reform legislation authorizes funding to increase training opportunities for primary care residents in community health centers (21). Collaboration with community members now exists in specialty education such as pediatric medicine (16). Innovative community placements for psychiatry residents such as court settings or faith-based clinics for uninsured are developing in Rochester. These programs build on notions that community presence and sensitivity of health providers such as family and primary care physicians can reduce health disparities (22). Institutional barriers prevent community health center partnerships with medical training centers from taking root and flourishing. Major challenges are competing primary missions, chronic under-funding for programs that share missions of joint education and service, and navigating complex government and administrative institutional regulations (17).

PRIDE aimed to address such barriers to clinical and public health training effectively addressing community health concerns. Traditions in the field of psychology provide a strong foundation to grow health disparities research training programs with various community partners (e.g., community psychology) (23). In contrast to biomedical training, psychology routinely emphasizes consultation competencies and the practicum experience; it requires internships to develop core competencies in various practice settings (24-26). Clinical psychology highlights prevention and health promotion implementation (24), but this competency may be less emphasized in medical center training contexts (2, 27). For instance, URMC's public psychiatry tradition maintains strong emphasis on clinical management of severe or persistent mental illness and behavioral health concerns such as substance use within community institutions serving low-income populations.

METHODS

PRIDE is an innovative, experiential model for research and health disparities education. In its fifth year, it aims to inspire and prepare trainees to engage in clinically relevant community-based research. Main objectives are to enhance academic-community team engagement skills and knowledge in research, and address junior clinical scientists' unique developmental and psychosocial challenges. The R25 National Institute of Mental Health (NIMH) research education grant mechanism provides fellowship stipends, research expenses for trainees and training sites, and special training events to licensure-enabling programs in psychology and medicine. Table 1 describes the community-based research projects, approved by a human subjects review board, and completed in 2011. Projects emphasize trans-disciplinary health phenomena such as healthy living and social adversity such as women exposed to violence. Trainees' pilot research projects on health promotion are collaboratively designed to varying degrees with scientific mentors and site preceptors. Imposing particular research projects on community partners is discouraged. PRIDE-sponsored research projects must blend trainees' research interests with community partners' needs and have appropriate scientific mentors. Peer-review criteria of pilot project proposals stresses both academic and community significance.

Table 1. Community-based Research Projects Completed by PRIDE Post-Doctoral Fellows

Research Projects Completed by Each Fellow	Community Agency
Spirituality in psychotherapy Mental health service use among African American church members: A pilot study	Strong Behavioral Health – Ambulatory Program
Examining beliefs about stress and well-being in individuals diagnosed with type II diabetes	Outreach Community Center
A pilot study of group interpersonal psychotherapy for depressed women with histories of intimate partner violence	Alternatives for Battered Women
Mindfulness-based stress reduction for low-income women with histories of interpersonal trauma	St. Joseph's Neighborhood Center
Behavior change through the health empowerment program	St. Joseph's Neighborhood Center
Success in achieving goals among participants of a healthy living program in an undeserved community health center	Westside Family Medicine

Trainees' need to complete projects provides context for academic-community joint mentoring of collaborative clinical research (broadly defined) that aims to promote community health. Working closely with academic scientists and community mentors to conduct research on specific community-relevant topics is a cornerstone. Expert local community- and faith-based health and human service providers who target health disparities join with PRIDE's academic-based faculty to educate clinical health professional trainees as research fellows. Competencies stressed include cultural competence, collaboration, and responsiveness to community needs and norms. Both community and academic mentors ensure trainees' service and research projects evidence: a) culturally and community relevant knowledge and skills in broad health promotion, and b) conceptualization, assessment or treatment of mental health disorders in diverse community-based contexts. Community partners' goals for trainees are in Table 2. Academic programmatic aims are in Table 3.

Some projects have led to second-generation academic initiatives such as a career development award proposal and a novel clinical services intervention for women with histories of partner violence. Community agencies may experience longer-term benefits. St. Joseph's Neighborhood Center, for instance, has received additional program grants and adopted research infrastructure to sustain trainees' efforts. This is not always the case. Other agency partners did not sustain delivery of a novel program without their fellow's time and expertise.

Table 2. Community-centered Training Goals

1.	Develop academic researchers with specific skills and knowledge for patient- and community-centeredness.
2.	Develop skills in co-designing research questions from the biopsychosocial paradigm around mental health, disease mechanisms, illness processes and health promotion.
3.	Teach trainees to aid in health promotion and prevention programs.
4.	Build community capacity to integrate research with practice among the medically underserved.
5.	Build a racially and ethnically diverse health professional community locally and nationally.

Table 3. Academic Program and Trainee Outcomes

Aim	Major Outcome Indicators
1. Establish research training partnerships with community agencies in a manner that facilitates trainee research	• Research training partnerships initiated for community-based research with tangible benefits among community partners • Adequate participant flow into pilot research projects • All research proposals pass IRB
2. Implement a collaborative mentoring-precepting program on conducting research in community settings	Mentors and preceptors regularly meet with trainees, advise on conducting research in community settings and draw in perspectives among underserved members of local communities
3. Monitor training outcomes as well as the a) dissemination of findings to academic audiences, and b) sustainability of locally delivery of the product.	• 19 trainees in medicine & psychology recruited • Trainees presentations are accepted at professional meetings (e.g., 2011 annual meeting of the American Psychological Association) • Trainees' research proposals successfully peer reviewed by PRIDE's ad-hoc peer review committee • PRIDE agencies access resources to sustain health promotion initiatives delivered by PRIDE trainees

PRIDE began first by embedding a specialized research track into preexisting, American Psychological Associated accredited, Adult Psychology internship and post-doctoral experiences. Psychology post-graduate fellows are engaged, halftime, in community-based and community-co-defined service-learning and research activities in one of several community agencies serving the medically underserved. PRIDE's psychology interns draw on elective time to pair with fellows in further developing projects. In 2010, "year-out" tracks for medical students and family medicine residents began. Common training contexts are presented in Figure 1.

The PRIDE Seminar

Medical and psychology trainees' didactic seminar is a weekly multidisciplinary training context about race and poverty in urban health, including community-based research in health improvement. Complimentary consultative monthly seminars help trainees unpack issues arising such as transitions to community sites, roles and relationship development, conflict resolution and best practices integrating research and health promotion with racial and ethnic minorities.

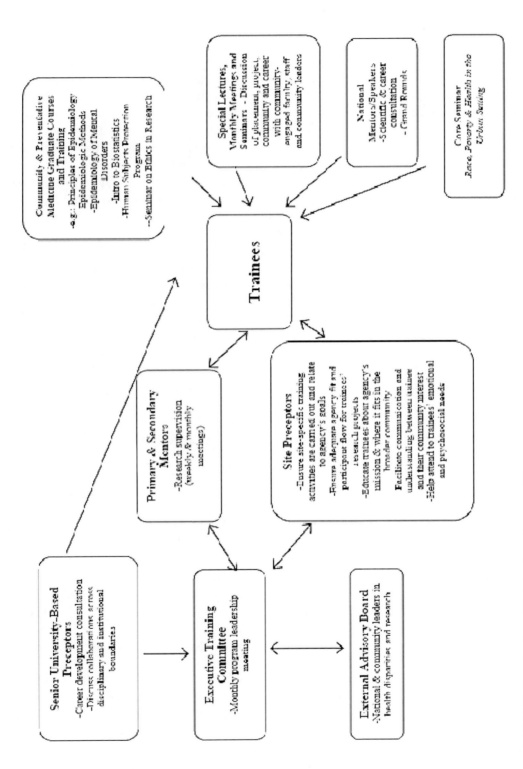

Figure 1. PRIDE's Organization of Training Experiences and Resources.

Community-based preceptors

Trainees are paired with site preceptors to develop collaborative relationships with one in a subset of small-to-midsized nonprofit agencies serving as de facto health care delivery systems. Community leaders with long-standing reputations of successfully engaging Rochester's underserved minority communities in alternative health-care delivery venues and/or health-promoting activities founded these agencies. These community settings address community health needs unmet by the University's academic medical center, such as faith-informed substance use counseling or food insecurity programs. Structural and other barriers to care seeking can lead many community members to stay away from URMC—even when they live in close proximity. Trainees placed at non-traditional sites buttress responsiveness of health professional education and research infrastructure to patterns of under-utilization of health services among racial and ethnic minorities.

For one to two years, trainees report to community agencies each week to jointly design and conduct hands-on research experiences. Mentors, preceptors and trainees initiate mutually beneficial action-research projects that meet organizations' health and research goals while aiming to maintain scientific rigor and integrity of trainees' research interests. For instance, one community preceptor asked a trainee to develop and implement a healthy eating training to address diabetes concerns in the community. This fellow then drew on observations from these sessions in designing a subsequent research project to generate an emic account of the relationship between mental health and diabetes. Trainees strive to pass on databases and data management skills to agency staff, as directed by site preceptors.

Academic mentors: Scientific, organizational, national and historical

PRIDE deliberately reinforces the partnership nature of its program and seeks to maintain long-term relationships via placement of newly recruited trainees. Longitudinal patterns of research projects prove difficult with completing fellows departing for job opportunities or the pull to return home. Trainees' projects often established research linkages between PRIDE's scientist mentors and partner agencies, and expanded service-oriented collaborations preceding PRIDE's genesis. PRIDE organizes annual celebrations to mark trainees' project and program completion and to express appreciation of PRIDE agencies and preceptors. This allows for public discussion about the future of the collaborative research agendas.

In addition to ensuring that scientific mentors are available to support fellows' research interests, each fellow is also assigned an institutional mentor who assists in such situations as negotiating career development issues. Site preceptors also discuss institutional norms that have historically contributed to racism and poverty, hindered community partnership development and minority engagement in research in Rochester, or "handcuffed" one's community responsiveness. National mentors and advisors periodically present leading mental health disparities research, or discuss career and program development with trainees and faculty. Local clergy and history experts help lead seminars sessions. Topics include relevant historical contexts such as minority engagement in mental health services and research, or local action agendas to address racism. All mentors help trainees prepare to work across systems and socio-cultural communities. They guide on priorities, issues and cultures among departmental, medical center, university, state, national, and historical structures in

Rochester and replicated in other communities. For instance, local experiences of civil unrest to combat racism and poverty are reviewed as these generated lasting effects and linked to national movements such as Saul Alinsky's community organizing among urban poor.

RESULTS

PRIDE reinforces key principles of community-academic collaborative research partnerships that facilitate health disparities research among community-based organizations (13, 28-30). Building on this literature, the results of PRIDE's featured partnership development elements, that helped transform existing training systems to sustain community-centered health improvement efforts, are described below.

Autonomy and authority of each partner alongside mutually held vision and goals: Balancing community and academic priorities

Constant attention is given to partners' goals and remaining true to agencies' core values for engaging their constituencies and employees (13, 29). Shared decision-making by trainees with site preceptors, and shared responsibility, accountability and resources are featured as key ingredients of successful projects. As different priorities of academic and community mentors emerge, trainees are encouraged to seek satisfactory resolution across mentorship teams and with emphasis on social components of successful academic-community partnerships (e.g., trust, authenticity and persistent commitment or responsiveness). Highly individualized training interventions to advance skills dictated by researched phenomena is a cornerstone. Novel exploration and diverse information gathering develops fellows' practice and research to be responsive to agencies' specific interests, questions and goals (31). Varied expertise among trainees is expected as unique community agencies require differential expertise, and as different communities are engaged.

Partnership success is threatened by outside and time-varying influences. For instance, research ethics board review schedules delay initiation of programs past community partners' desired start dates based on client needs. Also, negative beliefs persist that are barriers to community member engagement with URMC. Such issues listed in Table 4 are discussed in PRIDE-based interactions. PRIDE fellows respond, in part, by striving to deliver real, not deferred, benefits of academic-community collaboration. Trainees are encouraged to consider how to produce community benefits – such as sustainable community health improvement programming past their personal involvement.

PRIDE trainees acknowledge the importance of communication, a basic partnership-building skill. Fellows are encouraged to identify and navigate structures within partner agencies, to rely on agency leaders, to interface with staff, to regularly update agencies whether on- or off-site, and to draw on agency representatives and consumers when identifying needs. Site preceptors convene opportunities for trainees to explain research and interests beyond those immediately involved. Trainees draw on boundary-setting skills emphasized in psychology to negotiate roles and expectations fitting their time economy.

Table 4. Community barriers to partnerships in research

- Mistrust or fear of harm through research
- Concerns about exploitation of the Black community for the University's sole financial gain
- The belief that grants do not trickle down and benefit the community economically
- Seemingly endless construction projects threatening the integrity of residential areas and the loss of affordable housing
- Inequities in past and present hiring practices
- Disingenuous University interest in the community as projects lack follow-up or sustainability ethics after a lapse in research funding
- Inadequate reporting back to the community
- Cultural insensitivity of health care staff
- Major marketing and media campaigns that are seen as hypocritical
- Research participants being utilized as commodities that drive access to federal and private research resources
- Research participant compensation

Trainee and mentor socialization

Interpersonal communication and interactions are theorized as main catalysts of PRIDE's transformative learning goals (32). Collaboration reshapes one's professional role. New questions, knowledge, skills and attitudes that push beyond traditional research and intervention norms are expected. For a literature review and training recommendations, see Tricet and Espino, 2004 (29). Observation and practice of new competencies and knowledge generates reflective discussions about discontinuities and necessary accommodations (33). For instance, each program year trainees discuss key narratives in Rochester's history. One powerful presentation involved community members providing first-person accounts of being among the youth and young leaders at the center of Rochester's 1960s race "rebellion" (and aftermath). This period of intense civil unrest emerged in response to community-wide racial discrimination in police and housing practices. PRIDE faculty members similarly recount family members' experience with ethnic or religious discrimination decades earlier in Rochester.

To increase cultural sensitivity of both trainees and academic mentors, PRIDE stresses reciprocal teaching and learning with community partners, features that may prevent academia's potential "pro-innovation bias." (29,34) That is, striving to infuse new norms without full understanding of how such goals may undermine traditional practices that maintain mental health, or how some community leaders stand to lose face by accepting support from agencies, like URMC, perceived to be foreign to their community. PRIDE emphasizes cultural knowledge and autonomy of agencies – with trainee as humble visitor. One community partner noted the importance of this attitude to training they seek to impart, as prior experiences demonstrated medical student volunteers naively expecting to be seen as an "expert" upon arrival to their agency.

Increasing trainees and mentors' knowledge about the relevance of local and historical contexts to health care is an important building block. For instance, topics discussed include the mid-twentieth century migration of African-Americans to work in northern factories including those in Rochester, as well as racial segregation in patient care settings present at that time within URMC. Novel community settings such as domestic violence shelters broadens clinical science doctoral training in psychology and medicine beyond common work settings of medical centers, community mental health centers, academia such as college settings, hospitals and health care practices (31). This highlights competencies needed by health professionals, and their mentors, in novel community practice settings such as "adaptive expertise skills" (25) of being flexible, creative and open to new ways of knowing. For instance, one trainee began to regularly attend an agency's youth leadership council to become more a part of its group norms, functioning and to know its members. This responded to a direct challenge of these youth, when they asked the trainee: what makes you an expert on my life or what people my age need to know? This emphasized the need for meta-competencies of working collaboratively – such as forming good relationships and effective work-alliances with clients, employees and partners beyond the trainee-agency relationship. Another trainee's project triggered the need for a mediator to resolve interagency conflict with a different university-based partner. This fellow observed how their partner community agency maintained its long-standing relationship with another university partner when disputes arose (e.g., about competing priorities of increasing community access versus maintaining intervention fidelity).

PRIDE aims to increase community awareness of uses and benefits of research. The availability of community preceptors with academic partnership expertise and of agencies with strategic plans that include research facilitates this reciprocal learning goal. Trainees discuss research principles and constraints, and how to impart this information, with site preceptors.

DISCUSSION

The need for program models that bring local knowledge and cultures into academic medical centers' medical and psychology training systems cannot be overlooked (29). PRIDE offers a novel example of modifying existing education structures to address and explore barriers such as professional control, lack of means for dealing with conflict (29), and personal experience with discrimination. PRIDE's organization around such barriers facilitated community members designing and leading in-depth curricula and training within a medical center. Modifying trainees' research processes similarly, to foster community partnership in science, can potentially help sustain community-based interventions. For instance, time-honored community practices that maintain health (35) – and that residents may feel are waning in Rochester's minority communities - can become the subject of intervention research and perhaps further validated by robust scientific testing (36).

Novel clinical training benefits may emerge as secondary benefits of PRIDE. A primary target of health care reform is mental health, as fifty to seventy percent of all visits to primary care can be due to psychological factors (37). Rochester's health systems are also exploring new managed care contexts that emphasize accountability and cost-control. This may drive psychologists and other mental health professionals together with primary care doctors to offer lower-cost mental health services and to better reach underserved communities and reduce mental health disparities. PRIDE offers one model for shifting existing educational structures to coalesce future medical and mental health professionals to prepare for new working contexts.

Sustainability is a commonly cited challenge to community-based training innovations (38). The R25 grant mechanism can support modest research education programs, but not long-term clinical or research training infrastructure. As PRIDE's grant twilights, we are not yet submitting another R25 proposal due to NIMH's changing fiscal climate plus a lack of supporting R01s. Case-by-case, we can attend to linking partners' on-going evaluation research-related needs with university resources. For instance, the need for ongoing data management can be met by supervising undergraduate students seeking research experience. External funding will remain needed to sponsor trainees' time and to deepen clinical health disparities research training infrastructure in community settings.

PRIDE's sustainability and growth into a long-standing tradition is dependent on broader institutional and community factors. Ad-hoc approaches to developing research projects, and a limit of senior scientific experts, restricted PRIDE's accumulation of additional recruits or "next generation" research projects from trainees' original pilot studies. Future projects, if funded at R01 levels, could support additional research post-doctoral fellows and be means to expand PRIDE. Other limiting factors include: faculty recruitment and promotion patterns; desired geographical location among trainees; funding realities that keep community agencies small- and medical center business models that emphasize bottom line benefits of partnering in T1 translational research versus community health promotion and dissemination research.

Rapid and sustainable community development in research to reduce health disparities is also limited. Environmental challenges consistently arise that are barriers to this and to trainees' growth in these areas. Two common examples are the: a) availability of academic or minority research mentors to match recruits' interests, and b) differential availability of community preceptors to address daily trainee and research needs given the realities of running small agencies and the need for community preceptors to attend to their own professional development as a vehicle for their agency's development. Other barriers include: a) academic mentors' propensity for seeking to design efficacy as compared to effectiveness studies, or at minimizing formal evaluation of partnership development as part of the pilot grant (e.g., to measure community benefit), and b) community preceptors' scientific process naiveté While PRIDE helped fuel an explicit department-wide culture change in URMC's Psychiatry, any legacy in broad medical center changes can only be discerned in the future. Moving beyond boutique training program status will depend on broader academic contexts embracing its components and assigning top priority to eliminating health disparities in its local communities.

ACKNOWLEDGMENTS

The authors wish to thank Eric Caine, Nathan Franus, Nicole Mason, David Mowry, Jessica Poweski, Alice Wu and URMC's Laboratory of Interpersonal Violence and Victimization. Funding from the National Institutes of Health [R25MH074898] supported this work.

REFERENCES

[1]   Liyanage S, Wink R, Nordberg M. Managing path-breaking innovations: CERN-ATLAS, Airbus, and stem cell research. Westport, CT: Praeger, 2007.

[2]   Davidson L, Jefferson F, Shuherk C. Improving faculty recruitment and retention at the University of Rochester: A diversity and inclusion initiative. Rochester, NY: University Rochester, 2009.

[3]   Leshner A. Outreach training needed. Science 2007;315:161.

[4]   The Clinical and Translational Science Award (CTSA) Consortium's Community Engagement Key Function Committee and the CTSA Community Engagement Workshop Planning Committee. Researchers and their communities: the challenge of meaningful community engagement. Durham, NC: Duke Center Community Research, 2008.

[5]   Council of Public Representatives (COPR) to the Director of the National Institutes of Health. Role of the Public in Research Work Group, Presented to NIH Director; 2008 Oct. [cited 2011 Mar 10]. Available from: http://copr.nih.gov.ezpminer.urmc.rochester.edu/reports/Definitions_of_CE_ and_PP_Revised_508.pdf

[6]   National Institutes of Health. National Institute on Drug Abuse (NIDA) Health Disparities. NIH-Health Disparities Definition. [Internet]. 2011. [cited 2011 Mar 10]. Available from: http://www.nida.nih.gov.ezpminer.urmc.rochester.edu/about/organization/healthdisparities/about/nihh ealthdisparities.html.

[7]   Substance Abuse and Mental Health Services Administration, Center for Mental Health Services. Mental health: culture, race, and ethnicity - a supplement to Mental health: a report of the Surgeon General. Washington, DC: US Department Health Human Services; 2001.

[8]   Niederhauser VP, Stark M. Narrowing the gap in childhood immunization disparities. Pediatr Nurs 2005;31(5):380-6.

[9]   Green LW, Mercer SL. Can public health researchers and agencies reconcile the push from funding bodies and the pull from communities? Am J Public Health 2001;91(12):1926-9.

[10]   Baldwin JA, Johnson JL, Benally CC. Building partnerships between indigenous communities and universities: lessons learned in HIV/AIDS and substance abuse prevention research. Am J Public Health 2009;99(Suppl 1):S77-82.

[11]   Wallerstein N. Commentary: challenges for the field in overcoming disparities through a CBPR approach. Ethn Dis 2006;16(1):1.

[12]   Wallerstein N, Duran B. Using community-based participatory research to address health disparities. Health Promot Pract 2006;7:312-23.

[13]   Israel BA, Schulz AJ, Parker EA. Review of community-based research assessing partnership approach to improve public health. Annu Rev Public Health 1998;19:173-202.

[14]   Parmington B. Dr. Charles Terrell Lunsford. UR Research 2008. [cited 2011 Jun 25]. Available from: http://hdl.handle.net/1802/6338.

[15]   Morgan A. The experiences of African American males at the University of Rochester School of Medicine and Dentistry, 1940-2007. Warner Abstract E-Journal 2010 [Internet]. 2010. [cited 2011 Jun 25]. Available from: http://hdl.handle.net/1802/9401.

[16]   Paterniti DA, Pan RJ, Smith LF, Horan NM, West DC. From physician-centered to community-oriented perspectives on health care: assessing the efficacy of community-based training. Acad Med 2006;81(4):347-53.

[17]   Morris CG, Chen FM. Training residents in community health centers: facilitators and barriers. Ann Fam Med 2009;7(6):488-94.

[18]   McIntosh S, Block RC, Kapsak G, Pearson TA. Training medical students in community health: a novel required fourth-year clerkship at the University of Rochester. Acad Med 2008;83(4):357-64.

[19]   Badner V, Ahluwalia KP, Murrman MK, Sanogo M, Darlington T, Edelstein BL. A competency-based framework for training in advanced dental education: experience in a community-based dental partnership program. J Dent Educ 2010;74(2):130-9.

[20]   Gordon BA, Datema MR, Slager D, Martin JT, Vander Werf MC. Community participatory research: student nurses collaborate to reduce lead exposure by educating paint retailers. Nurs Educ 2009;34(1):43-6.

[21]   Patient Protection and Affordable Care Act (PPACA). PL 111-148. 111th Congress; 2010 Mar.

[22]   Lie DA, Lee-Rey E, Gomez A, Bereknyei S, Braddock I, C.H. Does cultural competency training of health professionals improve patient outcomes? A systematic review and proposed algorithm for future research. J Gen Intern Med 2011;26(3):317–25.

[23]   Shinn M. Expanding community psychology's domain. Am J Community Psychol 1987;15(5):555-74.

[24]   Masters KS, France CR, Thorn BE. Enhancing preparation among entry-level clinical health psychologists: recommendations for "best practices" from the first meeting of the Council of Clinical Health Psychology Training Programs (CCHPTP). Training Educ Prof Psychol 2009;3(4):193-201.

[25]   Hatcher RL, Lassiter KD. Initial training in professional psychology: the practicum competencies outline. Training Educ Prof Psychol 2007;1:49-63.

[26]   Rodolfa E, Bent R, Eisman E, Nelson P, Rehm L, Ritchie P. A cube model for competency development: implications for psychology educators and regulators. Prof Psychol 2005;36(4):347-354.

[27]   Nestro, C, Lynch, M. Embracing a mental "health" paradigm in the provision of outpatient psychiatric services: what you see just might be what you get. Paper presented at: Sixth World Conference on the Promotion of Mental Health and Prevention of Mental and Behavioral Disorders; 2010; Washington, DC.

[28]   Pinto RM. Community perspectives on factors that influence collaboration in public health research. Health Educ Behav 2009;36(5):930-947.

[29]   Trickett E, Espino S. Collaboration and social inquiry: multiple meanings of a construct and its role in creating useful and valid knowledge. Am J Commun Psychol 2004;34(1-2):1-69.

[30]   Minkler M, Wallerstein N, eds. Community-based participatory research for health. San Francisco, CA: Jossey-Bass, 2003.

[31]   McFall RM. Doctoral training in clinical psychology. Annu Rev Clin Psychol 2006; 2:21-49.

[32]   Vygotski LS. Mind and society: the development of higher psychological processes. Cambridge, MA: Harvard University Press, 1978.

[33]   Piaget J. The equilibration of cognitive structures: the central problem of intellectual development. Chicago, IL: University Chicago Press, 1985.

[34]   Miller RL, Shinn M. Learning from communities: overcoming difficulties in dissemination of prevention and promotion efforts. Am J Commun Psychol 2005;35(3/4):169-83.

[35]   Hermann H, Saxena S, Moodie R. Promoting mental health: concepts, emerging evidence, practice. Geneva: World Health Organization, 2005.

[36]   White AM, Funchess M, Sellars C, Nestro C, Coveny I, Brown N, Smith C, Caine E. Neighborhood natural helpers as community-based participatory research partners: mental health promotion and violence prevention in urban neighborhoods. Paper presented at: Sixth World Conference on the Promotion of Mental Health and Prevention of Mental and Behavioral Disorders; 2010; Washington, DC.

[37]   Heiby EM. Concluding remarks on the debate about prescription privileges for psychologists. J Clin Psychol 2002;58:709-22.

[38]   Andrus NC, Bennett NM. Developing an interdisciplinary, community-based education program for health professions students: the Rochester experience. Acad Med 2006;81(4):326-31.

Submitted: November 15, 2011. *Accepted with Revisions:* April 15, 2012. *Revised:* May 14, 2012.

In: Public Health Yearbook 2013
Editor: Joav Merrick
ISBN: 978-1-63321-095-0
© 2014 Nova Science Publishers, Inc.

Chapter 27

NUTRITION EDUCATION AND THE COST OF HEALTHY FOOD – DO THEY COLLIDE? LESSONS LEARNED IN A PREDOMINANTLY BLACK URBAN TOWNSHIP IN SOUTH AFRICA

Moïse Muzigaba*, MPH and Thandi Puoane, DrPH
Faculty of Community and Health Sciences,
School of Public Health, University of the Western Cape, Belleville,
South Africa and The Heart and Stroke Foundation, South Africa

ABSTRACT

The cost of healthier foods has been shown to contribute negatively to individuals' food choices in developed societies. However, there is a dearth of knowledge regarding this phenomenon in low to middle income countries, particularly in Africa. This study explored community members' experiences in buying healthier food options and compared their perceived cost of selected healthier and less healthy foods with actual market costs. The study was conducted amongst 50 adult health club members in Khayelitsha in the Western Cape Province of South Africa, using both quantitative and qualitative research methods. Data were gathered in three phases: The first phase involved interviews with all the 50 participants. The second phase involved in-depth interviews with ten purposively selected members. In the third phase, food price audits were conducted in supermarkets and convenient stores in the study setting. Quantitative data were subjected to descriptive statistical analysis, while content analysis was used to analyze qualitative data. Our quantitative findings showed that most of the members were illiterate, unemployed, and largely dependent on government grants. Qualitative findings showed that low household incomes, inability to read and interpret nutritional information and personal food preferences contributed to community members' unhealthy food-purchasing behavior. From both local store audits and participants'

---

* Correspondence: Moïse Muzigaba, Faculty of Community and Health Sciences, School of Public Health, University of the Western Cape, Private Bag X17 Bellville, 7535, South Africa. E-mail: mochemoseo@gmail.com and The Heart and Stroke foundation South Africa, POBox 15139 Vlaeberg 8018, Cape Town, South Africa. E-mail: moise@heartfoundation.co.za.

perceptions, healthier foods tended to be more expensive than their less healthy options. Low income was a major factor militating against participants' healthy food-purchasing behavior. Future research studies are needed to assess how trends in food prices over time affect individuals' healthy food purchasing behaviors.

Keywords: Public health, food, health, food retail milieu, South African Township

INTRODUCTION

Increasing evidence in some developed countries highlights the importance of examining the influence of individual-level (compositional) socio-economic and environmental (contextual) factors on healthy food-purchasing and consumption behaviour. Various studies around this subject have emerged mainly in some European countries (1-3), the USA (4, 5), Canada (6) and Australia (7, 8). Although there have been contradictory findings, much of this work consistently corroborates the view that the locally available retail outlets in addition to the socio-economic status of individuals influence food-purchasing behaviour. This suggests that in addition to individual responsibilities towards their health, the contextual forces which shape decisions people make and the behaviours in which they engage should not be underestimated if the complex world of food-purchasing behaviour is to be clearly understood. Figure 1 which we remodeled based on previous work by White (9) and Story et al., (10) illustrates a theoretical framework of inter-relationships of compositional and contextual factors which may act singly or collectively to influence food-purchasing behaviour at the household level.

The broad logic of this theoretical framework is that socioeconomic position- which may itself be determined by such factors as the family background, inherited wealth, educational achievement and employment status amongst other things – may determine the perceptions individuals have towards their ability to access and/or afford healthy foods. Similarly, the socioeconomic position may dictate individual's ownership of material resources (e.g., own transport, certain cooking utensils, a fridge, etc.) necessary to easily access, prepare, and/or store healthier foods. This model also argues that the less educated people are, the less likely they will be able to make healthy food purchasing decisions.

However, the framework also acknowledges the role that environmental parameters play in shaping food purchasing decisions that individuals make based on their socioeconomic positions. For example, the differences in cost and availability between healthier foods and their less healthy options, and the relative ease of access to retail outlets which sell these foods may all determine the healthiness of the food people buy.

In South Africa, there is still a dearth of evidence concerning the cost and availability of healthy food. Although some researchers (11-16) have begun to explore this area, there is still a need for evidence that substantiates and complements their findings. Public health efforts geared towards promoting healthy food consumption behaviour - such as the development and implementation of the South African Food-base Dietary Guidelines (SAFBDGs) may have little relevance in settings where there is poor access to affordable healthy foods and as such, nutrition education is likely to have little effect.

To substantiate this supposition, we conducted the current study based on an earlier interventional study in which a community-based model was developed to address lifestyle factors that contributed to the burden of non-communicable diseases in Khayelitsha (17), a predominantly black urban township in Cape Town, South Africa. During this intervention, community health workers (CHWs) first received training on the prevention of risk factors for non-communicable diseases focusing on diet and physical activity and on how to run a community-based health club. They then recruited individuals from the surrounding communities to join a health club in which nutritional education based on the SAFBDGs and physical activity sessions were conducted on a regular basis (17).

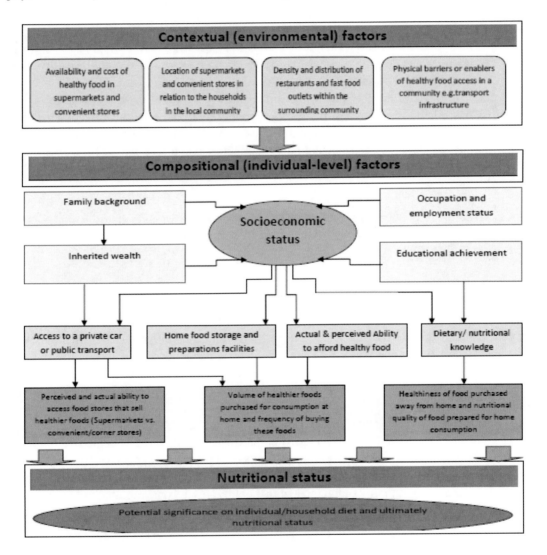

Figure 1. A theoretical framework of inter-relationships of compositional and contextual factors that may influence food-purchasing behaviour at the household level.

Despite these efforts however, some of the health club members (HCMs) still made unhealthy food choices. We then sought to investigate and describe HCM's experiences in buying healthier food items and to compare respondents' perceived cost of selected healthier foods and their less healthy counterparts with actual market costs in a South African township. In this paper, we present the results and the lessons learned from this investigation. The study involved three phases. The objectives of the initial phase were to:

- To describe the socio-economic and demographic characteristics of the HCMs;
- To assess the HCMs' sources of food and food purchasing patterns; and
- To determine if there were differences in "perceived "and "actual" market prices for various pairs of healthier foods and their less healthy options.

The second phase sought:

- To identify the least-compliant HCMs (with respect to self-reported healthy food consumption and purchasing patterns);
- To further explore the following dimensions with the least-compliant group of HCMs: Their perceived ability to afford healthy food and how this affects what food they purchase and how the local selection of the retail outlets affected their food-purchasing patterns and selected individual factors that affected their food choice.

Lastly, the third phase sought:

- To compare the percentage price differences between various pairs of healthier foods and their less healthy counterparts within different food retail market types located in the study setting.

METHODS

A cross-sectional descriptive study using quantitative and qualitative research methods was used. This study was undertaken in Harare in Khayelitsha district in the Western Cape Province in South Africa. In 2006, Khayelitsha had a population of about 330,000 people and of the 52% of economically active population, only 25% were employed (18). Educational attainment was also generally poor.

The sampling procedure involved three stages. Fifty of the HCMs who had been trained by CHWs about healthy eating were included in the first phase in which quantitative data was collected. After the quantitative analysis was complete, a purposive sample of ten HCMs was selected to participate in the second phase. This sample involved participants who scored lower percentages after their compliance with healthy food consumption and purchasing patterns were assessed. The process used for this sampling method is described in the analysis section.

The food retail environment in Harare was also assessed. The food stores (large, medium/small) identified in the quantitative phase as the most frequently visited by HCMs were targeted. These included the only nearby local supermarket, four randomly selected medium/small grocery stores (locally referred to as 'spazas') and three randomly selected street vendors.

Data collection

A survey questionnaire was designed based on literature and relevant established research tools. The questionnaire was administered to HCMs to collect data on HCMs' socio-economic and demographic characteristics, patterns of healthy food-purchasing and consumption behaviour, frequency of acquiring food from various food retail outlets and perceptions about relative market prices of various pairs of healthier foods and their less healthy options.

Qualitative phase

This phase involved in-depth individual interviews with selected club members. An interview guide was developed with semi-structured questions. Data collected included HCMs' opinions about their day-to-day experiences buying healthier food options, an exploration of their perceptions about the cost of healthier foods within food retail outlets in their community and how this affected the kinds of food they usually buy.

Food costing phase

In order to compare price differences between healthier foods and their less healthy options, only foods which were packaged and whose weights were indicated were subjected to costing. An attempt was also made to audit the prices of the cheapest brands of each food category available. Foods that were 'on sale' were not included. Since weight variations between packets of foods may have an influence on their respective prices, we established a standard unit price by calculating the cost of each food item per gram or per litre/millilitre, to enable comparisons to be made between the two options. The potential contribution of the packaging material to the overall price of each food item was not accounted for, however. The percentage price differences between healthier foods and their less healthy counterparts were then calculated. The list of food items audited is provided in Table 1.

Table 1. Food items audited, categorized into healthier and less healthy/regular options

Food category	Healthier type	Less healthy/regular option
Bread	Whole meal/brown bread	White bread
Orange fruit juice/drink	100% pure orange juice with no added sugar	Orange fruit drink with added sugar
Milk	Low fat milk	Full cream milk
Rice	Whole meal rice (brown)	Regular white rice
Chicken	Chicken thigh fillet (no skin)	Chicken thigh fillet with skin
Spaghetti	Whole meal spaghetti (brown)	Regular spaghetti (white)
Cooking oil	Sunflower vegetable oil	Animal cooking oil e.g., chicken or pork-derived fat

Healthier foods in this report have a comparatively *higher fiber* content and *lesser fat, salt* and *sugar* than their less healthy/regular counterparts.

They were selected arbitrarily based on the literature on foods traditionally known to be consumed by individuals in similar settings (11-14) and the South African FBDGs (19). Food items were paired in such a way as to reflect what would be a healthier choice and what would be a regular / less healthy one. Where possible pairing was done using food items from the same brand name to do away with "inter-brand" measurement bias.

Ethical clearance

Ethical clearance to conduct the study was obtained from the University of the Western Cape (UWC) Ethics Committee. Participants were requested to sign consent forms after the purpose of the study was explained. Owners/managers of the food retail businesses were also asked for permission before food cost audits were conducted. Quantitative data was collected from mid to end of October 2009, whereas qualitative interviews as well as retail food price audits took place throughout November in 2009. In both cases, interviews were held at respondents' households using IsiXhosa local language. All in-depth interviews were tape-recorded, and each took about 45 minutes to an hour to complete.

Data analysis

Data was analyzed using SPSS (Statistical Package for the Social Sciences) software Version 17.0 as well as Microsoft Excel for Windows 2007. Data was subjected to descriptive statistical analysis using means, frequencies and proportions. The qualitative interviews were transcribed verbatim and translated into English for analysis. The thematic content analysis technique described fully elsewhere (20) was used to analyse qualitative data. The percentage price differences between the healthier foods and their less healthy counterparts were calculated using the following formula (adapted from a similar study conducted in Australia (21):

> Price of the healthier food choice – the price of less healthy alternative/ the price of the less healthy alternative × 100

Selection of the qualitative sample

Qualitative sampling was guided by the questions describe in table 2. These were informed by a review of literature which identified 17 indicators of typical healthy food-purchasing behaviour and consumption pattern in an average South African household.

A question "I can say that in our household we" was first stated, followed by these 17 assertions. Participants were required to respond using a graded Likert-scale ('Never', 'Sometimes', 'Regularly', and 'Always'), graded from 1 to 4. For some assertions, 'Never (=1)' implied bad compliance and 'Always (=4)', good compliance.

Table 2. List of assertions to which participants answered

Eat fruits for a snack
Try new ways of preparing vegetables
Buy new kinds of fruits and vegetables
Hardly eat fruits for dessert
Eat salad or other vegetables for lunch
Drink 100% pure fruit juice instead of fizzy drinks (e.g., Coke)
Have at least three meals a day
Often don't have our meal at home
Cannot easily access healthy food for consumption at home in the community where we live
Can afford healthy food for consumption at home
Always buy healthy and nutritious food in shopping outlets where we buy food for consumption at home
Buy fast food for consumption at home
Eat fried meat with fat
Eat brown bread instead of white bread
Try to buy food that is low in fat when buying food for the family
Need to spend a lot of money to buy healthy and nutritious food
Have a diet that consists of healthy and nutritious foods.

For other assertions however, it was the opposite pattern whereby 'Never (=1)' implied good compliance and 'Always (=4)' bad compliance. This was done to avoid report bias which would potentially have resulted from leading questions posed in a unidirectional pattern. Scores were developed for each response category with an assumption that no assertion was more important than another. Three points were allocated for better compliance and a zero for bad compliance. Two points were allocated to indicate relatively good compliance whereas one point suggested inadequate compliance.

Since there was no literature available to support the ranking of the assertions in order of importance, instead of a weighted analysis, individual scores for all assertions were added up to constitute a value. This was compared to the total possible score each respondent could have attained in order to fall under the category of 'better compliance' (see formula in box 1).

Box 1

After all scores had been summed up, percentage scores were calculated for each individual. Table 3 highlights percentage score categories and the darker-shaded area indicates the categories from which the qualitative sample was drawn.

> - Total possible points attainable = 3 (maximum score possible per assertion) × 17 (number of assertions) = 51 points
> - Percentage score per individual =
> $$\frac{\text{(Total points scored)} \times 100}{51 \text{ points}}$$

Table 3. Distribution of percentage scores among the 50 participants

Compliance categories	Categories of percentage scores (%)	Number of responses (n)	Proportion of responses%
Less compliance			
	50 ≥	*0*	*0*
	50-54	*2*	*4*
	55-59	*10*	*20*
Moderate compliance			
	60-64	*13*	*26*
	65-69	*11*	*22*
	70-74	*6*	*12*
Good compliance			
	75-79	*3*	*6*
	80 ≤	*2*	*4*
	Missing	*3*	*6*
	Total	50	100

Table 4. Participants' socio-economic and demographic characteristics

Characteristics		n (%)
Gender		
	Male	3 (6.4)
	Female	44(93.6)
Age in years		
	<40	7(14)
	40-49	18(36)
	50-59	23(46)
	>60	2(4)
Level of education attained		
	Standard 5/Primary	16(35.6)
	Standard 7	15(33.3)
	Passed matric	13(28.9)
	Tertiary education	0(0)
	No education	1(2.2)
Marital status		
	Single – Never married	11(24.4)
	Married-Monogamy	22(48.9)
	Married-Polygamy	0(0)
	Widowed	7(15.6)
	Divorced- separated	5(11.1)
	Co-habiting	0(0)
Employment status		
	Paid full/part time job	15(32.6)
	State pension/grant	19(41.3)
	Unemployed	3(6.5)
	Retired	2(4.3)
	Contribution from others	3(6.5)
Kind of grant/pension		
	Child support grant	19(43.2)
	Elderly pension	5(11.4)
	Disability pension	10(22.7)
	Foster care grant	10(22.7)

RESULTS

Phase 1: Quantitative findings

The monthly household income for most participants was R940 (67%) with only one individual reporting a monthly income of R8,900. About 30% had reported household incomes of less than R900, the minimum being R550. Nearly two thirds (68.9%) had completed standard 7 or less (nine years of school), with half of these (35.6%) having only completed primary school (seven years of school). Other socio-economic and demographic characteristics are shown in table 4 below.

Table 5 shows that both 'spaza' shops and supermarkets were frequently utilized by CHMs. Ninety nine percent of participants purchased food from 'spaza' shops, and 95.7% from supermarkets. However on a weekly basis, more participants visited 'spaza' shops more often than they visited supermarket (63% and 8%, respectively).

As shown in figure 2, there was a clear perceived distinction between the price of an orange fruit drink with added sugar (regular type) and 100% pure orange juice with no added sugar (healthier type) - the latter being perceived by 91% of participants as more expensive. About 78% of the participants thought the healthy type of both cooking oil and rice categories were more expensive to purchase than their regular counterparts. Healthier bread was perceived by 60% as more expensive to purchase whereas only 28% perceived healthy milk as being more expensive.

Table 5. Participants' frequency of acquiring food from various food outlets

food outlets	% participants who obtained food from each outlet		Frequency of purchase of food from each outlet					
	Yes	No	At least five days a week	At least once a week	At least once a month	At least once six months	Less than once a year	Never
Supermarkets	95.7	4.3	8.7	19.6	67.4	0	0	4.3
'Spaza' shops	97.8	2.2	63	22.6	2.2	0	0	2.2

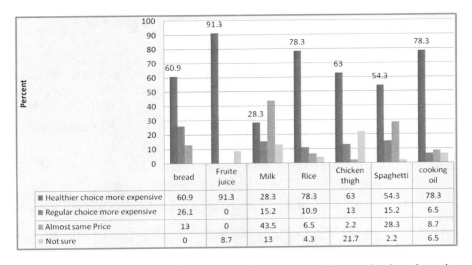

Figure 2. Comparison of various pairs of food items with respect to their perceived market price.

Price audits of these foods in the only one supermarket located around the study area revealed that generally healthier food options were, in fact, more expensive than their regular counterparts by between 3% and 22 % (see table 6). It was not possible to determine percentage price differences of most of the foods among medium/small stores because there was either no healthy or regular choices of each food category available for comparison.

Table 6. Percentage price differences between purposefully selected healthier foods and their regular options in one supermarket and four medium/small grocery stores in Harare – Khayelitsha

Foods		Objective price audits of the supermarket (n=1)	Objective price audits of medium/smaller grocery stores(n=4)
Food category	Food type (the cheapest option available)	Percentage price difference between the recommended and regular food types (%)[1]	Average percentage price differences between the recommended and regular food types (%)[2]
1. Bread	*Whole-wheat brown bread*	*4*[3]*	*8.04*
	Regular white bread		
2. Orange juice	*Orange fruit drink with added sugar*	8.47*	*Healthy choice not available*
	100%pure orange juice with no added sugar		
3. Liquid milk	*Full cream milk*	3.05*	*Healthy choice not available*
	2% fat milk		
4. Rice	*Whole meal rice*	9.75*	*Healthy choice not available*
	White rice		
5. Chicken breast	*Chicken breast fillet with skin*	12*	*Healthy choice not available*
	Chicken breast fillet without skin		
6. Cooking oil	*Animal cooking oil e.g., lard*	*Regular choice not available*	22*
	Sunflower vegetable oil		

Phase 2: Qualitative findings

A number of key themes emerged in the participants' responses. These were unbalanced diet due to food insecurity; their inability to afford healthy food; their inability to read and interpret food labels; family preferences; the relatively high cost of healthier foods in 'spaza' shops compared with supermarkets. Examples of what they said and a summary of responses is given in the table 7.

---

[1] Only one supermarket was audited (the only one located in the study area) therefore there was no need for finding an average.

[2] There were four medium/small grocery stores that were audited for price differences therefore an average was determined.

[3] Asterisked figures indicate by how much % the healthier choice was more expensive than its regular type and the one that is not asterisked indicates otherwise. Shaded areas indicate that there was absence of either the healthy type or its regular counterpart for comparison to be done.

Table 7. Key themes and illustrative quotes showing participants' responses

Key themes	Illustrative quotes from HCMs	Summary of responses
Unbalanced diet due to food insecurity	*"Hahahahah I laughed because we didn't eat because we didn't have food to eat".* *"During the day we didn't eat food other than bread and egg in the morning and potato chips for supper".* *"We always eat bread in the morning sometimes rice and stiff pap in the evening with chicken".*	Most respondents reported a diet with lack of diversity, and the number of meals eaten by majority varied from nothing to two meals on a particular day. Furthermore, diet included carbohydrates and not enough consumption of any kind of vegetables or fruits.
Ability to afford healthy food such as fruit and vegetables	*"I spend R500.00 on food and pay debts with other money that I borrow to Mashonisas (money paid with interest)".* *"It is very expensive. So we try and eat what we can afford".* *" I buy vegetables, but I only buy them when I have money".* *"Vegetables and fruit don't last, if it's finished I borrow money to other people if they don't have it, I wait for the end of the month". "I have to borrow money on credit in order to buy other stuff. After I borrow money, I buy vegetable and meat".*	Although participants were generally able to purchase basic food items for household consumption, majority relied on a meager income if one is to consider their household size and needs. This resulted in a limited amount and quality of food they could afford. Almost every respondent reported that their financial position was not good enough to enable them to buy healthy food as regularly as they require
Inability to read and interpret food labels	*"I just buy without looking what is written there. I don't know how to look".* *"I don't even look at that I just buy, the children choose without looking".* *"No I don't have time but I know those foods which have a heart on them are good for us".*	Majority of respondents indicated a disinclination to take some time checking for nutritional values and content of foods they buy. Participants' justification for this behaviour was centered on their inability to interpret the labels due to the fact that they do not have sufficient formal education on nutrition and health in general
Family Influences	*"No except me they eat everything whereas my husband eats meat and bread... "* *"We eat what is available except the young children like umvubo (bread with milk)"* *"I cook porridge and Corn flake for children's"*	Some respondents reported that particular individuals in their households influenced what kind of food they have to buy for consumption at home. Either the children or the respondents themselves had unique food consumption patterns which had an influence on what they have to buy
The relatively high cost of healthier foods in 'spaza' shops compared with supermarket	*"Spazas are not so clean and so expensive compared to bigger shops but convenient because you don't have to pay transport".* *"The spaza's are expensive and malls they have "sale" ".*	Majority of HCMs subscribed to the view that bigger chain retail outlets in their communities stock cheaper food items than do smaller Spaza shops and yet the later are more easily accessible and they don't have to pay transport money

DISCUSSION

The findings of the current study provide corroborative evidence as well as provocative insights into some socio-economic as well as market-related characteristics that have been reported in other studies to influence healthy food purchasing behavior.

The lowest aggregate monthly household income was R550 (about US$78) and the most frequently reported was R940 (Approximately US$134). Almost half of HCMs received child support grants and about 25% depended on disability grants. Furthermore, the mean age of respondents was 53 years, meaning that some respondents were in a less productive age category even if they had been able to find employment. These three parameters may be an indication of limited income potential. With such low incomes, it is probable that few households will own facilities such as refrigerator which may determine the frequency with which they shop for perishable foods such as fruits and vegetables and the amount of such foods they can bring home and safely store for later consumption.

Educational attainment may well impact directly or indirectly on dietary behaviour. During the qualitative enquiry, some HCMs reported that they were not in a position to read and interpret food labels despite their awareness of basic healthy eating tips. This might well impact on the healthiness or/and types of the food the HCMs purchase from food retail outlets (e.g., fat and salt content, presence and amount of "empty" calories, presence of unhealthy additives and other preservatives, etc.). A study that attempted to establish the link between the level of education and ability to read food labels as an indicator of food choice did not, however, confirm this likely relationship (22). Comparison of the findings from this Irish survey and the current study may however be a lot more complex. In order to explain the discrepancies between the two studies over and above the level of formal education, it may be important to consider the lack of language proficiency, in this case English, the proficiency of which was poorer among individuals who participated in our study.

Although most HCMs were less educated, it was interesting to learn that most of them could recognize healthy foods by the presence of a picture of a heart, a fork or a knife on the food package. This shows the likely impact interventions that use food labeling by means of pictorial messages would have in educating illiterate people about how to recognize healthy foods.

Participants' low socio-economic status can help to explain the prevailing food insecurity in most of the households surveyed. The types of food that had been consumed at home by the majority of study subjects a few days prior to the study lacked variety as well as enough fruits and vegetables. There was also inadequate frequency and consumption of certain types of foods as recommended in the SAFBDGs. Similar findings have been reported in the South African context. A study by Bourne et al. (16) on food and meal patterns in the urban African population of the Cape Peninsula and another study by Vorster et al. (23) which analyzed the nutrient intake of South Africans established that meal patterns in low socio-economic groups were confined to a relatively narrow range of foods. Bourne and colleagues (16) further argued that poverty, lack of knowledge and social instabilities in the black population militate against healthy eating practices.

Positive individual behaviour to make healthy food choices may not occur without supportive environments wherein there is availability of, and access to, affordable healthy foods. In their study on why Americans eat what they do, Glanz and colleagues (24) found that the cost of food was the second most important determining factor of food choice, after food taste. In South Africa, a study conducted by Temple and colleagues (12) to investigate the availability of healthier food choices and whether a healthier diet costs more than a diet commonly eaten by low-income families also established that healthier foods typically cost between 10% and 60% more than their regular options when compared on a weight basis (Rand per 100g). The findings of the latter study complements those from our study, that healthier food options were more expensive than their regular counterparts by between 3% and 22%. Even more striking was the fact that almost all healthier food options included in the study were not available for price audits in convenient stores ('spazas') which, interestingly, are the food retail outlets most frequently visited by study participants for food purchases.

Subjective measurements of differential food prices from study participants also seemed to substantiate the market-based objective measurements. The majority of subjects who were asked to compare the perceived market price of healthy food items and their regular counterparts indicated that healthy options were the most expensive to purchase. This may suggest that an individual on a meager income might have to forgo the costly yet healthier choice and opt to buying what is more affordable despite the fact that it is less healthy, as was the case for some participants in our study. A study by Blisard et al. (25) also showed that low income families are more likely to spend less on healthy food such as fruits and vegetables than high income families.

In our study, the major deterrent of frequent consumption of fruits and vegetables and other healthier foods was the lack of money. Borrowing money from friends and family or foregoing other groceries necessary for home use were some of the predictors of what kind and quantities of healthy food health club members could purchase for household consumption. These findings point to the importance of promoting food purchasing power in addition to increasing availability of and access to healthy food items, in order to foster healthy food-purchasing and consumption behaviour of individuals who are reasonably knowledgeable about healthy eating such as the participants in our study.

Variability in the price of, and access to, foods between larger and smaller food stores is also another important determinant of food-purchasing behaviour. A study in the USA (4) established that in areas served by smaller retail shops such as those in low income settings, access to healthier food alternatives is limited and a healthy food basket is more expensive. The current study also showed that some subjects perceived healthier food options in smaller convenient shops ('spazas') in their communities to be generally more expensive than in large retail outlets and yet the frequency of food purchase in 'spaza' shops was higher compared to supermarkets. This may be of concern. There is only one supermarket serving this community which is not easily accessible to everyone and there are numerous and yet easily accessible 'spaza' shops which, in addition to being expensive, also have few healthy food types available.

Previous work by Puoane et al. (17) undertaken in a similar setting of Khayelitsha showed that in such situations there is a tendency to resort to buying energy-dense foods which contain higher levels of sugar and fat as a coping mechanism to save money. This study established that community members sometimes prefer to buy cheap foods that have high fat content, such as fried meat and fat-cooks (equivalent to donuts). As such, continued failure to access healthier food at relatively cheaper price from the food stores immediately surrounding the community members could, in the long run, lead to poor diet and health.

Some findings from this study should however be interpreted cautiously. Not all the foods subjected to price audits are purchased by all study participants for household consumption. The study only gives a picture of the kinds of foods participants are exposed to and at what price they can purchase them. We also recognize the fact that prices of foods may fluctuate from time to time. Future research studies are needed to assess trends in food prices over an extended period of time and how this is related to food purchasing and consumption patterns. A wider, more socioeconomically and demographically diverse study population should also be considered for future research in order to capture variations in demographic and socioeconomic parameters as they relate to healthy food cost and purchasing behaviour.

Although the design of the current study does not allow for generalization of the findings to the larger population in Khayelitsha and beyond, it extends and complements the evidence from earlier works that have investigated the same subject matter.

The findings of this study may nevertheless be relevant to developers of public health interventions and policy makers. If the compositional and contextual factors highlighted in this study are explored at causal level in similar and wider communities in South Africa, this may lead to an increased understanding of the complexities regarding communities' access to healthy food, in terms of its availability and affordability, thereby providing the possibility of a more realistic platform upon which individual healthy food choices can be fostered.

ACKNOWLEDGMENTS

Special thanks are extended to Sybil Xapha and two community health workers – Mati and Sisi for their assistance during data collection. Our thanks also go to Ms Lungiswa Nkoki for her initial technical input during the conceptualization of this research which formed the basis of the Author's Masters in Public Health Thesis. This was an independent study and received no specific funding towards its completion.

REFERENCES

[1]   Barratt J. The cost and availability of healthy food choices in southern Derbyshire. J Hum Nutr Diet 1997;10:63-9.

[2]   Cummins S, MacIntyre S. A systematic study of an urban food landscape: The price and availability of food in Greater Glasgow. Urban Stud 2002;39:2115–30.

[3]   Darmon N, Ferguson EL, Briend A. A cost constraint alone has adverse effects on food selection and nutrient density: An analysis of human diets by linear programming. J Nutr 2002; 132:3764–71.

[4]   Jetter K M, Cassady DL. The availability and cost of healthier food alternatives. Am J Prev Med 2006;30(1):38–44.

[5]   Morland K, Diez Roux AV, Wing S. Supermarkets, other food stores, and obesity: the atherosclerosis risk in communities study. Am J Prev Med 2006;30:333–9.

[6]   Cummins S, Macintyre S. Food environments and obesity—neighborhood or nation? Int J Epidemiol 2006;35:100–4.

[7]   Turrell G, Blakely T, Patterson C, Oldenburg B. A multilevel analysis of socio-economic (small area) differences in household food-purchasing behavior. J Epidemiol Commun Health 2004;58:208–15.

[8]   Giskes K, Turrell G, Patterson C, Newman B. Socio--economic differences in fruit and vegetable consumption among Australian adolescents and adults. Public Health Nutr 2002;5(5):663–9.

[9]   White M. Food access and obesity. Obes Rev 2007;8(Suppl 1): 99-107.

[10]   Story M, Kaphingst M K, O'Brien R R, Glanz K. Creating healthy food and eating environments: policy and environmental approaches. Annu Rev Pub Health 2008;29: 253-72.

[11]   Temple NJ, Steyn NP. Food prices and energy density as barriers to healthy food choices in Cape Town. J Hunger Environ Nutr 2009;4:203–13.

[12]   Temple NJ, Steyn NP, Fourie J, De Villiers A. Price and availability of healthy food: A study in rural South Africa. Nutrition 2011;27(1):55-8.

[13]   Labadarios D, Steyn N, Maunder E, MacIntryre U, Gericke G, Swart R, et al. The national food consumption survey (NFCS): South Africa. Public Health Nutr 1999;8(5):544-43.

[14] Love P, Maunder E, Green M, Ross F, Smale-Lovely J, Charlton K. South African food-based dietary guidelines: Testing of the preliminary guidelines among women in KwaZulu-Natal and the Western Cape. South Afr J Clin Nutr 2001;14:9-19.

[15] May J. Experiences and perceptions of poverty in South Africa. Durban: Praxis Publishing. Accessed 2009 Dec 29. URL: http:experiences+and+perceptions+of+poverty+in+south+Africa.

[16] Bourne LT, Langenhoven ML, Steyn K, Jooste PL, Nesamvuni AE, Laubscher JA. The food and meal pattern in the urban African population of the Cape Peninsula. The BRISK Study. Cent Afr J Med 1994;40:140–8.

[17] Puoane T, Zulu J, Tsolekile L, Bradley H, Hughes G. Promoting healthy lifestyle: Community health workers' intervention program for primary prevention of non-communicable diseases in Khayelitsha, an urban township in Cape Town. Cape Town: School Public Health, University of Western Cape, 2007. [South Africa]

[18] Information and knowledge Management Department: Socio-economic Profiling of Urban Renewal Nodes – Khayelitsha and Mitchell's plain., Cape Town2006. Accessed 2011 Jan 16. URL: http://www.capetown.gov.za/en/stats/CityReports/Documents/Urban%20Renewal%20Programme/URP_Socio--Eco_Exec_Summary_228200612631_359.pdf

[19] Gibney M, Vorster H. South African food-based dietary guideline. South Afr J Clin Nutr 2001;14(3): S1-S80.

[20] Burgess R. Qualitative data analysis for applied policy research. In: Bryman A, ed. Analyzing qualitative data. New York: Routledge, 1994:164-80.

[21] Giskes K, Van Lenthe F J, Brug J, Mackenback JP, Turrell G. Inequalities in food purchasing: the contribution of respondent-perceived and actual (objectively measured) price and availability of foods. Prev Med 2007;45:41-8.

[22] Kearney M, Kearney JM, Dunne A, Gibney MJ. Socio--demographic determinants of perceived influences on food choice in a nationally representative sample of Irish adults. Public Health Nutr 1999;3(2):21-6.

[23] Vorster HH, Jerling JC, Oosthuizen W, Becker P, Wolmarans P. Nutrient intakes of South Africans: An analysis of the literature. SANSS group report to Roche Products. Potchefstroom: Roche, 1995;41.

[24] Glanz K, Basil M, Maibach E, Snyder D. Why Americans eat what they do: Taste, nutrition, cost, convenience, and weight control concerns as influences on food consumption. J Am Diet Assoc 1998;98:1118–26.

[25] Blisard N, Stewart H, Joliffe D. Low-income households' expenditures on fruits and vegetables. Agricultural Economic Report No833. Accessed 2011 November 3. URL: http://www.ers.usda.gov/publications/aer833/aer833.pdf

In: Public Health Yearbook 2013   ISBN: 978-1-63321-095-0
Editor: Joav Merrick   © 2014 Nova Science Publishers, Inc.

Chapter 28

MALARIA INFECTION AND ENVIRONMENTAL HEALTH PRACTICES AMONG WOMEN IN SELECTED RURAL COMMUNITIES IN NIGERIA

*Femi Tinuola, PhD, MSc, BSc**

Department of Sociology, Faculty of Social Sciences,
Kogi State University, Anyigba, Nigeria

ABSTRACT

This study investigates the incidence of malaria infection, knowledge of symptoms and causes of malaria infection and environmental health conditions in malaria endemic rural communities. Data were obtained from eight selected rural communities in East Senatorial District of Kogi State, Nigeria. The communities were selected on purposive sampling using Demographic Parameters. The instrument of data collection is a structured questionnaire which contains 90% closed ended questions on issues relating to the malaria infection and environmental health. The instrument was administered by Field Health Workers deployed to the rural areas under a WHO health surveillance program. Data were analyzed using Predictive Analytical Software. Findings show a high level of malaria infection, poor understanding of the symptoms, poor knowledge of the causes of malaria. The situation is worsened by the poor environmental health conditions and the inability of the existing health care systems to respond appropriately to the incidence. Malaria remains a serious threat to the health and wellbeing of the people. The need for a more proactive effort in preventive and curative measures is recommended to ensure a healthy rural population.

Keywords: Malaria, women, disease, health, infection

---

* Correspondence: Femi Tinuola, PhD, Department of Sociology, Faculty of Social Sciences, Kogi State University, PMB 1008, Anyigba, Nigeria. E-mail: adufem2000@yahoo.com.

INTRODUCTION

Malaria is one of the oldest recorded diseases in the world since the 18th century. It existed in parts of the United States from colonial times to the 1940s (1). One of the first military expenditures of the Continental Congress, around 1775, was for $300 to buy quinine to protect General Washington's troops. More than an estimated 600,000 cases of malaria occurred in the US in 1914. From 1956 to 1969, the United States, through the U.S. Agency for International Aid, (USAID) gave $790 million to the Global Eradication of Malaria Program (2).

Mortality arising from malaria varies across regions. In the past 100 years, nearly 150 million to 300 million people are estimated to have died from the effects of malaria, accounting for 2-5% of all deaths globally. Malaria remains the world's most devastating human infection, with 300-500 million clinical cases and 3 million deaths every year (3).

Malaria is a vector-borne infectious disease caused by protozoan parasites. It is widespread in tropical and sub-tropical regions, including parts of the Americas, Asia, and Africa. Each year, there are approximately 350–500 million cases of malaria, killing between one and three million people, the majority of whom are young children (4). In the sub-Saharan Africa, malaria is one of the most common infectious diseases and constitutes an enormous public health problem with 90% percent of malaria-related deaths occurring in the region.

Only *Anopheles mosquitoes* can transmit malaria, and they must have been infected through a previous blood meal taken on an infected person. When a mosquito bites an infected person, a small amount of blood is taken, which contains microscopic malaria parasites. About one week later, when the mosquito takes its next blood meal, these parasites mix with the mosquito's saliva and are injected into the person being bitten (5)

Malaria has infected humans for over 50,000 years, and malarial protozoa may have been a human pathogen for the entire history of the species (6). Malaria causes about 250 million cases of fever and approximately one million deaths annually. The vast majority of cases occur in children under 5 years and pregnant women (7). Despite efforts to reduce transmission and increase treatment, there has been little change in which areas are at risk of this disease since 1992. Precise statistics are unknown because many cases occur in rural areas where people do not have access to hospitals or the means to afford health care. As a consequence, the majority of cases are undocumented (8).

Malaria is presently endemic in a broad band around the equator, in areas of the Americas, many parts of Asia, and much of Africa; however, it is in sub-Saharan Africa where 85–90% of malaria fatalities occur. The geographic distribution of malaria within large regions is complex, and malaria-afflicted and malaria-free areas are often found close to each other (9). In drier areas, outbreaks of malaria can be predicted with reasonable accuracy by mapping rainfall (10). Malaria is more common in rural areas than in cities; this is in contrast to dengue fever where urban areas present the greater risk. For example, the cities of Vietnam, Laos and Cambodia are essentially malaria-free, but the disease is present in many rural regions. By contrast, in Africa malaria is present in both rural and urban areas, though the risk is lower in the larger cities (11).

Symptoms of malaria include fever, shivering, arthralgia (joint pain), vomiting, anemia hemoglobinuria, retinal damage and convulsions (12). The classic symptom of malaria is cyclical occurrence of sudden coldness followed by rigor and then fever and sweating lasting four to six hours, occurring every two days in P. vivax and P. ovale infections, while every three days for P. malariae. Malaria has been found to cause cognitive impairments, especially in children. It causes widespread anemia during a period of rapid brain development and also direct brain damage. This neurologic damage results from cerebral malaria, to which children are more vulnerable (13).

Prevention of malaria may be more cost-effective than treatment of the disease in the long run, but the capital costs required are out of reach of many of the world's poorest people. It has been argued that, in order to meet the Millennium Development Goals (MDGs), money should be redirected from HIV/AIDS treatment to malaria prevention, which for the same amount of money would provide greater benefit to African economies.

Brazil, Eritrea, India, and Vietnam have, unlike many other developing nations, successfully reduced the malaria burden. Common success factors included conducive country conditions, a targeted technical approach using a package of effective tools, data-driven decision-making, active leadership at all levels of government, involvement of communities, decentralized implementation and control of finances, skilled technical and managerial capacity at national and sub-national levels, hands-on technical and programmatic support from partner agencies, and sufficient and flexible financing (14).

Mosquito nets help keep mosquitoes away from people and greatly reduce the infection and transmission of malaria. The distribution of mosquito nets impregnated with insecticides such as permethrin or deltamethrin has been shown to be an extremely effective method of malaria prevention, and it is also one of the most cost-effective methods of prevention. Insecticide Treated Nets (ITNs) have been shown to be the most cost-effective prevention method against malaria and are part of WHO's MDGs.

The cost of treating malaria is high relative to income and the illness results in lost wages. Mosquito nets are often unaffordable to people in developing countries, especially for those most at risk. Only 1 out of 20 people in Africa own a bed net. Although shipped into Africa mainly from Europe as free development help, the nets quickly become expensive trade goods. They are mainly used for fishing, and by combining hundreds of donated mosquito nets, whole river sections can be completely shut off, catching even the smallest fish (15). Nets are also often distributed though vaccine campaigns using voucher subsidies, such as the measles campaign for children. Another alternative approach uses spores of the fungus *Beauveria bassiana*, sprayed on walls and bed nets, to kill mosquitoes. While some mosquitoes have developed resistance to chemicals, they have not been found to develop a resistance to fungal infections.

Many researchers have found that education in recognizing the symptoms of malaria will reduce the number of cases in some areas of the developing world by as much as 20%. Recognizing the disease in the early stages can also stop the disease from becoming a killer. Education can also inform people to cover over areas of stagnant still water which are ideal breeding grounds for the parasite and mosquito, thus cutting down the risk of the transmission between people. This is mostly practiced in urban areas with high population density with higher likelihood of transmission.

Malaria is not just a disease commonly associated with poverty but also a cause of poverty and a major hindrance to economic development. Tropical regions are affected most, however malaria's furthest extent reaches into some temperate zones with extreme seasonal changes. The disease has been associated with major negative economic effects on regions where it is widespread. During the late 19th and early 20th centuries, it was a major factor in the slow economic development of the American southern states (16).

A comparison of average per capita GDP in 1995, adjusted for parity of purchasing power, between countries with malaria and countries without malaria gives a five-fold difference ($1,526 USD versus $8,268 USD). In countries where malaria is common, average per capita GDP has risen (between 1965 and 1990) only 0.4% per year, compared to 2.4% per year in other countries (17). Poverty is both cause and effect, however, since the poor do not have the financial capacities to prevent or treat the disease. The lowest income group in Malawi carries the burden of having 32% of their annual income used on this disease compared with the 4% of household incomes from low-to-high groups. In its entirety, the economic impact of malaria has been estimated to cost Africa $12 billion USD every year.

The economic impact includes costs of health care, working days lost due to sickness, days lost in education, decreased productivity due to brain damage from cerebral malaria, and loss of investment and tourism. In some countries with a heavy malaria burden, the disease may account for as much as 40% of public health expenditure, 30-50% of inpatient admissions, and up to 50% of outpatient visits (18).

On 25th September 2008, government, business and civil society leaders gathered at the United Nations to launch a global campaign to reduce malaria deaths, currently at more than 1 million each year, to near zero by 2015, with an initial commitment of nearly $3 billion. The Global Malaria Action Plan (GMAP) aims to cuts deaths and illness by 2010 to half their 2000 levels by scaling up access to insecticide-treated bed nets, indoor spraying and treatment, and achieve the near-zero goal through sustained universal coverage. Ultimately, it seeks to eradicate the disease completely with new tools and strategies.

Full implementation of GMAP will require $5.3 billion worldwide in 2009, $2.2 billion of it for Africa, and $6.2 billion in 2010, $2.86 billion for Africa, to expand malaria control programmes. An additional $750 million to $900 million per year is needed for research on vaccines drugs and other new tools.

Despite all efforts, malaria remains the highest killer disease in Nigeria with higher incidence in rural areas. The situation is compounded with poor environmental conditions and management occasioned by poor housing plans and poverty.

All efforts towards reducing malaria incidence and its socio-economic burden through programs can only be achieved if the vulnerable population is well informed on the etiology and management of its symptoms. This is necessary because of the role of environmental factors in prevention cannot be under-estimated. Most programs on malaria are directed towards prevention and treatment with little emphasis on environmental health education. The need therefore arises for a study to examine the level of knowledge of etiology of malaria and environmental health practices among people in malaria endemic rural areas in Nigeria. This study examines the incidence of malaria infection, knowledge of symptoms and causes of malaria infection and environmental health conditions in malaria endemic rural communities in Eastern Senatorial Districts in Kogi State.

METHODS

This study was conducted in East Senatorial District, Kogi State. The survey instrument is included in the Appendix. Data were obtained from eight rural communities selected by purposive sampling technique. The basis of the selection was the characteristic of rural areas as demonstrated by the interplay of demographic variables among the population. In all, 120 respondents were randomly selected from the 8 communities to respond to various questions on the subject under study. These communities are Itama, Ewune, Iyale, Ajogwomi, Emewe-Opada, Ajiolo-Abocho, Etutekpe, Ojikpadala-Egume. Respondents were selected among women of reproductive age, 15-44 years. The instrument of data collection is a structured questionnaire which contains mostly close-ended questions. The questionnaire is divided into the following sections: characteristics, incidence of malaria, symptoms of malaria, knowledge of causes of malaria and environmental health conditions. The instrument was validated with the use of Pearson Product Moment correlation co-efficient. The instrument was administered by a group of field health workers deployed to the various communities on a World Health Organisation Program. Data were collated, edited and analyzed with the use of Predictive Analytical Software. They are presented using frequency distribution while variables are cross tabulated with the use of chi-square technique.

Data were analysed with the use of Predictive Analytical software. Responses were transcribed, coded and keyed on the data and variable view of the Software, after which descriptive statistics was used to analyse ordinal variables and are presented in Tables for clarity. Data are presented in frequency/percent distribution. The hypotheses are tested using a bi-variate statistics (Chi-square) and are tested at 0.05 level of significance. The data obtained in this field work, for clarity, is divided into social characteristics of respondents, incidence of malaria infection, knowledge of symptoms and causes of malaria infection and environmental condition.

RESULTS

This study was conducted among women of reproductive age. The recent NDHS reports that menopausal age has reduced drastically to 40-44 years in Nigeria. This study adopts the upper age limit to determine the age cohort of respondents. About 43.3% were between 15-24 years, 32.5% within 25-34 while the remaining 24.2% are within 35-44 years of age. With this data, 75.8% of the samples were below 35 years. Under a normal circumstance, the reproductive performance of this population with this classification is enhanced, all other factors of infertility held constant. The average age of the total respondents in this study is 25.2 years. A great proportion of women aged 25.2 years in a population signifies high tendency for some demographic events such as marriages, procreation, naming ceremonies and high expectation for intensive reproductive performance and migration.

RELIGION

Respondents are fairly distributed over the three major religions in the area with just 4.2% who did not respond to the question on religion. While 45% were Christians, 33.3% were Muslims, 17.5% were adherents of African Traditional Religion. Traditional norms and values at times influence one's perception of the etiology and treatment of diseases.

Education

This study was conducted in Eastern senatorial Districts of Kogi, in Nigeria. With power as the value orientation, people's attitude and goals are more focused relatively on the acquisition of political power at the expense of Western education. Among the selected respondents, 37.5% had no formal education, 20.8% primary education, 29.2% secondary education while just 10.5% had post-secondary education. Over half of the total respondents (58.3%) had a maximum of primary education.

Occupation

Two-fifth were farmers, 41.7% were traders, 13.3% worked with government, while 5.5% were artisans. The report indicates that an overwhelming majority (81.7%) were farmers and traders, making farming and trading the prevailing occupations in the study areas.

Marital status

About 33% were singles while 67% were married. There were no cases of divorce and separations among the selected respondents.

The question "if married what is the number of children you have" was asked to ascertain the reproductive performance of the selected women. Apparently, data show that about 32% had no children since they got married. Inability to conceive and bear children could result from primary or secondary factors depending to a large extent on the age of couples, age at marriage and the reproductive health component of the body. In this survey, 18.3% had 1-2 children, 28.3% had 3-4 children while 21.7% had more than 4 children. The average number of children respondents had was found at 4.5. Culturally, there is preference for children among the Igala ethnic group where this study was carried out. Children are described as the "salt of the earth" to express high premium placed on the value of children.

Incidence of malaria

To examine this prevalence of malaria among the people living in the communities, a question was asked on whether they have ever had malaria infection or not. Data show that almost all the respondents (97.8%) reported ever having malaria infection for at least three times. This figure shows a high prevalence of malaria infection history in the rural communities under study. The proportion reported shows that malaria is endemic and urgent action should be taken in both preventive and curative measures to contain the trend.

Mortality arising from malaria is dependent on how the available health care delivery system manages the reported cases. This is dependent upon available health care equipment, doctor/patient population ratio, cost of treatment and accessible health care facilities. In the sub-Saharan Africa, malaria remains the highest killer disease ravaging a greater proportion of the population of pregnant women and children. Those who ever had malaria were asked the number of weeks they had the last malaria infection. It is also important to note that about 62% had infection in the previous 4 weeks preceding this survey, 26.7% experienced the infection within the last 8 weeks. This data shows new cases of the infection with malaria in the selected communities.

A question was asked on "how did you know you had malaria? At the onset of an infection, methods or means through which the patients ascertain the infection are important factors influencing places where treatments are sought and consequently, the nature of diagnosis. It is of interest to note that 6.7% indicated that they discovered they had malaria through personal experience and understanding of the symptoms. Ten percent of the women reportedly discovered malaria when they were examined by their husbands, the remaining 83.3% consulted with nurses/doctors for a medical test to discover the infection. In medical parlance, only the result of a medical laboratory test is reliable for ascertaining an infection. Results of scientific laboratory tests are required and recommended before administering any form of treatment. This report indicates the availability of primary health facilities in the rural communities.

Symptoms of malaria

Understanding the etiology of a disease and early symptomatic detection are products of the awareness and understanding of the associated illness behaviour. The understanding of the symptoms is one of the major determinants of early presentation of illness cases for treatment. In this study, questions were asked of the respondents to examine the level of their understanding of causes and symptoms for early detection and diagnosis. All the respondents (100%) acknowledged that cold is a symptom of malaria fever, about 64% of these people are also knowledgeable that 'cold' could also be a symptom of other diseases. Similarly, an overwhelming majority (91.7%) was aware that severe headache could result from malaria infection, 8.3% were not aware of any link between headache and malaria. About 42% indicated that malaria could not result in stomach ache while over half (54.2%) reported that, in some cases, malaria infection could result in troubled stomach. About 90% believed that malaria infection could only aggravate pains resulting from menstruation but could not be a direct consequence. An overwhelming majority (80%) linked vomiting with the early stage of malaria, 100% stressed that malaria infection could cause inability of the infected to eat well, weakness of the body (95.8%) bad dreams (82.5%), eating in the dream (50%) and black tongue (25.8%), respectively.

Knowledge of causes of malaria

The knowledge of the etiology of disease is one of the major determinants of response to the illness and treatment seeking outlets. Apart from factors such as income, occupation, level of occupation, availability of health infrastructure and cost of treatment, the level of knowledge of the causes of a particular disease determines patients' perception of the severity of the problem and their health seeking behavior. For example, those who perceive that an ill state is caused by witchcraft may likely seek help from spiritual sources than those who perceive their ill state results from biological malfunctioning of the body system. However, the time and place where people seek help when ill are major determinants of treatment patterns and response to the administration of cure/care.

In this study, various questions were asked to examine the level of knowledge of the rural dwellers of factors causing malaria. It is revealing that 40% linked malaria infection with the activities of witchcraft. These respondents indicated that witches can bewitch an individual with malaria, whereas 79.2% acknowledged that malaria fever is caused by mosquito infection. Other risk factors of malaria infection identified by the sample include bad water (82.5%), bush around the house (90.8%) and rainfall (95%).

Environmental health

The nature of the environment one lives is one of the major influences of the risk factors of diseases in human society. This places environmental health as one of the priorities in any discourse and attempt to addressing the state of human health. In the sub-Saharan Africa region, poor environmental conditions have contributed to the relatively high state of disease that is currently ravaging a greater proportion of the human population. This has contributed to the burden of ill patients being experienced by the available health care facilities. Previous efforts aimed at addressing malaria infection have failed because of poor environmental conditions. In this study, the researcher examines the condition of the house of each of the respondents as a major factor in environmental health. Data shows that about 72% had bush surrounding the house, with about 55% having bad ventilation. Findings corroborate the data reported above. In Greenwood and Mutabingwa's studies, the duo discovered that 85-95% of malaria facilities occur in most countries of the sub-Saharan Africa because of the geographical distribution of houses and poor housing policies (19).

As a result, this environment has made outbreaks of malaria unpredictable. Associated with housing condition is the availability of ordinary window net and better still, ITNS. Just 13.3% had ordinary nets fixed on their windows to prevent mosquitoes from gaining entrance. Experience during the research shows that most of these window nets are old and torn due to the influence of hot weather and reptiles. The efficacy of the window nets in preventing mosquito gaining entrance may be low. In recent times, the introduction of ITNS is intended to reduce mosquito bites and infection with malaria. In fact, mosquito nets help keep mosquitoes away from humans and greatly reduce the infections and transmission of malaria. In the study areas, only 18.3% could acquire ITNS. Reasons respondents reported include relatively non-availability of ITNs and the inability to afford the cost in places where they are available. The finding of this study is in agreement with the report of *The Economist* (2007) that ITNS are often unaffordable to people in developing countries, especially for those at risk and that only 1 out of every 20 people in developing countries own a bed net. The 18.3% possession rate of ITNs reported in this study is an improvement on the 5% possession rate earlier reported by *The Economist* (2007). Notwithstanding, mosquito nets offer one of the cheapest means of malaria prevention.

The type and condition of toilet facilities in a living apartment are factors determining the state of environmental health. In the rural communities where this study was carried out, less than 30% had modern toilet facilities for faeces disposal. About 62% defecate in the nearby bush due to lack of modern toilet facilities. This may have increased the chance of spread of communicable diseases that worsened human health and pose serious pressures on the existing health care facilities. Generally, only 25% had an incinerator for human waste disposal while less than 10% has pit latrines for defecation.

Mosquitoes, the major transmitter of malaria infection, are found to breed on stagnant pools of water. This indicates that any environment where a body of water can be found is a breeding ground for mosquitoes. Because of the non-existence of tap water and bore holes in the study areas, most people who could not afford to buy kegs of water supplied by Malams depended mostly on water from streams for consumption and household uses. Over 65% built and lived in houses very close to the streams, to have greater access to water. Consequently, they fetched water into drums uncovered for many days. These drums of water are reserved for several days just in case there is scarcity from the stream. Both the streams and the reserve water are untreated and remain uncovered in drums for many days which could serve as mosquito breeding sites. This may have contributed to increased mosquito bites resulting in malaria infection in most rural communities in Kogi State.

This is extremely dangerous and risky in communities where 62.5% of the houses are made of mud, no fixed doors (72.5%), no environmental sanitation (67.5%), bush around the house (71.7%) and only 19.2% of the selected respondents could afford insecticides once in three months. The source of water for consumption is another serious public health issue of concern in these malaria endemic communities where 87.5% depended on water from the streams, lake (18.3%), rain (70.8%) and only 3.3% could afford to buy borehole water from those who offer them for sale.

Cross Tabulation

In this section, various variables are cross tabulated to examine the nature of how such relationships could assist in determining the knowledge and environmental health practices in the rural communities where the study was carried out. Data obtained are discussed under various subheadings as follows:

Age/ever had malaria

Age of respondents was cross tabulated with responses on "Ever had malaria" to explore the relationship between age and malaria incidence. It intends to answer "could malaria incidence be distributed over age? If yes, what age cohort of the population is prone to a higher incidence than the other? Data obtained in the study are cross tabulated with the use of chi-square. The result of the chi-square was found at 3.11 while the table value $X2t = 4.50$. The result shows that X2c < X2t. We accept and confirm the null hypothesis while we reject the alternative position. Therefore, there is no significant relationship between age of the respondents and the tendency to be infected with malaria. This indicates that the infection with malaria is not distributed per specific age. The incidence cuts across all ages of the selected respondents.

Level of education/Where people seek treatment

The level of education of respondents was cross tabulated with where people seek treatment for malaria. This was done to examine whether the level of education of a patient influences where he seeks treatment. This is founded on the belief that one of the factors influencing perception of the etiology of a disease is its knowledge which may be acquired through education. Consequently, one's perception of a disease is a major influence of places where he seeks treatment. In this study, respondents identified five places where they sought help when infected with malaria. The Chi-Square shows that $X^2_c = 8.39$ while the table value $X^2_t = 8.44$. $X^2_c < X^2_t$. The degree of freedom is equal to 14 and when tested at 0.05 level of significance, the result shows that the null position is accepted and confirmed. This indicates that level of education is not a determinant of where people seek medical treatment. Earlier report on the education shows that a greater proportion of the respondents had a maximum of secondary education.

Ever had malaria/Have mosquito net

The hypothesis was framed to examine the relationship between possessing a mosquito net and the tendency to have infection from mosquito. Mosquito nets are distributed / sold to prevent mosquito bites. This cross tabulation shows whether there is a direct relationship. The $X^2_c = 2.29$ while the $X^2_t = 1.304$. The degree of freedom = 2. Since $X^2_c < X^2_t$, there is a significant indirect relationship. Those who had ITNs may not likely report frequent cases of malaria infection compared to those without ITNs. Mosquito nets are to keep mosquitoes away from the people and reduce the transmission of malaria. The distribution of ITNs is judged an effective and affordable method of malaria. This data evidently corroborates various earlier reports on the efficacy of ITNs in the prevention of malaria. In the rural communities where this study was carried out, people do not have free access to ITNs as a significant proportion complained of their inability to afford the cost of procuring it as a factor of non-use.

Ever had malaria/Environmental sanitation

The quality of the environment is judged one of the major determinants of breeding space for mosquitoes. Various studies have linked poor and an unhygienic environment to incidence of malaria fever. In this study, various questions were asked to determine the quality of the environment and a hypothesis was framed to establish any possible link between environmental sanitation and incidence of malaria infection. Using chi-square, the calculated value was found at $(X^2_c) = 18.4$ while the table value equals 15.2. The data shows that there is a significant relationship between participation in environmental sanitation and incident of malaria infection. Those who reportedly participated in community initiated monthly environmental sanitation recorded low cases of malaria.

DISCUSSION

This study recognizes that malaria is one of the highest infectious diseases arising from insect bites. The incidence, as reported by the respondents, is high and remains the most common infection in the study areas. Generally, the knowledge of the causes of malaria is relatively high but the situation is compounded by poor environmental health and the non-existence/non-implementation and enforcement of environmental sanitation laws. The commercialization of ITNs distributed freely by the government has reduced its usage, thereby making malaria prevention through ITNs non-accessible. The water supply situation has further compounded the availability of breeding space for mosquitoes. With respondents depending primarily on the stream as a source of water for household uses, the tendency to preserve water in open space conducive for mosquito breeding is high. The inability of the existing health care facilities in the areas to meet the challenges of the epidemics may have led to the increase in morbidity arising from the infection.

In the light of the above findings, the following recommendation will assist in reducing and curtailing malaria infection in the study area and other rural communities of similar characteristics in Nigeria.

1. There is the need for adequate health education geared towards malaria prevention and cure.
2. The water supply system in the communities requires a total over-hauling towards achieving the supply of potable water for the people.
3. The price of Insecticide Treated Nets should be subsidized so that it can be affordable for the people.
4. The existing health care delivering system in the areas should be improved and equipped with relevant drugs to manage the reported cases of malaria infections.
5. Formulate and implement environmental law to improve the quality of environment.

APPENDIX

Questionnaire of knowledge and environmental health practices among women of reproductive age in malaria endemic rural communities in Kogi State.

Number: / / /
Social characteristics
1. Age: 15-24 ( )25-34 ( )   35-44( )

2. Religion: Christian ( )   Islam ( ) ATR ( )

3. Education: No formal education ( )   primary ( ) Secondary ( ) Post-secondary ( )

4. Occupation: Farming ( )   Trading ( )   Govt. ( ) Artisan ( )

5. Marital Status: Single ( )   Married ( )

6. If married, number of children: 1-2 ( )   3-4 ( ) above 4 ( )

Incidence of malaria
7. Ever had malaria: Yes ( )   No ( )

8. How long did you have malaria: 4 weeks ( ) 6 weeks ( ) 8 weeks ( ) above ( )

9. How did you know you had malaria? Myself ( ) Husband ( ) Nurse ( ) Doctor (

Knowledge of symptoms of malaria
10. The followings are symptoms of malaria

Response	Yes	No
Cold		
Headache		
Stomach Ache		
Menstrual Pain		
Running Stomach		
Swollen tormy		
Vomiting		
Running nose		
Inability to eat		
Weakness of body		
Bad dreams		
Eating n the dream		
Black tongue		

Environmental factors

11. *Condition of the house*

Please tick as appropriate	Yes	No
Bush around the house		
Good ventilation		
Window net		
Modern toilet facilities		
Mosquito net		
Drums contain water		
Modern waste disposal system		
Pool of water		
Stream very close		

Mud houses		
Well-fixed doors		
Environmental sanitation		
Trees around the house		
Have insecticides		

12. *Source of water for household uses*

Please tick	Yes	No
Stream		
Lake		
Borehole		
Rain		
Tap		

13. *Toilet facilities*

Please tick	Yes	No
Bush		
Pit latrine		
Water system		

14. *Causes of malaria*

Causes of malaria	Yes	No
Exposure to sun and rain		
Witches		
Mosquito		
Bad water		
Bush around the house		
Refuse		

Health seeking behaviour

15. In case you have malaria, where do you normally seek treatment?

   a.   Church prayer   ( )

   b.   Mosquito-prayer   ( )

   c.   Herbalist   ( )

   d.   Leaves and herbal concoction   ( )

   e.   Self-medication   ( )

   f.   Clinic   ( )

REFERENCES

[1]   Cox F. History of human parasitology. Clin Microbiol Rev 2002;15:595–612.

[2]   Desowitz RS. The malaria capers. More tales of parasites and people. Research and reality. New York: Norton, 1991.

[3]   Breman J. The ears of the hippopotamus: manifestations, determinants, and estimates of the malaria burden. Am J Trop Med Hyg 2001;64(1-2 Suppl):1–11.

[4]   Snow RW, Guerra CA, Noor AM, Myint HY, Hay SI. The global distribution of clinical episodes of Plasmodium falciparum malaria. Nature 2005;434(7030): 214–7.

[5]   Yoshida S, Shimada Y, Kondoh D. Hemolytic C-type lectin CEL-III from sea cucumber expressed in transgenic mosquitoes impairs malaria parasite development. PLoS Pathog 2007;3(12):192.

[6]   Joy D, Feng X, Mu J. Early origin and recent expansion of plasmodium falciparum. Science 2003;300(5617):318–21.

[7]   Greenwood BM, Bojang K, Whitty CJ, Targett GA. Malaria. Lancet 2005;365: 1487–98.

[8]   Hay SI, Snow RW. The malaria atlas project. Developing global maps of malaria risk. PLoS Medicine 2006;3(12):473.

[9]   Greenwood B, Mutabingwa T. Malaria in 2002. Nature 2002;415:670–2.

[10]   Van BB, Vanwambeke S, Khantikul N, Burghoorn-Maas C, Panart K, Oskam L, Lambin E, Somboon P. Spatial patterns of and risk factors for seropositivity for dengue infection. Am J Trop Med Hyg 2005;72(2):201–8.

[11]   Keiser J, Utzinger J, Caldas de Castro M, Smith T, Tanner M, Singer B. Urbanization in sub-Saharan Africa and implication for malaria control. Am J Trop Med Hyg 2005;71(2 Suppl):118–27.

[12]   Beare NA, Taylor TE, Harding SP, Lewallen S, Molyneux ME. Malarial retinopathy: a newly established diagnostic sign in severe malaria. Am J Trop Med. Hyg 2006;75(5):790–7.

[13]   Boivin MJ Effects of early cerebral malaria on cognitive ability in Senegalese children. J Dev Behav Pediatr 2002;23(5):353–64.

[14]   Barat L. Four malaria success stories: how malaria burden was successfully reduced in Brazil, Eritrea, India, and Vietnam. Am J Trop Med Hyg 2006;74(1): 12–6.

[15]   The Economist. Traditional economy of the Kavango. Economist Documentary. Available on http://www.economist.com.na/2002/15mar/03-15-22.htm

[16]   Humphreys, M. Malaria: poverty, race, and public health in the United States. Baltimore, MD: John Hopkins University Press, 2001.

[17]   Rowland M, Durrani N, Hewitt S, Mohammed N, Bouma M, Carneiro I, Rozendaal J, Schapira A. Permethrin-treated chaddars and top-sheets: appropriate technology for protection against malaria in Afghanistan and other complex emergencies. Trans R Soc Trop Med Hyg 1999;93(5):465–72.

[18]   Hoffman SL, Goh LM, Luke TC. Protection of humans against malaria by immunization with radiation-attenuated plasmodium falciparum sporozoites. J Infect Dis 2002;185(8):1155–64.

[19]   Mockenhaupt F, Ehrhardt S, Burkhardt J, Bosomtwe S, Laryea S, Anemana S, Otchwemah R, Cramer J, Dietz E, Gellert S, Bienzle U. Manifestation and outcome of severe malaria in children in northern Ghana. Am J Trop Med Hyg 2004;71(2):167–72.

In: Public Health Yearbook 2013
Editor: Joav Merrick

ISBN: 978-1-63321-095-0
© 2014 Nova Science Publishers, Inc.

Chapter 29

USING APPROPRIATE COMMUNICATION STRATEGIES FOR HIV PREVENTION EDUCATION IN RURAL COMMUNITIES IN GHANA

Patricia Anafi, PhD, Mphil, BA,*
Ebenezer Asiamah, MSc, DipHEd
and Irene Akua Agyepong, DrPH, MCH, MBChB

Department of Public Health, School of Public Health and Health Sciences, University of Massachusetts-Amherst, United States of America and Greater Accra Regional Health Directorate, Ghana Health Service, Accra Ghana and Dangme East District Health Administration, Ghana Health Service, Ada Foh, Ghana

ABSTRACT

The paper presents both qualitative and quantitative data gathered from a rural Ghanaian district to examine existing HIV/AIDS communication channels and strategies and determine the appropriate communication strategies for effective HIV preventive education. Radio, TV, neighbors, teachers, pastors, health workers and print media were found to be the major channels for HIV/AIDS education and communication. However, respondents did not consider existing HIV/AIDS communication channels to be very accessible as their messages are not usually in the local language. They expressed needs for more detailed information, with illustrations and in their local language. Local people noted that community involvement in HIV/AIDS communication and education has been low, but felt that they could have an important role to play. They suggested involving heads of households and parents, individuals, and setting up community-based groups to improve current HIV-communication efforts in rural communities if HIV/AIDS education is going to have an impact on rural people's knowledge and behavior.

---

* Correspondence: Patricia Anafi, PhD, Mphil, BA, University of Massachusetts- Amherst, Department of Public Health, School of Public Health and Health Sciences, 325 Arnold House Amherst, MA 01003 United States. E-mail: patricia_anafi@hotmail.com.

Keywords: Appropriate communication strategies, HIV/AIDS prevention education, sexual behavior change, rural communities, Ghana

INTRODUCTION

Human Immunodeficiency Virus/Acquired Immune Deficiency Syndrome (HIV/AIDS) remains one of the world's most critical social and health problem. Globally, about 33 million people are currently infected with the disease, while over 20 million people have already died from the epidemic (1). There is no known cure for AIDS, but infected people are increasingly gaining access to anti-retroviral drugs, which are still costly and inaccessible to the majority of those infected. Although a global problem, HIV/AIDS has had its worst impact on Africa. About 68% of the people infected with HIV live in sub-Saharan Africa and nearly 80% of all AIDS-related deaths since the early 1980s have occurred there (1). The severe socio-economic impact of the epidemic in sub-Saharan Africa has been thoroughly documented and includes the rapid loss of human labor and capital, reduced productivity, socio-economic stagnation, poverty, hardship and misery. HIV/AIDS contributes immensely to the health burdens of African countries, depleting scarce resources and reducing household coping capacity (2-3).

In confronting HIV/AIDS crisis, many African countries have committed themselves to AIDS control and prevention programs (4-5). In Ghana, several communication strategies have been used to sensitize the public of the dangers of the HIV/AIDS and appropriate preventive behavior for many years. In year 2000, the "Stop AIDS Love Life" campaign was officially launched in Ghana. This campaign used various communication strategies such as the Love Life songs and videos to reach across the entire country with message about safe sexual behavior and to foster compassion toward those living with HIV/AIDS (6). Communication materials developed for the campaign included leaflets, question and answers booklets, stickers, posters, t-shirts and caps for HIV prevention education (6). Following this, the "Life Shield" campaign was launched in 2002. The main objectives of the "Life Shield" program were to increase the risk perception of HIV/AIDS in the workplace, promote compassion for people living with HIV/AIDS in the workplace and encourage the adoption of preventive behavior among formal employees (7).

The current HIV prevalence rate in Ghana is estimated at 1.7 percent—indicating that the country has a lower prevalence rate than most countries in the sub-Saharan Africa. However, there are wide regional variations in HIV prevalence rate with the Eastern region having the highest rate of 4.7 percent, followed by the Greater Accra region with 3.0 percent and the Northern region with the lowest rate of 1.2 percent (1). In addition, despite the fact that HIV/AIDS is thought of as an urban phenomon, research has found that high HIV prevalence rate exist in rural communities in Ghana (8-9). Therefore, the question that needs to be asked is: Why do some regions and rural communities still have high HIV prevalence rates despite efforts at awareness creation and education for behavioral change in lifestyles that predispose individuals to HIV infection?

This study was carried out in the rural Dangme West district of Ghana, where HIV/AIDS reported cases remain relatively high. Previous studies conducted in the district have revealed that preventive messages on HIV have been conveyed to people, but these messages have not translated into actions as hoped to achieve (8-9). Thus, this current study sought to: (i) identify the existing HIV/AIDS communication channels and strategies in the district, (ii) assess the strengths and weaknesses of these channels and strategies, and (iii) determine the most effective communication strategies for HIV prevention education for sexual behavioral change in the rural district.

THE STUDY SITE

The Dangme West district is a rural district in the Greater Accra Region of Ghana. The Greater Accra region is one of the ten regions of Ghana. The Dangme West district has estimated mid-year population of 125,866 in 2007 and a land size of about 1700 square-kilometers (10). It lies in the coastal savannah and it is inhabited by the Ga- Adangme ethnic group. The inhabitants are predominantly fisher folks and farmers who use traditional non-mechanized, labor-intensive farming techniques. Until recently, traditional controls on adolescent sexual behaviors were strong. Indigenous cultural rites such as the 'Dipo' (puberty rites), which sought to suppress adolescent sexual expressions are no longer effective. The district has a current literacy rate of about 39% and the major local language spoken widely by residents is Ga-Dangme (11) Modernity, migration and new forms of social interactions have weakened traditional social norms. Young people in this culture are increasingly becoming sexually active at early ages (5, 12).

The district shares border with the Eastern region—the region with the highest prevalence rate of HIV infection in Ghana. There are no HIV sentinel surveillance sites in the district. Data on HIV/AIDS cases are obtained from 5 hospitals in districts that border on Dangme West. HIV/AIDS continue to be major health and social problem in the district and the residents still feel reluctant to talk openly about HIV/AIDS and they cover up their HIV/AIDS status for fear of stigmatization.

METHODS

The study used qualitative and quantitative research methods comprising focus group discussions (FGDs) and a pre-tested, structured questionnaire to gather data on HIV/AIDS and sexual behavior change communication channels and strategies. The study populations were adolescent (13-19 years) and adult (20 years above) males and females in the Dangme West district. Forty-two percent of this population was between 0-12 years, 50% between the ages of 13-49 years and 8% are 50 years and above based on the 2007 mid-year population estimates. Thus, the population targeted for the study represents approximately 58% of the district total population.

To obtain qualitative data, we held twelve FGDs in three communities with the highest reported incidence of HIV/AIDS in the study area. Six of the FGDs were held with adolescents ages 13-19 years. There were three separate FGDs each for adolescent male and female participants. We held the remaining six FGDs with adults: three with males and three with females. Each group comprised 8-10 participants. Key informants were used to recruit 8-10 adolescent males and 8-10 adolescent females from each of the communities. We repeated the same process for the adult FGDs in the three sampled communities. The FGDs were mainly conducted in the Ga-Dangme, the local language.

For the survey, we recruited 280 adolescents and 320 adults. We used close-ended questions administered in face-to-face interviews. Systematic random sampling was used to select 30 enumeration areas (EAs) or communities from the study site. The sampling frame was a list of all the enumeration areas in the district with their population count obtained from the 2000 national population census and household data report available at the Ghana Statistical Service. In each of the selected EAs, we randomly selected 10 households and in each household, we interviewed both adolescent and adult respondents. We selected the households by first locating the landmark of the enumeration area and we selected a household close to the landmark, then we moved on to the next until 10 households in each EA had responded. In a household, if we did not get either an adolescent or adult respondent to interview, we moved to the next household. We interviewed the first person we met in the target age range while visiting a given household. We achieved gender balance by alternating the sex of people interviewed.

In both the structured interviews and focus group discussions, information was sought on the following: existing channels and strategies for HIV/AIDS information; access to channels of communication for HIV/AIDS and sexual behavior change information; acceptability and perceived credibility of available channels and strategies, and ways to enhance effective HIV/AIDS communication and education strategies for sexual behavior change.

Data analysis

Data from the focus group discussions were analyzed using thematic analysis. Frequencies and cross-tabulations were used to analyze the survey data. All the focus groups tapes were transcribed from the local language into English and entered into Microsoft Word and the data was cleaned together with the field notes. We used thematic content analysis to categorize the data into common themes. The data were given unique quotes as we read through the transcripts and sorted them out into common themes. Based on the objectives of study, we organized the data into five major themes: "Existing HIV/AIDS communication channels and strategies," "Access to HIV/AIDS communication channels," "Acceptability and credibility of HIV/AIDS communication channels and strategies," "Community role in HIV/AIDS and sexual behavior change communication" and "Parental role in HIV/AIDS and sexual behavior change communication."

We used the cut and paste method to rearrange text with similar codes under the theme headings. Using Microsoft word processor, we copied and pasted coded transcripts on the screen into a new document, with headings for each theme. We discussed, compared and identified issues as they emerged in the various categories. Quotes from participants were used to illustrate the issues raised in the focus group discussions. The close-ended questions were coded, entered into Microsoft Excel and transferred into Stata @ 5.0 for cleaning and analysis. Means, frequencies and cross-tabs are used to present the survey data.

RESULTS

The results show that the most common channel of communication for HIV/AIDS information available to the respondents was the radio (92% of adult respondents and 86% of adolescent respondents). Also frequently mentioned were television (40% of adults and 47% of adolescents) and neighbors/relations (24% of both adults and adolescents). Other channels included teachers, pastors, community elders, assembly members, health workers and prints. Table 1 summarizes the responses of both adult and adolescent respondents for communication channels available to them in their communities for HIV/AIDS information.

Table 1. Existing communication channels for HIV/AIDS information

Communication channels	Adult (%) N=320	Adolescents (%) N=280	Total (%) N=600
Radio	92.0	86.0	89.0
TV	40.0	47.0	44.0
Neighbors /Relations	24.0	24.0	24.0
Teachers	4.0	24.0	14.0
Pastors/Church elders	15.0	7.0	11.0
Health workers	14.0	7.0	11.0
Prints	11.0	8.0	10.0
Information Van	9.0	4.0	7.0
Drumming	6.0	4.0	5.0
Community Elders	9.0	4.0	5.0
Assembly members	5.0	3.0	4.0
Durbars/Forum	4.0	2.0	3.0
NGO	0.7	0.7	0.7
Imam	0	1.4	0.7

Table 2. Existing communication strategies for HIV/AIDS information

Communication strategies	Adults (%) N=320	Adolescents (%) N=280	Total (%) N=600
Radio News	43.0	38.0	41.0
Radio discussions	24.0	24.0	24.0
Radio advertisements	31.0	26.0	29.0
TV News	15.0	21.0	18.0
TV discussions	7.0	11.0	9.0
TV advertisements	20.0	18.0	19.0
Open talks/seminars/discussions	40.0	36.0	39.0
Teaching	3.0	16.0	9.0
Preaching	13.0	8.0	11.0
Dialogue	6.0	10.0	8.0
Story telling	0.6	4.0	2.0
Drama/Cultural display	2.0	4.0	3.0
Songs	1.0	1.0	1.0
Films/Photographs/posters	10.0	6.0	8.0
Cartoons/Comics	0	0.6	0.3

The major strategies for communicating HIV/AIDS information identified by the community members were radio news broadcasts (43% adults and 38% adolescents), radio discussions (24% adults and 24% adolescents) and radio advertisements (31% adults and 26% adolescents). These were followed by TV communication strategies. Adolescent respondents recorded higher percentages for TV news (21%) and TV discussion (11%) than the adults. Adolescents more frequently mentioned teachers than the adults. Only adolescents mentioned dialogue, storytelling, drama and cartoons. Songs, storytelling, cartoons and drama were the least common communication strategies for HIV/AIDS and sexual behavior change communication for both adult and adolescent respondents (see Table 2).

Access to channels of communication for HIV/AIDS

Respondents were asked to describe how difficult it is to get access to the communication channels and to access information on HIV/AIDS through the available channels. We looked at both economic and physical accessibility. From the FGD accounts, radio emerged as quite accessible and community members said they could tune in for information at any time. They also felt that radio is affordable and has wider coverage than any other communication channel. About 80% adult respondents and 84% adolescent respondents in the survey said that radio is easy to access in their communities. However, they thought that the numerous radio stations in the country made it difficult for them to tune to the appropriate channel for the right information at a given time. An adolescent girl explained the problem this way:

> "I do not know which program is being transmitted on which channel and I often not listen to important programs because I do not know which radio station is presenting what."

Most community members thought that TV sets are difficult to access and talked about their inability to buy them. The focus group discussions revealed that TV ownership in communities is low, unlike radios, and in many cases, people visit other homes to watch TV. They also said that some communities do not have electricity—making access to TV programs quite difficult for them. One FGD participant thus observed:

> "Not everyone can afford a television set because of poverty. There is no good work to do to earn some money to be able to buy television."

Other channels viewed by respondents as providing easy access to information include teachers, neighbors and relatives, pastors and church leaders, and community leaders (see Table 3).

With respect to how often people in their communities get HIV/AIDS information through these channels, 59% of the adults and 50% of adolescents responded that they hear HIV/AIDS and sexual behavior change educational information on radio daily. Forty percent of the adult and 29% adolescent respondents have access to HIV/AIDS educational information on TV daily. Only 6% of adult respondents and none of the adolescents get HIV/AIDS information from print media on a daily basis. However, 47% of adults and 44% of adolescents indicated that they occasionally received HIV/AIDS educational information in the print media (see table 4). The print media include books, brochures, posters and daily newspapers.

Focus group discussion data also showed that adolescents received HIV/AIDS information in their schools at least once in a week or fortnightly. This usually occurred during weekly morning worship services or in regular school lessons.

HIV/AIDS and information on sexual behavior change were rarely received through mobile information vans, because they do not come to these communities for health education at all. With regards to other channels, including local health workers and community members, the majority of respondents (both adults and adolescents) said that they receive HIV/AIDS information from them only occasionally. They survey findings revealed that there was no critical difference between adults and adolescents with respect to their sources of information on HIV/AIDS and sexual behavior change.

Acceptability and credibility of communication channels and strategies

The community members interviewed felt that information on HIV/AIDS that reached them through these existing channels is reliable. They noted that they understand the messages and believed them to be correct. Based on self-reports, they understand programs on HIV/AIDS covered in TV news, advertisements and discussions, especially when people see photographs of HIV/AIDS sufferers. In one of the FGDs, a participant maintained:

> "With the photographs, you could see that HIV/AIDS is real."

Another participant added;

> "We believe that what we are taught at school about HIV/AID is real and true. In addition, we read from books."

They emphasized that these channels of communication make them aware of the causes of HIV as well as how to protect oneself from infection. HIV/AIDS information given by health workers, teachers, neighbors, relations and other community members were reportedly very easy to understand. This was largely because respondents had the opportunity to ask questions on HIV/AIDS related issues. However, they complained that background illustrations and photographs accompanying TV programs and other visual messages on HIV/AIDS are not done well enough to help them understand messages. FGD participants acknowledged the importance of HIV/AIDS messages that they get through channels available to them and mentioned that these communication strategies for HIV/AIDS and sexual behavior change do not conflict with the traditional structures and norms in their communities. A community elder in one FGD session put it this way:

> "The channels and the strategies of communication for HIV/AIDS and sexual behavior change information do not conflict with our social norms and practice. They do rather promote good sexual behavior and reduce teenage pregnancy if young people take such messages more seriously."

Table 3. Respondents Access to communication channels for HIV/AIDS information

Communication channels (No. of respondents)	Adults			Adolescents			Total		
	Difficult (%)	Somewhat difficult (%)	Easy (%)	Difficult (%)	Somewhat difficult (%)	Easy (%)	Difficult (%)	Somewhat difficult (%)	Easy (%)
Radio (N=540)	7.5	12.6	80.0	5.5	10.2	84.3	7.0	11.0	82.0
TV (N=267)	21.1	22.6	55.5	11.5	30.0	58.5	17.0	26.0	57.0
Neighbors (N=177)	5.8	24.1	70.1	1.1	13.3	85.6	3.0	19.0	78.0
Print (N=74)	15.6	37.8	46.7	27.6	31.0	41.4	20.0	35.0	45.0
Gong-Gong/Drum (N=136)	6.4	15.4	78.2	6.9	15.5	77.6	7.0	15.0	78.0
Durbars/Forum (N=17)	16.7	16.7	66.7	0	20.0	80.0	12.0	18.0	70.0
Community elders (N=40)	11.1	18.5	70.4	0	4.6	95.4	6.0	12.0	82.0
Assembly members (N=44)	20.7	3.4	75.9	0	6.7	93.3	14.0	4.0	82.0
Teachers (N=54)	0	0	100.0	17.8	2.2	80.0	15.0	2.0	83.0
Health worker (N=35)	22.7	31.8	45.5	15.4	30.8	53.8	20.0	31.0	48.0
Pastors/church elders (N=50)	0	10.7	89.3	9.1	9.1	81.8	4.0	10.0	86.0
Imam ((N=7)	0	--	100	16.7	--	83.3	14.0	--	86.
Information van (N=69)	16.7	41.7	41.7	19.1	47.6	33.3	17.0	44.0	39.0

Table 4. Frequency of access to communication channels for HIV/AIDS information

Adult respondents (%)						Adolescent respondents (%)					
Channels	Daily	Weekly	Fortnighty	Monthly	Occasionally	Channels	Daily	Weekly	Fortnightly	Monthly	Occasionally
Radio (n=290)	58.6	28.2	1.4	0.7	10.7	Radio (n=238)	50.4	31.1	3.8	2.1	12.6
TV(n=137)	40.2	34.3	2.9	2.1	20.4	TV (N=131)	29.0	44.3	6.9	3.8	16.0
Prints (n=34)	5.9	38.2	5.9	2.9	47.1	Print s (N=23)	-	34.8	4.4	17.3	43.5
Neighbors (n=137)	18.1	15.3	6.9	1.4	48.4	Neighbors (n=62)	22.6	21.0	4.8	3.2	48.4
Health workers (n=43)	2.3	9.3	2.3	11.6	74.4	Health workers (n=20)	-	5.0	5.0	35.0	55.0
Teachers (n=13)	15.4	-	30.8	-	53.9	Teachers (n=63)	27.0	15.9	9.5	6.4	41.3
Church (n=46)	8.7	30.4	8.7	15.2	37.1	Church (n=20)	10.0	40.0	15.0	-	35.0
Durbars (n=10)	-	-	-	-	100	Durbars (n=5)	-	20.0	-	-	80.0
Drums (n=18)	5.7	5.7	11.1	11.1	66.7	Drums (n=11)	-	-	-	9.1	90.9
Assembly members (n=10)	-	8.3	8.3	16.7	66.7	Assembly member (n=10)	-	10.0	40.0	-	50.0
Elders (n=15)	-	20.0	6.7	6.7	66.7	Elders (n=16)	-	6.25	31.25	-	62.5
Mosque (n=4)	-	25.0	-	25.0	50.0	Mosque (n=0)	-	-	-	-	-
NGOs (n=3)	-	-	-	-	100.0	NGOs (n=3)	-	-	66.7	-	33.3
Information Van (n=23)	-	-	7.7	7.7	84.6	Information van (n=13)	7.7	-	-	7.7	84.6
Others (n=14)	14.3	7.1	7.1	14.3	41.8	Others (n=14)	14.3	7.1	-	14.3	64.2

More importantly, they felt that more action is needed on HIV/AIDS and sexual behavior change communication to enable communities to become more aware of HIV/AIDS, and understand the messages and their implication for sexual health. FGD participants thought that the major barrier in HIV/AIDS prevention education in their area was the language used in HIV education. According to them, English and Twi languages are most often used to communicate HIV/AIDS and sexual behavior change messages. The use of those languages often makes it difficult for many community members to understand the messages relayed. To assess the magnitude of language as a barrier in communicating HIV/AIDS and sexual behavior change information, the survey respondents were asked whether they would like to hear HIV/AIDS messages in English or not. Of the 320 adults and 280 adolescents interviewed, 53% adults and 35% adolescents indicated that they prefer not to receive messages in English. The main local language that they would prefer to hear HIV/AIDS information is Ga-Dangme (68% adults and 62% adolescents). About 82% of adult respondents and 88% of adolescent respondents felt that community members would prefer to hear HIV/AIDS and sexual behavior messages in Ga-Dangme.

Table 5. Language preference for HIV/AIDS and sexual behavior communication in rural communities

Language individual prefers for HIV/AIDS and sexual behavior change communication					
	Ga-Dangme (%)	English (%)	Ewe (%)	Twi (%)	Other (%)
Adults	68	10	9	10	3
Adolescents	62	22	8	8	1
Language community prefers for HIV/AIDS and sexual behavior change communication					
	Ga-Dangme (%)	English (%)	Ewe (%)	Twi (%)	Other (%)
Adults	83	1	8	5	3
Adolescents	88	0	8	3	1

Table 5 summarizes the findings on languages that respondents prefer for HIV/AIDS and sexual behavior change communication and education.

Community role in HIV/AIDS and sexual behavior change communication

The data gathered suggest that community members' involvement in HIV/AIDS and sexual behavior change communication in their communities was not high. The following comments made by an adult leader participant in one of the FGD sessions reflect the prevailing view:

> "I am aware of some of the channels and strategies for HIV/AIDS and sexual behavior change communication and education in the district, but I think that community members' involvement in sexual behavior change and HIV/AIDS communication is inadequate. More especially, I see parents' involvement to be small and they should be given the necessary information and encouragement to be able to pass on this information to children since they spend most of their time with their parents."

A pastor who participated in one of the FGDs likewise noted:

"I think community members' involvement is not enough because I am not aware of any community member direct involvement in HIV/AIDS education, but I have heard of some community based-organization yet to be set up in the district".

Findings from the survey indicate that community involvement in HIV/AIDS communication was limited. Only 19% adult and 21% adolescent respondents were aware of any community involvement in HIV/AIDS and sexual behavior communication; those involved were parents, teachers, pastors and opinion leaders. Others mentioned as participating in local HIV communication efforts include community-based organizations, drug vendors, assembly members, local committee members, and health volunteers trained several years ago by Plan Parenthood Agency, Ghana (PPAG) and some local NGOs. When asked about how individuals in communities could become more involved in HIV/AIDS communication and education, respondents reported that individuals could be involved in household HIV communication and outside the household (91% of adults and 90% of adolescents). Respondents suggested that parents and heads of families need training to improve their involvement in HIV/AIDS education and communication. They also thought that individuals should be encouraged to communicate HIV/AIDS and healthy sexual behaviors messages to other people in their communities. A health co-coordinator in one district school put it this way:

"For a more positive approach to HIV/AIDS and sexual behavior change communication, I think the participatory learning activity approach can be used where community members are made to be involved in designing, implementing, monitoring and evaluating communication strategies that they think will suit them for HIV/AIDS education."

In the survey, respondents frequently spoke of the need to set up community-based HIV/AIDS teams (27% adults and 36% adolescents) to visit community members on regular basis. They also felt that it is good set up community drama troupe (11% adults and 13% adolescents) and felt the need to organize community durbars or gatherings and campaign to educate community members (41% adults and 38% adolescents). It was also felt that communities should support HIV/AIDS communication efforts by way of mobilizing funds to complement the efforts of other agencies (5% of adult and 12 % of adolescent respondents). There were also those who felt that chiefs and community leaders should be responsible for HIV/AIDS communication (5% adults and 12% adolescents). Some community members felt that the struggle for survival makes involvement in HIV/AIDS and sexual behavior change communication and education very difficult. As one FGD participant noted:

"Because there is no meaningful work for people to do, they always go out to look for what they will eat. They do not have time to be involved in HIV/AIDS communication and education, and it will be difficult to organize something like this here."

Yet another participant maintained:

"The poverty has eaten so much into the people that gathering of this nature on HIV/AIDS will be of no use to them. Here people are thinking first of how to survive."

Respondents generally agreed that individuals would listen to HIV/AIDS and sexual behavior change information and put what they hear into practice when members of their communities were involved. There were also those who felt that few people would put what they hear into practice (28% of adults and 27% of adolescents). Only very few of the interviewees consider community involvement in HIVAIDS communication and education as less relevant.

Parental role in HIV/AIDS and sexual behavior change communication

Data from both FGDs and survey support the need for parental involvement in HIV/AIDS and sexual behavior change communication. All the adolescent groups felt that parents and guardians should be more serious about and take responsibility for communicating sexual health and HIV/AIDS information. Young people thought that the ability of parents and their children to talk about sexual behavior and its implications for sexual health was central to HIV/AIDS communication. However, in most cases, parents were reportedly very reluctant to talk to their children about sexual behavior. Young people also maintained that those parents and guardians who muster the courage to tell children about sexual behavior and its impact on sexual health often do it in the wrong way. One adolescent girl revealed:

"They always shout at us that we would be pregnant and my mother does this to me."

Another girl asserted:

"My aunt always shouts warnings of pregnancy and insults for everybody to hear when she sees me moving with boys who are friends."

During the focus group with adolescents, an animated discussion revolved around how to talk with young people and how parents should be actively involved in sexual health and sexual behavior change communication but not infringe on the rights of young people. Interestingly, the adults also felt that parents must come out of their shells and talk to their children about sexual reproductive health issues. When adolescent respondents in the survey were asked how best parents and guardians should communicate HIV/AIDS and appropriate sexual behavior practices to their children, 83% felt that they should be spoken to alone, when other relations or siblings are not around. Young girls felt that they want their mothers to talk to them without the involvement of fathers. Many girls said they would be shy if their fathers were part of sexual health and sexual behavior communication. Some of them are averse to having such messages communicated to them when family or other relations are around (12%). The rest (5%) said that young people deserve access to books and magazines on HIV/AIDS and sexual behavior change. They also thought that young people need biblical or Quran-based instructions as well as the opportunity to watch and attend programs on sexual health and appropriate sexual behavior.

Similarly, the majority (70%) of adult respondents felt that parents should make the effort to talk to their children. They felt that the best approach to communication would be to guarantee young peoples' privacy. Thus, parents and guardians should have an attitude of talking to their children quietly and politely on this subject. Others also thought that young people need teaching on what is good and bad and the consequences with each action (13%). They also believed that books, pamphlets and magazines on HIV/AIDS and sexual behavior should be made available to young people and regular education based on the Bible or Quran be given to them at all times.

DISCUSSION

There is a wide range of communication channels and strategies in the district for HIV/AIDS education. The radio is the readily available medium, followed by television and neighbors. Others include teachers, pastors, health workers, prints and assembly members. However, for radio and television, there are no proper program guides available for people to see and select programs. There is the need to have more programs in local languages rather than in English. Our results show that the radio is the most accessible of all the communication channels. The findings support other studies that found radio ownership to be very high in the rural Africa because they are inexpensive to acquire and maintain (13-14).

The findings also revealed the radio is a highly acceptable channel and convenient in rural settings even where electricity supplies is limited. The radio is the medium from which people most often get information on HIV and AIDS and other health related messages. Television came second on the list; TVs are, however, not as accessible as radio. They are not as affordable. These findings suggest that the usefulness of the radio for HIV/AIDS prevention and sexual behavior change communication and education cannot be underestimated. Thus, any attempt at behavior change communication should rely on the radio to channel health education messages (15). Radio could use strategies like songs, poems, storytelling and drama, which were recognized as less common for HIV/AIDS prevention education in the study site—but which are likely to make lasting impact on audience. Using songs, drama, storytelling and many others in these ways for HIV/AIDS education have yielded successful results in many places in Sub-Saharan Africa (16-17).

Other strategies such as discussions, health talks, advertisements should be made more common for HIV/AIDS education on radio so that people hear these messages more often. The use of print media was limited in the communities studied. In many rural communities, the literacy rate tends to be low (18). In this study, access to and use of print media by adults and adolescents were very low probably due to low literacy rate among people. Others reasons are that people are unable to afford daily newspapers and many communities could not even be reached with these materials. Therefore, if print media are to be used for HIV/AIDS education, they should be in the local language and designed in ways that would convey more visual messages for HIV/AIDS.

Emerging from this study is evidence that community members accept existing communication channels and strategies for HIV/AIDS education and information. They also tend to believe the messages that they hear as well as the sources of the information. However, language is a major barrier to their understanding of these messages. Most information that they hear is in English and Twi, which are not understood by many people. More than 80% of both adults and adolescents in the study prefer the use of their local language for HIV/AIDS and sexual behavior communication and wish there could be a kind of communication strategy that would make use of the local, indigenous language. Studies have confirmed that the use of local language in Ghana (19) and elsewhere (20) in supplying important health information has produced positive outcomes. The results of the study also provide information on the need for the use of more background illustrations and visuals to accompany HIV/AIDS and sexual behavior messages.

The study has demonstrated that, although community members are currently not highly involved in HIV/AIDS education, they present an underutilized resource. The findings revealed that only 19% adults and 21% adolescents were aware of community members' involvement in HIV/AIDS education and communication. Moreover, ways suggested for community involvement in HIV/AIDS communication included setting up community teams, community drama troupes and community durbars for HIV/AIDS communication and education. It was also recommended that heads of households become more involved in HIV/AIDS communication and education. These findings agree with earlier studies in the developing world (21-22) where community members suggested similar ways for health education, health promotion and disease prevention.

In Dangme West and many other communities, parents' inability to communicate effectively with their children on many issues adversely affects children's future life (23-24). This appears most typical in the area of adolescent reproductive health (25). Many parents are reluctant to talk about reproductive health with their wards because of the cultural framing of sexuality as belonging to the realm of secrecy (24). However, there is evidence from the present study that parents appear to realize the need for their effective involvement in communicating HIV/AIDS and sexual health and sexual behavior messages to their children—which offers opportunities for adolescents' sexual behaviors to become safe. Over 80% adolescents said that they want parents to communicate sexual health and HIV/AIDS information to them directly. Similarly, teachers emerged as important channels for reaching adolescents with HIV/AIDS and sexual behavior change messages. All these indicate young people's readiness to learn. Studies done elsewhere have shown that the involvement of parents and teachers in ensuring positive and healthy behavior lifestyles in children, for instance, has yielded encouraging outcomes since children need direct messages to motivate them to change certain lifestyle behaviors (26-27). Church elders, pastors, community elders and health workers are important in reaching adults; others that may be useful include neighbors and relatives.

In conclusion, the present study demonstrates that radio and TV are the most available channels in these rural communities. Community members accept current channels and strategies. They understand HIV/AIDS and sexual behavior messages through these channels. However, community members prefer more background illustrations and photos to accompany HIV/AID messages and feel that such materials will enable them to understand the issues better. They also prefer the use of local language for HIV/AIDS and sexual behavior change education and see community members as a potential resource for HIV/AIDS communication and education. Currently, however, the involvement of community members in HIV/AIDS education efforts in rural Ghana is limited. Future policy must ensure that the channels and strategies used in HIV/AIDS education and communication in rural Ghana must be those that reflect the needs and sensitivities of the expected beneficiaries of those activities.

ACKNOWLEDGMENTS

This study and the preparation of this paper were financially supported by the Ghana – Netherlands Health Research and Development Program and the Five College African Scholars Program, University of Massachusetts. We are also grateful to Professor David Ross Buchanan and Dr. Chimaroake O. Izugbara for their inputs in shaping the writing of this paper.

REFERENCES

[1]   UNAIDS. Report on Global AIDS Epidemic, 2010. Accessed 2011 September 20. URL: http://www.unaids.org/globalreport/Global_report.html.

[2]   Haacker M. Economic consequences of HIV/AIDS in Southern Africa. International Monetary Fund Working Paper WP/02/38, Africa Department, 2002.

[3]   WHO/UNAIDS. AIDS Epidemic Update, World Health Organization/United Nations Program on HIV/AIDS. 2006.

[4]   Anarfi JK. Under reaction to sexual behavioral change among the Youth in Ghana. In Agyei-Mensah S, Casterline JB, Agyeman DK. Reproductive Change in Ghana: Recent Patterns and Future Prospects. Accra: University Ghana Press, 2005:225-42.

[5]   Bertrand JT, O'Reilly K, Denison J, Anhang R, Sweat M. Systematic review of the effectiveness of mass communication programs to change HIV/AIDS-related behaviors in developing countries. Health Educ Res 2006;2(4):567-97.

[6]   Tweedie I, Boulay M, Fiagbey E. Stop AIDS love life in Ghana: Shatters the silences. Commun Impact 2003;Number 15.

[7]   Nimo KP, Wood S. Situational analysis on HIV/AIDS services within the private health sector in Ghana, World Health Organization, Ghana Office, 2005.

[8]   Garbrah-Aidoo, NA. Community perception of HIV/AIDS and other STDs: A study of two sub-districts of the Dangme West District. Master's Thesis. University of Ghana, 2000.

[9]   Integrated Community Development Limited. A survey on knowledge, attitude, beliefs and practices on HIV/AIDS in the Dangme West District. Ghana:Integrated Development Limited, Koforidua 2000.

[10]   Ghana Health Service. Greater Accra Region 2007 Review of Sector Performance, Ghana Health Service, Accra, April 2008.

[11]   Agyepong IA, Anafi P, Asiamah E, Ansah E et al. Evaluation of the impact of CQI on malaria control in the Greater Accra region, Ghana. Ghana Health Service, Dangme West District, 2003.

[12]   Nukunya GK. Tradition and Change in Ghana, Accra: Ghana Universities Press, 2003.

[13]   Benefo K. The mass media and HIV/AIDS prevention in Ghana. Journal of Health and Population in Developing Countries, 2004, URL: http://www.jhpdc.unc.edu.

[14]   Bajunirwe F, Muzoora M. Barriers to the implementation of programs for the prevention of mother-to-child transmission of HIV: A cross-sectional survey in rural and urban Uganda. AIDS Res and Theraphy 2005; 2:10. URL: http://www.aidsrestherapy.com/content/2/1/10.

[15]   McCombie S, Hornik RC, Anarfi JH. Effects of a mass media campaign to prevent AIDS among young people in Ghana. In: Hornik RC. Public Health Communication: Evidence for Behavior Change. Mahwah, New Jersey: Lawrence Erlbaum Associate, 2002; 147-162.

[16]   Panford S, Ofori Nyaney M, Opoku Amoah S, Garbrah Aidoo N. Using folk media in HIV/AIDS prevention in rural Ghana, Am J Public Health 2001;91(10):1559-62.

[17]   Klepp K, Ndeki S, Seha AM. AIDS education for primary school children in Tanzania: An evaluation study. AIDS 1994;8:1157-62.

[18]   Vaughan PW and Rogers EM. A staged model of communication effects: Evidence from an entertainment-education radio soap opera in Tanzania. Health Commun 2000;5:203-27.

[19]   Obeng-Ouaidoo, I. Assessment of experience in the production of messages and programs for rural communication system: the case of the Wonsuom project in Ghana. Gazette 1999;42:53-67.

[20]   Minja H, Schellenberg JA, Mukasa O, Nathan R. et. al. Introducing ITN in the Kilombero Valley, Tanzania: The relevance of local knowledge and practice for an IEC Campaigns. Trop Med Int Health 2001;6:614-23.

[21]   D' Cruz-Grote, D. Prevention of sexual transmission of HIV/STDs in developing countries: Experiences and concept. Frankfurt: Gasellschaft, 1997.

[22]   Evian C. Community Theater and AIDS education in South Africa. Progress Report on Health and Development in Southern Africa 1992; Spring- Summer: 32-29.

[23]   Botchway AT. Parent and adolescent males' communication about sexuality in the context of HIV/AIDS: A Study in the Eastern Region of Ghana. University of Bergen, 2004.

[24]   Babalola S, Tambashe OB, Vondrasek C. Parental Factors and Sexual Risk-Taking among Young People in Cote d'Ivoire. Afr J Repr Health 2005;9: 49-65.

[25]   Wamoyi J, Fenwick A, Urassa M, Zaba B, Stones W. Parent-child communication about sexual and reproductive health in rural Tanzania: Implications for young people's sexual health interventions. Repr Health 2010; 7:6, Accessed 2011 June 12. URL: http://www.reproductive-health-journal.com/content/7/1/6.

[26]   Bora ST, Kelly L, Shirreff MB, Greiger CJ. Developing health messages: Qualitative studies with children, parents and teachers to help identify communication. opportunities for healthful lifestyle and prevention of obesity. Am Diet Assoc 2000;103:721-8.

[27]   Cullen WK, Baranowski T, Rittenberry L. Social-environmental influences on children's diet: Results from focus groups with African-Euro-Mexican- American Children and their parents. Health Educ Res 2000;15(5):581-90.

In: Public Health Yearbook 2013
Editor: Joav Merrick

ISBN: 978-1-63321-095-0
© 2014 Nova Science Publishers, Inc.

Chapter 30

The 'Il Ngwesi-ICA Canada Approach': Lessons learned in supporting local leadership to address HIV/AIDS in North Central Kenya

Katharine Hagerman*, MPH
and Suzanne Jackson, PhD
Health Economics and HIV/AIDS Research Division (HEARD),
University of KwaZulu-Natal in Durban,
South Africa and Dalla Lana School of Public Health,
University of Toronto, Canada

ABSTRACT

The predominant policy response to HIV/AIDS in Sub-Saharan Africa focuses on individual behaviour change, often with insufficient attention to its underlying structural, cultural and social determinants. The Il Ngwesi Afya Program in north central Kenya is a community-led HIV/AIDS intervention designed to address these root drivers of the epidemic. It was developed in partnership with the Institute of Cultural Affairs (ICA) Canada to support a 'sense of community ownership' and subsequently, a culturally inclusive and contextually responsive HIV/AIDS program for the community. This paper presents key findings that articulate how this 'sense of community ownership' was created and supported, and how it has contributed to program success. The analysis includes information collected from key informant interviews (n=15) and focus groups (n=10). The research was conducted within a participatory action research framework.

Keywords: HIV/AIDS, Community Responses, Community Development, Health Promotion, Participatory Research

* Correspondence: Katharine Hagerman, MPH, POBox 505, Haliburton ON K0M 1S0, Canada. E-mail: kghagerman@gmail.com.

INTRODUCTION

The dominant policy response to HIV/AIDS in Sub-Saharan Africa (SSA) has focused on biomedical and individual behaviour change (IBC) interventions, albeit with little scientific evidence of success. This is in part due to their failure to account for the social and political contexts of vulnerable groups (1,2). For many 'hard-to-reach' populations the prevailing policy response inadequately addresses structures of social inequality, termed 'structural violence' (3-5).

Conscious community involvement in HIV/AIDS initiatives, termed "community participation" is a strategy for addressing this gap. Supporting local leadership in developing and implementing effective HIV/AIDS interventions has become a priority of key global actors such as the joint United Nations program on HIV/AIDS (UNAIDS) and the United Nations Development Program (UNDP) (6). Yet without critical examination, this strategy risks facilitating the inclusion of marginalized groups using existing socio-economic structures, rather than transforming them (7). Community-led responses that focus on ownership, empowerment and partnership as means to redistribute power within systems, thereby mitigating risk and vulnerability to HIV/AIDS are emerging (2, 8-9). Critically examining strategies that can respond to and change the community contexts of the epidemic is key to an effective HIV/AIDS response. The Il Ngwesi-ICA Canada Approach, emerging from the Maasai community of Il Ngwesi in north central Kenya, is one such strategy. The approach formed the basis of research about the Il Ngwesi Afya Program and provides a case study of the impacts of community-led, partnership-supported approaches to HIV/AIDS programming.

Context of the study: Il Ngwesi and the Afya Program

Il Ngwesi is a rural community located on the edge of the Great Rift Valley in north central Kenya. Approximately 9 500 semi-nomadic Maasai pastoralists live in a 50km2 area around a collectively owned group ranch, which includes a profitable eco-tourism lodge. Risk and vulnerability to HIV/AIDS in Il Ngwesi is heightened by limited access to public infrastructure, conservative cultural practices and quickly eroding environmental conditions that affect traditional pastoral livelihoods. There are two partially equipped nursing stations in the area, but prior to the program's inception, little access to HIV/AIDS testing, counseling or treatment.

The Il Ngwesi Afya Program began in 2006 after an intensive period of facilitated community strategic planning with the Institute of Cultural Affairs (ICA) Canada, a non-governmental organization (NGO) invited by community leaders to partner in program development. Program strategies were implicitly based in theories of participation, community organizing and community building, as described by Minkler and Wallerstein (10). The program's goals were that:

- HIV/AIDS is under control in Il Ngwesi
- The model and methodology developed to inform the community-led HIV/AIDS initiatives are sustainable, comprehensive and enhance regional and national

strategies to make a lasting impact in communities underserved by government and other agencies

Having HIV/AIDS 'under control' was defined as an infection rate close to zero and that all people infected or affected by HIV/AIDS were receiving adequate supports to live a healthy life. The core program strategies are:

- Mobilization, HIV/AIDS Awareness and Education
- Access to Core Services: VCT and Follow-up care
- Community Building and Participation
- Replication and Expansion

Since 2008 the program has expanded into seven surrounding Group Ranches, with concerted efforts to support community leaders to adapt the program to their own needs. The observed program successes in Il Ngwesi prompted calls for research to assess program impacts and explore the approach to supporting community ownership of the intervention. This research was undertaken with the aims of improving program design and informing future replication and expansion efforts.

There were two key evaluation and research questions of interest to stakeholders: "What have been the program impacts on individual and community-level behaviour related to HIV prevention and the support and treatment of people living with HIV/AIDS (PLWHAs) in the community of Il Ngwesi?" and "What aspects of the approach to program design and implementation facilitated these impacts?"

METHODS

A community-based participatory (CBPR) approach was utilized to examine program outcomes and methods used in building community ownership. CBPR emphasizes community ownership of and participation in, research. It catalyzes social change through the research process and the application of findings (11) by engaging participants throughout the process. This builds community research capacity and increases uptake of the findings. Health promotion researchers advocate for complex, reflexive and inclusive approaches to evaluation that highlight multiple perspectives (12, 13). As such, a research and evaluation system was developed to address these questions using three measurement instruments: a community household survey, focus group discussions (FGDs) and key informant interviews. The first research question was addressed through a community household survey and FGDs with peer educators and program staff across Il Ngwesi. These results are reported in a separate article (Hagerman, Jackson, and Steele, forthcoming). The focus of this paper is the second question – what facilitated the impacts reported by the participants? To explore this research question, FGDs and key informant interviews were conducted.

Focus Group Discussions (FGDs)

Ten FGDs were conducted with two participant groups and co-facilitated in English, KiMaasai and KiSwahili. Two FGDs were held with program staff (n = 13) and eight were held with volunteer peer educators (n=5-10 per group) across Il Ngwesi. The FGDs reflected on program successes and challenges, the degree of and impact of 'community ownership' of the program in Il Ngwesi and scaling up activities to date. One FGD was held in the neighbouring Makurian community, into which the program had been scaling-up for the last year. The peer educator FGDs were separated by gender to ensure all participants felt comfortable sharing their views and experiences. The exceptions were in two neighbourhoods, where at the request of participants, the meetings were held with men and women together.

Interviews

In-depth interviews were held with key stakeholders (n=15), engaging participants in a reflective conversation about the approach to program development and factors contributing to success. These responses provide contextual understanding of the FGDs and survey results. Interviews were conducted in English, as all participants were fluent speakers.

All FGDs and interviews were audio-recorded. Summative notes of the translations of the FGDs were taken. Information was entered into tables using Word and the audio-recordings were transcribed and checked against the notes for quality. Inclusivity and accessibility were emphasized throughout the research process. Implementation of FGDs was planned in consultation with community members in order to be sensitive to the cultural, gendered and age-related challenges to participation. The primary investigator led the thematic coding of qualitative data. Dissemination was participatory and action-oriented, taking place in the district capital of Nanyuki, across Il Ngwesi and in Toronto, Canada. Program staff designed and implemented a dissemination plan for participants and stakeholders.

Focus groups and interviews were analyzed separately and then combined to assess key areas of success, challenges and the role of community ownership. The summative notes and interview transcripts were read three times before identifying themes by observing patterns, repetition and relationships between concepts. The thematic analysis identified key program successes and challenges, as well as the underlying factors respondents felt contributed to success.

RESULTS

Although not the focus of this paper, it is important to note that the evaluation, (Hagerman, K., Jackson, S. and Steele, S. Forthcoming) demonstrated positive impacts in a number of key areas. It also assessed challenges, articulated program strengths and provided recommendations for moving forward. The areas where positive impacts were demonstrated are presented below to highlight the comprehensiveness of both the program and the evaluation framework. Indicators of success were demonstrated in:

- HIV/AIDS knowledge
- Widespread individual behaviour change in: sexual behaviour, accessing voluntary counseling and testing (VCT) services, and changes in traditional practices, i.e., the use of sterile instruments in both male and female circumcision practices and an increasing number of women choosing to give birth in a clinic.
- Capacity building in: facilitation, peer education and program management
- Creating safe social spaces for dialogue (decreasing stigma)
- Development of a strong body of committed and trained community program volunteers
- Provision of integrated and accessible health services
- Co-operation with voluntary organizations in prevention and care
- Community members playing key roles in service provision
- Building solidarity within Il Ngwesi to get HIV/AIDS under control
- Building confidence in local strengths
- Promoting ownership and responsibility
- Scaling-up: strengthening, replicating and expanding for sustainability
- Building of a comprehensive, long-term and sustainable program

Necessary program elements

The focus of this paper is to explore what facilitated these positive impacts, as reported by participants. An analysis of the impact evaluation results with the interview and focus group data articulated a relationship between the positive impacts and the underlying approach to program partnership and development: wherever success was demonstrated in the evaluation, the following four "program elements" (see figure 1) were present: Capacity building, informational content, access to core services and a sense of community ownership.

Once these four program elements were identified, the focus group and interview data were reviewed to explore how program participants and key informants described the connections between the results they observed and the 'sense of community ownership'. One example is the role played by community ownership in decreasing HIV/AIDS stigma and encouraging widespread community participation in training and program activities. Having community leaders at the forefront of the program's development facilitated the design of culturally inclusive and accessible peer education strategies and training a cross-section of volunteers, resulting in increased access to HIV/AIDS knowledge and prevention services. One respondent described it as:

> "They decided to do an initial volunteer training with community members, to train on basic HIV knowledge, and also a focus on what it means to be a community volunteer. This emphasis was critical in that it created an atmosphere within the project where these young people were engaged, really cared about the project, had gained a lot of knowledge and were focused on making it work. Participatory methods were woven in –i.e., figuring out as a group, how you would do peer education in various settings, such as having a conversation with an elder –this set a great tone for future trainings, it emphasized that it was community owned, allowed the stigma about talking about HIV to come down a little. A series of peer education trainings with various community members followed."

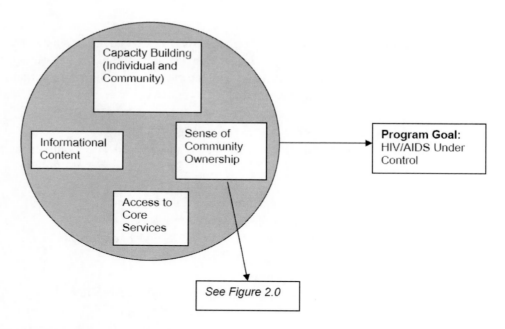

Figure 1. Necessary Program Elements.

In each program strategy area, presented above (Mobilization, HIV/AIDS Awareness and Education; Access to Core Services: VCT and Follow-up care; Community Building and Participation; Replication and Expansion", respondents spoke about the importance of a 'sense community ownership' in successful program impacts. One respondent stated: "It was a 'home grown' solution for the problem. We baked it here, took our culture into consideration – that's why it was successful. If we had imported ideologies, it wouldn't have worked."- FGD Participant.

Il Ngwesi-ICA Canada Approach, creating a sense of community ownership

"Locally, there is a really strong pride that they were doing it themselves, the idea that it was "our project" was critical to making it work." – Interview participant

Analysis of FGDs and interviews highlighted the integral role community ownership has played in getting HIV/AIDS under control. The fundamental approach described in Figure 2 outlines the story of how this sense of community ownership was created and supported in Il Ngwesi.

A number of "Pre-Existing Conditions" played important roles creating the sense of community ownership and contributed to the program's success. The community's commitment to change and 'state of readiness' to deal with HIV/AIDS were indicated through the invitation to ICA Canada, and the support of the community leadership to develop a community symbol and anti-stigma declaration. Respondents spoke about the importance of the community initiating the program.

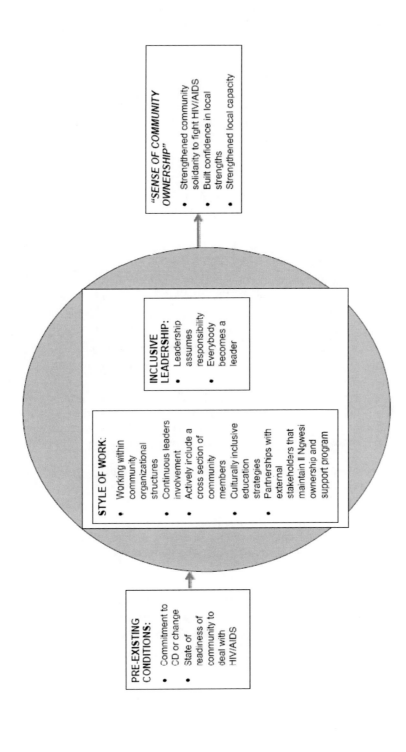

Figure 2. *The Il Ngwesi- ICA Canada Approach,* Creating a Sense of Community Ownership.

"This organization has come as a felt need from the community, owned by the community – it is their own project, the community itself made a decision that they needed this work done"- FGD Participant

A key informant articulated why the initiative from the community was so important in the program's success,

"They (community leaders) need to have the approach to it that they're all ready to be tested and to work on it (HIV). They need a huge determination and enthusiasm to deal with it—there's no way any outsider to a community can convince them to have this determination, it has to come from within. This is where government interventions sometimes get into trouble, they try to impose and convince. We didn't do that at all, it doesn't make sense to try and convince people. The initiative has to come from the local interest" – Interview participant

The qualitative analysis articulated a "Style of Work", described in figure 2 and identified five aspects: working within the existing community organizational structures; the continuous involvement of leadership; actively including a cross-section of community members; cultural respect and inclusion; and partnerships that supported Il Ngwesi's ownership of the program.

Key informants noted the critical importance of working within the existing community organizational structures for effective partnership and program development. One respondent shared what has been learned through initial expansion activities: the importance of working within the Group Ranch (GR) structure for Il Ngwesi and other Maasai communities.

"The approach of entering has been the same with that of Il Ngwesi, meaning, we first of all recognize the setup of a GR, Because the group ranch belongs to the people. I can choose not to talk to the councilor, or the chief for five years. But I don't think many people, or if any, person chooses to be not a member of their own GR." – Interview Participant

The importance of continuously involving leadership throughout the program's development and implementation was described as:

"Involvement of community leaders – if you involve them and have them on your side makes it easy to reach the community but the moment you alienate them from this exercise, it's not going to be easy for you to reach the community people."- FGD Participant

Respondents articulated the approach of: including a cross-section of community members in program development; and how that was integral to propelling social changes forward: "Il Ngwesi has been going about addressing HIV/AIDS with the total involvement of the community...to make sure its children, adults, men, women, old men or women, they're involved."- Interview participant. And:

"The individual is key to community-wide change. With enough individual behaviour change, it can become a critical mass, and then becomes a community-level change. The project has been successful because it really worked at that critical mass. We did repeated trainings for some, incorporated new participants into each new training (and retraining some). –Interview Participant.

Key informants described how working from a stance of cultural respect and inclusion deepened ownership and uptake of program activities in the community:

"The lifestyle of the people and culture must be understood before anybody has started. Because whenever you take new things, which might be conflicting with culture, you'll be met with resistance. They'll be saying, 'this is their project, not ours'. I think it's good that people, the project initiators, must understand people's lives, their needs, and when it comes to planning of any project, it must be planned with the people who this project is going to affect. So they're going to give a lot of input. So people actually have solutions to their problems. When they give solutions, they'll take up their solutions, not the solutions being given by others." – Interview participant

Partnerships that supported Il Ngwesi were emphasized as critical to fostering the 'sense of community ownership' whilst supporting program development. The partnership with ICA Canada was described as:

"Other programs sit on their own and come to us with everything arranged. This one, they came to us without anything arranged and we did it together."- FGD Participant

This experience has had a profound impact on the approach to expansion and replication activities of Il Ngwesi leaders into neighbouring communities. One respondent advised that,

"When you move to another group ranch, it should always be with a very clear mind that you're going there to help these people form their own HIV program. I think with that, then in my opinion, it could really develop sustainable projects." – Interview participant

The intersection of these five aspects of the program's work resulted in meaningful community participation, which increased accessibility of information to the broader public and decreased HIV/AIDS stigma. Including a cross section of community members, particularly women and youth as leaders, was reported to positively impact their self-efficacy.

"Inclusive Leadership" has played multiple roles in program success. Involving both formal and informal leaders built sustainability by increasing community participation. Community leaders played important roles in initiating, planning and implementing the program, decreasing stigma and increasing HIV/AIDS awareness through their participation. As 'cultural gatekeepers' they 'spearheaded' the program. The idea that "leadership assumes responsibility" has been a key component of the program approach. "Community members have been involved right from the beginning. The leadership's presence instigated the whole process. The community was very interested in doing something about HIV – they recognized the need" -Interview participant.
"There has been total community involvement. The leadership has been involved. Not only the Maa community but also even government leaders have been involved. You know like when you include the chief in your committee, you have actually gone a long way towards mobilizing the community. You know the chiefs and the elders, they're opinion makers and shapers—what they say is listened to. So the involvement of the leadership has been a very positive step towards creating a community acceptance, enhancing community ownership of the project."--- Interview Participant

In addition, the inclusive understanding of leadership taken by program members has been critical to its success. One respondent explained it as:

"Because in our program, everybody seems to be a leader- whomever we involve is a leader. Because we recognize a women's group leader is a leader of women, a youth group leader is a leader. So when I talk of 'leadership assumes responsibility', I don't only mean the Group Ranch leadership, I want to mean the leadership in all levels."- Interview Participant

These approaches to program development and implementation were supported by partnerships that recognized and valued the role of community ownership over processes and outcomes, and contributed to the "Sense of Community Ownership", shown to be such an integral component of the overall program approach.

"The idea of this program was started by the leadership of Il Ngwesi. So you can say that this is their project. Decision-making, all these things are done by the Il Ngwesi community, so it's owned by them." -Interview participant

Another result has been a strengthened solidarity to fight HIV/AIDS in Il Ngwesi and beyond, demonstrated by the ongoing expansion and replication efforts of community members:

"The reception of the leadership (in new communities) has always been great. Because this is something that a brother is bringing to you. We get to them and say, in Il Ngwesi we've got this concept, we have friends who've helped us, we did this with our people. In Maasai culture we say, 'you cannot eat an elephant and finish until even the tail'. So we decided we cannot finish and keep quiet. So we've come to the leadership and said 'listen, you guys, we've done this, this is the approach and we are ready to help you as a Group Ranch fight HIV/AIDS" -Interview participant

Another respondent spoke of the understanding of solidarity and collective action in fighting HIV/AIDS,

"Because fighting HIV means you cannot fight as an individual. It's a group kind of collective responsibility to make sure that we come up, we join our hands together and do It." – Interview participant

In addition to this solidarity, respondents articulated the increased capacity and confidence of community members to affect change in their lives, even beyond HIV/AIDS. Such as:

"In meetings, people use our example 'yeah we can do it like the HIV/AIDS program'- people think anything can be possible, if talking of this life-taking disease is possible, why not other things like creating water, which is a positive thing from the beginning?"- Interview Participant.

Another noted that,

"This project is very good because it helps to build the capacity of the community to be able to perform, even to do other things apart from health."–Interview Participant

While other respondents spoke to the empowering processes of program involvement for community members,

"These community members are demonstrating empowerment, in that they are dramatically transformed just by the process of standing up in front of other groups (including government) and sharing their story and their experiences." --Interview participant.
"Because we (community members) are experienced now, we're experts of our own way."- Interview participant

DISCUSSION

Analysis of focus group and interview data highlighted the complex relationships amongst program components and shed new light unto how community ownership of HIV/AIDS programming can contribute to a program's success. One could say that underlying each area of the program's success was the use of the 'Il Ngwesi-ICA Canada Approach' to creating a sense of community ownership (see figure 2). The 'Il Ngwesi-ICA Canada Approach' has supported the people of Il Ngwesi to respond to and address the determinants of risk and vulnerability to HIV/AIDS in their community. This finding supports strategic policy and practice directions that would promote community-led responses to HIV/AIDS programming. By playing the central role in collectively identifying and addressing the drivers of HIV/AIDS within their own lives, community members are responding to and changing these structural conditions. By articulating this approach, in conjunction with the evaluation research demonstrating the positive program impacts, lessons for building community capacity to address HIV/AIDS can be learned from the Il Ngwesi experience for communities across Kenya and possibly Sub-Saharan Africa.

Further study is needed to assess how this approach would work in different contexts such as urban, high-prevalence and/or with different cultural groups. Nevertheless, lessons from the Il Ngwesi experience could inform approaches elsewhere. The 'Pre-Existing Conditions' of figure 2 may be used as starting points in other community settings. Lessons from the 'Style of work' and the 'Inclusive Leadership' elements of the approach can be applied to community work in a variety of settings. In the Il Ngwesi context, the involvement of traditional leaders as an entry-point proved integral to the program's success and community mobilization. The importance of such traditional leadership structures may vary across contexts but the idea of working within existing organizational structures is of central importance to mobilizing widespread community participation.

Although not analyzed in this report, data collected also included challenges faced in the development of the approach and program implementation. Respondents noted that 'ownership and empowering processes' in partnership with program funders need to be consistently addressed and evaluated to ensure progress. While funding in the initial phases of program development was flexible and responsive to community needs, the current funding agreements are much more restrictive. Respondents cited difficulties in: obtaining adequate funding supports to address broader contextual challenges and to adequately support 'scaling-up' of the 'Il Ngwesi Approach' in other communities.

CONCLUSION

This study demonstrates how creating and supporting a sense of community ownership in Il Ngwesi has resulted the successful implementation of a comprehensive HIV/AIDS program, the 'Il Ngwesi Afya Program'. Success was contingent on a combination of four program elements: Capacity Building, Informational Content, Access to Core Services and a Sense of Community Ownership. This sense of community ownership was created and supported by assessing a set of pre-conditions and adopting a specific 'Style of Work' that engaged a diversity of community leaders. The consistent application of the 'Il Ngwesi-ICA Canada Approach' to creating a sense of community ownership throughout all stages of program development and implementation has been integral to its success.

ACKNOWLEDGMENTS

This study was made possible by collaboration between Il Ngwesi Program staff, the Institute of Cultural Affairs (ICA) Canada and the University of Toronto. Thanks to Miriam Patterson, Christine Cullen, Saaya Tema Karmushu and Dr. Suzanne Jackson for their supervision. Special thanks to Il Ngwesi Program staff and community volunteers for their logistical support during data collection. ICA Canada, Abbey North and private donations funded this study.

REFERENCES

[1]   Barnett T, Whiteside A. AIDS in the twenty-first century: Disease and globalisation. Basingstoke: Palgrave, 2006.

[2]   Campbell C, Nair Y, Maimane S. Building contexts that support effective community responses to HIV/AIDS: A South African case study. Am J Commun Psychol 2007;39(3-4):347-63.

[3]   O'Manique C. Neo-liberalism and AIDS crisis in Sub-Saharan Africa: Globalization's pandemic. New York: Palgrave McMillan, 2004.

[4]   Parker RG, Easton D, Klein CH. Structural barriers and facilitators in HIV prevention: a review of international research. AIDS 2000; 14(Supplement 1): S22-S32.

[5]   Campbell C, Jovechelovitch S. Health, community and development: Towards a social psychology of development. J Appl Commun Psychol 2000;10:255-70.

[6]   Gueye M, Diof D, Chaava T, Tiomkin D. Community capacity enhancement strategy note: The answer lies within: UNDP: HIV/AIDS Group, Bureau for Development Policy, 2005.

[7]   Mohan G. Beyond participation: Strategies for deeper empowerment. participation: The new tyranny? London: Zed Books, 2006:153-67.

[8]   Evans C, Lambert H. Implementing community interventions for HIV prevention: Insights from project ethnography. Soc Sci Med 2008;66(2): 467-78.

[9]   Baylies C. International partnership in the fight against AIDS: Addressing need and redressing injustice? Rev Afr Polit Econ 1999; 26(81):387-94.

[10] Minkler M, Wallerstein N. Improving health through community organization and community building. In: Glanz K, Rimer B, Lewis F, eds. Health behaviour and health education, 3rd ed. San Francisco, CA: Jossey-Bass, 2002.

[11] Israel BA, Eng E, Schulz AJ, Parker EA. Methods in community-based participatory research for health. San Francisco: Jossey-Bass, 2005.

[12] Nutbeam D, Harris E. Theory in a nutshell: A practical guide to health promotion theories. North Ryde, Australia: McGraw-Hill, 2005.

[13] Potvin L, Gendron S, Bilodeau A, Chabot P. Integrating social theory into public health practice. Am J Public Health 2005;95(4): 591-5.

In: Public Health Yearbook 2013
Editor: Joav Merrick

ISBN: 978-1-63321-095-0
© 2014 Nova Science Publishers, Inc.

Chapter 31

AN INTERPROFESSIONAL COMMUNITY-BASED SERVICE DELIVERY MODEL FOR THE MANAGEMENT OF CHILDREN WITH BURNS LIVING IN CHINA

Lorna M Hayward*, EdD, MPH, PT,
Ann L Charrette, PT, DPT, MS, PCS, NCS, Li Li, PT, DPT
and Brecken Chinn Swartz, PhD

Department of Physical Therapy, Bouve College of Health Sciences, Northeastern University, Boston, Massachusetts, United States of America

ABSTRACT

In China, burns are a major cause of morbidity and mortality with large societal and economic ramifications. Burn injuries exhibit greater prevalence in: children under age 3, males, and people living in rural settings. After 1979, the Maoist social welfare system collapsed and China experienced a dramatic health care reform resulting in a movement away from a socialist centralized, government funded system to one that is privatized, fragmented, and underfunded. The Chinese government has devoted significant resources to advance the surgical management of burns, but rehabilitative services are in extreme shortage with respect to quality and quantity. Rehabilitation is a critical element for the successful management of a patient who has been burned. A recent trend in China is the blending of eastern and western medicine which has particular relevance for rehabilitative services. The purpose of this case report is to present a community based model: the HandReach Starfish which relies on a five pronged, interprofessional, rehabilitative approach and to describe the experiences of an American rehabilitative team who during 2010 co-treated 65 patients and reciprocally shared knowledge with Chinese medical personnel about the International Classification of Functioning, Disability and Health (ICF) model and management of burns in children. Lessons learned included: while a fundamental philosophy difference existed, American and Chinese clinicians are uniquely position to blend eastern and western medical philosophies. A challenge for American clinicians is to promote a paradigm shift from an impairment

---

* Correspondence: Lorna M Hayward, EdD, MPH, PT, Northeastern University, Bouve College of Health Sciences, Department of Physical Therapy, 6 Robinson Hall, Boston, MA, USA. E-mail: l.hayward@neu.edu.

perspective to a functional and evidenced based approach for burn rehabilitation in China.

Keywords: Global health, interprofessional, community-based rehabilitation, burns in children, ICF Model, China

INTRODUCTION

Burns are devastating injuries due to the resulting high mortality rates and life altering physical and psychological aftermath experience by survivors. Severe burns pose a considerable financial burden for both families and society due to the medical treatment, surgical intervention, and long rehabilitative process required for the management of scar formation, joint deformities, psychological needs, and return to function for the patient (1). While burn injuries are devastating for anyone, "95% of burn-related deaths occur in developing or low and middle income countries" such as China (2). While the Chinese population experiences a high incidence of burns, there is a paucity of literature available describing the epidemiology, effective treatment approaches, and prevention strategies (2).

When examining the existing literature regarding the epidemiology of burns in Chinese children, a consistent picture emerges. Research suggests that burn injuries exhibit greater prevalence in: children under age three, males, and people living in rural settings. Injuries occur predominately at home (71-86%), or at industrial locations. An explanation for these statistics is that the rural population is slightly greater, accounting for 50.5% of China's 1.37 billion people, both parents may work with children cared for by alternative providers, and that parents are less educated regarding burn-prevention strategies (3, 4). In a study retrospectively examining over 20 years' worth of data on the epidemiology of burns in 1494 Shanghai residents, children under age three represented 63.3%, and males 61% of all burns documented. Moreover, scalding accounted for 84.3% of pediatric burns, 86.5% occurred in domestic settings, with a migrant rural population accounting for 46% of all burns. Common body areas affected included the anterior trunk, head, neck, and right lower limb. Forty-four percent of the 1494 cases required surgery (5). A recent work describing the epidemiology of burns treated in Chinese military hospitals revealed the highest incidence was in children under age five (29.4%), with males and scalding accounting for 95% of cases (2). In summary, research demonstrates that burn injuries in children are a significant public health problem in China. These data support the need for rehabilitative care, educational initiatives regarding burn prevention, and for research on the effectiveness of both.

Burn rehabilitation is complicated, expensive, and is financially overwhelming for families and society. In China, after 1979, the Maoist socialist health care system collapsed (6, 7). As a result, the centralized, government funded program that had provided free or low cost health care to all citizens disintegrated and what system remained was privatized, fragmented, and underfunded (7-9). This organizational change caused a dramatic shift regarding the financing of and access to health care for Chinese citizens (9, 10). Without government funding, the current health care system became predominately a self-pay model. In addition, physician's salaries became linked to the income they generated, which has resulted in practice habits consisting of over prescription of pharmaceuticals, a propensity for performing expensive diagnostic tests, and an increase in hospital based care (7, 9). To compound this problem, over 50% of urban Chinese, who are non-governmental employees, are without health insurance or the finances to pay for care which greatly limits access (7). Prior to 1980, a community based system of "barefoot doctors" provided basic medical care to the rural farming population. However, with the transition to a market driven structure, the system of "barefoot doctors" disintegrated. Now, 60-70% of the rural population has either limited access to or is unable to afford basic health care (7, 9, 11). Currently, leadership in China is financially promoting the development and expansion of an urban health infrastructure, while devoting minimal attention to health care needs of the rural community (7, 11).

Another trend within Chinese health care is that since the late 1950's, western medicine has become increasingly integrated with traditional Chinese medicine (TCM) (7, 12). Today, at all levels within the health care system, western medicine and technology is routinely used in conjunction with TCM approaches (12). The blending of eastern and western medicine has particular relevance for rehabilitative services. Chinese rehabilitative care may include TCM such as massage, cupping, acupuncture, moxibustion, and herbal therapies. The western rehabilitative approaches most utilized in China include occupational (OT) physical (PT) and speech therapy (ST) (13). Since 1989, the training of rehabilitative therapists (OT, PT, and ST) has consisted of yearlong courses provided at medical schools (14). However, as of 2002, only 6,000 rehabilitative clinicians existed in China and access to equipment and services is especially limited in rural areas (12).

Rehabilitation is a critical element for the successful management of a patient who has been burned. Currently, rehabilitative services for burn care in China include OT and PT and clinicians rely on the use of modalities such as ultrasound, paraffin treatment, massage, and rudimentary manual therapy techniques. While the Chinese government has devoted significant resources to advance the surgical management of burns, rehabilitative services are in extreme shortage with respect to quality and quantity (13, 15).

Western rehabilitative care for the management of burns in a pediatric population is complex and involves a combination of medical, surgical, physical, and psychological approaches (1, 16). Rehabilitative personnel in the United States (US) are highly trained with preparation for PTs, OTs, and ST at either the clinical doctorate or master degree level (17-19). Occupational and physical therapy intervention commences once a patient is admitted to the hospital and involves splinting, positioning, mobility, functional training, strengthening, and use of pressure garments to combat scar formation and joint contracture. The overall goal of rehabilitation is to promote functional independence in a patient (16).

The philosophy of clinical care in the US has evolved from a disability based model to the International Classification of Functioning, Disability and Health (ICF) approach (20, 21). In 2001, The World Health Organization (WHO) endorsed the ICF model which defines disability and function as related to: body function and structure; activities of daily living experiences; and environmental factors that impact these experiences (20). Conversely, the philosophy of burn care management in China is impairment based and preparing individuals with disabilities to live independently has not been encouraged as it is culturally acceptable for a disabled person to live with one's family (14).

A need exists to explore the efficacy of rehabilitative services in China for children who have been burned. Efforts are indicated to address: 1) promoting a functional based philosophy for rehabilitative care; 2) promoting inter-professional collaboration with other medical specialties; and 3) educating the public about the benefits of rehabilitative services

(13, 15). Therefore, the purpose of this case report is to describe a community based model, the HandReach Starfish, and process for providing inter-professional rehabilitative care for children suffering from burns in China. The model is informed by the ICF philosophy which encourages activity and participation in society using a multi-dimensional approach. The case report will share lessons learned from a two week east-west medical exchange that includes the perspectives of both US and Chinese clinicians.

Model description-HandReach Starfish

Recognizing the fiscal, administrative, and cultural norms that have traditionally separated the functioning of various departments in developing world hospitals, the Boston-based 501(c)(3) nonprofit organization, HandReach, launched its Children's Healing Initiative in 2007. The initiative brings together clinicians capable of developing and promoting clinical training and practice protocols that integrate surgery, rehabilitation, nursing, orthopedics, and psychosocial care in the healing of trauma-injured children. Using a metaphorical "starfish" to characterize the five-pronged model, HandReach seeks to equalize the importance of each specialization and create channels of communication about rehabilitative care, both within a US-based team and cross-culturally (see Figure 1).

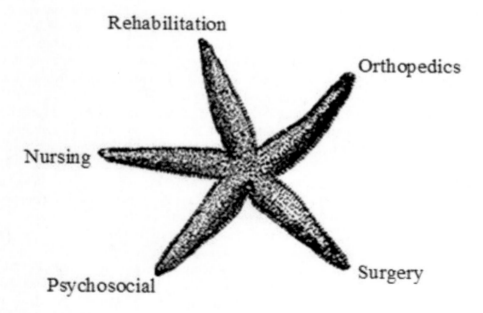

Figure 1. HandReach Starfish Model.

In the model, the five "arms" of the starfish must be developed, and integrated within a coherent inter-professional treatment approach (22). The HandReach model is aligned with the WHO mission, which recognizes inter-professional collaboration as an innovative strategy for mitigating the global health workforce crisis and for enabling clinician teams to provide best practice (23, 24).

Burn care within the Chinese hospital setting

Currently, Chinese patients suffering burns are treated primarily through reconstructive surgery and post-operative nursing in the Burns and Plastics Department within local hospitals. Each line item of a patient's care, from surgical procedures to pain medication, is billed directly to the patient, and families are often unable to afford these costs and therefore only pay for needed surgeries. Nursing care is abbreviated, and patients are discharged before wounds are healed and function restored. Most patients cannot afford rehabilitative or orthopedic care, so these services are rarely included in post-operative treatment. Pediatric patients, in particular, return home without splints or other rehabilitative techniques to prevent joint contracture and scaring, which limits their return to independent function. Needed prosthetics for limb amputations must be procured, not from hospitals, but directly from factories. Psychosocial care is largely non-existent, China, making it impossible to address patients' post-traumatic stress, social rejection, and overall feelings of hopelessness.

Rehabilitative team approach-US

In June 2010, a HandReach team of eight clinicians, two graduate students—one each in OT and PT--and three music therapists spent one week each at the JianShe Hospital located in Changsha (Hunan province), and at the Air Force General hospital in Beijing, China working alongside Chinese surgical and rehabilitative clinicians—PT and OT. Chinese military hospitals are among the best medical facilities with resources dedicated to the treatment of burns (2). Rehabilitative clinicians included physical, occupational, prosthetic, music, and child life therapies. The June, trip was a follow up to the January 2010 Medical Volunteer effort, which established a foundation for the future HandReach trips to China.

Interprofessional burn care provided by the US team included scar management, splinting, play therapy, sustainable therapeutic exercise, functional mobility programs, and strategies for psychosocial challenges. Therapeutic drumming was utilized to build community and reinforce the PT and OT functional goals regarding active movement of the upper extremities, and for pain management. To promote a shift from an impairment model to an active treatment approach, inservice education was provided through lecture/presentation for the Chinese clinicians on the ICF model, theory supporting contemporary western rehabilitative therapies for burn care, and information on how rehabilitation can augment surgery (24). During the two week stay, between the two clinical sites, the HandReach team co-treated 65 patients (40 in Changsha and 25 in Beijing) from rural, underprivileged backgrounds ranging in age from 1 to 21, many with significant burns (up to 95% total body surface area).

For each patient, the HandReach team used the ICF model approach to emphasize participation and activity level goals, versus focusing on the impairments. For example, the team worked with an 8 year old boy who had suffered burns affecting both of his legs and part of his trunk—approximately 40% total burn surface area. The injury prevented him from transferring from sit to stand, ambulation, independent dressing, and the patient was emotionally withdrawn. His care was addressed by the rehabilitation team at all three levels of the ICF model: participation, activity, and impairment (21). To address his emotional concerns, the child life therapist used strategies to help him articulate his fear and pain related to his injury. Then, the team worked to address his rehabilitative needs. The child had a passion for racing, so he was provided with a scooter in the clinic that he could sit on and propel primarily with his upper extremities (see Figure 2). However, to move the scooter forward, it also required lower extremity involvement which increased passive and active knee and ankle motion. Using this strategy, the participation goal of mobility was initiated through the activity of play (scootering) allowed the boy to independently propel himself and interact with other children in the clinic. At the same time, the activity served to improve ambulation and addressed the impairment level restriction of decreased knee and ankle mobility and strength. The US team approach differed from the customary Chinese method which would have addressed the impairment—restriction of knee and ankle mobility and strength-- with modalities such as massage and manual stretching aimed at improving range of motion and pain relief while not attending to the promotion of function and social interaction using a modality such as a scooter.

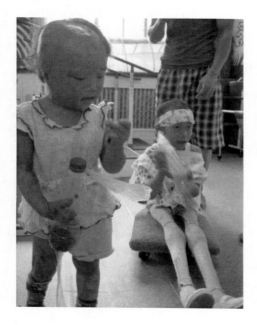

Figure 2. Scooter Example.

RESULTS AND DISCUSSION

To gather information regarding the perception of the US-Chinese rehabilitative partnership, informal feedback was gathered via discussion with the community partners—family and clinicians-- by three individuals on the HandReach team. One team member was the PT graduate student who was originally from the Sichuan province, fluent speaking both Mandarin and English, and intimate with the Chinese culture. A second team member was a Beijing native who lived in China during the Cultural Revolution. She was fluent in both languages and well versed in the Chinese culture. The third member was the HandReach executive director, an American, also fluent in Mandarin and familiar with the culture.

Lessons learned- Community perspective

The collaboration between the JianShe hospital, the Air Force General Hospital, and HandReach team was viewed positively by the local Chinese burn survivors' community. In both settings, the burn survivors and their families gathered at the Air Force General Hospital and JianShe hospital to enthusiastically welcome the US team. The families expressed hope that the US team would "help" their children recover from devastating burn injuries. Volunteers from a Chinese philanthropic group, the AngelMom Foundation, demonstrated extraordinary hospitality and offered translation services between patients/families and the US clinicians. The Chinese clinical team expressed their sincere desire to learn from the US interprofessional model despite the overwhelming demand to simultaneously manage their heavy patient caseload. The exchange of information between health care practitioners was facilitated through two formal inservice presentations relying on lecture followed by a question and answer session. Information was provided to the Chinese clinicians on the ICF model, theory and research supporting contemporary western rehabilitative therapies for burn care, and information on how rehabilitation can augment surgery (24). Translation was provided by the HandReach multilingual PT graduate student and the Beijing native who served as a bridge to optimize the cultural and rehabilitative knowledge exchange. Sharing information is critical as global citizenship and learning is fostered through "interaction and cross-cultural dialogue" (25).

Finally, the US team's visit to the Air Force General Hospital was the subject of two Chinese news media reports—one in January and one in June. The purpose of the reports was to feature the US-China collaboration, raise awareness on burn prevention, and the need for psychosocial support for burn survivors (26, 27).

However, during the visit, several concerns were voiced by the Chinese families. These concerns pertained to: 1) not having time to do therapy because they spend so much time just trying to survive; 2) if "play therapy" really works; 3) if PT is just play, why does it cost money?

The Chinese rehabilitation clinicians indicated that their metrics for productivity were tied to the use of modalities that were billable. When asked about the use of outcome measures to document improvement in patients such as range of motion, stretching, exercise and other active activities, the Chinese therapists indicated that their job performance was not based on these criteria.

Lessons learned- US team

Team members were curious and amazed by the history of TCM and the Chinese rehabilitation approach to burn care. Through visits to four clinical sites—two hospitals and two smaller rehabilitation clinics—the team witnessed TCM—cupping and acupuncture--integrated into traditional rehabilitative care. The team realized that a fundamental rehabilitation philosophy difference exists between the eastern and western cultures. Bed rest, passive modalities, and symptom relief were common practice after an injury or surgery in China while the US approach consisted of early mobilization, functional rehabilitation, and an active patient role. A critical element with respect to rehabilitation differences was the timing of interventions. For example, in the US, functional splinting occurs immediately after surgery. Splinting, a hand for example, after surgery, is critical for full functional recovery. However, splinting is not used after surgery in China. So while the surgery is a success, the patient is left with a non-functioning hand.

To process their experiences, the US team participated in reflective dialogue before, during, and after travel. Interaction and cross-cultural discussion, followed by reflection is essential for a deeper understanding of perplexing phenomena (28, 29) which in our example pertained to cultural issues in medicine (25). Cross cultural understanding, with respect to medicine, was facilitated by assuming the following perspective: respect the TCM and rehabilitation philosophy differences yet promote evidence based practice (30) and functional rehabilitation and the ICF model (21).

The primary objective of US team was to share knowledge with the Chinese clinicians regarding the importance of: 1) functional splinting immediately post-surgery; 2) early rehabilitation to prevent joint contracture; and 3) functional mobility once the patient is medically stable. However, the major challenges faced by the team included: 1) an impairment based philosophy of rehabilitation; 2) Chinese therapists with only two years of college education who were without the academic background required for higher level critical thinking; 3) an absence of objective outcome measurements to monitor rehabilitation progress; 4) lack of education for patients and family regarding rehabilitation goals and home exercise prescription; 5) patients of low–socioeconomic status without sufficient education to comprehend the complexity rehabilitative care; and 6) a language barrier and an insufficient number of interpreters. At departure, a lingering concern for the US team pertained to the sustainability of the teaching imparted and how to evoke a rehabilitation paradigm shift.

Limitations

A major limitation of this case study was the absence of formal evaluation methods to explore the perceptions of the both the Chinese community and the clinicians on the impact of the interprofessional collaboration on the rehabilitation of children with burns. A major question for the US clinicians was if we could make a difference despite the cultural and practice differences. However, with limited time in country, the clinicians believed that the medical needs were primary. A future visit is planned for June 2012 and at that time, formal assessment strategies will be utilized for collecting survey and interview data on the various constituent perspectives and on specific outcomes related to therapy.

Global relationships must be cultivated and trust is established over time. With repeat visits, the potential grows for global partnerships to evolve into solid collaborations involving research and teaching. Global collaborations are maintained because they provide sustained learning opportunities and intellectual stimulation for participants and address.

CONCLUSION

Creation of an interdisciplinary model enabled a U.S. rehabilitative team to co-treat and reciprocally share knowledge with Chinese medical personnel about current management of burns in children. The collaboration between Air Force General and JianShe Hospitals and

HandReach is viable and evolving. Both teams are committed to creating a sustainable program for pediatric burn care despite the cultural, medical, and rehabilitation practice differences. American and Chinese clinicians are uniquely position to blend eastern and western medical philosophies and promote a paradigm shift in burn rehabilitation. Mutual understanding can only benefit outcomes, adherence, and sensitivity to existing cultural practices. Research is needed to formally explore the impact of interprofessional education and clinical effectiveness.

ACKNOWLEDGMENTS

We would like to acknowledge Qi McIntosh for her translation and organizational support of the HandReach mission.

REFERENCES

[1]　Meyer W, Blakeney P, Russell W, Thomas C, Robert R, Berninger F, Holzer C. Psychological problems reported by young adults who were burned as children. J Burn Care Rehabil 2004;25(1):98-106.

[2]　Yao Y, Liu Y, Zhou J, Qiu J, Zhang L, Yuan D, et al. The epidemiology of civilian inpatients' burns in Chinese military hospitals, 2001-2007. Burns 2011;37(6):1023-32.

[3]　China Health and Medicine. Accessed. 2011 Sept 11. URL: http://www.chinatoday.com/health/health.htm.

[4]　Yang LK, Zhao-Fan X, Luo-Man Z, Yi-Tao J, Tao T, Wei W, et al. Epidemiology of pediatric burns requiring hospitalization in China: a literature review of retrospective studies. Pediatrics 2008;12(2):132-41.

[5]　Xin W, Yin Z, Qin Z, Jian L, Tanuseputro P, Gomez M, et al. Characteristics of 1494 pediatric burn patients in Shanghai. Burns 2006;32(8):613-8.

[6]　Burke A, Wong Y, Clayson Z. Traditional medicine in China today: implications for indigenous health systems in a modern world. Am J Public Health 2003;93(7):1082-84.

[7]　Haley DR, Zhao M, Nolin JM, Dunning K, Qiang S. Five myths of the Chinese health care system. Health Care Manager 2008;27(2):147-58.

[8]　Xu W, Sheiman I, van de Ven WPMM, Zhang W. Prospects for regulated competition in the health care system: what can China learn from Russia's experience? Health Policy Plann 2011;26(3):199-209.

[9]　Hesketh T, Zhu WX. Health in China: the healthcare market. BJM 1997; 314(7094): 1616.

[10]　Akin JS, Dow WH, Lance PM, Loh C. Changes in access to health care in China, 1989-1997. Health Policy Plann 2005;20(2): 80-9.

[11]　Blumenthal D, Hsiao W. Privatization and its discontents: the evolving Chinese health care system. New Engl J Med 2005;353(11):1165-70.

[12]　Hesketh T, Zhu W. Traditional Chinese medicine: one country, two systems. BMJ 1997;314:1616.

[13]　Zhao M, Haley R, Nolin JM, Dunning K, Wan J, Sun Q. Serving billions: a pilot study on clinician-perceived efficacy of rehabilitative services in China. Health Care Manager 2008;27(3):252-8.

[14]　Zhang HN. An evolving rehabilitative service delivery system in the People's Republic of China [internet]. J Rehabil 2001; 62. Accessed. 2011 October 18. URL: http://findarticles.com/p/articles/mi_m0825/is_3_67/ai_79741187/.

[15]　Zhao M, Haley R, Nolin JM, Dunning K, Wan J, Sun Q. Utilization, cost, payment, and patient satisfaction of rehabilitative services in Shandong, China. Health Policy 2009;93(1):21-6.

[16]　Herndon DN. Total burn care, 3rd ed. Philadelphia, PA: Saunders Elsevier, 2007.

[17]   American Physical Therapy Association. Accessed 2011 October 18. URL: http://www.apta.org/ PTEducation/Overview/.

[18]   The American Occupational Therapy Association. Accessed 2011 October 18. URL: http://www.aota.org/Students/Schools.aspx.

[19]   American Speech-Language-Hearing Association. Accessed 2011 October URL: http://www.asha.org/ careers/professions/slp.htm.

[20]   Rosenbaum P, Stewart D. The world health organization international classification of functioning, disability, and health: a model to guide clinical thinking, practice and research in the field of cerebral palsy. Seminars in Pediatric Neurology 2004;11(1): 5-10.

[21]   World Health Organization. International Classification of Functioning Disability and Health. Accessed 2011 October 18. URL: http://www.who.int/classifications/icf/en/.

[22]   HandReach. Accessed 2011 September 13. URL: http://www.handreach.org/.

[23]   Mickan S, Hoffman SJ, Nasmith L. Collaborative practice in a global health context: common themes from developed and developing countries. J Interprof Care 2010;24(5):492-502.

[24]   Rodger S, Hoffman SJ. Where in the world is interprofessioanl education? A global environmental scan. J Interprof Care 2010;24(5):479-91.

[25]   Bringle RG, Hatcher JA. International service learning. In: Bringle RG, Hatcher JA, Jones SG, eds. International service learning: conceptual frameworks and research. Sterling, VA: STYLUS, 2011.

[26]   China Daily. Accessed 2011 November 11. URL: http://www.chinadaily.com.cn/cndy/2010-07/12/ content_10092286.htm.

[27]   China Daily. Assessed 2011 November 11. URL: http://www.handreach.org/images/ china_daily_ Jan_10.jpg.

[28]   Dewey J. How we think: a restatement of the relation of reflective thinking to the educative process. Chicago: DC Heath,1993.

[29]   Schon DA. The reflective practitioner: how professionals think in action. New York: Basic Books, 1983.

[30]   Sackett DL, Rosenberg WM, Gray JA, Haynes RB, Richardson WS. Evidence based medicine: what it is and what it isn't. BMJ 1996;312(7023):71–2.

In: Public Health Yearbook 2013
Editor: Joav Merrick

ISBN: 978-1-63321-095-0
© 2014 Nova Science Publishers, Inc.

Chapter 32

THE GRAND-AIDES® PROGRAM IN BAOTOU, INNER MONGOLIA: A REVOLUTIONARY HEALTH CARE WORKFORCE

Christiana G White, Elizabeth S Bowles, Gordon M Carver IV,
Forrest B Compton, Thomas A Eschenroeder Jr,
Mary M Van Meter, Michael Marquardt, MBA
*and Arthur Garson Jr, MD, MPH**

Jefferson Public Citizen Program and the Center for Health Policy, University of
Virginia, Charlottesville, Virginia, US

ABSTRACT

The Grand-Aides® Program is an innovative health care workforce model designed to help provide personalized health care to all by increasing access to care. This program trains grandparents and senior citizens as medical care workers in order to provide less expensive, more accessible, and more appropriate health care to patients from a trusted community member. The program aims to increase access to care while alleviating health care professional shortages and crowding in hospitals and community clinics. University of Virginia students traveled to the Inner Mongolia region of China to collect baseline data for a pilot study to determine the effectiveness of a future Grand-Aides program. The collected data suggested that 53% of all patients visiting the clinic and/or hospital over a period of one year could have been cared for by a Grand-Aide and supervisor, with children's visits showing an even higher percentage of symptoms treatable by a Grand-Aide at 74%. These results suggest that once successfully implemented, the Grand-Aides program will be able to have a significant impact on the health care system in Baotou, Inner Mongolia.

Keywords: Community health worker, primary care, health care workforce

* Correspondence: Arthur Garson, Jr, MD, MPH, Director, Center for Health Policy, University of Virginia, Charlottesville, VA 22903 United States. E-mail: atg2n@virginia.edu or cgw4u@virginia.edu.

INTRODUCTION

Many people in Inner Mongolia live within walking distance of health care clinics; however, these clinics often have long waits and inconsistent care. As a result, these people may opt to remain untreated in an effort to avoid long lines and poor service. The only other option for care for the large, relatively poor population in this area is the emergency department. Emergency care is meant to stabilize patients with acute health problems, not provide consistent primary care or ongoing care for chronic diseases. Grand-Aides seeks to circumvent this problem by providing an intermediary source of personalized medical attention in the form of trained grandparents. We expect Grand-Aides will increase patient welfare, reduce overall hospital expenses, utilize resources more efficiently, take advantage of an eager pool of labor, and galvanize change that will further improve health care and increase both standard of living and life expectancy.

Grand-Aides was founded in 2008 with the idea that an experienced grandparent can successfully treat many of the medical cases presented in hospitals and health clinics worldwide. Since the formal establishment of Grand-Aides, pilot programs have been initiated domestically in Houston, Texas and Harrisonburg, Virginia and internationally in Shanghai and Baotou, Inner Mongolia with the prospect of starting more both nationally and abroad. While the Grand-Aides workforce model is currently undergoing pilot programs to gauge operational effectiveness and financial performance, research of the potential Grand-Aides utilization in international healthcare systems demonstrates high potential program impact. Continued interest from world leaders indicate a strong global belief in the benefits that Grand-Aides has to offer.

Regardless of the location of the program, every Grand-Aide must have the equivalent of a high school education, or significant health care experience, and successfully complete Grand-Aide training. The training program is customized to each program location, but usually it is divided into two-month sections punctuated by testing. Training of the primary care Grand-Aides begins in the classroom, where trainees learn about basic medical care and primary care protocols customized to medical practice in the region. Next, they enter a period of additional classroom training with a specific focus on fieldwork procedures followed by a period of supervised fieldwork, during which they begin to meet their patients and work according to their newly learned protocols. Finally the Grand-Aides enter a period of primary care fieldwork with an assessment every six months (1).

Once practicing, Grand-Aides care for 200 to 250 families as paid professionals. They will either make home visits (if available, using telemedicine that they bring with them such as Skype on a mobile phone) or give advice over the telephone if a family member complains of symptoms. Health professionals such as nurses or physicians supervise the Grand-Aides during these calls and visits (the supervisor is on the phone and available whenever the Grand-Aides are working), ensuring quality while also allowing greater individual patient attention. Patients will still have access to physicians if needed, but this added level of primary attention will increase access to care so that symptoms do not remain untreated due to lack of access to care. In an effort to promote healthy behavior, Grand-Aides will also make home visits to teach preventative care and early management of primary care conditions (2).

Since Grand-Aides is a new program, it must be assessed and practical methods for implementation must be developed to determine the actual need for Grand-Aides in each area. With this in mind, the research team traveled to Baotou, Inner Mongolia, to begin the pilot project there by assessing the need for Grand-Aides and helping develop the methodology for the future assessment of the program's success.

The research goal was to determine the potential demand for Grand-Aides in a specific part of the Qingshan District in Baotou that is served by the Fourth Affiliated Hospital of the Inner Mongolia Medical College (IMMC). This community has three forms of health providers: the hospital clinic, a local community clinic, and an emergency department. In order to determine the demand, the research team reviewed medical records for the one-year period dated from January 1, 2009, to December 31, 2009 and answered the research question, what percentage of patients that visited these three venues could have been cared for by a Grand-Aide? Through analysis of the data in these medical records with methods explained below, the team numerically gauged the local need for Grand-Aides by determining what percentage of the population that visited the three venues could have been cared for by Grand-Aides instead. This data will also be used as a baseline for future studies on the success of the Grand-Aides program in Baotou.

In addition to this specific research goal, the research team conducted interviews with health care providers, the Grand-Aides, and members of the community in order to develop recommendations for the adaptation of the Grand-Aides program for this specific community. Grand-Aides is a program that has the potential to be particularly successful in communities where elders are truly valued, trusted members of society as they traditionally are in China.

When the team from University of Virginia (UVA) arrived in Baotou, the six Grand-Aides participating in the pilot study had already been chosen and were beginning their training. The team worked with Dr. Garson and medical professionals in China to adapt the training materials for this specific region and to determine which diagnoses Grand-Aides would be allowed to treat. The Grand-Aides program is easily adaptable to different needs in different countries and environments through collaboration with local health care providers and community members.

METHODS

Data collection involved compiling all available medical records from the emergency department, hospital clinics, and community clinics in a specific neighborhood in Baotou. In total, 50 medical record books were utilized for the study, containing 35,148 individual patient visit entries. With a full calendar year of data, the research team was confident that the collected data was representative of the health care utilization trends of the Baotou community because any seasonal trends could be recognized and accounted for in the results. With a large and random sample, the data could be used to determine the future demand for Grand-Aides in the area.

All of the medical records were hand written in Chinese; therefore, data were collected after translation from Chinese to English. Each member of the research team from UVA paired with an IMMC student to translate medical records and record the relevant patient data in English. The following data variables were collected: patient visit location, date, sex, age, and diagnosis. The patient diagnosis was reported by clinical condition name if the patient had one of the 28 common conditions that could be potentially cared for by a Grand-Aide, as listed in Table 1. If the patient did not have one of the 28 common conditions, then "not applicable" was recorded in the patient visit entry. A patient entry was completely omitted if any part of the entry was illegible, as determined by the IMMC student. The project received a waiver from the Institutional Review Board of the University of Virginia.

Table 1. List of 28 Common Conditions Potentially Cared for by a Grand-Aide

Common Cold	Nausea, Vomiting, Adult
Congestion	Nausea, Vomiting, Child
Cough	Abrasion
Earache, Drainage	Insect Bite
Headache	Rash, Adult
Sore Throat	Rash, Child
Abdominal Pain, Adult	Back Pain
Abdominal Pain, Child	Joint Pain, Swelling
Constipation	Breastfeeding Problems
Diarrhea, Adult	Spitting Up, Infant
Diarrhea, Child	Diaper Rash
Gas, Belching	Excessive Crying
Gas, Flatulence	Fever, Adult
Indigestion	Fever, Child

Data were collected and analyzed using Microsoft Excel. The research question was analyzed by calculating the count and percentage of pediatric and adult cases that Grand-Aides could have potentially cared for at the Community Clinic, Hospital Clinics, and Hospital Emergency Department. In determining the percentages of patient visits that could have been treated by Grand-Aides, we assumed that Grand-Aides could care for all patients affected by the 28 common conditions (See Table 1).

The resulting analysis determined the percentage of patients with one of the 28 common conditions divided by the total number of patient visits collected from each of the three health care provider locations.

In addition to the qualitative research, the team conducted informal interviews, translated by the Chinese partners, with Grand-Aides and community members about how the program would be received once it began later in the year. The results of these interviews were used to develop recommendations for the initial implementation of the program.

RESULTS

A total number of 35,148 patient visits were observed at three different locations: a community clinic, hospital clinic, and hospital emergency department. Results are summarized in Figure 1 below.

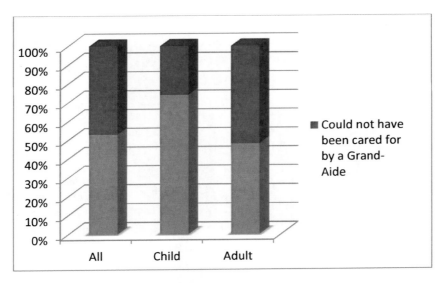

Figure 1. Total Percentage of Patient Visits Potentially Cared for by a Grand-Aide.

	All	**Child**	**Adult**
Total Percentage	53% (n=18,625)	74% (n=5076)	48% (n=13,549)

In total, 18,625 patients were diagnosed with 1 of the 28 common conditions potentially cared for by a Grand-Aide. Therefore, roughly 52% of the annual patient visits at these locations could have been at least initially cared for by a Grand-Aide and supervisor. About 74% of pediatric patients and 48% of adult patients could have been cared for by a Grand-Aide and supervisor. A breakdown of the results by location is shown in Figure 2 below.

At 64%, the community clinic had the highest percentage of patients diagnosed with 1 of the 28 common conditions. The community clinic had the highest percentage of pediatric patients potentially cared for by a Grand-Aide at 87%. They also had the highest number of adult patients with 1 of the 28 common conditions at 62%.

In the hospital clinics, 46% of the patients were diagnosed with 1 of the 28 common conditions. As in the community clinic, categorizing patients by age within the hospital clinics showed a significant variation between pediatric and adult patients: 75% of pediatric patients and 32% of adult patients had diagnoses that could potentially be cared for by a Grand-Aide and supervisor.

Similar to the hospital clinics, 49% of the patients visiting the hospital ED were diagnosed with 1 of the 28 common conditions. Variation by patient age was minimal, with 47% of pediatric and 49% of adult patients potentially cared for by a Grand-Aide and supervisor.

From the informal interviews, the research team found that for adult care, the community was receptive to the idea of calling a trusted community member before going to the doctor. The overall impression in the community was that people did not find the hospital or clinic visits pleasant and would prefer to talk to a neighbor they trust: confidentiality concerns were not high.

Interestingly, the team found that parents are extremely protective of their children in this community, leading to frequent doctor visits and a strong reluctance to accept the idea of trusting a Grand-Aide over a physician in the care of a child.

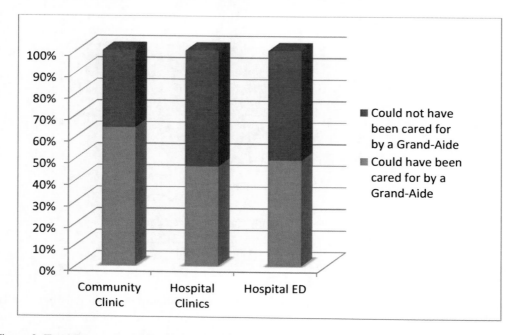

Figure 2. Total Percentage of Patient Visits Potentially Cared for By a Grand-Aide at Each Location.

	All	Child	Adult
Community Clinic	64% (n=7593)	87% (n=6648)	62% (n=945)
Hospital Clinics	46% (n=7007)	75% (n=3860)	32% (n=3147)
Hospital ED	49% (n=4025)	47% (n=271)	49% (n=3754)

DISCUSSION

The goal of this project was to determine the applicability and the need for Grand-Aides in Baotou, Inner Mongolia. The results of the study showed that almost half of adults and nearly three quarters of children went into a clinic or emergency department for symptoms that could be treated by a Grand-Aide with basic health care training. Therefore, the Grand-Aides Program could significantly improve both the quality of and access to health care in this region of Baotou while decreasing the cost of care.

Introducing Grand-Aides would improve this community's health care system in several ways. First, it would increase access to health care: another level of care would be available to all patients. Rather than having to miss work and wait in line at a clinic or emergency room, patients would be able to call a Grand-Aide and receive the care they need right away. The Grand-Aides program could also greatly improve the quality of care patients receive. Grand-Aides would have more time to spend with patients than doctors, so they could form closer patient-caregiver relationships, be able to do house calls, and keep their patients on track through treatment plans. This level of care could greatly improve the quality of available health care. The high percentage of cases that could be treated by a Grand-Aide means that this program could have a profound impact by decreasing the overcrowding and waiting time in clinics and hospitals and by allowing doctors to focus more on the patients who really need a higher level of training in order to be treated.

The idea of adding community health workers (CHWs) to the health care workforce is not a new one. It has been both highly criticized and successfully implemented around the world, depending on the structure and organization of the program. Similar programs to Grand-Aides, for example, Brazil's *Programa Agente Comunitário de Sáude* and Ghana's National Community Health Worker Programme, have had great success with using CHWs to deliver primary care, curative treatments, and health education, much like a Grand-Aide would (3). In Brazil in 1994, just five years after adoption of this national program, infant mortality dropped by 32% and from 2003 - 2006 hospitalization dropped from 52 to 38 people per 10,000 (4). In Ghana, after 6 years of starting its nationwide program, there was a 33% reduction in child mortality (5). The successes of these similar programs in decreasing mortality rates and improving health outcomes of their populations suggest that Grand-Aides could have similar success.

Because community health worker programs exist in different forms in many countries, the World Health Organization (WHO) completed a report in 2007, *Community Health Workers: What do we know about them?,* where they identified four main statements about community health workers there seemed to be a consensus about based on a thorough review of many of the programs in existence at the time. They found that first, "CHWs *can* make a valuable contribution to community development and, more specifically, can improve access to and coverage of communities with basic health services: there is robust evidence that CHWs can undertake actions that lead to improved health outcomes" (4, p.26). Grand-Aides will be trained to perform the types of actions that lead to both improved outcomes and access to care. Second, in order for programs to work effectively, their members must be "carefully selected, appropriately trained and – very important – adequately and continuously supported" (4, p.26). Grand-Aides follows this paradigm by specifically selecting older members of the community for their wisdom and respect from society and training them to become part of a primary health care team working towards the best interests of all of its patients. Third, the WHO is careful to highlight that because of the training, support, and management necessary for a successful program, "CHW programs are neither the panacea for weak health systems nor a cheap option to provide access to health care for underserved populations" (4, p.26). In the Grand-Aides program, the community health worker, the Grand-Aide, leverages the capabilities of the current health care system by increasing the number of patients the team as a whole is able to take care of; it requires a health system to support it. Finally, the WHO cautions that "CHW programs are vulnerable unless they are driven, owned by, and firmly embedded in communities themselves" (4, p.26). The Grand-Aides program is inherently owned by its community: Grand-Aides are already the leaders in the community and are now trained to provide an even greater service to their neighbors. Based on these four WHO findings in combination with the specific needs suggested by this study, Grand-Aides is set up to be a great success in Baotou.

LIMITATIONS

Our results suggest an overwhelming need for Grand-Aides in Baotou; however, there were some noteworthy limitations on the data used. In order to perform this research, researchers collected all of the hand-written ledger books for a full calendar year from the three desired locations. The entire year was used in order to have a statistically significant number of records in each location and to be sure that the data would not be affected by the inherent seasonality of certain illnesses (for example, more people are likely to get the flu during flu season).

The data from this experiment were not complete, however, because some ledger books had been lost over the year and others were written such that they were illegible to the Chinese students who were translating them. Although some of the data were missing, the results were still statistically significant because the data that were missing were determined to be random (from different time periods and clinics) and there was still a large enough data set.

Another problem with our data was that it was all written in Chinese, so it had to be translated before it could be recorded into Excel. There could have been some translational errors that occurred, but each translator learned English at the same school and was given the same training as to how to complete this study, so any errors that did occur should have occurred consistently throughout the process. There was ongoing dialogue between the translating students and the research team, so the likelihood of translational error is minimal.

Finally, health care records in the clinics visited in this study were not as consistent or thorough as those in the United States. Often, patients would have a single symptom listed, "headache" for example, and there would be no further information. Since "headache" is one of the conditions that Grand-Aides will be trained to treat, this would be listed as a patient that could have been cared for by a Grand-Aide. However, this patient could have had additional, more complex symptoms or diseases that were simply not recorded in the records. Because of the potential incompleteness of these records, the percentages found in this study could be higher than the actual percentages of patients that could be cared for by a Grand-Aide. This problem, however, does not have strong implications on the implementation of Grand-Aides in Baotou: even decreasing the number of patients who go to the clinics by 10% would greatly improve the access and quality of health care.

CONCLUSION

The results from this study show that the Grand-Aides program would not only succeed in Baotou, but could improve the health of this population. The health of this population suffers from the overcrowding and long wait times in clinics and hospitals. This study shows that a high percentage of the patients in these clinics and hospitals could be taken care of by a Grand-Aide instead. In addition to helping solve overcrowding problems, Grand-Aides will be able to provide higher quality primary care by spending more time with patients and providing more personal, individualized care. Six Grand-Aides began training in the summer of 2010 in Baotou. The Grand-Aides pilot project in Baotou is now in need of government funding, which has been applied for, in order to continue. Once funding is received and the project continues, the results from this study will be used as a baseline to compare with later data on hospital and clinic visit numbers and symptoms as Grand-Aides are introduced into their health care system. Hopefully, Grand-Aides will generate results within the community showing increased access and quality of health care, decreased costs, and improved overall health of the population.

The Grand-Aides program is easily adaptable to different cultures and communities as it is inherently a community-based program aiming to improve health care by training trusted community members. The goal is to allow these figureheads of society to increase their role in the health of their communities by becoming valuable members of the health care team. Because of its potential for success in both rural and urban settings, both internationally and abroad, the Grand-Aides program is quickly spreading to over ten countries including pilots in Bangladesh, Indonesia, and Australia and over fifteen sites in the US including Houston, Boston, and New York City. This revolutionary health care workforce team-based model has extremely high potential to improve access to and quality of health care while decreasing costs; it gives communities responsibility for their own health by granting ownership to its most respected members.

ACKNOWLEDGMENTS

Funding for this research team was through a grant from the Jefferson Public Citizen program at the University of Virginia; funding for the Grand-Aides program in Baotou, Inner Mongolia was through the Dreyfus Health Foundation.

We would like to thank all of the individuals who contributed to this project. We would particularly like to thank: Dr. Garson for his vision of Grand-Aides and for including us in his research team, the Jefferson Public Citizen program for making this project possible, Hsin-Ling for arranging our accommodations in Baotou and ensuring we were well taken care of throughout our stay, the staff members of the Fourth Affiliated Hospital of the Inner Mongolia Medical College for their cooperation and transparency, the Grand-Aides for their participation in this program, and the IMMC students for being such clear translators and hospitable friends. This project would not have been possible without you all and we are extremely grateful for your help.

REFERENCES

[1]   Grand-Aides. Grand-Aides flow chart. 2010. Accessed January 8, 2011, URL: https://docs.google.com/viewer?a=v&pid=sites&srcid=ZGVmYXVsdGRvbWFpbnxncmFuZGFpZGV zfGd4OjI2NmM1NDEzODk0YmE3MjI.

[2]   Grand-Aides. What does a grand-aide do? 2010. Accessed November 8, 2011. URL: http://www.grand-aides.org.

[3]   Giugliani C, Harzheim E, Duncan MS, Duncan BB. Effectiveness of community health workers in Brazil: A systematic review. J Ambul Care Manage 2011;34(4):326-38.

[4]   Lehmann U, Sanders D. Community health workers: what do we know about them? Geneva: World Health Organization, 2007.

[5]   Christopher JB, Le May A, Lewin S, Ross DA. Thirty years after Alma-Ata: a systematic review of the impact of community health workers delivering curative interventions against malaria, pneumonia and diarrhea on child morality and morbidity in sub-Saharan Africa. Human Resources Health 2011;9:27.

In: Public Health Yearbook 2013
Editor: Joav Merrick

ISBN: 978-1-63321-095-0
© 2014 Nova Science Publishers, Inc.

Chapter 33

TYPE-2 DIABETES IN BELIZE: A CROSS-SECTIONAL STUDY AND HOLISTIC APPROACH TO INCREASING HEALTH EDUCATION

Shelley M Brown, MPH*, Anna Monahan, MS, Jena E Daniels, BS and Tracy R Burton, RN

Department of Health Sciences,
College of Health and Rehabilitation Sciences Sargent College,
Boston University, Boston, Massachusetts, US

ABSTRACT

In May 2011, sixteen undergraduate students from Boston University organized and staffed health clinics, implemented diabetes education within school systems and screened for type 2 diabetes risk factors in Punta Gorda, Belize. Two types of health clinics were created, where willing adults participated from communities surrounding Punta Gorda. The first was mobile where students travelled to remote residences in six villages to screen for diabetes. The second was a walk-in clinic, located within schools and in town centers. There were stations set up for height and weight, as well as tables with three Boston University students recording other variables. We discovered the prevalence of type 2 diabetes to be higher in the more rural communities where the diet is more limited. Of the participants, 181 had complete data. The average blood glucose level was 143 (mg/dL). Blood glucose levels of 126 (mg/dL) or above are classified as high, which means that 52.6% of the participants had high levels. Of these individuals, less than 5% self-reported feeling symptomatic. Among the interesting findings was a lack of relationship between body mass index and blood glucose levels, irrespective of the most significant risk factors for type 2 diabetes. The prevalence of type 2 diabetes is rising at alarming rates in Belize. This cross-sectional study aimed to increase the general public's knowledge regarding overall health as it relates to diabetes. Boston University has transformed this pilot trip into a sustainable annual project.

* Correspondence: Shelley M Brown, MPH, Clinical Instructor of Health Sciences, Faculty of Sargent College of Health and Rehabilitation Sciences at Boston University, Room 441, 635 Commonwealth Avenue, Boston, MA, 02215 United States. E-mail: shelleyb@bu.edu.

Keywords: Type 2 diabetes, positive lifestyle choices, health clinics, risk factors, low socioeconomic cohorts, and sustainability, Latin America, diet

INTRODUCTION

Type 2 diabetes is a metabolic disorder that is characterized by insulin resistance. Cells fail to use insulin properly, while in some cases, there is complete insulin deficiency. The defective insulin action, insulin secretion, or both, cause the presence of hyperglycemia. Hyperglycemia can lead to significant mortality, morbidity, and significant costs of rehabilitation and tertiary care (1,2). In recent years, type 2 diabetes has become the leading cause of deaths Belizeans, as of 2005 (2). This trend is evidenced by the quality of care that patients receive who are experiencing the disorder, suffer from one or more other chronic conditions, or both.

The prevalence of Type 2 diabetes is rising in Belize due to an increase in obesity and physical inactivity, aging, population growth, and urbanization (3). The modifiable risk factors that are independent of each other are low physical activity and obesity (4). In a holistic approach to combat these two aspects, the present cross-sectional study took part in increasing the general public's knowledge regarding overall health by hosting health care clinics and educational booths, distributing culturally appropriate handouts to targeted communities, implementing educational programs in the school systems included in the study, and testing willing participants for Type 2 diabetes.

Boston University undergraduate students, in collaboration with faculty and a registered nurse from Winchester Hospital, hosted healthcare clinics that were both mobile and stationary. With the traveling clinics, the sample size became more diverse and education expanded beyond the school systems. The stationary clinics were organized in the center of the town of Punta Gorda where the majority of individuals participated in the study. Other sites included school classrooms, health clinics, and other health care facilities. Supplementing the testing at clinics, an education booth, staffed by Boston University students and faculty, was available. Culturally specific and appropriate information was distributed regarding type 2 diabetes care and prevention, culturally relevant diet-based prevention, and educational materials on other public health issues common to the region. Contact information for the local primary care physicians was also made available.

Concluding each testing session at the clinics, participants were handed an index card containing all of the data recorded for the study with a recommendation section. In correspondence with the trauma nurse that travelled with the students to each clinic, the recommendation section of the card clearly stated if there was a significant need to visit a local doctor, diet and exercise alterations, as well as indications for high or low blood pressure and/or blood glucose levels.

The other major component to increase the public's awareness of type 2 diabetes and its precursors was focused on the school system, where the undergraduate students taught in elementary-aged classrooms about health, nutrition, exercise, stress and hygiene. Depending on the age level and working knowledge of various topics, each lesson plan was tailored according to NEEMA principles from the Journal of National Medical Association (10). The outline of the Belizean study stems from the core of NEEMA. In addition, the school systems were targeted for their lack of available healthy food choices and specific educational programs. The intention of the implementation of educational programs, where previously they were lacking, is to target the modifiable risk factors for type 2 diabetes and positively influence the students to make healthier lifestyle choices. The principals and classroom teachers also participated with the children in the various health-related activities and lesson plans. Participation by the administration demonstrates the commitment of the local community to support healthier choices for students and their families.

With the ability to personalize and tailor the lesson plans in the classrooms and focus the health care clinics on specific common health disparities in Belize, transformation to a unique community-focused program occurred. The flexibility allowed positive outcomes for the public health issues being considered. Educating elementary aged students about health, nutrition, and type 2 diabetes, will positively influence their diet decisions and will potentially decrease the prevalence of type 2 diabetes in future generations. For example, in the classrooms, a Belizean-tailored food pyramid was incorporated.

There were adjustments to various food groups to their accessibility and affordability to the population. What is reasonable in terms of cost was not always nutritionally beneficial. Lack of resources, access and underemployment in the surrounding communities introduced restrictions for applying what was taught in the holistic approach to everyday life since it is not attainable for the majority. It was not necessarily that children or families willingly choosing to eat various types of food, but that they were not offered those options in the homes, mostly due to the cost of food products.

There is a need to focus on increasing the education levels in low socioeconomic countries. Equal access to healthcare and health information is imperative to affect positively the general health of all individuals (6). The common denominators for the major risk factors of type 2 diabetes are obesity, sedentary lifestyle, an unhealthy diet, and genetics (2). Although there is no way to influence some of these factors, there is a way to affect the prevalence of type 2 diabetes, to some extent, by targeting the lack of education on the necessary nutrition an individual needs (7). Poor general health often is associated with a notable lack of education and lack of resources (6, 7). Research on this topic alludes to the necessity of higher education for poverty-stricken areas; however, few programs have actually been initiated (6, 7). The implementation of such programs is a simple intervention that would be very cost effective with minimal training for those involved. Funding of this approach would provide coverage for wide ranges of cohorts and positively influence societies about their health. With these practices and increased knowledge of proper dietary requirements, the virulence of Type 2 diabetes on an individual level as well as the prevalence and incidence rates would likely decrease.

This requirement for further knowledge leads to questions of how to implement the programs how will such programs be funded, and what type of programs and information should be assigned. Expanding general knowledge in regards to overall health in low socioeconomic societies would also lead to decreasing severity, and possibly prevalence, for other diseases where nutrition is a key risk factor as well.

The evidence base suggests that a major challenge for diagnosis and treatment of diabetes in low resource settings, in particular Latin American countries, is that many individuals with diabetes related health issues and Type 2 diabetes, are asymptomatic and therefore often do not seek treatment and are diagnosed at more advanced stages of diseases (8). Adding to this challenge is the estimation that the impacts will only worsen in the future, as many young individuals continue to lead unhealthy lifestyles and the healthcare systems within Latin American countries, including Belize, are ill-equipped to handle the increasing burden (8). Later diagnosis can lead to both more expensive treatments and negative health consequences. The evidence suggests the gold standard of the medical community in the asymptomatic phases, based on a consensus reached by 17 Latin American countries, which is to adopt a nutrition program consisting of healthy eating habits, exercise and reduction in other lifestyle behaviors which could impact health (8).

The consensus recommends behavior modification as a solution to address challenges unique to Latin American countries, especially in consideration of distinct cultures, beliefs, and religions coupled with low resource settings (8). The aims of this Boston University pilot project were to form a multi-faceted approach to address the persistent public health problem of obesity and diabetes in the diverse urban and rural towns surrounding Punta Gorda, Belize.

METHODS

Two faculty members from Boston University and a registered intravenous nurse accompanied sixteen undergraduate students. The students ran two types of health clinics where 234 willing adults participated from communities surrounding Punta Gorda and consulted the faculty members and nurse when necessary. The first type of health clinic was mobile where the students travelled from residence to residence in six villages surveying those that were willing to participate in diabetes screening. The second type of clinic was a walk-in clinic that was held at the local schools and in the town center of Punta Gorda. Signs were posted describing the purpose of the clinics and participants willingly volunteered. There were stations set up for height and weight, as well as tables with three Boston University students recording blood glucose levels (mh/dL), blood pressure, age, gender, and time from last meal. In both clinics, students provided an index card to the participant that included all of the recorded data and had a special section where recommendations were written (i.e., see local physician, include more fruits or vegetables in diet, high/low blood pressure, high/low blood glucose levels, etc.)

Participants

Punta Gorda was the main host district for this study. Aside from Punta Gorda, data was collected from five other surrounding towns. The minimum age requirement was 18 years; otherwise, there were no restrictions in terms of participants. Adolescents were not the targeted age population due to the increased incidence rate in individuals over the age of 25 years (4) and under age 18 constitutes a vulnerable population group. There was no documentation of past or present health concerns, be it physical, mental, or biologic, tobacco and alcohol consumption, nor were there recordings of normal physical activity levels. Participants were given explanations for the testing and results.

Evaluation measures

Diabetes is the leading cause of death in Belize, among all low-income and middle-income countries, with an average prevalence for this metabolic condition of 80% for both sexes (4, 5). As a low-income, Central American country, Belize possesses the smallest population density and is one of the only countries where English is considered the official language and where Kriol and Spanish are secondary (4).

RESULTS

The prevalence of type 2 diabetes is higher in the more rural communities where their diet is more limited than to the community in Punta Gorda. There were 234 surveyed participants; however, 181 of them had complete data. The average age was 38 years old, the average blood glucose level was 143 (mg/dL), the average weight was 151 lbs, and the average blood pressure was 129/77. Blood glucose levels of 126 (mg/dL) or above are classified as high levels. 52.6% of the participants had high levels of glucose in their blood. The highest blood glucose level was over 600 (mg/dL) and the highest BMI was 40. Of those that were above normal blood glucose levels, less than 5% said they felt symptomatic.

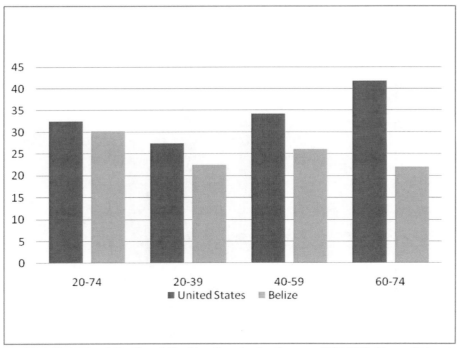

Sources: CDC/NCHS, National Health and Nutrition Examination Surveys, 2007-2009, Boston University Belize Pilot Study 2011.

Figure 1. Prevalence of obesity in men aged 20-74, by age group: United States 1988-1994 and 2007-2008 and Punta Gorda, Belize 2011.

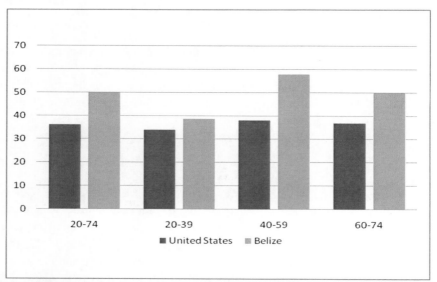

Sources: CDC/NCHS, National Health and Nutrition Examination Surveys, 2007-2009, Boston University Belize Pilot Study 2011.

Figure 2. Prevalence of obesity in women aged 20-74, by age group: United States 1988-1994 and 2007-2008 and Punta Gorda, Belize 2011.

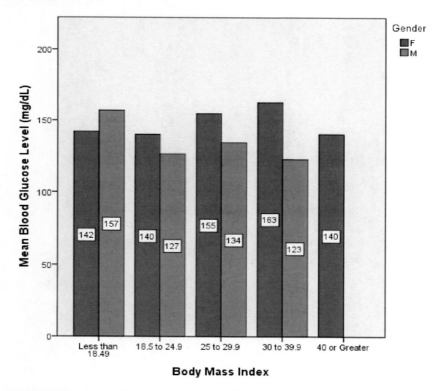

Figure 3. Mean Blood Glucose level in women and men 18-80, by BMI category: Punta Gorda, Belize 2011.

Body mass index

Of our population sample, results for body mass index (BMI) were separated into five categories according to 2007-2008 National Health and Nutrition Examination Survey (NHANES): underweight, normal weight, overweight, obese, and extremely obese (9) (see figures 1 and 2). Of our random population sample over the age of 20 years, 4% are classified as extremely obese. Mimicking the United States' standards, most of the Belizean population falls into the overweight and obese categories. However, our results indicate 41.6% are overweight and 77.8% of the population is overweight, obese or extremely obese and 22.2% are normal or underweight (see figures 1 and 2). Of the population studied, 23.9% of the women are classified as overweight, in terms of their BMI, whereas 17.7% of the men are overweight (see figure 3). For a BMI greater than or equal to 30, 27.2% were females and 8.8% were males. In the United States, 36.2% of women and 32.6% of men have greater than or equal to a BMI of 30. The overall prevalence of obesity in the United States is 34.4% and in Belize, it is 36.5%.

Blood glucose levels

There is a slight relationship with blood glucose levels and BMI where there is some related increase in BMI and blood glucose levels for the categories normal weight, overweight, and obese. Unexpectedly, however, there is a decrease in blood glucose levels in extreme obese participants.

Blood pressure

According to our results, there was no relationship between blood pressure and BMI, blood pressure and age, or blood pressure and blood glucose levels.

CONCLUSION

In Belize, type 2 diabetes has become more prevalent and those that have above normal blood glucose levels are more likely to be asymptomatic. Individuals lack health education and therefore are unaware of the severity of their health status. Limitations to this study include lack of consistent data with specified time of food intake, asking and documenting if participant has previous or present health concerns or has been diagnosed with a medical problem, small sample size, only significant data for adults, and not considering racial or ethnic factors in data. There are possibilities for human error in blood pressure and height data as well.

Considerations for pre-diabetes, when blood glucose levels were taken and genetic variations need to be taken into account for this study and its results. There was no documentation for when and/or if any medication was being taken or prescribed to a participant. According to our data analysis, there is surprisingly no relationship between participants BMI and their blood glucose levels. With this interesting finding, could suggest even a potential genetic component or variation in the type of diabetes in this region.

There was no significant relationship between BMI and blood glucose levels, even though it was expected. These conclusions call for further research. There was, however, significant data for BMI for the entire population; 77.8% of our sample size was categorized as being overweight. There was also significant data for men and women in regards to BMI. Roughly four times more women were obese than men. This could be due to the gender roles and culture, men typically work in the fields while women stay at home, care and cook for the family. It could also be due to study limitations. In general, though, results from this cross-sectional study are comparable to the United States (9). With over three quarters of the population overweight to some extent, concerns for long-term complications arise for future health disparities. There was no further data collected on obesity and after analyzing the data, more specific data is required. There is also opportunity here for supplementary understanding of this population in regards to race, ethnicity, and gender. Considerations for studying the younger population are another route for future studies. In any regards, the limitations that have been outlined need to be minimized to maximize results and relationships between BMI, blood glucose levels, blood pressure, age, ethnicity and race, as well as time of food intake.

REFERENCES

[1]   Wild S, Roglic G, Green A, Sicree R, King H. Global Prevalence of diabetes: estimates for the year 2000 and projections for 2030. Diabetes Care 2004; 27:1047–1053.

[2]   Andrewin A, Castillo N, Hoare M, Morey F, Perez J, Barneyy B, Thompson L. Managing diabetes in primary care in Belize. Caribbean Health Research Council and the Pan American Health Organization, Office of Caribbean Program Coordination 2010;7-66.

[3]   Cabrera-Freitag P, Escalada J, Goikoetxea MJ, Laguna S, Sanz ML, Gartaminza G. A severe case of lipoatrophy due to human insulin and insulin analogs in a patient with diabetes: is an immunological mechanism involved? J Invest Allergol Clin Immunol 2011;21:410-21.

[4]   World Health Organization. Burden: mortality, morbidity, and risk factors. In: Global status report on NCDs 2010. WHO 24/7 2010;9-11. Accessed 2011 Nov 14. URL: http://www.who.int/ nmh/ publications/ncd_report_chapter1.pdf.

[5]   World Health Organization. Health experts accept use of HbA1c for diagnosing diabetes. WHO 2011. Accessed 2011 Nov 14. URL: http://www.who.int/diabetes/en/.

[6]   Kumar A, Mittal S, Orito S, Ishitani K, Ohta, H. Impact of dietary intake, education, and physical activity on bone mineral density among north indian women. J Bone Mineral Metabol 2010;28(2):192-201.

[7]   Borges TT, Rombaldi AJ, Knuth AG, Hallal PC. Knowledge on risk factors for chronic diseases: A population-based study. [Conhecimento sobre fatores de risco para doencas cronicas: estudo de base populacional] Cadernos De Saude Publica / Ministerio Da Saude, Fundacao Oswaldo Cruz, Escola Nacional De Saude Publica 2009;25:1511-1520.

[8]   Guzmán JR, Lyra R, Aguilar-Salinas CA, Cavalcanti S, Escaño F, Tambasia M, Duarte E, ALAD Consensus Group. Treatment of type 2 diabetes in Latin America: a consensus statement by the medical associations of 17 Latin American countries. Rev Panam Salud Publica 2010;10(6). ACCESSED 2011 Nov 15. URL: http://dx.doi.org/10.1590/S1020-49892010001200008.

[9]   Ogden CL, Carroll MD. Prevalence of overweight, obesity, and extreme obesity among adults: United States, trends 1960-1962 through 2007-2008. CDC 2011;6:1-2.

[10] Shaw-Perry M, Horner C, Trevino RP, Sosa ET, Hernandez I, Bhardwaj A. NEEMA: A school-based diabetes risk prevention program designed for African-American children. J Natl Med Assoc 2007;(4):368-75.

[11] Banegas JR, Cruz JJ, Rodrı´guez-Artalejo F, Graciani A, Guallar-Castillo´n P & Herruzo R. Systolic vs diastolic blood pressure: community burden and impact on blood pressure staging. J Hum Hypertension 2002;16:163–7.

[12] MacMahon S, Alderman MH, Lindholm LH, Liu L, Sanchez RA, Seedat YK. Blood-pressure-related disease is a global health priority. Am J Hypertens 2008;21(8):843-4.

In: Public Health Yearbook 2013
Editor: Joav Merrick

ISBN: 978-1-63321-095-0
© 2014 Nova Science Publishers, Inc.

Chapter 34

A PICTURE IS WORTH A THOUSAND WORDS: EVALUATION OF THE ARTMAIL SENIOR ART PROJECT AMONG SENIORS WITH COGNITIVE LIMITATIONS IN NORTH CAROLINA

S Sudha, PhD*, Lia Miller, Emma H Thomas and Edward Chia

Department of Human Development and Family Studies, University of North Carolina at Greensboro, Creative Aging Network-NC, Greensboro, North Carolina, United States of America

ABSTRACT

Participating in structured art programs is said to improve physical and mental health and social functioning of older adults including those with dementia. However, research on this subject is fairly new, and awareness of these programs is limited. Feedback for improved program design and delivery is also needed. In a partnership between UNC Greensboro and the Creative Aging Network-NC, we conducted a pilot project in North Carolina (USA) in 2011 to evaluate whether participating in a 10 week art exchange project called ARTmail improved mood and social connectedness among seniors. Although 60 seniors took part in the ARTmail program, most of them with a cognitive limitation, only 31 seniors took part in the evaluation, mostly because the legal representative of many cognitively limited seniors did not give permission for them to participate in the evaluation. We collected baseline and endline information on socio-demographic background, physical health, functional status; and depression, loneliness, and mood / connectedness scales appropriate for dementia and non–dementia groups. We also conducted qualitative interviews with selected site staff, volunteers, and participants, and performed field observations. Our findings suggested that among seniors with cognitive limitations, the mean of mood scores at endline was lower than at baseline, suggesting improved mood (approaching significance at the .10 level). A larger sample would likely have shown significant results. We conclude with a discussion of

* Corresponding author: Associate Professor Sudha Shreeniwas, PhD, Faculty of Human Development and Family Studies, Department of Human Development and Family Studies, The University of North Carolina at Greensboro, 248 Stone Building, Greensboro, NC 27402 United States. Email: s_shreen@uncg.edu.

observations and suggestions from staff, volunteers, and participants, on experiences with the program and suggestions for improved implementation in future.

Keywords: Older adults, dementia, ARTmail evaluation, positive aging development, structured arts program

INTRODUCTION

As the older population increases in size and proportion worldwide, the numbers of persons diagnosed with dementia or other age-related cognitive impairments is projected to increase rapidly. In the US alone, current estimates show that about 5.4 million Americans of all ages, including about one in eight persons aged 65 and older, and nearly half those aged 85 and above, have been diagnosed with Alzheimer's disease (1). Thus, designing and delivering services for persons living with this condition is emerging as an extremely important priority in public health and human services fields. Though reviews of evidence-based service initiatives to improve quality of life for those with Alzheimer's disease have identified the importance of psychosocial interventions including engaging in pleasant activities as important, there is greater emphasis and evidence on practical issues related to medication, behavior management, caregiver support, and care programs (13). Programs that keep cognitively limited seniors creatively engaged and improve their mood have received comparatively little attention for reasons including preconceptions of the limitations of seniors with cognitive diagnoses, difficulties in finding appropriate programs, and lack of recognition by funding agencies.

Gerontology studies show that participating in professionally conducted multi modal cultural or arts programs improves physical and mental health and social functioning of older adults including those with dementia (2-5). The mechanisms by which such participation improves wellbeing of older adults includes improved sense of control or mastery, positive pathways in psycho-neuro-immunology (mind-body connection and brain plasticity), and social engagement (3). In light of such findings, practitioners and researchers are beginning to design and deliver structured arts and culture programs for seniors with varying levels of physical and cognitive ability. However, these efforts are newly emerging, and more evidence is needed on their feasibility and efficacy across a wide range of settings.

In the present study, we conducted a small scale, pilot evaluation of the ARTmail program, which offers a structured art creation and exchange program for seniors in North Carolina. The ARTmail art exchange project is designed to encourage freedom of expression and creative growth for older adults across a wide range of abilities, skills, and comfort levels. Participants and staff at each site who assist in administering the project learn new visual arts skills, develop relationships, and increase their understanding of the value of the creative process. These activities will, it is hoped, promote psychosocial wellbeing among the participants.

The ARTmail project and evaluation study were conducted by a partnership between faculty and students at the Department of Human Development and Family Studies at the University of North Carolina Greensboro (UNCG), and the Creative Aging Network-NC (CAN-NC), a state wide community based network that designs and delivers creative arts programming for seniors. CAN-NC designed and delivered the ARTmail program, the UNCG faculty designed and conducted the evaluation, and UNCG students served as volunteers to assist in program completion. This partnership addresses an important conjunction of interests in the field of gerontology and that of community programming, emphasizing the collaborative connection that enables better program design and delivery to underserved groups along with exploring and documenting the effect on seniors of participating in structured arts programs.

Our pilot study presents: a) an evaluation of whether participating in ARTmail improved mood and social connectedness among seniors and b) lessons 'from the field' about improving the design and delivery of this structured arts program and conducting an evaluation in a community setting. Specifically, we examined:

- whether older adults who participate in a structured art program report improved mood at endline compared to baseline
- whether older adults who participate in a structured art program report decreased loneliness at endline compared to baseline
- how practical aspects of the design and delivery of the structured arts program, and the associated monitoring and evaluation, can be improved.

The first two objectives are measured through survey assessments of seniors at baseline and at the conclusion of the project supplemented by field observations and in depth interviews of selected key informants among staff, volunteers, and participants, and the third objective through the field observations and in-depth interviews. We expected that those involved in this weekly participatory art exchange project would express more positive responses on mental health measures, less loneliness, and more engagement with activities and peers at the end of the 10 week project.

ARTmail art program

The ARTmail art exchange program uses the inside surface of a cardboard box as the canvas and the postal system as a means of exchanging the art between partners at the participating sites (see figure 1). The art form used in this project is Abstract Expressionism, which values individuality, spontaneity, and the exploration of the self, with no requirement for 'correct' representation of recognizable images. Working in an abstract style enables older adults to connect both with themselves and their partnering artists in a way that words alone cannot (see figure 2). As an integral part of the ARTmail activity, seniors are encouraged to write a short narrative called a Box Story to accompany their art. The artwork is exchanged back and forth between partners over a 10 week period (see figure 3). At the end of this period, CAN-NC recommends a public exhibition of the collective artworks and a reception with family and friends to celebrate the senior artists' achievements (see figure 4).

Through the ARTmail project, CAN-NC aims to bridge gaps among older adults of diverse cultural and socio-economic backgrounds by providing creative, nonverbal opportunities that can be experienced by all, overcoming language and memory barriers.

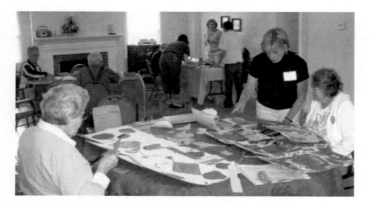

Figure 1. Group creating art boxes.

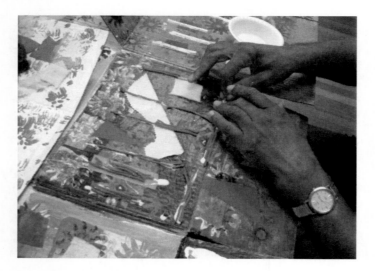

Figure 2. A participant creating art.

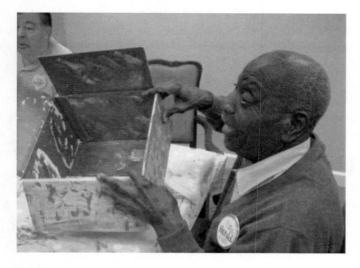

Figure 3. Participant receiving and opening a box.

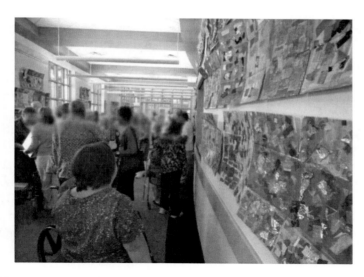

Figure 4. Exhibition at the end of the project period.

The role of art is essential in exploring the emotional dimensions of life experiences and in shaping public discourse about critical issues (in this case aging) both for the artists and the audiences. By giving voice through the arts to older adults, the aim is to educate the community about who they are, their past achievements, and what they are still capable of achieving. Exhibitions of the finished artwork showcase the talents and contributions of diverse older adults and educate the public about the rich histories of this population.

The ARTmail program is administered at each senior site by paid staff who provide space and serve as facilitators providing specific instruction for each class, and volunteers (one to two at each site) who assist the site staff. Both provide hands-on assistance as needed. Some sites had more than one staff person or volunteer for additional support.

METHODS

We conducted the evaluation in the six senior sites which invited the ARTmail program for their clients. Four of these are adult day care centers, and the majority of their clients have dementia or other cognitive diagnoses. The other two are residential sites serving clients who may or may not have cognitive diagnoses. At each site, a group of about 10 clients participated in ARTmail, and were recruited for the evaluation (a potential total of 60 participants for the evaluation). For those with cognitive limitations, their legally authorized representatives were contacted for informed consent. Unwillingness to participate in the evaluation did not affect eligibility to participate in ARTmail. Those who agreed to participate in the evaluation completed a baseline interview as described below. After the project, they were given an endline interview. Only about 31 ARTmail participants took part in the evaluation, mostly because among seniors with cognitive limitations, their representative did not consent for them to participate in the evaluation.

Study instruments

The baseline interview gathered standard socio-demographic information; measures of physical health and functional status; the Geriatric Depression Scale Short Form (for the non-dementia population) and the Cornell Scale for Depression in Dementia (for the dementia population); the UCLA Loneliness scale (for the non-dementia population) and the observed Engagement, Expression of Emotion, and Indicators of Self Esteem scale for the dementia population (6-8, 12). Most of those who agreed to participate in the evaluation were able to communicate. In most cases, site staff and site supervisors filled out the background demographic information based on patient records, and completed the mood and social connectedness scales by interviewing the seniors or by observing them based on the requirement of the scales. From these quantitative data, we used T-tests to compare mean scores on depression, loneliness, or connectedness measures at baseline and endline.

Supplementary individual qualitative interviews and field observations

A supplementary series of in-depth qualitative interviews was also conducted by the UNCG senior undergraduate student with selected key informants. Two senior site supervisors and site staff were selected based on convenience and availability, and two senior participants based on their ability and willingness to communicate. The question guides for these individual in-depth interviews were drafted jointly by UNCG faculty and CAN-NC senior staff. The questions focused on asking how the ARTmail process was experienced and how it could be improved; how the evaluation process had been conducted and how that could be improved; and what impact participating in ARTmail may have had on mood and social connectedness among the participants. The interviews were brief, usually lasting about half an hour each. The transcripts were read by the senior author, and emerging themes on the experience of participating in ARTmail and recommendations for improved program design and delivery were identified and explored.

Field observation of the process of ARTmail and the evaluation study was conducted by the senior undergraduate member of the research team, who was also a key volunteer with the ARTmail project. She volunteered at one site over the 10 week project period, assisting the group with creating art, observing and recording her impressions after each session. She also observed the evaluation process. Her field observations form part of the evidence presented in this study.

Research team

The research team comprised CAN-NC staff, and UNCG faculty and students. There were two parallel sets of activities that the research team was involved in, the ARTmail art project and the evaluation process:

- For the ARTmail art project, the CAN-NC staff co-ordinated senior site volunteers and staff conducted all activities related to the administration of the ARTmail project over the 10 week period February-May 2011. This included developing the training materials for ARTmail, communicating among multiple sites, and scheduling the 10 week project timeline. They provided an orientation for site staff and volunteers at each participating site. The CAN-NC staff provided assistance throughout the project as needed and documented segments of the project using photography and video, for promotional and archival needs (ARTmail participants signed waivers allowing their photographs to be taken and used). UNCG students formed part of the group of volunteers.

- The UNCG faculty applied for IRB approval for the evaluation data collection, designed evaluation research plans and data collection instruments, and oversaw data entry and the research, analyses, and dissemination process. UNCG student activities included volunteering at the sites to facilitate ARTmail, assisting in coordinating data collection, data entry for the evaluation, and one student conducted the key informant in-depth interviews and field observations. UNCG faculty, the CAN-NC director, and one UNCG senior undergraduate student and one graduate student participated in data analyses, report writing, and dissemination of the findings. The senior site staff also played an important role in completing the evaluation questionnaires. The Institutional Review Board of UNC Greensboro reviewed and approved the project.

RESULTS

Baseline and endline interviews among participants assessed their mood and social connectedness, including information on basic demographic, socioeconomic, and health status. Our initial target sample had been 60 older adults (10 participants at each of six sites) who took part in the ARTmail activity. However, only about 31 seniors participated in the evaluation study, mainly because the legally authorized representatives of the seniors with cognitive limitations did not allow them to take part. Four participants agreed to take part in the evaluation but dropped out of the activity and the study due to ill health.

Table 1 shows that most participants were aged 76 and above, a little over half were male, more than one-third were African American, almost two-thirds had completed High School or more. Almost three-quarters had some cognitive limitation. Most were evenly divided between widowed and married. Most lived in a private home at baseline.

In results not shown in tables, when participants were asked to rate their own physical health during baseline interviews, about three-quarters of them rated their health as good or better, with endline interviews showing an increase in the number of persons rating their health as good or better. When participants were asked if they received help or supervision with personal care or getting around the house, over half answered "yes," with a decrease in needing this type of assistance at endline. Over three-quarters of persons received help or supervision using the telephone, paying bills, taking medications, preparing light meals, doing laundry, going shopping, or managing money at the time of baseline interviews, with again a slight drop in the number of persons needing this type of assistance at endline. These figures are suggestive of a trend toward improved well-being, though the sample size was too small to yield a statistically significant result. Additionally, baseline numbers showed that approximately one-quarter of interviewees had been to an Emergency Room or Urgent Care in the last six months, while only one-tenth had visited these places in the ten weeks before the endline interviews. The majority of participants answered all questions on their questionnaires, although an increase in unanswered questions was noted in the endline data.

Since the majority of the group who participated in the evaluation (22 out of 31) had a cognitive limitation, we report the results only for this subgroup. We report changes in the mean of the Cornell Scale for Depression in Dementia to assess mood, and Engagement, Expression of emotion, and Indicators of Self Esteem scale to assess social connectedness. Table 2 presents changes in mood and social connectedness between baseline and endline (assessed by ANOVA techniques). Mean scores on both measures went down (indicating a lessening of symptoms, i.e., an improvement in status), though only the difference between the two means on the Cornell Score approached significance at the .10 level. Though our limited sample size did not provide sufficient statistical power, the results suggest a trend toward improvement (see Table 2).

Table 1. Information on some basic characteristics of the seniors

Participants' Characteristics (N=31)	Percentage
Age Group	
% Less than 55	12.9%
% 55-75	29.0%
% 76+	51.6%
% Did not Answer	6.5%
Gender	
% Male	51.6%
% Female	45.2%
% Did not Answer	3.2%
Race	
% White	54.8%
% Black	38.7%
% Other	3.2%
% Did not Answer	3.3%
Education Level	
% Completing High School	61.3%
% With less than High School	19.4%
% Did not Answer	19.3%
Population Member	
% with Cognitive Disabilities	71.0%
Baseline Marital Status	
% Single	16.1%
% Married	29.0%
% Divorced	16.1%
% Widowed	35.5%
% Did not Answer	3.3%
Living Arrangements	
% In a Private Home	71.0%
% In a Living Facility	25.8%
% Did not Answer	3.2%

Table 2. Change in mood and social connectedness between baseline and endline

Descriptive Statistics					
	N	Minimum	Maximum	Mean	Std. Deviation
Round 1 Cornell score*	22	.00	21.00	5.55	5.50
Round 2 Cornell score*	22	.00	15.00	4.18	4.87
Round 1 Domains score	22	21.00	42.00	31.40	5.52
Round 2 Domains score	22	17.00	37.00	30.68	5.08

* means significantly different between round 1 and round 2 at the .10 level.

Results from the qualitative interviews

Our original research plan was to use a qualitative technique called Photovoice with the seniors' art and accompanying box stories. Photovoice is a tool for participatory research in studies where participants are from marginalized or vulnerable populations (9-11), and is a process by which people can use a photographic technique to present rich descriptive information about their community based on their unique perspective (9,10). In addition to photographs, data can include interview and discussion transcripts (9). The box stories were intended in this vein. However, due to limited capacity of seniors with cognitive diagnoses to express themselves in writing, and structural difficulties administering the project among participants with cognitive limitations and with overburdened site staff, the Box Stories component did not get created. These issues are addressed in the recommendations and discussion section.

In depth interviews were conducted with selected key site staff, volunteers, and participants. Responses revealed that site staff and volunteers felt that improvements could be made in the structure and process of the ARTmail activity and the evaluation. Regarding the ARTmail project, site staff felt that there was not sufficient introduction to the project. One supervisor said "There was the intro meeting where we talked about the project ... then boom, here's the project and one volunteer, then done". Regarding process, they also felt that the demands of the project were great, on the cognitively limited participants and on the staff. "Next time, maybe have smaller boxes ... I would like to see some more volunteers come to help maybe some actual art students ... maybe break it down into tasks, one day practice, and next time glue the practice paper onto the box. ... I also was not able to do any box stories because I never had time to do them". Regarding outcomes, we asked if they had observed how participating in the project changed mood and social connectedness among participating seniors. The site staff indicated mixed results including difficulties and achievements. One staff member reported: "I think in the moment the majority of the participants were happy but some were frustrated ... some yelled and cried because they felt overwhelmed ... anyone who went on the field trip to see their art loved it. They did feel special". Regarding the ARTmail evaluation, the staff felt the process was overwhelming. One staff member noted that: "I also was very overwhelmed with the assessment forms. It would have been nice to have either been taught how to use them properly or had a student come in and do them". However, they were willing to do the project again.

Two senior ARTmail participants (one male and one female) were interviewed separately. Both of them were in the group that had cognitive diagnoses. Each is identified here by a pseudonymous initial (KL for the woman, and TM for the man). To probe the impact on mood, participants were asked how they felt while participating in ARTmail. KL said at first "I got pretty anxious about doing it". When probed by the interviewer why she felt anxious, she clarified "Just wanting to get back to it." Later she elaborated on her feelings: "Like I was doing something constructive … I was happier". The man, TM answered "I felt good … it gave me something to do", and "I was calm". Examining social connectedness required more probing, however, the participants did provide valuable insights in their replies. For example, when asked about how creating the ARTmail box had changed her as a person, KL replied "Well, I'm usually a shy person … and it didn't bring me out of my shyness … but it made me a less shy person". When asked whether she felt closer or more connected to the other participants, KL said "I looked at her [another participant's] box and wondered what it was going to look like". When probed further, she added that "I felt closer to … what's that crazy man … he's red-headed … a famous artist … they even had a half hour show on his artwork on public television the other day … he's dead now" who turned out to be Van Gogh. TM was much less forthcoming about whether the experience made him feel closer to the other participants, because he responded that "we ain't ever talk about it, you know". When asked about what suggestions they would have for improving the process of ARTmail, KL replied "having different materials … different kinds of materials". TM said "more time … more than once a week", which KL concurred with.

Results of the field observations

The senior undergraduate student author assisted in the fieldwork for the ARTmail project, and was actively involved at one site in the process of helping elder participants to begin their creative project each day and providing them with materials and emotional support. She documented her observations on the ARTmail and evaluation process from this site. During the course of ARTmail, she noticed a variation in attitudes toward the ARTmail project. At the beginning of the project, some seniors were excited to begin, while others were more hesitant - sometimes warming up to the process and displaying self-motivated creativity and concentration. In some cases, participants were proud of the art they created, while others never achieved this sense of pride. In most cases, participants were calm and appeared to enjoy making their art; their mood seemed positive. Most participants created their art in silence and with a great deal of concentration. Conversation between participants was limited and discussions were usually between participants and staff members about supplies such as paint and glue.

Staff at the care center experienced some obstacles and stress during the course of the project, particularly regarding the administering of evaluation interviews or the recording of box stories. Staff members noted that they were understaffed and it appeared that their lack of time to conduct uninterrupted interviews was due to a shortage of human resources needed to complete other tasks simultaneously. She also noted that in many ways, the staff members found the recording of participants' demographic and other information necessary for the evaluation to be burdensome. The staff members seem to recognize the value of the art project portion, but some expressed a reluctance to assist with the evaluation in the future due to the frustrations and complications of the non-art portions of the evaluation data collection. Overall, staff members enjoyed the ARTmail project and some participated in painting a box of their own, but they also appeared to be stretched thin by the requirements of the project.

DISCUSSION

The older age group is the most rapidly growing demographic segment across the world. While the needs of this group are rapidly growing, and the incidence and prevalence of dementia and other age-related disorders is likely to rise, programs that improve the psychosocial wellbeing and quality of life of this group are lacking, because of a greater focus on medical management and physical health needs. Participating in structured arts programs is argued to improve psycho social wellbeing of older adults, e.g., improved mood and social connectedness, which in turn has a positive impact on care givers. Improved quality of life, mood, and social connectedness may play a role in allowing seniors to delay institutionalization.

However, design and delivery of such programs too often exclude seniors, because of lack of awareness and documentation, and more resources being targeted toward youth. Thus, further exploration and documentation of benefits of structured arts programs for seniors, and improvements in their design and delivery, are needed. The University-community organization pilot partnership for evaluating the ARTmail program described in the present study aimed to address this gap. The partnership represents a significant collaboration between the community partner and the University, where the former designed and delivered the art activity, and the latter designed the evaluation and facilitated student volunteers to assist with the art project and the evaluation. The results of the project assist in building the capacity of the partner organization to improve design and delivery of the activity, and also document its beneficial effects on participants which may strengthen applications for funding support.

While the pilot quantitative evaluation was under powered and thus could not generate statistically significant results, the findings did suggest a trend toward improvement. The overall effort yielded rich insights which can be used to improve all aspects (design and delivery of the program, and the accompanying evaluation) of the effort in subsequent endeavors. The suggestions and recommendations for building capacity to improve the program include the following:

- Art activities such as ARTmail are enjoyed by seniors, including those with cognitive limitations. Site staff and seniors said they would like to be involved again.
- Structural issues with program design and delivery:
  - To make it easier for staff to successfully administer the activity, there needs to be increased volunteer support: at least 3 volunteers per site who remain consistently throughout the project, to support a group of ten participants.
  - For seniors with cognitive limitations and for the staff assisting them, the art activity needs to be broken down into smaller steps. The ARTmail manual needs to be revised to simplify the activity.

- To successfully complete key aspects of the art project, such as the Box Stories, staff and volunteers are needed to specifically solicit descriptions from seniors and record what they say. This is specifically needed for seniors with dementia or other cognitive diagnoses, who may have difficulty with written communication, but who nonetheless have much to communicate. Their direct input is not often incorporated into research that is conducted "on" them, rather than "with" them.
- Structural issues related to senior site staff and workload:
  - To successfully complete art activities, senior sites need to budget one and a half hours per session. Many sites' time is structured so that only one hour blocks are available for activities, thus each ARTmail session was limited to one hour, which seemed to limit participants' creativity.
  - Staff needs to be involved in the art activity planning process so that their recommendations can be taken into account from the start.
  - The site staff who are asked to provide hands-on assistance with the ARTmail project or evaluation activities, including filling evaluation forms and recording Box Stories, must be appropriately compensated since they are being asked to undertake additional complex work. These staff are already over worked and under paid, and their investment in the project is key to success. This implies that funding support for ARTmail and evaluation activities need to budget for this.
- Evaluation design and implementation
  - Sample recruitment is key to a successful monitoring and evaluation component. The quantitative component of the current evaluation study was statistically under powered because many legally authorized representatives of the participating seniors gave consent for them to participate in ARTmail, but not in the evaluation component. Future efforts should make outreach and awareness raising among family members of cognitively impaired seniors a high priority.
  - The evaluation process itself needs a higher level of planning and support, that incorporates senior site staff perspectives from the outset. There needs to be enough trained volunteers (perhaps through collaboration with area Universities and Colleges) to assist with completing the baseline and endline assessment forms.
  - There needs to be more time spent on training, and on support throughout the project, which would promote staff understanding the various aspects of the project and lowering the rate of unanswered questions on the assessment form. Time needs to be devoted to promoting the understanding of the value of creative programming for seniors.

In conclusion, our pilot evaluation partnership results indicated that ARTmail is an activity that is enjoyed by seniors with cognitive limitations, and may improve their mood. The pilot partnership also yielded significant lessons to promote successful implementation and evaluation of this program in future: including the need for additional training, volunteers, and budget to compensate site staff. Creative programming is an under-explored activity that can improve the enjoyment and quality of life of seniors with cognitive limitations through non-pharmacological methods. As the population with dementia and related conditions is likely to expand greatly in the coming decades, programs and activities that improve seniors' quality of life beyond the needs of medical management, and that do not rely on pharmacological interventions, are vitally necessary. The ARTmail activity and its ongoing monitoring and evaluation are efforts toward increasing community capacity to meet that goal.

ACKNOWLEDGMENT

We thank the School of Human Environmental Sciences, and the Office of Leadership and Service Learning UNCG, for pilot funding for the evaluation. We thank all the student and community volunteers who enabled ARTmail. We are grateful to all the site staff for facilitating this activity for seniors and the evaluation. We are grateful to all the senior participants of ARTmail and the pilot evaluation.

REFERENCES

[1]   Alzheimer's Association. Alzheimer's disease facts and figures. Alzheimers Dement 2003;7(2).

[2]   Cohen GD, Perlstein S, Chapline J, Kelly J, Firth KM, Simmens S. The Impact of professionally conducted cultural programs on the physical health, mental health, and social functioning of older adults. Gerontologist 2006;46(6):726–34.

[3]   Cohen GD. Research on creativity and aging: the positive impact of the arts on health and illness. Generations 2006;XXX(1):7-15.

[4]   Greaves CJ, Farbus L. Effects of creative and social activity on the health and well-being of socially isolated older people: outcomes from a multi-method observational study. Perspect Public Health 2006;126(3): 134-42.

[5]   Rusted J, Sheppard L, Waller D. A multi-centre randomized control group trial on the use of art therapy for older people with dementia. Group Analysis. 2006;39(4):517-36.

[6]   Hays RD, DiMatteo, MR. A short-form measure of loneliness. J Pers Assess 1987;51(1):69-81.

[7]   Kinney JM, Rentz CA. Observed well-being among individuals with dementia: memories in the making, an art program, versus other structured activity. Am J Alzheimers Dis Other Demen 2005;20(4): 220–7.

[8]   Sheikh JI, Yesavage JA. Geriatric depression scale (GDS): recent evidence and development of a shorter version. In: Brink TL, ed. Clinical gerontology: A guide to assessment and intervention. New York: Haworth, 1987:165-73.

[9]   Catalani, C, Minkler M. Photovoice: a review of the literature in health and public health. Health Educ Behav 2010;37:424-51.

[10]   Wang C, Burris MA. Photovoice: concept, methodology, and use for participatory needs assessment. Health Educ Behav 1997;24:369-87.

[11]   Wiersma, EC. Using photovoice with people with early–stage Alzheimer's disease: a discussion of methodology. Dementia 2011;10: 203-16.

[12]   Alexopoulos GA, Abrams RC, Young RC, Shamoian CA. Cornell scale for depression in dementia. Biol Psychol 1988;23:271-84.

[13]   Logsdon RG, McCurry SM, Teri L. Evidence-based interventions to improve quality of life for individuals with dementia. Alzheimers Care Today 2007;8(4):309–18.

In: Public Health Yearbook 2013
Editor: Joav Merrick

ISBN: 978-1-63321-095-0
© 2014 Nova Science Publishers, Inc.

Chapter 35

PARTNERING TO ADDRESS THE RELENTLESS STI EPIDEMIC: A UNIQUE COLLABORATION BETWEEN THE JAIL, LOCAL AND STATE HEALTH DEPARTMENTS, AND AN ACADEMIC HEALTH CENTER IN DOUGLAS COUNTY, NEBRASKA

Ruth Margalit, MD[1]*, Mary Earley[2], Jillian Fickenscher[1], Raees Shaikh[1], Austin Person[1], Kari Simonsen[1], Monirul Islam[1], Kathy Kaiser[3], Uriel Sandkovsky[4], Adi Pour[5], Elizabeth Berthold[5] and Mark Foxall[2]

[1]Service Learning Academy, College of Public Health, University of Nebraska Medical Center, Nebraska Medical Center, Omaha, Nebrask, US
[2]Douglas County Department of Corrections, Omaha, Nebraska, US
[3]UNMC Department of Community-Based Health, College of Nursing, University of Nebraska Medical Center, Omaha, Nebraska, US
[4]UNMC Division of Infectious Diseases and HIV Clinic University of Nebraska Medical Center, Nebraska Medical Center, Omaha, Nebraska, US
[5]Douglas County Health Department, Douglas County Midtown Campus, Omaha, Nebraska, US

ABSTRACT

Douglas County, Nebraska, has high prevalence of sexually transmitted infections (STI) with Chlamydia trachomatis (CT) and Neisseria gonorrhoeae (NG) rates 30% and 88% higher than the rest of the nation, respectively. The local jail emerged as a crucial public health partner, positioned to facilitate interventions to reduce STI rates within its high

* Corresponding author: Ruth Margalit, MD, Associate Professor and Director Inter-Professional Service Learning Academy, Room 2038, Maurer Center for Public Health, University of Nebraska Medical Center, 986075 Nebraska Medical Center Omaha NE 68198-4375 United States. Email: rmargalit@unmc.edu.

risk population, joining the effort to combat the high STI prevalence in the region. Criminal justice populations are at disproportionately higher risk for STI, with less access to STI screening. Objective: Develop an innovative program addressing the problem, through collaboration between the jail, local health departments, public health agencies, and the Service Learning Academy at the College of Public Health. Methods: Health-profession students offered STI education, screening and treatment to jail inmates. They coordinated their peers, interacted directly with jail authorities and the local and state health departments, provided education and treatment under clinical supervision. Students used a succession leadership plan to ensure continuity and sustainability of the program. Over 1500 inmates have been provided education and over 1000 screened so far. Conclusion: Strong commitment, multi-sectorial expertise, and effective collaboration have ensured the implementation of this program, which is intended to test and disseminate best practices for universal screening in jails and assist in establishing effective policy. The program presents an opportunity for health professions students to develop public health knowledge, along with organizational, communication and leadership skills, while engaging in hands-on interprofessional education and practice, ultimately leading to personal and professional growth.

Keywords: Sexually transmitted infections, jail, screening, service learning, collaboration

INTRODUCTION

It started with a phone call; Deputy Director Mark Foxall, now current Director of the local jail said: "We need to talk! There is an STI epidemic in the city, we see the most risky population passing through our facility, and you are doing various service learning projects. My Captain Mary Earley is on board and will facilitate the process. When can we work together?" So we scheduled a meeting and got together at the jail. At the urging of the local Douglas County Health Department Health Director, this group had met several times to discuss the problem and was now ready for action.

The population of incarcerated individuals in jails and prisons in the United States represent a unique group of underserved and medically-vulnerable individuals, which poses a challenge for public health within the correctional system. Inmates are more at-risk for multiple health problems due to limited access to health care both prior to incarceration and following release, variable disease specific maintenance practices, and social stigma (1). Incarcerated individuals especially carry a disproportionately high risk of sexually transmitted infections (STI) due to precarious sexual behavior, lack of access to routine screening, and lack of access to treatment (2). Accessing this high-risk population provides unique opportunities for health promotion and disease prevention within incarceration facilities. Creatively utilizing the relatively short length of stay for inmates in correctional facilities (an average of two to three months in jails, ranging from a few hours to over one year), effective programs for prevention education, screening, diagnosis, and treatment within these settings have the potential to reduce the rates of diseases not only within the facilities, but also, and importantly, in the communities they serve (3). However, many correctional centers do not have stand-alone capacity to implement comprehensive programs such as STI screening and treatment for their population (4). This paper describes a unique partnership developed to address the high STI rates in the County, reflecting on lessons learned in building capacity to address this persistent public health problem in our area, and providing recommendations for future direction.

The incarcerated population

Today there are approximately 2.3 million people incarcerated in United States jails and prisons, compared to just 500,000 in 1980 (5). This group typically lack regular medical care while at higher risk than the general population for many diseases (6). The incarcerated population is primarily male (about 90%) with a growing female segment (1). A disproportionate number of the incarcerated individuals come from racial and ethnic minority groups, with African-Americans and Latinos being especially over-represented (3, 5, 7). Many sources note that of these 2.3 million, a vastly disproportionate number come from low social economic status, face poverty circumstances, unemployment, and have low education or literacy levels, with 68% having no high school degree(1,8). Wang et al. (1) noted that 11% of inmates were homeless prior to incarceration, and were more likely to have been a victim of sexual assault (9). Additionally, many inmates lead a risky lifestyle prior to incarceration such as drug and/or alcohol abuse and unsafe sex practice (3). These compounded risk factors make it even more significant to have screening, treatment, and education programs for STI available at correctional facilities like jails.

STI rates in jails and prisons

Despite the publication of several studies measuring and monitoring the prevalence of STI in jail and prison systems, Sosman et al. (10) noted that STI systematic national surveillance is lacking in incarcerated settings. Summarized data from smaller local and regional studies indicate that the prevalence rate for human immunodeficiency virus (HIV) is 4 times higher for incarcerated persons than for the general US population; the hepatitis C virus (HCV) rate is 9 to 10 times higher, and STI rates at the time of intake into jail or prison were as high as 35% (10). Approximately 30% of all new hepatitis B virus (HBV) infections occur in individuals with a history of incarceration (10) (11). Nevertheless, Barry et al. (12) noted that even with these high rates and documented high-risk behaviors, incarcerated adults might not be screened because of limited access and multiple barriers to adequate health care, inside and outside of the jail system.

In 1996, the Centers for Disease Control (CDC) began monitoring the prevalence of major STI in various large correctional facilities in the United States, which became known as the 'Jail Sexually Transmitted Disease(STD) Prevalence Monitoring Project' (13, 14). These data from the CDC and various other smaller studies in the U.S. showed that among inmates, prevalence of the three most commonly reported bacterial STI – chlamydia, gonorrhea, and syphilis – was far greater than in the general population (14). Per a CDC report in 2010, the overall chlamydia positivity among adult men and women entering corrections facilities in 2009 was 6.6% and 7.2%, respectively. The overall Gonorrhea positivity for men and women entering adult corrections facilities in 2009 was 1.2% and 1.6% respectively (15). Kraut-Becher et al. (16) reported much higher prevalence ranges for chlamydia (1-27% in women and 1-21% in men) and gonorrhea (0.2-17% in women and from 0.1-32% in men) compared to the non-incarcerated population, but these vary depending on the baseline prevalence in the local community population, and with the type of screening tests that are used.

Mertz et al. (2) importantly note that while the prevalence of STIs in the incarcerated population is very high, most of these infections are asymptomatic and therefore cannot be detected without routine screening. Analysis of data from the CDC's 'Jail STD Prevalence Monitoring Project' showed that of all males who tested positive for Chlamydia, only 2.7% of adolescent boys and 2.9% of adult men reported any symptoms, and of males who tested positive for Gonorrhea, only 7.3% (adolescents) and 9.6% (adults) reported symptoms (2). Consequently, if STI testing is performed only for those who report symptoms, over 90% of these infections will go untreated, leading to a subsequently increased transmissions to the sexual partners in the community (2).

Realizing the potential benefit to screening and prevention programs within correctional centers, National Screening Guidelines for Correctional Health Care Systems were developed by the CDC that call for routine universal screening of adolescent and adult females up to age 35 (but not males) for Chlamydia and Gonorrhea at the time of admission to juvenile detention or jail facilities (8). The National Commission on Correctional Health Care (NCCHC) recommends "offering universal, routine screening to all inmates in corrections facilities regardless of behavioral risk profile for STI (14).

Despite these well-supported recommendations, the implementation of these guidelines remains elective and varies from state to state (1). Only 17% of prison systems and 4% of jail systems have mandatory or routine Gonorrhea screening, and 20% and 4% provide Chlamydia screening, respectively (4). The more common approach to testing for STI in correctional facilities is testing only those who are symptomatic. However, this approach is not sufficient since the majority of these infections are asymptomatic and therefore likely to go undetected, untreated with the risk for ongoing transmission (2,8).

STI rates in Douglas County, Omaha Nebraska (NE):

Chlamydia trachomatis (CT) and Neisseria gonorrhoeae (NG) have been a concern for public health officials in Douglas County, Nebraska for the greater part of the last decade. According to the Douglas County Health Department (DCHD) statistics (17), the CT rate in Douglas County in 2009 was 527.5 per 100,000 population as compared to 305.2 for the state and 409.2 for the nation.

Similarly, the rate for NG was 186.6 per 100,000 population for the Douglas County (when Nebraska was - 77.2 and the US - 99.1 per 100,000 population respectively). In the majority of zip codes in the county, average CT rates have remained at =500 per 100,000 population and NG rates at =100 per 100,000 population for the past five years (17).

Since 2004, the Douglas County Board of Health declared epidemic rates of both CT and NG, with rates in 2009 more than 30% and 88% higher respectively than the rest of the nation (17), and including significant disparities in infection rates, with almost 62 % (585/940) of NG infections reported among African Americans, compared to 17% among whites and 4% among Hispanics. Similarly, 45.4% reported CT infections, were in African Americans, 27.9% in Whites, and 9.4 % in Hispanics (17).

STI in the Douglas County Department of Corrections (DCDC)

The DCDC serves the greater Omaha metro area with a population of over 1 million citizens. The facility provides secure detention for local arrestees and per diem housing for surrounding counties, the United States Marshall and Immigration and Customs Enforcement detainees. The DCDC has the capacity to house an average daily population of over 1500. According to DCDC health records (17) there is an average prevalence rate of 6.1% for CT

2.5 % for NG, 0.2% for HBV and about 10% for HCV. These rates are based on the current system wherein individuals are tested for STI and HIV only when they self-identify high risk behaviors, known exposure, and/or complain of symptoms. No real prevalence has been obtained.

Currently, all DCDC inmates receive a medical intake screening within two hours of their arrival. The screening serves to identify overall health status as well as urgent/emergent and non-urgent medical, dental, or mental health conditions that require follow-up care. The DCDC also offers an optional education program for STI and HIV, but no universal screening for CT/NG is currently available, thus true prevalence cannot be determined.

Because jails have a high turnover rate of inmates coming and going out of the community (3), correctional health care holds the potential for significant public health impact. Within their system, jails screen, educate and treat large numbers of individuals, with a high-risk for STI who may have little access to testing anywhere else (18). Awareness of the STI epidemic in Omaha coupled with the vision for the role of the jail in promoting the public's health, the DCDC staff was challenged by the local health director to partner and help address the persistent public health problem in Douglas County, considering new collaborations, new policies, and devoting significant resources to this effort.

The DCDC STI Project and pilot universal screening

In March of 2008, the DCDC Director initiated communication with the Service Learning Academy (SLA) that operates from and is supported by the College of Public Health at the University of Nebraska Medical Center (UNMC). The question posed was how the jail, in concert with the academic health center and the public health practice, could take a role in leading a collaboration to address the county's unrelenting high rates of STI. With this program, students and faculty from medicine, nursing, pharmacy, allied health, public health and informatics collaborated on the development and implementation of the education, screening, and treatment program. In over two months of intense meetings, a unique partnership was formed and included the following members: Douglas County Department of Corrections, the Douglas County Health Department (DCHD), NE Department of Health and Human Services (NDHHS), the NE Public Health Laboratory (NPHL), Correct Care Solutions (CCS – DCDCs contracted medical provider), Nebraska Aids Project, University of Nebraska Omaha (UNO), College of Information Science and Technology, the Service Learning Academy with student leaders and faculty advisors from the academic medical center, UNMC. Funds for CT and NG laboratory testing for this project were provided by Nebraska Department of Health and Human Services in collaboration with Douglas County Health Department and Nebraska Public Health Laboratory. Treatment medications were provided by NDHHS.

With a commitment to reduce rates of STI in the jail population and ultimately in the community, the OPT-IN program for education, screening, and treatment for CT and NG, was initiated. The program was developed as an educational experience for students, under the umbrella of the SLA, with students, faculty, jail, and other organizations involved in management and collaborative leadership. It has quickly grown into a noted exercise in public health and community collaboration, providing health professions' students with valuable clinical and public health experience. The collaborative planning process helped to establish a strong foundation for an effective sustainable partnership.

To date, over 120 students have made more than 50 visits to the jail, providing education to over 1500 inmates, and testing over 1000 individuals. Infection rates within this opt-in program were measured at 5.5% for CT and 0.8% for NG. When positive, inmates were treated accordingly by the students, with clinical supervision. In addition, those participating in the education session but who opted out of testing were surveyed to better understand their decision for not participating.

All students were required to go through a background check and complete a four-hour orientation course at the jail, after which they received a 'blue badge'. The blue identification badge provides access to the secure side of the jail and permits students to enter and leave the jail without an officer to escort them. On Saturday mornings, teams of three to 16 health professions student volunteers enter the jail housing units (with 30-62 inmates in each unit) to deliver STI education, followed by opt-in collection of urine samples for CT/NG screening. Education topics during the sessions include STI transmission, preventive measures, signs and symptoms of infection, and treatment options. Collected urine samples are then processed by the students at the jail medical department and sent to the NPHL. Results are retrieved from the Electronic Lab Information Report in Technology (ELIRT) in 2-4 days. Students offer treatment and individual counseling to those tested positive, with supervision of clinical faculty. A new data management system where inmate data are securely collected, was developed with assistance with the University of Nebraska Omaha, College of Information Science and Technology faculty and students. The secure database also allows tracking of re-admissions in order to prevent unnecessary testing.

Even though the rates found in voluntary testing within the DCDC were higher than the epidemic rates in the surrounding community at large, this screening program did not provide the true prevalence of STIs in DCDC, but represented a convenient sample of those opting-in for testing at various housing units. Thus, the concerned partners sought input from experts around the country who have experience with similar programs in the jail setting and developed a pilot program: This program was designed to provide an estimate of the actual STI rates in DCDC, provide information on risk factors for STI (such as drug abuse and sexual behavior among inmates), and to test the feasibility of such a universal program at the jail. Over a one-week time frame urine CT/NG screening was completed for every inmate who entered the jail at the time of admission. During this one week universal STI screening program implemented by the jail, a total of 310 inmates participated. Ongoing testing was implemented round the clock and was incorporated into the flow of the regular intake process. Thirty inmates (10%) tested positive for CT and 3 inmates (1.3%) tested positive for NG. The results from this week were much higher than in the opt-in program and further demonstrated the need for and the potential public health impact of universal screening and treatment within the county jail. The jail is using this data as a first step in determining feasibility for universal STI screening.

Lessons learned

The whole experience was very interesting to me. I would like to learn more about how we could help this population once we get their vital statistics. I would like to learn more about the role of the nurses in that particular setting. I would like to learn more about why the population has such an STD problem, which motivational strategies are lacking. (Nursing student)

A key element in health care quality improvement is to enhance communication between professions. One strategy used in our medical center is interprofessional service learning. Service-Learning (SL) is a structured learning experience that combines community service with preparation and reflection. Students engaged in SL provide community service in response to identified concerns and learn about the context in which service is provided, the connection to their academic coursework and their role as citizens. SL benefits both the provider and the recipient and is often called reciprocal learning. Perhaps the greatest value of this program is found in its mutually beneficial nature. Through this project, students are able to develop skills that are difficult to master, such as taking a sexual history. In addition, students hone presentation and patient education skills in discussing sensitive topics like sexually transmitted diseases with inmates who may have little or no health literacy; and in the event of a positive infection, students learn how to provide a patient with difficult or unwelcome news, explain treatment and administer it. From testing to treatment, ordering to sample processing, dispensing to administering medications, students engage in every aspect of the care that these patients receive. As the impact of this project has grown, so has campus interest in participation. Following the lead of UNMC leaders and administrators, this project has sought to create more of a collaborative environment by making it more interprofessional and including students from multiple pre-professional programs on campus. Recently, background check forms were filled out and returned to jail administrators by more than 60 new students interested in participating from UNMC professional programs.

Sufficiently addressing the STI epidemic locally will require support for universal screening. Health professions students can participate in such service, working together with jail and public health authorities while gaining a valuable experience. The program presents a tremendous opportunity for health professions students to develop public health knowledge, expanding specific knowledge of STI (prevention, screening, treatment), and developing organizational, communication, and leadership skills. Through this project, students also have the opportunity to engage in hands-on interprofessional education and practice leading to personal and professional growth. Inmates benefit from the exposure to medical profession students who are enthusiastic, idealistic, and ready to learn firsthand about determinants of health, ridding of stereotypical beliefs about inmates, and gaining skills necessary to collaborate with various professions. Community academia partnership (i.e., jail, health department and the medical center) proved to be a powerful vehicle to address complex public health issues.

> This was an eye opener for me, the experience to see what a jail is like and how healthcare fits into the jail population. I should not judge the people in jail for being dangerous people because many of them didn't necessarily do dangerous things to get them there. I need to keep in mind that not everyone in jail will have an STD. It's a common thing in society to see people in jail as "dirty". (Nursing students)

Challenges and barriers to care in the correctional system

Even with guidelines and recommendations for STI screening in place, many correctional facilities face challenges and barriers to providing ideal prevention and health care within their system. Most correctional facilities do not consider public health activities to be part of their mandate (2) and many face a shortage of staff, space, laboratory facilities, ability for partner notification, and other logistic and financial barriers for such activity (1, 19). Current budget restrictions can also significantly impact a facility's ability to provide much needed services.

> As a result of this experience, I will be more aware of the health care needs of the jail population. (MPH student)

RECOMMENDATIONS

The primary future goal of this initiative is the development of a universal OPT-OUT STI program, including HBV/HCV, and HIV education, screening, testing, and vaccination at DCDC, with a linkage to care for released individuals. The program will continue to build on the existing and ongoing OPT-IN pilot screening program, which helped establish a strong collaborative and effective partnership among the participants. The plan is to develop a secure specialized interactive information system, facilitating efficient coordination between all components, processes, and participants of the program, allowing quick retrieval of data necessary for patient follow-up and treatment planning, as well as providing timely reports to assist in the facilitation of in-time programming, monitoring, and evaluation of both the OPT-IN and OPT-OUT programs. The idea is to utilize small mobile devices that can be used in the screening area, housing units, or medical department of the DCDC. This comprehensive strategy will only be realized with a combination of funding sources, including extramural granting agencies, and ongoing collaborative, and in kind support from the current cadre of partners and stakeholders.

The collaborative, community-focused nature of this program lays the foundation for moving this initiative outside the DCDC and into other community-based agencies or partnerships which likewise share the vision of improving the public's health, through the reduction in the rates of STI in our community.

CONCLUSION

The current OPT-IN strategy is already making a difference for inmates, who have been educated, tested, and treated through the DCDC STI program, and possibly their partners. Individuals who would otherwise have been difficult to reach, or may not have been aware of their risk or able to seek care for STI, have been identified, tested and treated by the volunteers in this program. The increase in student participation over the years exemplifies the interest and dedication to continuing this effective program.

The pilot feasibility screening project has demonstrated that even greater numbers of infected persons can be identified and treated with a routine testing strategy. The epidemic rates of STI in our community highlight the importance of assisting correctional facilities to align with the CDC recommendations calling for universal testing and treatment of STI. The broad-based support and collaboration from our myriad partners, including health professions student participation, demonstrated the dedication to providing the care necessary to improve the health of the incarcerated patient as well as the community.

ACKNOWLEDGMENTS

We are grateful for the vision, trust, dedicated effort, and the relentless commitment of the following members of our team: Barbara Glaser – Douglas County Department of Corrections Education and Programs Manager; Chris Brown MPH – founder student Board president; Jessica Ott MD candidate - past student Board president; Brady Fickenscher MD candidate - past student Board president; Tammy Bursovsky – Health Services Administration, Correct Care Solutions, Douglas County Department of Corrections; Dean Collier PharmD, past faculty supervisor; each and every committed medicine, nursing, pharmacy and public health students who participated early Saturday mornings and late Thursday nights, despite their hectic schedule and pending exams. Thanks to this program we have learned to know and appreciated each other's role and now have a stronger commitment to public health.

Hearing the officer talk about the inmates was good because it helped me to realize how in need this population is. I believe this realization was important for me because it took me out of the role of feeling like a student that is trying to complete an assignment and began to help me transition into the role of being a health professional. I was surprised to learn that though a general structure had already been devised, we were all encouraged to look for ways to make improvements. We were going to have an opportunity to mold this into something we could be proud of. I am excited for the months ahead in the jail. This is an awesome opportunity to impact a real life public health issue. Medical Student)

REFERENCES

[1]   Wang EA, White MC, Jamison R, Goldenson J, Estes M, Tulsky JP. Discharge planning and continuity of health care: Findings from the San Francisco County Jail. Am J Public Health 2008;98(12):2182–4.

[2]   Mertz KJ, Voigt RA, Hutchins K, Levine WC. Findings from STD screening of adolescents and adults entering corrections facilities: Implications for STD control strategies. Sex Transm Dis 2002;29(12):834.

[3]   Goldenson J, Hennessey M. Correctional health care must be recognized as an integral part of the public health sector. Sex Transm Dis 2009;36(2):S3.

[4]   Hammett TM. Sexually transmitted diseases and incarceration. Curr Opin Infect Dis 2009;22(1):77.

[5]   Minton TD. Jail inmates at Midyear 2010. Statistical Tables, 2011.

[6]   Beckwith CG, Zaller ND, Fu JJ, Montague BT, Rich JD. Opportunities to diagnose, treat, and prevent HIV in the criminal justice system. J Acquir Immune Defic Syndr 2010;55(Suppl 1):S49-55.

[7]   US Census Bureau. US Quick Facts–US Census Bureau. Retrieved from http://www.prb.org/Articles/2002/JustHowManyBabyBoomersAreThere.aspx 2011.

[8]   Workowski KA, Berman SM, Warts G, Proctitis P. Sexually transmitted diseases treatment guidelines, 2010. MMWR 2010;59(RR-12):1-110.

[9]   Barry PM, Kent CK, Scott KC, Goldenson J, Klausner JD. Is jail screening associated with a decrease in Chlamydia positivity among females seeking health services at community clinics?-San francisco, 1997-2004. Sex Transm Dis 2009;36(2 Suppl):S22-8.

[10]   Sosman J, MacGowan R, Margolis A, Gaydos CA, Eldridge G, Moss S, et al. Sexually Transmitted Infections and Hepatitis in Men With a History of Incarceration. Sex Transm Dis 2011;38(7):634.

[11]   Spaulding AC, Arriola KR, Hammett T, Kennedy S, Tinsley M. Rapid HIV testing in rapidly released detainees: next steps. Sex Transm Dis 2009;36(2 Suppl):S34-6.

[12]   Barry PM, Kent CK, Scott KC, Goldenson J, Klausner JD. Is jail screening associated with a decrease in Chlamydia positivity among females seeking health services at community clinics?-San francisco, 1997-2004. Sex Transm Dis 2009;36(2 Suppl):S22-8.

[13]   Kahn RH, Mosure DJ, Blank S, Kent CK, Chow JM, Boudov MR, et al. Chlamydia trachomatis and Neisseria gonorrhoeae prevalence and coinfection in adolescents entering selected US juvenile detention centers, 1997-2002. Sex Transm Dis 2005;32(4):255.

[14]   The health status of soon-to-be-released inmates, A report to Congress, 2002.

[15]   Centers for Disease Control and Prevention (CDC). Disparities in diagnoses of HIV infection between blacks/African Americans and other racial/ethnic populations--37 states, 2005-2008. MMWR 2011;60(4):93-8.

[16]   Kraut-Becher JR, Gift TL, Haddix AC, Irwin KL, Greifinger RB. Cost-effectiveness of universal screening for chlamydia and gonorrhea in US jails. J Urban Health 2004;81(3):453-71.

[17]   Douglas County Department of Health. STDs in Douglas County. 2010; Available at: http://www.douglascountyhealth.com/disease-a-immunization/sexually-transmitted-diseases. Accessed 02/05, 2011.

[18]   Barry PM, Kent CK, Scott KC, Snell A, Goldenson J, Klausner JD. Optimising sexually transmitted infection screening in correctional facilities: San Francisco, 2003–5. Sex Transm Infect 2007;83(5):416.

[19]   Chow JM, Joesoef MR, Kent C, Weinstock H, Fenton K. Responding to the burden of STD, HIV, and viral hepatitis in correctional populations through program collaboration and integration. Sex Transm Dis 2009;36(2):S1.

In: Public Health Yearbook 2013
Editor: Joav Merrick

ISBN: 978-1-63321-095-0
© 2014 Nova Science Publishers, Inc.

Chapter 36

THE MARTHA'S VINEYARD PUBLIC HEALTH SYSTEM RESPONDS TO 2009 H1N1

Melissa Ann Higdon and Michael A Stoto, PhD[*]

Department of Society, Human Development, and Health,
Harvard School of Public Health, Boston, Massachusetts and Department of Health
Systems Administration, Georgetown University, School of Nursing and Health Studies,
Washington DC, United States of America

ABSTRACT

The 2009 H1N1 pandemic required a concerted community response, involving public health agencies, health care providers, and other components of local public health emergency preparedness systems. This case study of the island of Martha's Vineyard (MV) in Massachusetts is based on a review of local newspapers, interviews with key stakeholders including local health agents; the MV hospital officials, and the MV school superintendent. This review illustrates the challenges of managing the distribution of vaccine when the timing and amount of vaccine to be delivered was uncertain and identifies a number of lessons about community resilience. In particular, it shows the need to balance precise policies with flexible implementation as well as the importance of local involvement in decision-making and increasing the transparency of communications. There were notable successes in the handling of the H1N1 epidemic on the Vineyard, especially with regards to mass dispensing of influenza vaccine. By pooling vaccine, sharing resources such as vaccination teams that would go from one school to another in a region and other means the Vineyard demonstrated the importance of strong community-wide partnerships. This case illustrates the importance of building community capacity to address persistent public health problems.

Keywords: Public health system, public health emergency preparedness, regionalization, H1N1, pandemic influenza

[*] Corresponding author: Michael A Stoto, PhD, Professor of Health Systems Administration and Population Health, Georgetown University School of Nursing and Health Studies, 3700 Reservoir Road, NW Room 236, Washington, DC 20057-1107 United States. Email: stotom@georgetown.edu.

INTRODUCTION

The Institute of Medicine defined the public health system as the "complex network of individuals and organizations that have the potential to play critical roles in creating the conditions for health" (1). For public health emergency preparedness (PHEP), this system includes not only federal, state and local health departments, but also hospitals and healthcare providers, fire departments, schools, the media, and many other public and private organizations (2). The 2009 H1N1 pandemic required a concerted effort from the entire US PHEP system, from the federal government down to local areas. Given the isolation of the community, residents of Martha's Vineyard (Islanders) were pressed to use existing community resources to address the H1N1 outbreak on the Vineyard, and the response involved several public health agencies, health care providers, and other components of local public health emergency preparedness systems.

This case study examines the community response in an island community. Limited resources, such as school nurses, were shared across the six diverse towns to enhance the community's capacity when responding to the outbreak. The school system came together with the hospital, town local public health entities, and organizations such as the Visiting Nurses Association to protect the health of Vineyard residents. These practical solutions that the Islanders on their own demonstrate the community resilience that is necessary to respond effectively to public health emergencies.

We present our analysis in three sections. First, to set the stage and provide context, we describe the Vineyard community and public health system that serves it. Next, we describe the system's response to the H1N1 pandemic, primarily in the Fall of 2009. We conclude the results section with an "after action analysis" of the response on the Vineyard. The discussion section that follows identifies five lessons that are potentially generalizable to other similar communities.

METHODS

This case study is based on a review of local newspapers and interviews with key stakeholders. First, we reviewed the two local newspapers, *The Martha's Vineyard Gazette* and the *Martha's Vineyard Times*, between May and December, 2009. We also reviewed *The Boston Globe* for H1N1 related material involving Massachusetts, Cape Cod, or Martha's Vineyard. We also draw on the Massachusetts H1N1 After Action Report/ Improvement Plan, which the authors helped to prepare.

We also interviewed key stakeholders on the Island in May 2010 and June 2011. The majority of the Martha's Vineyard (MV) local health agents were interviewed in a group, including the health agents from the towns of Tisbury, Edgartown, and Chilmark. We also interviewed the Chief Executive Officer, the Chief Nurse Executive, the lead Pharmacist, and the Employee Health and Infectious Disease Nurse from Martha's Vineyard Hospital. Finally, the MV School Superintendent was interviewed, as the schools had a large role in the island's vaccination program.

RESULTS

The Martha's Vineyard public health system

Martha's Vineyard is a 90 square mile island in Massachusetts with a year-round population of approximately 16,000. As one can see from Exhibit 1, the island is composed of six towns that, together with the town of Gosnold (population 75) on a separate group of islands, make up the entirety of Duke's County, Massachusetts.

While the Vineyard has a reputation based on its wealthy summer visitors, the year round population is comprised of mostly agricultural and service workers, with relatively low income and education in comparison to the rest of the state. A substantial number of the year-round residents are Brazilian and speak Portuguese as their primary language, and there is also a Native American community on the island known as the Wampanoag Tribe of Gay Head, located predominately in Aquinnah, the island's smallest and most rural town.

The public health system on the island is both formal and informal. Unlike in many other parts of the United States, Massachusetts counties have no role in public health or most administrative matters, meaning the six town boards of health have the primary responsibility for public health matters. The largest towns have a full-time Health Agent and up to two other staff members and the smallest towns have less than one full-time equivalent worker.

The 19-bed Martha's Vineyard Hospital (MVH), which is affiliated with the Massachusetts General Hospital (MGH) in Boston, is the only hospital on the island. Housing several hospital-owned physician practices (including the only obstetrics practice on the island) as well as one independent practice (Vineyard Pediatrics) and the Windemere nursing home, MVH is a major part of the island's public health system. The Vineyard Nursing Association (VNA) also plays a role in the local public health system, contracting individually with each town, with the exception of Aquinnah, for standard public health nursing services including immunizations and epidemiology.

The Wampanoag Health Service, which provides programs and services to members of the federally-recognized Indian tribe is another part is the island's public health system. The service's contract health program provides assistance to tribal members with purchasing comprehensive health services such as inpatient and outpatient care, hospital medical office visits, and pharmaceutical services. In 2009, Mr. Ron MacLaren managed the tribe's health affairs.

The Martha's Vineyard Regional High School (MVRHS) serves the entire island, as does one charter school that includes kindergarten through 12th grade. Five elementary schools exist on the island, ranging in size and composition. Tisbury, Edgartown, Chilmark, and Oak Bluffs each have one school and a regional elementary school in West Tisbury. Anticipating the second wave of H1N1 in the Fall of 2009, the school superintendent, Dr. James Weiss, appointed Dr. Michael Goldfein from Vineyard Pediatrics as the school system physician on a consulting basis.

Emergency preparedness efforts on Vineyard have been both formal and informal. In 2002, the Massachusetts Department of Public Health (MDPH) established seven regions and 15 sub-regions to coordinate emergency preparedness efforts (3). As one can see from Exhibit 2, The Cape and the Islands Emergency Preparedness Coalition, part of Region 5, encompasses Barnstable County (Cape Cod), Martha's Vineyard, and Nantucket.

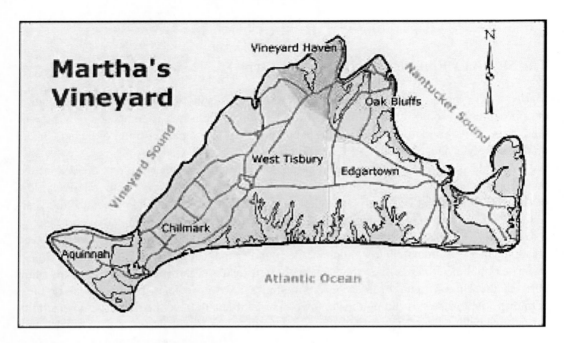

Exhibit 1. Map of Martha's Vineyard (12).

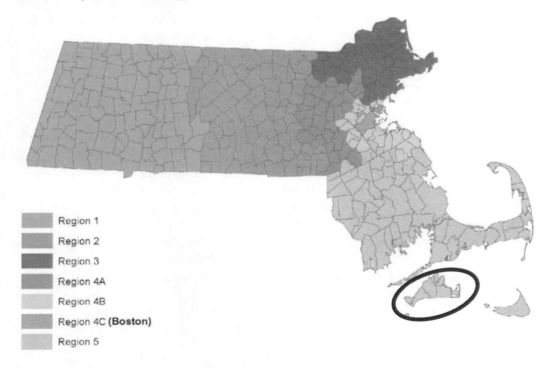

Exhibit 2. MDPH Emergency Preparedness Regional Coalitions (3).

In addition to the six town health departments, MVH was represented in the coalition's hospital preparedness efforts mainly through Carol Bardwell, the Chief Nurse Executive. The

Coalition has been the primary vehicle for Vineyard health departments and the hospital to access federal public health and hospital preparedness funds.

In addition, around 2005 the six towns and the Wampanoag Health Service formed the informal Martha's Vineyard Public Health Coalition (MVPHC) to strengthen communication among the six towns on the Vineyard and the Wampanoag tribe. In addition to regular meetings, the MVPHC's major activity has been to organize an annual island-wide seasonal influenza vaccine clinic, usually on the Veterans Day holiday (November 11).

MVH, VNA, and town emergency management agencies are brought in to the MVPHC's activities as needed. The Vineyard's public health system is characterized by the many informal connections that one finds on a small island. For instance, in addition to participating in the Cape and Islands Emergency Preparedness Coalition efforts, MVH Chief Nurse Executive Carol Bardwell is also a member of the island's Medical Reserve Corps (MRC) board, as are representatives of each of the six towns. Dr. Michael Goldfein, the leading practitioner at Vineyard Pediatrics, also serves as the school system physician. And Mr. David Caron, the MVH Director of Pharmacy also serves as a member of the Oak Bluffs board of health.

The public health response to 2009 H1N1

The first Massachusetts cases of H1N1 were seen in late April 2009 in Boston, shortly after the pandemic emerged in Mexico, California, and New York City (4). Because children seemed to be particularly at risk for infection, these and subsequent cases triggered a wave of school closings in Massachusetts and throughout the U.S. (5)

A second wave of the H1N1 epidemic was predicted for the fall, with children, young adults, and pregnant women to be most affected by the virus, triggering a national vaccination campaign (4). Vaccine deliveries were expected by late September or early October (4). In July, the Centers for Disease Control and Prevention's (CDC) Advisory Committee on Immunization Practices (ACIP) identified the following priority groups for the vaccine: pregnant women, children aged six months through 24 years, caregivers of children aged less than six months, and high risk/chronically ill individuals (6).

As the summer progressed, CDC encouraged the state health departments to develop plans for administering vaccine at the local level in their states (7). In late August, MDPH expanded its vaccine distribution program by building on the existing Vaccine for Children (VFC) program for pediatric vaccines and urged hospitals and other health care providers not already in the system to register to be able to receive H1N1 vaccine (8). In the registration process, MDPH asked for the number of individuals that would be vaccinated, but not more specific details such as the number of children. MDPH also alerted local health departments at this time to prepare mass dispensing plans (8).

Delays in vaccine production announced in late August and early September 2009 prompted MDPH to announce more specific "tiers" within the CDC priority groups (7). The first tier included pregnant women, children aged six months to five years old, caregivers of children aged less than six months, and healthcare workers (8). The second tier covered the remainder of CDC's priority groups: children aged five years old to 24 years old, emergency medical technicians, paramedics, and adults aged 25 to 65 in poor health (8).

In August, a 26-year-old Vineyard man of Brazilian descent developed severe flu-like symptoms and was treated at Martha's Vineyard Hospital. The diagnosis was not initially clear and tularemia, which is endemic on the Vineyard, was considered. MVH initiated a web-enabled consultation with physicians at their affiliate Massachusetts General Hospital, and as the patient's conditioned worsened, he was transferred to MGH, where he ultimately died on August 14 (9).

In September, in response to MDPH's recommendations, the Vineyard health agents collaborated with the VNA to register as one entity for five of the six towns on the island, and the Wampanoag Health Service registered for the tribe and the town of Aquinnah, where most tribal members live. MVH registered for its staff as well as the physician offices owned by the hospital. Vineyard Pediatrics, an independent physician practice co-located at the hospital, was previously registered to receive vaccine separately through the pre-existing childhood immunization system.

In addition, the town health agents and the VNA chose a single island-wide vaccination clinic at the regional high school, where previous seasonal flu clinics had been held, to administer both H1N1 and seasonal flu vaccine. As the planned date for the island-wide clinic neared, however, vaccine production delays were announced, and the clinic was postponed first until October 24th and eventually until November 11th, when only seasonal vaccine was administered.

In the last week of October, students at Martha's Vineyard Regional High School started to come down with flu-like symptoms. Absenteeism increased throughout that week and the next, and health officials assumed that this reflected students with influenza or students kept home by their parents out of concern they would be infected. The worst day for student absences was on Friday, October 30, when approximately 140 out of the 800 total MVRHS students were absent (10).

H1N1 vaccine started arriving on the island in late October, but only in small batches (8). Faced with a very different vaccine availability situation than had been expected, the Vineyard Public Health Coalition switched tactics. In a series of meetings in October with school superintendent Dr. James Weiss and the school system physician Dr. Michael Goldfein, a school-based approach was adopted. School officials chose to vaccinate students at their own school when it was in session to reach the most students. Because the schools did not have enough staff to vaccinate every student in a day, the MVPHC assembled "shooter teams" consisting of health officials and emergency medical services (EMS) staff from every town on the island as well as from the VNA that would go from school to school. The smaller schools – the Chilmark School and the Public Charter School – were done first, beginning November 9, when the amount of vaccine available was not sufficient for the larger schools. The larger schools were done later, when more vaccine became available.

Martha's Vineyard Hospital, meanwhile, had used its first doses of vaccine at a hospital-wide flu clinic on October 29, at which 209 hospital and Windemere nursing home staff were vaccinated. Rather than waste vaccine in multi-dose vials that had been opened, MVH also vaccinated emergency medical technicians and paramedics at this time (8). Having observed a fatal case at close range in August, the hospital CEO, Mr. Tim Walsh, wanted to be sure that the vaccine was used as soon as it became available. Because he assumed (incorrectly, as it turns out) that the towns were waiting to assemble enough vaccine to hold the island-wide clinic, MVH also took on the responsibility of vaccinating the pregnant women on the island (as the only obstetrics practice on the island was based at the hospital) and pre-school children on Saturday, October 31.

After action analysis

Overall, there were notable successes in how the Vineyard handled the H1N1 epidemic. Perhaps the most important achievement was the way the towns, the hospital, the tribe, the schools, and others came together as a resilient public health system and shared personnel and other resources across towns to protect the health of those on the island. For instance, with regard to mass dispensing, the decision to share personnel and resources across towns to constitute "shooter teams" was essential in vaccinating school children in a timely manner. Moreover, the decision to vaccinate the children attending smaller schools first and the children at larger schools as vaccine became available was easy to explain to the general public and was well accepted. It also represents an adroitly flexible response to uncertainty about when vaccine would arrive.

Despite concerted efforts, however, there were a number of problems that emerged as more vaccine became available in November. MVH, for instance, originally assumed that since it housed the island's only obstetrics practice, all pregnant women were covered in the hospital's October 31 clinic. Town health officials pointed out that some women received their prenatal care off island or were not covered at all. Vineyard Pediatrics, which had registered to receive vaccine separate from the hospital and the towns, committed to vaccinating its own patients. Confusion arose, however, about whether this should include the patients of Dr. Melanie Miller, who works at Vineyard Pediatrics but is a hospital employee. Although these problems were quickly resolved, they created confusion and frustration.

Many of these problems were the result of incomplete "situational awareness," that is knowledge of the scope of the outbreak and who had received vaccine supplies, as well as making assumptions about what others were planning to do with the vaccine they had. Despite best efforts, communication and coordination within the Vineyard public health system did not always run smoothly. Throughout the Fall, some of those involved felt that the hospital maintained a level of independence from the MVPHC. Town health agents, the VNA, the tribe, the schools, and public safety officers were generally represented at coalition meetings, but a hospital representative was less consistently present. Some health agents and school representatives felt there was a "one way relationship" with the hospital and the coalition. For instance, coalition members were frustrated when the hospital would ask the coalition for information about the location and number of H1N1 cases that they came into contact with, but would not provide information from their records to the coalition. The hospital sometimes cited the Health Insurance Portability and Accountability Act (HIPAA) Privacy Rule as a barrier to discussing the number and locations of H1N1 cases despite the Rule's public health exemption. This experience highlights the need to build trust within the public health system. If MVH and Vineyard Pediatrics had been more formally involved in the coalition's planning and response efforts, perhaps the response would have been better coordinated and its legitimacy higher in the public's eye.

MDPH's vaccine allocation process also contributed to situational awareness problems. Faced with an urgent need to rapidly increase the number of potential vaccinators, MDPH chose to adapt an existing registration system designed for the federal Vaccines for Children program. In this system, the allocation of vaccine to communities and registered vaccination sites was not determined by a public formula or algorithm. Rather, MDPH assessed the number of doses and formulation of each dose in the shipments received, and assigned them to registered vaccination sites based on the estimated numbers of people in priority groups eligible for the vaccine available. This approach allowed MDPH to use its judgment to ensure that allocation followed the epidemiology and was equitable (8). The downside of this approach was a lack of transparency. Sites compared the amounts of vaccine they received to the amounts received by neighboring providers but did not always understand why a particular site received more vaccine than they did. In addition, the resulting *ad hoc* system did not adequately account for the diversity of the sites to which the vaccine was being distributed. Dealing with approximately 4,500 registered sites state-wide, it was difficult for MDPH to know that the VNA had contracted to vaccinate children in the Vineyard schools rather than the elders that are typically served by visiting nursing associations. In addition, given that the hospital and Vineyard pediatrics were also registered, it also may not have been clear that the VNA was responsible for all of the island's school children since most Massachusetts towns registered individually. This became an issue when vaccine was in short supply and available in batches of 100. If the five towns had registered separately they might have received one batch each, whereas the VNA only received one. Thus another lesson from this experience is that more clarity is needed about the purpose of the registration process, as well as the implications for the amount of vaccine supplied to each registered site. Moreover, in the future more detailed demographic information on the population served by the registered site should be collected from the point of registration.

More generally, this experience reflects MDPH's inability to recognize informal regional public health systems (3) even if they are "natural" like the island of Martha's Vineyard. For instance, Vineyard officials could have coordinated their efforts better if they knew how much and what kinds of vaccine were coming to the island. Even though Ron MacLaren, director of the Wampanoag Health Service, became known as the voice of the Vineyard, the state health department was not able to report on the amount of vaccine that had been delivered to the island. Rather, the MDPH vaccine distribution system produced reports only for the formally-designated emergency preparedness regions such as the Cape and the Islands Coalition.

DISCUSSION

Overall, there were five lessons suggested by the H1N1 experience on the Vineyard. First, the case illustrates the challenges of managing a public health crisis under uncertain conditions. For instance, Vineyard officials, as in many other state and local public health systems, had been preparing for years for mass dispensing of vaccines or other counter measures in public health emergencies. Consistent with such planning, and based on federal and state assurances in the summer and early fall that vaccine would be produced and delivered in large amounts starting in early October, MDPH adopted a mass-dispensing approach to the 2009 H1N1 vaccination effort by sharply increasing the number of registered vaccination sites and trained vaccinators (8). Initially, the Vineyard planned to use a single Island-wide mass dispensing site, as called for in public health emergency plans. The reality, of course, is that vaccine did not arrive nearly as quickly or in as large numbers as had been promised, and demand waned after the perception developed that the crisis has passed. Since some future public health emergencies may be more like 2009 H1N1 than the acute events on which many planning assumptions are based, plans should be developed for situations emerge over extended periods of time and are characterized by uncertainty.

The second lesson is the need for more community involvement in decision-making and program management. In order to maximize H1N1 vaccine delivery capacity, MDPH rapidly expanded the number of sites registered to receive vaccine in the summer of 2009 (8). They achieved this by building on an existing system used to allocate state-purchased childhood vaccines under the federal Vaccines for Children program, which was used to distribute vaccines to over one thousand registered sites shortly after it arrived in the state (8). As the Vineyard case demonstrates, though, the downside of this approach is that the registration system did not include complete information on the population served by each registered site or provide any information on the number and types of vaccine that had been delivered to the Vineyard. As a result, no one either at MDPH or on the Island had the information they needed to coordinate local efforts to share vaccines or to ensure that the available vaccine was going where it was most needed.

The third lesson is the need to balance clear and precise policies with flexible implementation, taking into account the local situation. When the H1N1 vaccine was in short supply, clear definitions of priority groups were essential to ensure that the available supply went to those most in need. The case illustrates how Vineyard officials were grateful that MDPH established tiers within CDC's vaccine priority groups (7). On the other hand, lack of clarity about the definition of "healthcare worker" or the intended uses of vaccine allocated to hospitals caused problems. Should opened batches of vaccine left over at the end of a school clinic be used for the emergency medical services (EMS) workers who helped with the clinic, even if they are not in MDPH's first tier? The entire PHEP system – from the federal and state level down to the local level – needs a shared understanding of the situation and situational awareness. Similarly, the fourth lesson is the critical importance of increasing both the transparency and clarity of communications. Beyond the issues of the vaccine allocation process, the case also illustrates the importance of not assuming that informal communication channels are either accurate or complete. For instance, MVH believed that MVPHC was still planning a single island-wide H1N1 clinic even after the focus had switched to school-based plan. In addition, parents were confused about whether their children should be immunized at school, at the hospital's preschool clinic, or by Vineyard Pediatrics and whether it mattered which doctor's patient they were.

Finally, the Vineyard case provides many examples of the fifth lesson, which is how trusting relationships can enhance – and their absence impede – an effective public health emergency response. Trusting relationships are also central to the effectiveness of regional activities, as discussed above in the discussion of "local" involvement in decision-making and program management. For instance, the Vineyard experience illustrates the importance of encouraging and enhancing relationships among all of the organizations connected with health, including school nurses, hospitals, and EMS. The Island's approach to pooling resources in the form of vaccine as well as "shooter" teams that moved from the small to the larger schools as vaccine came available, would not have been possible without everyone involved trusting that this was the most appropriate way to ensure that the most populations were best protected.

CONCLUSION

Although the specifics of the Vineyard's public health "system" are unique, it clearly illustrates both the challenges posed by 2009 H1N1 and lessons learned in building community capacity to address persistent public health problems. By pooling vaccine, sharing resources such as vaccination teams that would go from one school to another in a region, and other means the Vineyard demonstrated the importance of strong community-wide partnerships. It is of course impossible to know what would have happened if the system had responded in a less coordinated way, but it seems likely that public concerns might have been greater and the public health system's credibility undermined. In particular, this case illustrates the need for clear and precise policies that can be implemented flexibly, taking into account the local situation.

The entire PHEP system – from the federal and state level down to the local level – needs a shared understanding of the situation and situational awareness. More generally, the challenges of managing under uncertainty coupled with the need to coordinate regionally, call for improvements in the public health's system's social capital, "networks of interpersonal trust and norms of mutual aid and reciprocity ... that act as resources for individuals and facilitate collective action" (11). Although far from perfect, the Vineyard's collective response to 2009 H1N1 pandemic illustrates both the value of previous investments in building social capital as well as the need for more.

April 21-27	CDC and Mexico issue alerts regarding novel influenza virus strain, WHO raises pandemic threat level
May 1	First Massachusetts H1N1 cases diagnosed in Boston
May	Vaccine production begins, CDC announces that the first doses are expected to be delivered in late September or early October
June 2	First case of H1N1 confirmed on Martha's Vineyard
July 29	CDC ACIP issues priority groups for 2009 H1N1 vaccine
August 14	26 year-old Vineyard man dies of H1N1
August 27	MDPH encourages as many sites as possible to register to receive H1N1 vaccine, alerts local health departments to prepare mass dispensing plans
September 14	MDPH issues guidance identifying two tiers within the ACIP high priority group
September 26	Planned island-wide seasonal and H1N1 vaccine clinic postponed
October 24	Planned island-wide seasonal and H1N1 vaccine clinic postponed
October 28	First noticeable H1N1-related school absenteeism on Martha's Vineyard
October 29	MVH and VNA vaccine staff and EMS workers with direct patient contact
October 31	MVH hold vaccine clinics for pregnant women and pre-school children
November 9	H1N1 vaccine clinics held at the Chilmark, West Tisbury and Martha's Vineyard Public Charter Schools
November 11	Island-wide vaccine clinic conducted with seasonal vaccine only
November 20	H1N1 vaccine clinic held at Tisbury School

Exhibit 3. 2009 H1N1 timeline.

ACKNOWLEDGMENTS

This article was developed with funding support awarded to the Harvard School of Public Health under a cooperative agreement with the US Centers for Disease Control and Prevention (CDC) grant number 5P01TP000307-01 (Preparedness and Emergency Response Research Center). The content of this publications as well as the views and discussions expressed in it are solely those of the authors and do not necessarily represent the views of the CDC or the US Department of Health and Human Services nor does mention of trade names, commercial practices, or organizations imply endorsement by the US Government.

The authors are grateful to the Martha's Vineyard officials interviewed for this case study, and for those who commented on earlier drafts of this report. In particular we would like to thank Maura Valley, the Assistant Health Agent from the town of Tisbury; Matthew Poole, the Health Agent from the town of Edgartown; and Marina Lent, the Health Administrator and Health Inspector from the town of Chilmark. We also thank the Martha's Vineyard Hospital staff that were interviewed, including Tim Walsh, the Chief Executive Officer; Carol Bardwell, the Chief Nurse Executive; David Caron, the lead Pharmacist; and Donna Enos, an Employee Health and Infectious Disease Nurse; MV School Superintendent, Jim Weiss; and John Grieb from the MDPH Emergency Preparedness Branch.

Another version of the events and analysis in this report will appear in a teaching case study in a book edited by Isaac Weisfuse and Linda Landesman: "Preparing public health to respond to disaster: Case studies" published by Jones and Bartlett Publishers, Burlington, MA.

REFERENCES

[1]   Institute of Medicine. The Future of the Public's Health in the 21st Century. Accessed 2011 July 15. URL: http://www.nap.edu/catalog.php?record_id=10548.

[2]   Institute of Medicine. Research Priorities in Emergency Preparedness and Response for Public Health Systems. Accessed 2011 July 18. URL: http://www.nap.edu/catalog.php?record_id=12136

[3]   Koh HK, Elqura LJ, Judge CM, Stoto MA. Regionalization of local public health systems in the era of preparedness. Annu Rev Publ Health 2008; 29:205-18.

[4]   Centers for Disease Control and Prevention. H1N1 Meeting the Challenge: A New Virus. Accessed 2011 July 11. URL: http://www.flu.gov/timeline/#event2

[5]   Massachusetts Department of Health and Human. H1N1 (Swine) Flu. Accessed 2011 August 5. URL: http://www.mass.gov/?pageID=eohhs2onlineservices&L=7&L0=Home&L1=Provider&L2=Guideline s+and+Resources&L3=Guidelines+for+Services+%26+Planning&L4=Diseases+and+Conditions&L5 =Influenza&L6=H1N1+%28Swine%29+Flu&f=H1N1+%28Swine%29+Flu_more&sid=Eohhs2

[6]   National Center for Immunization and Respiratory Diseases. Use of Influenza A (H1N1) 2009 Monovalent Vaccine Recommendations of the Advisory Committee on Immunization Practices. Accessed 2011 July 8. URL: http://www.cdc.gov/mmwr/preview/mmwrhtml/rr58e0821a1.htm/.

[7]   Centers for Disease Control and Prevention. 2009 H1N1 Vaccination Recommendations. Accessed 2011 July 13. URL: http://www.cdc.gov/h1n1flu/vaccination/acip.htm

[8]   Massachusetts Department of Health and Human Services. Guidelines for the Vaccination of Employees of Licensed Clinics, Dialysis Centers, Hospitals and Long Term Care Facilities Against Seasonal Influenza and Pandemic Influenza H1N1. Accessed 2011 August 5. URL: http://www.mass. gov/Eeohhs2/docs/dph/quality/hcq_circular_letters/dhcq_0908521_attachment.pdf

[9]   Massachusetts Department of Health and Human Services. State Health Officials Announce Eleventh
         Death. Accessed 2011 August 5. URL: http://www.mass.gov/?pageID=eohhs2pressrelease&L=4&L0
         =Home&L1=Government&L2=Departments+and+Divisions&L3=Department+of+Public+Health&si
         d=Eeohhs2&b=pressrelease&f=090817_h1n1_deaths&csid=Eeohhs2.

[10]   Seccombe M. Flu Hits High School Hard. Accessed 2011 July 7. URL: http://mvgazette.com/PDF1/
         VineyardGazette110609-1.pdf

[11]   Lochner K, Kawachi I, Kennedy BP. Social capital: a guide to its measurement. Health Place
         1999;5:259–70.

[12]   Hostel's International. Map of Martha's Vineyard. Accessed 2011 July 25. URL: http://www.
         hihostels.com/dba/hostels-HI---Martha-s-Vineyard-060011.en.htm

SECTION FOUR – HEALTH PROMOTION

In: Public Health Yearbook 2013
Editor: Joav Merrick

ISBN: 978-1-63321-095-0
© 2014 Nova Science Publishers, Inc.

Chapter 37

CHALLENGES, OPPORTUNITIES AND STRATEGIES IN MENTAL HEALTH PROMOTION IN CHINA: LITERATURE REVIEW OF MENTAL HEALTH PROMOTION MODELS

Jing Sun, PhD[1] and Nicholas Buys, PhD[2]*

[1]School of Medicine and Griffith Health Institute, Griffith University, Gold Coast campus, Parkland, Gold Coast, Australia
[2]School of Human Services and Social Work, and Griffith Health Institute, Griffith University, Parkland, Gold Coast, Australia

ABSTRACT

This paper reviews the issue of high levels of mental health problems among Chinese children. It argues that current strategies used to address these problems are inadequate. As an alternative it explores the potential for a socio-ecological approach, focussed on mental health promotion and prevention, to address resilience—an emerging area to promote mental health. A key insight in this paper is that mental health is determined by not only qualities of the individual child (i.e., cognitive and social competences) but also the characteristics of the systems in which children develop (i.e., a good sense of connectedness to family, peers and school community). The socio-ecological model, focussing on building children's skills, and placing greater emphasis on changing contexts and strengthening relationships, is seen as an effective approach to improve children's resilience, hence mental health. It is suggested that the socio-ecological approach should be used more widely in China to improve children's resilience and social and emotional wellbeing.

Keywords: Mental health promotion, resilience, China

---

* Corresponding author: Jing Sun, PhD, School of Medicine, Griffith University and Griffith Health Institute, Griffith University, Gold Coast campus, Parkland, Q4222 Australia. Email: j.sun@griffith.edu.au.

INTRODUCTION

In 1948, the World Health Organisation defined health as a 'state of complete physical, mental and social wellbeing and not merely the absence of disease of infirmity' (1). Unfortunately, this visionary conception did not guide research or service delivery in human health in China. Instead, the past half century showed a persistent focus on health from an illness and disease perspective, ignoring issues of psychological and social wellness. For example, during the period 1950 to 1990, public health efforts mainly focused on effective control of fatal communicable and infectious diseases, severe endemic diseases, severe infectious diarrhoea, infant pneumonia, and high morbidity and mortality caused by severe malnutrition. There is no doubt that this focus has resulted in a dramatic decrease in infant mortality and morbidity rates (2). However, we argue that mental health and social and emotional well-being should now be major components of health delivery, especially given the decline in communicable and infectious diseases in the more developed social-economic areas of China.

CURRENT MENTAL HEALTH PROBLEMS AND STRATEGIES IN CHINA

The burden of mental health problems appears to be increasing in China, adversely affect individuals, families and communities. This increase is associated with the rapid social and economic development and changes that have taken place over recent years (3). Mental health problems in China now rank fourth in morbidity after diseases such as cardiac diseases, diabetes, and cancer (4). Suicide, in association with depression, is now the primary cause of death for youth, with an increasing incidence in lower age groups as well. (5). The incidence of students who have mental health problems is now 16.4% for primary school students, and 14.2% for secondary school students (6).

Mental health issues for Chinese children relate to social and emotional problems and inability to adapt change and challenges (7). Poor relationships between children and parents and students and teachers compound feelings of loneliness and anxiety, and exacerbate hostile behaviour in children (7,8). However, such issues remain largely neglected as priorities for mental health service delivery, Considering the large youth population in China and the heavy burden on family and society of childhood mental health problems, this situation can no longer be ignored,

Traditional treatment and therapy, such as clinical psychological diagnosis and treatment, behavioural therapy, and individual education programs, do not effectively deal with many of these problems. Although scientific advances have led to aetiological discoveries and improved diagnostic tools, thereby reducing the severity and number of mental health problems (3), this has not led to the widespread alleviation of suffering. Clinical services provided by Chinese Mental Health Research Centers (i.e., the Child Mental Health Research Center in Nanjing) are limited due to the overwhelming numbers of people who require assistance. Efforts to prevent mental health problems and promote mental health and well-being have received little recognition in society. Prevention therefore remains an unrealised tool in China.

Causes of mental health problems in Chinese children

One of the ongoing debates in the literature has focused on whether the criteria to measure adaptation should include *both* internal adaptation and daily challenges (positive psychological well-being versus distress, depression, and anxiety) and external adaptation to changing environment and various cultural contexts. This debate reflects the dual nature of living systems (9,10). Human individuals are living organisms that must maintain coherence as a unit and also function as part of larger systems, such as families, communities, and society. From a perspective that views children's developmental success as grounded in the surrounding social conditions of their development, the fact that a significant number of children are not doing well in terms of their academic achievement, social and behavioural choices, and mental health suggests serious problems not only within children themselves but also across the broader cast of adults, families, institutions and policy context charged with helping them become full members of society. This was the view of Erikson (11) who believed that successful identity development in children involves the overall configuration of ego needs and the social ethos and contexts of families, schools and communities during a particular moment in life. The quality of fit between the developmental needs of children and the nature of the social opportunities afforded them by adults and communities may provide answers to the question of why some Chinese adolescents have academic, social, and emotional success, whereas a substantial minority of young Chinese children do not.

The problems facing millions of Chinese children are rooted in debilitating social and environmental conditions that include poor school organisational structures, overly demanding school curricula, inadequate mental health services, insufficient focus on social and emotional development, loneliness and anxiety due to the lack of peer interactions, high expectations from parents and society, and the absence of after-school and community recreational programs for children (12,13). Such conditions undermine the fulfilment of basic children and adolescent physical and physiological development needs (e.g., play, leisure, and safety) and also their basic psychological needs for trusting and accepting relationships with adults and peers, for self-expression and exploration, and for developing their academic and social competencies in the direction of viable occupational and social outcomes (11).

Often the key criterion of judgement of success for a young person in China is to graduate from university and gain the education and occupational skills needed for financial independence. In line with cultural traditions, children are also expected by their parents to outperform their peers in terms of academic achievement. In order to fulfil their expectations, parents invest their time, energy, money and intellect in the development of the one child, often neglecting their specific personal interests, talents and feelings. School curricula is often arranged to prepare children for examinations, rather than being centred on the developmental needs of the child. Resilient children and youth manage to meet these expectations, even though they may have faced more significant obstacles to success in life than children in most developed countries. However, the increasing numbers of children who have social, emotional and mental problems indicate that they are not able to cope, and therefore require a substantial support from health, psychological and social services.

Emerging area to promote children's mental health

In research relating to children over the past three decades, the concept of resilience has emerged from the studies on individuals who adapt to extraordinary circumstances, achieving positive and unexpected outcomes in the face of adversity (9, 14). Resilience is inferred because two major judgements are required to identify individuals as belonging in this class of phenomena. First, individuals are judged as to whether they are 'doing OK' or 'better than OK' with respect to a set of expectations for behaviour and second, they are judged as to they thrive even when there have been extenuating circumstances that posed a threat their good outcomes. For example, some children survive without developing serious problems even though they are exposed to hostile environments (15). Resilient children seem to have a self-correcting capacity, an ability to respond with resourcefulness and tenacity when confronted with challenges or adversity. Resilience is a dynamic response to a multiplex of biological, psychological, social, and other environmental influences. For children, resilience is closely tied to development. The skills and competence that characterise resilient functioning at one point in time may thrive in the face of new developmental challenges or new contingencies in the environment.

Studies on school-aged children's positive development have found that children who develop well have several variables in common. These include, firstly, good *internal strengths*, such as sufficient personal assets and competencies, high self-esteem, an internal locus of control, optimism and clear aspirations, achievement and goal-orientation, reflectiveness and problem solving capacity, respect for the autonomy of themselves and others, and healthy communication patterns. Secondly, they include effective *external nurturance and support* from the social environment, such as nurturing and supportive family, school and community environments. These resources, recognised as protective factors, contribute to their positive development and protect them from stress and dysfunction (10,14). Protective factors are "the quality of persons or contexts that predict better outcomes under high-risk conditions" (10). Protective factors predict future outcomes. Protective factors modify risk by directly reducing a disorder or dysfunction, and they mediate risk in chains of risk and protective factors (16). Sometimes, too, they provide resistance to risk by moderating the relationship among risk factors and problems or disorders (17). The latter usually is called a "buffering" effect, because it buffers an individual against the full effect of risk. Protective factors are important because they provide clues for designing more effective social programs. They identify potentially targetable influences that, if fostered by a program, may directly affect a problem or moderate a risk related to a problem (18). Protective factors that refer to individual characteristics (i.e., an easy-going temperament, high self-esteem and self-efficacy) are often recognised as human capital or personal strength. Group or community factors, such as family factors (i.e., parental warmth and supervision), or extra-familial conditions (i.e., having a network of supportive friends) are often referred to as components of social capital in the resilience literature (10,14).

MENTAL HEALTH EFFECTS FROM INDIVIDUAL CHARACTERISTICS

Individual characteristics allow the option of maximizing opportunities in the context of personal limitations and environmental adversity. Generally, individuals characteristics include positive psychological characteristics, such as positive affection and emotion, high self-esteem, and competent social emotional abilities, tend to be physically, socially, and mentally active (19). Also, contemporary researchers emphasise that it is the process of striving for goals—rather than goal attainment *per se*—that is crucial for positive psychological development (19). Myers and Diener (20) conclude that satisfaction with life grows from involvement in valued activities and progress toward one's goal rather than from passive experience of desirable circumstances. Following this argument, it is essential that we perceive these things to be important and as representing goals that are well worth pursuing. The details of mental health effects from individual characteristics, such as, positive affection and emotion, high self-esteem, optimism, and self-efficacy, are discussed below.

Positive affection and emotion

Experiencing positive emotions such as joy, interest, contentment, love, and the like significantly contribute to optimal functioning. Experiments on humans and animals found that positive traits and states and behaviours linked with positive states-such as play –lead to increases in physical, intellectual, and social resources. Furthermore, positive emotions also produce improved well-being. For example, if positive emotions broaden the scope of cognition and enable flexible and creative thinking, they also should facilitate coping with stress and adversity. By broadening people's modes of thinking and action, positive emotions should improve coping and thus build resilience. Increments in resilience should in turn, predict future experiences of positive emotions (21).

Self-esteem

In resilience research on human strengths, self-esteem is thought of as a sign of well-being for two reasons. First, reasonably good self-esteem provides an indication that mood is working within optimal limits to motivate and caution human action. Self-esteem is a measure of the person's expectation of positive events, and accordingly, her or his willingness to approach objects and others. Second, and more broadly, good self-esteem is indicative of a positive and integral personal and social identity (22)—that is, a sense that one is located securely in the social world, competent to meet its challenges, ready to participate in life with others, and able to balance social demands and personal desires. Effective ways to achieve good self-esteem must recognise a number of conditions, namely: acceptance within a social context, a sense of security, cultural competence, and the capacity to reconcile personal goals and social expectations. Hewitt (23) proposed that the individual and the good of the community should be reconciled. Individuals are products of their community but also its creators. When people experience self-esteem, they are living in the affective link between individual and community.

Optimism

Optimism is the expectation people have that good things will happen to them. Studies on optimism found that optimists experience less distress than pessimists when dealing with difficulties in their lives. People who are confident about the future exert continuing effort, even when dealing with serious adversity (24). Optimists use more problem-centred coping than pessimists. They also used a variety of emotion-focused coping techniques, including working to accept the reality for difficult situations and putting the situations in the best possible light. These findings indicate that optimists may have a coping advantage over pessimists even in situations that cannot be changed.

Self-efficacy

Self-efficacy is defined as beliefs about the ability to attain desired goals in particular domains and circumstances. It is not concerned with beliefs about the ability to perform specific and trivial motor acts but with beliefs about ability to coordinate and orchestrate skills and abilities in changing and challenging situations. Self-efficacy is influenced primarily by two interacting factors. First, it is influenced by the development of the capacity for symbolic thought, particularly the capacity for understanding cause-and-effect relationships and the capacity for self-observation and self-reflection. Children must learn that one event can cause another event; that they are separate from other things and people; and that, they can be the origin of actions that affect their environment.

Second, self-efficacy is influenced by the responsiveness of the environment, especially social environments, to the infant or child's attempts at manipulation and control. Environments that are responsive to the child's actions facilitate the development of efficacy beliefs, whereas nonresponsive environments impair this development. Thus, children usually develop a sense of efficacy from engaging in actions that manipulate the people around them, which then generalizes to the non-social environment (25). Parents can facilitate or hinder the development of this sense of efficacy not only by their response to the infant's or child's actions, but also by encouraging and enabling the child to explore and master his or her environment. A sense of control over our behaviour, our environment, and our own thoughts and feelings is essential for happiness and a sense of well-being, together with meeting life's challenges, building healthy relationships, and achieving personal satisfaction and peace of mind.

MENTAL HEALTH EFFECTS FROM SOCIAL CAPITAL

Social capital is related to family and community support and structure that promote personal competence including self-esteem, self-efficacy, problem-solving, or providing guidance at points of life transition.

School social climate

A school's social climate, reflected in the sense of connectedness to others and support from the social environment, are well-established correlates of resilience and contribute to numerous positive outcomes for children (26). The sense of the positive classroom climate affected school satisfaction directly and indirectly through its influence on stress and psychological distress. For example in the Baker et al. (27) study, classroom environments that are perceived as friendly, supportive and free of harassment, are associated with school satisfaction and perceived quality of teacher-student relationships from both teacher and child perspectives. This also predicts student school-related outcomes and behaviours (28). The teacher-student relationship has been identified as a significant influence on overall school and behavioral adjustment (28). Teachers who "provide emotional support, reward competence, and promote self-esteem" (p.10) are considered to be one of the factors that decrease the vulnerability of high-risk students in response to stressful life events (29).

Classroom structures, goals, and practices

Specific classroom practices are associated with positive school attitudes (30). Tasks that provide optimal levels of challenge, feedback that is informational rather than judgemental, recognition of mastery efforts rather than relative performance, and minimisation of interpersonal competition, are all associated with enhanced academic motivation. Classroom practices that afford students opportunities to feel competent and to exercise developmentally appropriate autonomy are associated with a positive appraisal of school. Some developmental models of school reform afford a view of the linkages between school practices and positive school attitudes.

Peer influence

Children's peers play an important role in their positive development and wellness. Friendships serve as an important context for students' comfort and support and have been considered an important part of social context for human development (31). Peer groups also serve to socialize children, causing them to adopt similar goals and attitudes to their peers. Wentzel (32) found that children who felt their peers supported them, adopted prosocial and socially responsible goals within the classroom, such as aiding classmates in classroom activities. In contrast, socially rejected adolescents who are actively disliked by many peers perceive less social support within the classroom and exhibit less positive psychosocial, behavioural, and academic outcomes. Some evidence suggests a link between peer relationships and a sense of school connectedness. Chen et al. (31) found that Chinese students in China who had more friends and had high quality of friendships have more positive attitudes toward school, school-related competence, and academic achievement. As in the classroom climate area, social contexts that are characterised by positive attitudes and lack negative ones are associated with increased school satisfaction.

Family influence

The influence of the family is pervasive on children's development. For example, home environment predicts significant positive changes in children's overall adjustment (33), and predicts increased positive expectations for the future (34). Specifically, families influence positive adaptation in many ways including modelling academically oriented behaviours, socializing an achievement orientation and values regarding education, and direct teaching and structuring of the home so that school tasks are prioritised, emphasized and accommodated (35). The active involvement of home with schools provides continuity across these two critical developmental settings and extends opportunities for learning activities outside of school (36)). Parental involvement in school has been found to be a better predictor of school adjustment and engagement, and children's well-being than other measures of parenting behaviour including monitoring and expectations (36). This probably is because parents demonstrate their care and concern for the children and provide opportunities for direction and encouragement by knowing a lot about the life of their children.

In summary, it can be concluded that there are two effects deriving from the protective factors discussed above. The first effect is a compensatory protective effect, typically directly reducing a problem or disorder. One usually thinks of a compensatory protective effects as a statistical main effect. That is, it does not affect risk but rather exerts a direct effect on a problem or disorder. In a study of over 36,000 seventh-through 12th grade students in Minnesota, compensatory protective effects for externalising problem behaviours were found for family, school connectedness, plus low exposure to poverty, parental unemployment, parental substance abuse, and domestic violence (37). Werner (38) identified protective factors which included significant relationships with kin, intimate partners, and mentors, such as coaches or teachers, who supported their efforts, believed in their potential, and encouraged them to make the most of their lives. Wolin and Wolin (39) identified seven protective factors which included insight, independence, fulfilling relationships, initiative, creativity, humour, and the capacity to distinguish good from bad. These are conceptualised as directly altering the chances of negative future outcomes.

The second effect of protective factors is interactional. With the advance of more complex conceptualisation of protective factors, Rutter (14) proposed that the developmental outcome of a human is whole person and behaviour as a function of person in interaction with environment. He has argued that protective factors are defined both by compensatory effects and perhaps more importantly by interactional effects i.e., those effect that moderate risk. This interactional perspective does not exclude a possibility that a factor exerts an important influence on people who are not at risk. To be an interactional protective effect, a factor must exert an even stronger, positive effect on children who have been exposed to adversity.

Unlike research in vulnerability, which focuses on children in high-risk settings, the study of resilience encompasses all children and focuses on positive development. It has been found that the socio-ecological model with its orientation towards to community development to enhance child outcomes and focus on building positive adjustments in children allows for new insight into mental health promotion amongst young people in China. As a 'settings' approach to health promotion, it has the potential to promote resilience since it is based on the inclusive, participatory and democratic principles shown to be necessary for the development of resilience at the broader community level. The model illustrates this potential through two mechanisms. The first is processes that are characterized by inclusivity and the meaningful, active participation of the diverse range of members that make up a school community as well as equal 'power' relationships, or equal partnerships among community members, parents and school staff. The second are structural mechanisms such as school policies, school organisation and the school's physical environment, reflect the values of participation, democracy and inclusiveness and/or that promote processes based on these values. These processes and structures typified by the socio-ecological model, and located in the broad school environment and the immediate classroom environment collectively has potential to promote resilience in the school setting.

SOCIAL ECOLOGICAL FRAMEWORK TO PROMOTE MENTAL HEALTH

The theoretical development of mental health promotion research is underpinned by the notion that mental health is the transactional product of individual attributes and environmental contingencies. Adaptational response is often tied to skills and competences in problem solving, interpersonal attributes, coping, as well as an ability to act in a planned way. Such attributes are considered to be core elements of resilience (40), but they also interact with and often depend on familial and extra-familial resources. Because the contexts in which individual develop play an influential role in promoting their adaptation and adjustment (26), the degree to which schools function as psychologically healthy environments is a key issue within resilience research as applied to children.

The Social Ecological Model draws on this notion. For example, a fundamental concept of this model is that being autonomous and in a position to choose to function well is necessary to maximise health potential. It follows from this fundamental concept that the promotion of health is facilitated by the promotion of student functioning. The primary mechanisms through which schools promote student resilience and hence health, are through the influence of school system including school organisation, curriculum development, and educational practices on pupil development. This notion is supported by a variety of World Health Organization documents that argue that in order to promote health, the health promotions needs to shift from focusing on the modification of individual risk factors or risk behavior to addressing the "context and meaning" of health actions and the determinants that keep people healthy. School as a health promoting setting should not neglect their management structures, internal and external relationships as well as teaching and learning (41). Others support this focus arguing that in order to be health promoting, social institutions such as schools should focus on their organisational systems and human interaction within the organisation (42,43).

The Social Ecological framework is multidisciplinary, using a population based approach which acknowledges the range of influences on mental health and wellbeing. These include biological, psychological and social factors and more broadly, their interactions with environmental and economic factors (44). Unlike research on psychoanalytic or behavioral therapy which focuses on the diagnosis, deficiency treatment and illness therapy of individuals, the socio-ecological approach focuses on the prevention of mental health problems and early intervention to promote mental health and well-being. It emphasises building up individual and community strengths and capacity to respond with resourcefulness and tenacity in the face of adversity and challenges. The socio ecological health promotion Model specifically addresses: social determinants of health, enhancement of human capital, and enhancement of social capital.

Social ecological health promotion model and social determinants of health

The socio ecological health promotion approach has been proven to be effective at aggregate, population or community levels of action (45-47). By focusing on the settings where people congregate, lead their daily lives and interact on a regular basis, health promotion professionals can work with communities to help create environments that positively affect the behavior that occurs in the setting, and intervene to create change in aspects of those settings that foster behavior with negative consequences. Within these perspectives, children are seen as genetic contributors to their own development. As they interact with social settings, children construct meaning about themselves, others and the nature of school. The meanings children derive from the environment influence their beliefs about themselves as individuals, as learners, and about the purpose, nature and goals of those that they meet in the school and the formal educational processes that take place. These beliefs, in turn, affect children's engagement and participation in school. The school thus influences development because their climate characteristics affect children's appraisals of the school environment, their sense of belonging and connectedness. This in turn affects children's cognition about school, their school-related behaviours, and hence well-being (48). For example, practices that extend a sense of classroom community are likely to be appraised as supportive by students, resulting in increased satisfaction and school engagement (27). Schools also directly affect development because their structure and practices exert a socialising influence on student. For example, there are significant differences in school attitudes and academic outcomes between students in academic and non-academic "tracks", suggesting that educational practice may be a significant factor associated with student's differential outcomes.

Schools are likely to have a positive influence on children's development if there is a good fit between the developmental needs of students and the school environment. Self-determination theory may be used to guide the understanding of student's needs. This theory posits that individuals have three fundamental developmental needs: to be meaningfully connected to others, to have developmentally appropriate choice and self-direction, and to perceive themselves as competent in their endeavours (49). Schools that afford opportunities for students to satisfy these needs would promote student health and well-being (43).

Promotion of individual characteristics

The notion that individual characteristics can be enhanced is based on the assumption that the power of human adaptational systems can be mobilized. These strategies aim to mobilize fundamental protective systems for development. Efforts have been made to influence processes that will change a child's life rather than simply remove risk or adding assets. In terms of increasing the sense of connectedness within the school environment there is good evidence to indicate that this promotes mental and emotional well-being (50-52) and is protective against health risk-taking behaviours related to substance use, violence and early sexual behaviour (51,53). Evidence also indicates that a sense of belonging and connectedness also contributes to improved academic achievement and engagement (50,54,55) as well as to reducing crime (56, 57). As a significant protective factor for several health, academic, and social outcomes, school connectedness has enormous potential to contribute to child and adolescent health and development into adulthood (58-60).

A wide range of programs have been designed to improve the quality of attachment and build self-esteem, self-efficacy to succeed in life, such as the Social and Emotional Learning program in New Haven, Connecticut, public schools (61), and the Resolving Conflict Creatively Program (RCCP) that began in the New York city public schools (62). The program goals include increasing awareness of the different choices available to children for dealing with conflicts; developing skills for making these choices, encouraging children's respect for their own cultural background and the background of others; teaching children how to identify and stand against prejudice; and increasing children's awareness of their role in creating a more peaceful world. A follow-up program, Peace in the Family, trains parents in conflict resolution strategies.

Promotion of social capital

The notion that the social capital can be built up is on the basis of the assumption that the number or quality of resources or social capital can be improved and that whilst the human capital conceptualisations recognise the importance of individual attributes associated with resilience, the school as a social institution involves multiple actors and agencies. The notion of social capital helps to remind us of the importance of links to other social systems such as the family environment and the broader community environment, including health services and community agencies, that have an enormous impact on the health of children and adolescents within the school (63) and on the effectiveness of the school as an educational institution (64-67).

It has been argued that a clearer insight into the nature of school connectedness can be provided by conceiving it as an ecological concept (68). This allows a more complete recognition of the nature and associated processes of the school environment and recognises valuable social systems such as the family environment and the broader community. These systems influence on the health of children and adolescents and on the general effectiveness of the school.

In China, the school context can be understood as: competition for places, stern teaching style, and strict classroom control. Although more than 20% of students can have the opportunity to go to university, the struggle in Chinese society for school success and employment is intense nowadays. The pressure to succeed is relentless and exerts a considerable toll in student anxiety and depression, not to mention family pressure around the doing of homework. Class sizes are large because resources are often scarce, but more importantly because the Chinese believe that "on one mountain, there cannot be two tigers", in other words, competition will better enable the best student to get to the top, thereby proving that the best choice has been made. There is little opportunity for individual instruction in class, examinations are frequent and grading is based almost exclusively on their outcomes. Students respond to teachers as to a stern parent—with attention, silence, and fear. They do not question teachers, or challenge their judgements. In classroom, great amounts of time are devoted to academic activities, and most of the class time is devoted to activities where the teacher is in charge. Such a school context is opposite against to the notion of resilience and the socio ecological approach outlined above.

From socio ecological theoretical perspective, a teachers' perception of their own ability to handle challenging behaviours and to establish positive relationships has a possible influence on the quality of teacher-student relationship. High teacher self-efficacy and low teacher stress has been linked to a variety of positive outcomes, such as positive classroom environments, and better relationships with students (28).

Positive peer relationships provide an avenue to meet student's developmental needs for connectedness to others, thus enhancing their positive adjustment and well-being at school. Children in China are generally discouraged from participating in informal peer groups because they may threaten adults' authority. Parents and teachers may be particularly concerned about negative influences of deviant peers and thus likely exert high control and supervision on children's peer groups (69). Evidence indicates that the percentage of students in Chinese schools (70%) involved in peer groups is substantially lower than what is typically reported in Western cultures (about 85-90%) (70).

Studies examining the antecedents and determinants of the quality of school life have also explored mental health variables such as self-esteem, depression, and stress. Due to the scarcity of the quality of school life literature in China, examining mental health variables associated with life satisfaction from western research is useful. Research suggests there are strong interrelationships between psychological and environmental variables that influence quality of school life. For instance, Baker (27) found that school climate had a significant indirect effect on school satisfaction by influencing psychological variables such as psychological distress and self-concept. Furthermore, internal locus of control mediated the relationship between negative life experiences and quality of school life, indicating the contribution of both psychological and environmental variables to quality of school life. The interplay of these variables implies the necessity of optimising many aspects of children's lives in order to promote their quality of school life.

SOCIAL ECOLOGICAL FRAMEWORK AND CHINESE CHILDREN'S MENTAL HEALTH

We have argued that the school environment and climate does not seem to meet students' psychological needs in China. School systems in China will clearly need to change or be modified if they are on the one hand to help promote mental health and well-being yet, on the other hand remain true to cultural characteristics. The increasing level of mental illness amongst young people is a pressing and significant problem, and prevention efforts must be prioritised in order to limit and reduce the impact of this problem. The socio ecological approach uses a comprehensive methodology which allows for multi-strategy efforts to address the problem. Such efforts will be mutually supportive and involve all those with whom young people come into contact in the school setting. This approach may help China to solve a number of mental health problems that students, family and school community currently confront.

An orientation toward positive development and building on strengths has significant implications for research using a social ecological approach in China. This perspective challenges China to consider markers of positive adjustment rather than diagnosis of developmental problems and to engage in preventative rather than reactive models of practice. Considering not just the prevention of dysfunction but the promotion of adjustment is a critical feature of socio ecological approach to school-based practice. This type of research recognises the reality of health as an integral part of everyday life, and the added complexities when studying the influence of environmental features.

China's economic development poses a challenge to the thousand year tradition of the Confucian family where the role of the person is fundamentally to submit and adapt. As China continue to modernise, Chinese people are facing with the challenge of serving both as a force and recipient of change in their social world, including larger society, school community, family unit and individual. As this change will occur at varying speeds for different members and in different context, what once was a more static social world is likely to become more dynamic, changing and challenging. These challenges have brought already and will inevitably bring about disequilibration for the individual, family and community, and propose an essential question for the mental health of Chinese peoples.

Environments are complex in China, and include multifaceted entities that create numerous theoretical difficulties for research. Careful conceptual analysis of the potentially reciprocal, hierarchical, and embedded nature of relationships between children, school, community and social environments need to be considered. Despite these concerns, it is believed that socio ecological approach has an important place in the research of Chinese children's resilience and mental health. The perspectives that development is transactional and that environments play key roles in shaping or constraining development are important as theory unfolds in this area. The sensitivity to the effects of socio ecological approach on children's development encourages us to look critically and creatively at environmental contributors to Chinese children's resilience.

REFERENCES

[1]   WHO. World Health Organisation constitution. Geneva: 1948.
[2]   Zhu ZH. Strengthen micro-health concepts and draw up the plan of prevention and health in new millennium. China Hospital Management 1998;14(6):322-6.
[3]   Zhou Y, Yang X, eds. Second Sino-American mental health conference. 2000; Beijing, China.
[4]   Murray CJL, Lopez AD. Global mortality, disability, and the contribution of risk factors: Global burden of disease study. Lancet 1997;349(1436-42).
[5]   Parker G, Gladstone G, Chee KT. Depression in the planet's largest ethnic group: The Chinese. Am J Psychiatry 2001;158(6):857-64.

[6] Liu X, Kurita H, Guo C, Miyake Y, Ze J, Cao H. Prevalence and risk factors of behavioral and emotional problems among Chinese children aged 6 through 11 year. J Am Acad Child Adolesc Psychol 1999;38(6):708-71.

[7] Yang B, Ollendick TH, Dong Q, Xia Y, Lin L. Only children and children with siblings in the People's Republic of China: Levels of fear, anxiety, and depression. Child Dev 1995;66:1301-11.

[8] Liu X, Sun Z, Neiderhiser JM, Uchiyama M, Okawa M, Rogan W. Behavioral and emotional problems in Chinese adolescents: Parent and teacher reports. J Am Acad Child Adolesc Psychiatr 2001;40(7):828-36.

[9] Masten AS, Coatsworth JD. Competence, resilience, and psychopathology. In: Cicchetti. D, Cohen. D, eds. Developmental psychopathology. New York: Wiley, 1995:715-52.

[10] Masten AS, Reed MJ. Resilience in development. In: Snyder CR, Lopez SJ, eds. Handbook of positive psychology. New York: Oxford University Press, 2002: 74-88.

[11] Erikson EH. Identity, youth and crisis. New York: Norton, 1968.

[12] Chen Y. Chinese classification of mental disorders (CCMD-3): Towards integration in international classification. Psychopathology 2002;35:171-5.

[13] Ying YW, Zhang X. Mental health in rural and urban families: The role of intergenerational personality discrepancy and family solidarity. J Comparative Fam Stud 1995;26(2):233-9.

[14] Rutter M. Psychosocial resilience and protective mechanisms. Am J Orthopsychiatry 1987;57:316-31.

[15] Smith CA, Lizotte AJ, Thornberry TP, Krohn MD. Resilience to delinquency. Prev Res 1997;4(2):4-7.

[16] Coie JD, Watt NF, West SG, Hawkins JD, Asarnow JR, Markman HJ, et al. The science of prevention: A conceptual framework and some directions for a National Research Program. Am Psychol 1993;48:1013-22.

[17] Bryant KJ, West SG, Windle M. Overview of new methodological developments in prevention research: Alcohos and substance abuse. In: Bryant. KJ, Windle. M, S. G. W, eds. The science of prevention: Methodological advances from alcohol and substance abuse research. Washington, DC: American Psychological Association, 1997:xvii-xxxii.

[18] Burt MR, Resnick G, Novick ER. Building supportive communities for at-risk adolescents: it takes more than services. Washington, DC: American Psychological Association, 1998.

[19] Watson D. Mood and temperament. New York: Guilford, 2000.

[20] Myers DG, Diener E. Who is happy? Psychol Sci 1995;6:10-9.

[21] Fredrickson BL. Positive emotions. In: Snyder. CR, Lopez SJ, editors. Handbook of Positive Psychology. Oxford: Oxford University Press, 2002:120-34.

[22] Hewitt JP. The myth of self-esteem: Finding happiness and solving problems in American. New York: St. Martin's, 1998.

[23] Hewitt JP. The social construction of self-esteem. In: Snyder. CR, Lopez. SJ, eds. Handbook of positive psychology. Oxford: Oxford University Press, 2002:135-47.

[24] Carver CS, Scheier MF. Optimism. In: Snyder CR, Lopez SJ, eds. Handbook of positive psychology. Oxford: Oxford University Press, 2002:231-43.

[25] Bandura A. Self-efficacy: The exercise of control. New York: Freeman, 1997.

[26] Masten A, Best KM, Garmezy N. Resiliency and development: Contributions from the study of children who overcome adversity. Dev Psychopathol 1991;2:425-44.

[27] Baker JA. Teacher-student interaction in urban "at-risk" classrooms; Differential behaviour, relationship quality, and student satisfaction with school. Jf Elementary Educ 1999;100:57-70.

[28] Yoon JS. Teacher characteristics as predictors of teacher-student relationships: Stress, negative affect, and self-efficacy. Soc Behav Pers 2002;30(5):485-93.

[29] Werner EE. Protective factors and individual resilience. In: Meisels. SJ, Shonkoff. JP, eds. Handbook of early childhood intervention. New York: Cambridge University Press, 1990:97-116.

[30] Roeser RW, Eccles JS, Sameroff AJ. School as a context of early adolescents' academic and social-emotional development: A summary of research findings. Elementary Sch J 2000;100(5):443-549.

[31] Chen X, Chen H, Kaspar V. Group social functioning and individual socioemotional and school adjustment in Chinese children. Merrill-Palmer Quart 2001;47(2):264-99.

[32]   Wentzel KR. Family functioning and academic achievement in middle school: A social-emotional perspective. J Early Adolesc 1994;14(2):268-91.

[33]   Dubow EF, Ippolito MF. Effects of poverty and quality of the home environment on changes in the academic and behavioural adjustment of elementary school-age children. J Clin Child Psychol 1994;23:401-12.

[34]   Dubow EF, Arnett M, Smith K, Ippolito M. Predictors of future aspectations of inner-city children: A 9-month prospective study. J Early Adolesc 2001;21:5-28.

[35]   Scott-Jones D. Parent-child interactions and school achievement. In: Ryan. BA, Adams. GR, Weissberg. RP, Hampton. RL, eds. The family-school connection. Thousand Oaks, CA: Sage, 1995:75-107.

[36]   Simons-Morton BG, Crump AD. Association of parental involvement and social competence with school adjustment and engagement among sixth graders. J Sch Health 2003;73(3):121-6.

[37]   Resnick MD, Harris LJ, Blum RW. The impact of caring and connectedness on adolescent health and well-being. J Pediatr Child Health 1993;29 (Suppl 1):S3-S9.

[38]   Werner EE. Vulnerable but invincible: High risk children from birth to adulthood. Eur Child Adolesc Psychiatr 1996;5(Suppl 1):47-51.

[39]   Wolin S, Wolin S. The resilient self: How survivors of troubled families rise above adversity. New York: Villard Books, 1993.

[40]   Hetherington EM, Stanley-Hagan M. The adjustment of children with divorced parents: A risk and resiliency perspective. J Child Psychol Psychiatry 1999;40:129-40.

[41]   World Health Organisation. Promoting health through schools. Report of a WHO expert committee on comprehensive school health education and promotion. Geneva: WHO Report Series 870, 1997.

[42]   Poland BD, Green LW, Rootman I, eds. Settings for health promotion: Linking theory and practice. Thousand Oaks, CA: Sage, 2000.

[43]   Markham WA, Aveyard P. A new theory of health promoting schools based on human functioning, school organisation and pedagogic practice. Soc Sci Med 2003;56:1209-20.

[44]   Bronfenbrenner U. Ecological systems theory. Ann Child Dev 1989;6:187-249.

[45]   King KA, Vidourek RA, Davis B, McClellan W. Increasing self-esteem and school connectedness through a multidimensional mentoring program. J Sch Health 2002;72(7):294-9.

[46]   Lee A, Tsang C, Lee SH, To CY. A comprehensive "Healthy Schools Programme" to promote school health: The Hong Kong experience in joining the efforts of health and education sectors. J Epidemiol Commun Health 2003;57(3):174-82.

[47]   Xu L, Pan B, Lin J, Chen L, Yu S, Jones J. Creating health-promoting schools in rural China: A project started from deworming. Health Promot Int 2000;15(3):197-206.

[48]   Baker JA, Dilly LJ, Aupperlee JL, Patil SA. The developmental context of school satisfaction: School as psychologically healthy environment. Sch Psychol Quart 2003;18(2):206-21.

[49]   Connell JP, Wellborn JG. Competence, automomy and relatedness: A motivational analysis of self-system processes. In: Gunnar M, Sroufe LA, eds. Minnesota Symposium of Child Psychology. Minneapolis, MN: University of Minnesota Press, 1991:43-77.

[50]   Rutter M, Maughan B, Moretimore P, Ouston J, A. S. Fifteen thousand hours: Secondary schools and their effects on children. London: Open Books, 1979.

[51]   Resnick M. Protecting adolescents from harm: Findings from the national longitudinal study on adolescent health. JAMA 1997;278(10):823-32.

[52]   Hawkins J, Catalano R, Kosterman R, Abbot R, Hill K. Preventing adolescent health-risk behaviours by strengthening protection during childhood. Arch Paediatr Adolesc Med 1999;153(1):226-43.

[53]   Nutbeam D, C. S, L. M, Bauman A. Warning! Schools can damage your health: Alienation from school and its impact on health behaviour. J Paediatrics Child Health 1993;29(1):S25-S30.

[54]   Mortimore P, Sammons P, Stoll L, Lewis D, Ecob R. School matters: The junior years. Wells: Open Books, 1988.

[55]   Hargreaves A, Earl L, Ryan J. Schooling for change: reinventing schools for early adolescents. London: Falmer, 1996.

[56]   Catalano RF, Hawkins JD. The social development model: A theory of antisocial behaviour. In: Hawkins. JD, ed. Delinquency and crime: Current theories. New York: Cambridge University Press, 1996:149-97.

[57]   Hawkins J, Catalano R, Miller J. Risk and protective factors for alcohol and other drug problems in adolescence and early adulthood: Implications for substance abuse prevention. Psychol Bull 1992;112(1):64-105.

[58]   Hertzman C. Population health and human development. In: Keating DP, Hertzman C, eds. Developmental health and wealth of nations, social, biological and educational dynamics. New York: Guilford, 1999:21-40.

[59]   Van der Gaag J. From child development to human development. In: Young ME, ed. From early child development to human development. Investing in our children's future. Washington, DC: World Bank, 2002:63-80.

[60]   Vimpani G, Patton G, Hayes A. The relevance of child and adolescent development for outcomes in education, health and life success. Research Report. Melbourne: Australian Institute Family Studies, 2002.

[61]   Shriver TP, Schwab-Stone M, DeFalco K. Why SEL is the better way: The New Haven Social Development Program. In: Cohen J, ed. Educating minds and hearts: Social emotional learning and the passage into adolescence. New York: Teachers College Press, 1999:43-60.

[62]   Lanrieri L, Patti J. Waging peace in our schools. Boston: Beacon, 1996.

[63]   Bronfenbrenner U. The ecology of human development: Experiments by nature and design. Cambridge: Harvard University Press, 1979.

[64]   Sanders MG. The role of "community" in comprehensive school, family and community partnership programs. Elementary Sch J 2001;102(1):19-34.

[65]   Gailmore R, Goldenberg C. Analysing cultural models and settings to connect minority achievement and school improvement research. Educ Psychol 2001;36(1):45-56.

[66]   Taylor L, Adelman HS. Connecting schools, families and communities. Professional Sch Couns 2000;3(5):298-311.

[67]   Sun J, Stewart D. How effective is the health promoting school approach in building social capital in primary schools? Health Educ 2007;107(6):556-74.

[68]   McNeely C, Nonnemaker JM, Blum RW. Promoting school connectedness: Evidence from the national longitudinal study of adolescent health. J Sch Health 2002;72(4):138-47.

[69]   Chen X, Chen H, Kaspar V, Noh S. Adolescent social, emotional and school adjustment in Mainland China. Int J Group Tensions 2000;29:51-78.

[70]   Kinderman TA. Natural peer groups as contexts for individual development: The case of children's motivation in school. Dev Psychol 1993;29:970-7.

In: Public Health Yearbook 2013
Editor: Joav Merrick

ISBN: 978-1-63321-095-0
© 2014 Nova Science Publishers, Inc.

Chapter 38

CHILD ABUSE, NEGLECT AND MALTREATMENT HEALTH SERVICE IN AUSTRALIA: A LITERATURE REVIEW

Jing Sun, PhD[1] and Nicholas Buys, PhD[2]*

[1]School of Medicine and Griffith Health Institute, Griffith University,
Gold Coast campus, Parkland, Gold Coast, Australia
[2]School of Human Services and Social Work, and Griffith Health Institute,
Griffith University, Parkland, Gold Coast, Australia

ABSTRACT

This paper reviews child abuse, neglect and maltreatment health service practice in Australia. Child abuse, neglect and maltreatment and the need to protect children from harm and prevent abuse and neglect has become a significant public health concern. This paper reviews current clinical and community practice in Australia in the following aspects: clinical governance, workforce development, early prevention and intervention, partnership, communication and coordination, and core activities development. It is recommended that the framework for child protection work should include the following: 1) Develop health service capacity with institution: Each health service district, hospital and departments need to develop service roles. 2) Develop district and department governance procedures. 3) Professional training provision. 4) Multi-disciplinary teamwork. 5) Develop personnel role and responsibilities package within each department 6) Stipulate clinical handover and care coordination procedures and 7) Develop early identification and early intervention strategies.

Keywords: Child abuse, neglect, maltreatment, health service

---

* Corresponding author: Jing Sun, PhD, School of Medicine, Griffith University and Griffith Health Institute, Griffith University, Gold Coast Campus, Parkland, Q4222 Australia. Email: j.sun@griffith.edu.au.

INTRODUCTION

Child abuse and neglect, and protection of children from the same, has become a significant clinical and community concern both in Australia and overseas (1-4). It is estimated that the prevalence of child physical abuse Australia ranges from 5-18% (5,6), prevalence of child neglect ranged from 2% to 12% (6,7). The prevalence estimates of child emotionally maltreated are quite different, ranging from 6% (8) to 17% (6); The prevalence of male child abuse was 1.4-8.0% for penetrative abuse and 5.7-16.0% for non-penetrative abuse, and prevalence rates female children was 4.0-12.0% for penetrative abuse and 13.9-36.0% for non-penetrative abuse (1-4). Given the significant impact of early experiences of violence, abuse and harsh parenting regimes on later development, it is important that children are protected effectively from potential harm.

Health services play a crucial role in recognising such harmful situations and taking immediate action to ensure the physical safety of children and minimize the long term emotional harm that accompanies abusive family, community, and social contexts. It is a common practice that Child Protection Health Services provide reporting and documentation to child protection service or child welfare services, assessing and diagnosing the children needing protection, investigating matters where a child is at possible risk of significant harm, and referral of children and families to social and health services that provide for the ongoing safety and well-being of the children. However, using an integrated approach to provide health services in child protection has not been evaluated. Physicians and nurses in many countries are legally required to refer suspicious child abuse or neglect cases to designated child welfare agencies. Reporting of child maltreatment is a challenging task (9,10), but protect children from harm becomes priority. Queensland Health, as a key stakeholder in the child protection work, has provided services in identification and reporting of suspected child abuse and neglect. To continue this role, a contemporary and effective service model to incorporate strategies and implementation plans in child protection is needed.

The aim of the Child Protection Service Delivery Project was to develop a comprehensive and effective health service model for a health district in Queensland Health. It is critical that this framework is evidence-based and informed by the best evidence and practices in child protection. This review of literature was undertaken in order to support the project team in service framework development and implementation.

Aims of the literature review

The main objective was to review the service delivery model in child protection in order to;

1. Inform and support the development of child protection service delivery framework in a Health Service District in Queensland.
2. Ensure the model is evidence-based and encompasses current best practice from other countries.

METHODS

An extensive national and international literature search was conducted during June 2007-June 2008 using a variety of databases including academic databases [Medline from 1966 to December 2007, ProQuest from 1980 to 2007, Science Direct 1980 to 2007, Balckwell Syndergy from 1966 to 2007], Australian databases [Australian Institute of Family Studies Library Catalogue, Australian Public Affairs Information Service, Australian Family & Society Abstracts, CINCH (Australian Criminology Database), National clearinghouses in the fields of child protection, health and domestic violence], and international databases [Care Data, Child Abuse, Child Welfare and Adoption (NISC), Educational Resources Information Clearinghouse, National Criminal Justice Reference Service, Sociological Abstracts, Social Services Abstracts].

Search words for identifying the research on organizational risk factors, management, recruitment and assessment included child and worker, staff and child, exploitation and institutions, recruitment and child, actuarial and child, and actuarial and risk and assessment. For identification of research on child-related and perpetrator-related risk factors, the search words included child abuse and child abuser. The key words "child abuse", "physical", and "neglect" were used to search the literature. The results published before 1980 and in language other than English were used. Articles identified in the search were subdivided into Clinical governance, Workforce development, Early Prevention and Intervention, Partnership, Communication and coordination, Core activities, and Culturally and diverse background population. Articles with core activities were sought with the terms "case management" or "risk assessment". Additionally, the Child Abuse Quarterly Review of research on child maltreatment and the journal "Child Abuse and Neglect" from January 1995 to December 2007 were also reviewed.

CURRENT KNOWLEDGE AND PRACTICES

No service framework at a district level was available either from literature review or from interstate. Therefore, the research team was required to determine relevant topics and issues to guide the selection and examination of the literature. After consultation with Child Protection Project team, the concept of Child Protection Service Delivery Framework was interpreted to have the following core dimensions:

1. Clinical governance
2. Workforce development
3. Early prevention and intervention
4. Partnership, communication and coordination
5. Core activities

CLINICAL GOVERNANCE

Clinical governance is the set of processes and systems that ensure the safety and highest quality of the process of care. It includes the systems for accountability, oversight and systematic improvement of care and a set of checks and reviews, whereby teams and communities of clinicians oversee and systematically improve the processes and practices of care (11). It was introduced in the 1990s in the National Health Service in the United Kingdom and has become popular in the UK, Canada and Australia (12).

Clinical governance is closely associated with functional health service units including the ward, unit, department, health centre and clinic. The governance of all units begins at the highest level, requiring the leadership to set up organisational agendas for corporate, district and clinical governance. Having adequate reporting mechanisms and reviewing clinical and organisational performance through accurate data on a regular basis are preconditions for effective leadership. Governing authorities need to ensure that the organisation is performing effectively, services are being delivered according to predefined standards, and mechanisms are in place to take remedial action when problems are encountered.

Describing the clinical governance framework for government, district and area service level in explicit terms is important for a number of reasons. First, it provides a clear and transparent communication of the organisation's intentions and expectations in relation to the delivery of care to all stakeholders. Second, it clarifies roles and responsibilities of consumers and staff across the organisation while explicitly demonstrating the value and contribution they bring to the service, and the interdependence of each person's roles and responsibilities. Third, it allows operationalization through the inclusion of relevant elements of the clinical governance framework in job descriptions, staff selection processes, performance review, education and training needs analysis, building of staff and service capacity, and testing and improvement of the framework's elements.

The Australian Council of Healthcare Standards (13), in 2004, defined clinical governance as *"the system by which the governing body, managers and clinicians share responsibility and are held accountable for patient safety, minimising risks to consumers and for continuously monitoring and improving the quality of care."* The application of clinical governance in a health care setting in Australia is new and the success of its implementation has not been evaluated. But a number of common principles have been proposed across Australia (14):

1. Collaborative relationship between clinicians and managers in which the specific roles and responsibilities of each are made explicit, are understood by the other and are complementary, and where the highly trained, skilled clinicians provide increasingly complex, evidenced-based care to high-risk patients in collaboration with managers who have the high level training and skills to manage and to change highly complex, high-risk health systems (15).
2. Safeguarding principles in clinical risk management, where doctors play a crucial role in protecting children from abuse and neglect (16). There is a legal and professional duty for all doctors to ensure that advice provided, either to the child or young person or to their parents or carers, is appropriate and has taken into account any impact that this may have on the ultimate safety of the individual (16).

3. Strengthening the roles and responsibilities of clinicians in clinical governance, which has been identified as the mechanism to systematically improve standards of clinical care (17). Its components are evidence-based practice, audit, risk management, mechanisms to monitor the outcome of care, lifelong learning among clinicians, and systems for managing poor performance.

4. Monitoring and clinical supervision of nurses, the importance of which has been emphasized in past decade in a range of United Kingdom government and professional policy documents (17).

5. Maintaining effectiveness in clinical governance, where the medical audits were the first type of activity implemented in the National Health Service in United Kingdom. It is a process that strives to improve patient care and outcomes through systematic review of care against explicit criteria, the implementation of change at an individual, team, or service level, and further monitored to confirm improvement of service delivery. However, opinions about its effectiveness are mixed in United Kingdom (18), many seeing audit solely as an educational exercise for junior doctors and having a limited contribution due to lack of methodological rigour and the poor quality of resultant recommendations. Those with a more positive view saw national audits as especially useful, particularly when they had been developed with clinical input. Others highlighted the benefits of audits that were able to identify areas of clinical risk or explored a problem arising from a clinical incident in detail. Audit meetings were one mechanism for bringing together departments on different hospital sites, providing a building block for standardisation of services. Effective audits were seen as those that involved the whole team, including other health care professionals, and had consultant input into both the conduct of the audit and the implementation of the recommendations (18).

6. Facilitation of a more conducive cultural climate by the use of a variety of approaches, including reviewing and aligning policies, structures and processes within a clear vision and framework of goals related to quality improvement, reviewing and celebrating positive behaviours, involving staff in the process of change with support for any training and development needs, improving the effectiveness of communication across the organization and providing teams with time and space to reflect upon their performance. All these have been shown to have a positive effect (19-21).

Clinical governance includes systems for accountability, oversight and systematic improvement of care (15), where the use of sound evidence as a basis for management of decision-making is been increasingly acknowledged. A vital focus in effective application of clinical governance principles to the development of enhanced systems of performance management for nursing, medical and technical staff, including staff appraisal and ensuring continued professional development (15). Clinical governance has been found critical to the successful development and implementation of an effective "system" approach to patient safety in health care (22). Developing clinical governance at corporate level rests on the core processes of clinical audit, clinical effectiveness, clinical risk management (CRM), quality assurance, and organisational and staff development. CRM is a key driver of patient safety processes within a clinical governance structure. There is a variation observed in the knowledge, beliefs and attitudes of experienced staff concerning clinical governance and CRM processes because;

- The clinical governance and CRM processes currently being operationalised in the Australian health care sector are relatively new in Australia;
- There is a lack of attention to these issues in the Australian child protection literature;
- There is a lack of educational opportunities at both undergraduate and post registration levels for nurses to develop knowledge and skills relevant to clinical governance and CRM;
- The predictable resistance of a minority of staff to change (12,23).

WORKFORCE DEVELOPMENT

Health care workers, ranging from clinical staff who are responsible for conducting specialist medical investigations, to nurses working the community in positions such as school nurses, midwives and health visitors, have been recognised as having a key role in the child protection service internationally and in Australia. While child abuse work may constitute one of many responsibilities, nurses and paediatricians are often the first professionals to identify children who have been or are at significant risk of child abuse and neglect. However, the potential for nurses and paediatricians to fulfil this role in many settings is hampered by a perceived lack of training around child protection (24). Most studies show that the training for child protection workforce is inadequate in many countries, and has highlighted the need for adequate for initial and continued training in the identification, assessment and intervention in child protection, for all health professionals in primary and tertiary health care in regular contact with children,(25-27).

The findings from inquiries and research suggest that in order to provide an effective child protection service, primary care workers need both the skills and knowledge to identify cases of child abuse and to know their roles and responsibilities, as well as how to liaise with other agencies involved in child protection. Fifty eight percent of services in United Kingdom did not have enough trained nurses (28). It is particularly important that front line nurses are well trained so that they can draw the attention of designated child protection staff to any cases of concern. Seventy percent of services nationally did not have enough trained nurses at this level. Eight-five percent of services in Accident and Emergency departments did not meet the standard training in child protection service (29). In the United Kingdom, with identification of training needs of already qualified nurses in the field of child protection (30, 31), it has been suggested that mandatory qualifying and in-service training should be provided to enable nurses to identify, assess and refer children for protection. The Royal College of Nursing (28) has produced guidelines with regard to the extent and level of training required by nurses in child protection.

Further, given the rising scale of expectations placed on general medical practitioners (GPs) in taking on responsibility for child protection, it is essential to provide them with the skill, knowledge, attitudes, and values in this area of practice. However, a survey conducted in Canada found that among 16 medical schools, only 3 programs had mandatory clinical training for residents, and nine programs offered electives in child protection which were taken during the previous year by only 4.7% of respondents (32). Overall, only 26.8% of the residents have had any kind of clinical instruction in child protection at any time during their medical training. Over 91% of residents and 85% of fourth-year residents have indicated their need of further training in this area.

Within Australia and New Zealand, advanced training in child protection workforce falls within the scope of Community Child Health. Recently, advanced trainees who work under the Specialist Advisory Committee for Community Child Health are required to complete 3 months of training in child protection. The child protection paediatrician may participate in multidisciplinary meetings, and participate in shared decision-making. In their clinical work, they may be called upon to advocate for the child for services and assess the development and behaviour of children who may have experienced abuse or neglect (9,33). One-third of CP paediatricians have reported receiving no training at all in child protection, and two thirds of CP paediatricians have received less than 4 months of training prior to completing their FRACP. Those paediatricians contribute to decision making with other child protection stake-holders in multi-agency meetings, and 50% of paediatricians indicated that they had less than adequate training for this role prior to FRACP (9, 33). Most paediatricians spend half of their allocated child protection time assessing children referred to the child protection system from health services. Only 13% of their working week is spent on the ongoing medical follow up of these children. In addition, only 50% of paediatrician continue to manage behavioural or developmental problems identified in these children beyond 6 months (9) suggesting that half these high-risk children receive long-term management elsewhere. Doctors who take on such tasks need additional opportunities for training and professional development, and a means of accreditation that confirms their expertise to clinical and forensic colleagues and to the judiciary.

Nurses in Australia, who have considerable contacts with children, such as midwives, school nurses and nurses in paediatric wards or acute hospitals did not provide services in child protection, reflecting the fact that these services are provided by other departments (24). The challenge to provide adequate training to nurses who have identified a need for further knowledge about child protection issues is great, especially given a lack of consensus among most groups of nurses as to what training they require.

EARLY PREVENTION AND EARLY INTERVENTION

The early identification of child maltreatment and early intervention to reduce the degree of harm in children is critical to child's physical and psychological development (29). The main strategies in early identification and intervention discussed in the literature are identification of children and parents who fall into high risk groups and identification of risk factors.

Child maltreatment is usually the result of interaction of many risk factors, such as presence of a disability (34), a parent with substance abuse and/or depression (35), intimate partner violence within the family (36), residence in dangerous neighbourhoods or poor recreational facilities, and poverty and associated burdens (37). The family, community and the health department are collectively responsible for the children's safety within their families. When the child maltreatment occurs and an adult fails his/her role to protect a child from harm, child protection system becomes responsible to provide service response by providing primary, secondary and tertiary services.

The goal of primary health services is to provide support and education for children and families before problems arise. In many cases, primary services prevent abuse and neglect occurring, are offered to everyone, and include ante-natal services, maternal and child health services and human relationship education in schools.

Community education and awareness programs focus on addressing community attitudes towards violence, children's rights and physical punishment which are associated with child abuse. These programs educate the public about alternatives to abuse, changing social attitudes towards violence, and encourage community debate about issues such as censorship, family violence, substance abuse and drug use, etc. Physicians can help prevent child maltreatment in several ways (38). Establishing a good relationship with a family provides opportunities to observe parent-child relationship and identify risk of potential harm from adults.

In many countries, all new births are notified to the nurses and they have a minimum of five contacts during the first year of life which take place at prescribed times, although in practice there may be more frequent visits if necessary (39). School- aged children are followed up through the school nursing service, which plays an important role in child protection due to the routine contact with all young children and their families (40). For example, in Ireland, a breakdown of time spent on domiciliary child development visits shows that 82% of time is given over to developmental checks, 1.5% to ante-natal care, 14.7% to visiting vulnerable families and 2.1% to family surveillance (41).

Parental education is useful to help with diminishing the risk of child abut and maltreatment. Hospital based programs can be developed to educate parents about infants behaviours and the parental methods to prevent abusive physical injury. Health check-up can provide opportunities to check psychosocial risks, such as parental depression, substance use, domestic violence, financial strains and stresses. However, the primary care role of advising and supporting parents to prevent poor child health care practices and child maltreatment has not yet been evaluated. Gough (42) in an extensive review of the literature on child abuse interventions suggests that interventions such as education and support may not be evaluated because of the difficulties inherent in measurement of their effectiveness.

Nurses can refer to statutory and voluntary agencies before any problems arise and they may play an effective role in primary protection of children (43). The Dublin-based Community Mothers' Programme provides an example of how nurses' work effectively through the identification of community needs, and initiation and referral of children and families to support programmes (43).

There are several types of service provision for child protection at a primary health care level (44):

- Universal (core) health visiting: The new birth visit was the cornerstone of the universal health visiting service, which predicted more postnatal home visits and more frequent group and community-based activities.
- Teamwork delivering core service: The core service was delivered, in most instances, by the health visitor in conjunction with others, including members of the wider primary care team. Where health visitors led a skill-mix team, fewer scheduled home visits occurred, but there were more group and community activities overall.

- Extra health visiting: Services included additional home visits by health visitors and by other team members for service provision with regard to postnatal depression, breast-feeding, parenting education, sleep or behaviour problems, domestic violence, drug users and support, menopause, weight management, men's health, language support, speech and language development, learning difficulties, mental health, multiple births, rural health and sexual health.

Secondary prevention is concerned with the early identification and appropriate referral of families once there is evidence of risk of child abuse and neglect. Secondary health services include in-home family support, counselling, respite care and various parenting and self-help groups. The secondary role of the nurses and paediatricians in early detection of families at risk is grounded in their expertise of normal emotional and physical development of children in the context of their families, as well as in an in-depth knowledge and awareness of injuries or behaviour likely to be non-accidental in nature (45).

Currently, reporting a child on an "at risk" is mandatory in Australia (45,46). In the presence of an 'at risk' reporting, there is a formal mechanism for differentiating between 'vulnerable' and 'at-risk' children. Consequently, a family may be protected from the situation as 'vulnerable' and/or 'at risk'. However, in many Western Countries, the need to differentiate these criteria remains largely unarticulated. This has led to nurses and paediatricians retaining responsibility for child protection in situations where specialist intervention is required.

Tertiary prevention deals with minimizing disabilities. Greenwalt, Sklare, and Portes (47) described the current practice of some mental health practitioners in the treatment of cases involving physical child abuse in America. The family is considered the primary client most frequently with the focus of the family therapy to stop the abuse and to improve family relationships. Whether this focus should be considered the primary therapeutic goal needs further longitudinal research on the abused child.

One would expect physically abused children to receive the help needed to stabilize their lives and become productive members of society as soon as possible.

However, while some authorities recognize the importance of providing treatment for the abused child (48), little can be found in the literature about the treatment actually provided to the victim (49). White (50) notes mental health services to the abused child only as a part of foster care, residential care, or day care but not in the context of health service. Greater emphasis appears to be placed on the treatment of the parents and the safety of the child (51) than on overcoming the effects of the abuse on the child.

PARTNERSHIP, COMMUNICATION AND COORDINATION

Interagency coordination and collaboration is a significant issue for the provision of child protection and family support services. A coordinated response to the problem of child maltreatment can produce more effective risk assessment, greater efficiency in the use of resources, improved service delivery by the avoidance of duplication and overlap between existing services, clarification of agency or professional roles and responsibilities in front-line problems and demarcation disputes, and the delivery of comprehensive services.

The structures or mechanisms that facilitate interagency collaboration and coordination are referral protocols, case conferencing, and the development of multidisciplinary teams. The formal referral protocols between health departments and social workers are mostly the primary means of communication. Informal linkages in conjunction with formal communication structures appear to be an effective partnership and coordination between agencies (52). The collaboration between medical evaluation for abused children and local child protection social (CPS) workers is needed, and to achieve agreement between paediatricians and CP workers are critical to identify the cases and improve the services (53).

Standardising decision making, information sharing, consensus decision making, mediation by an administrator in the absence of consensus, rational discussions among members of the team and supportive attitudes towards other members, leading role played by the persons with most first-hand knowledge about the case handled, and the decisions made are respected despite the status of the person in team, all lead to better service provision (54). In Queensland, where child protection and adult mental health are the responsibility of separate government departments-the Department of Communities and Queensland Health, workers engage in collaboration to provide a wide range of services and supports focusing on adult mental health, child protection, family counselling and support, child health and mental health, and legal and financial assistance (55). The provision of these various supports is delivered via a highly fragmented and decentralised network of over 100 government (federal, state and local) and community-based programs, services and agencies.

In some respects, the respondents' description of their experiences of interagency collaboration was encouraging. In half the cases reported, respondents identified that either no issues had arisen, or that collaboration had resulted in an improved outcome for the client or a positive collaborative process for the workers. This finding supports previous research, indicating that collaboration can be rewarding and beneficial for both workers and clients. However, in one-third of cases communication was cited as a problem and support previous findings (56-58) which indicate that information sharing, communication, and negotiating issues of confidentiality are crucial to a successful collaborative relationship. The second most commonly cited difficulty was the need for role clarity, including boundaries and leadership. This result supports the findings of Mizrahi and Rosenthal (59), which found leadership to be the most important factor for successful coalitions. This raises the questions of who the leader should be, how leaders should be chosen, and the scope of the authority to be bestowed.

It is evident that effective communication and collaboration between health professionals on child protection issues is related to organisational level strategies, case level strategies, inter-professional relationships, staff training and supervision, types of knowledge required, and understanding of the interdependent needs of parents and children (55). Policy and practice is closely linked to effective partnerships. With high incidents of child maltreatment in Queensland (60), the state department of health, hospital-based child protection teams, nurses, and medical practitioners are increasingly asked to evaluate and treat child abuse and neglect despite their lack of formal training. In an effort to manage increased caseloads, other disciplines have trained paraprofessionals and lay people such as parent aides, lay therapists, and lay health visitors to provide services to abusive families. These workers have been shown to be fully capable of identifying abusive situations, and have alleviated workloads and provided additional services.

In Australia, Departments of Health (DOH) plays a coordinating role in addressing child abuse and domestic violence through developing Mental Health Policy and Framework, and establishing partnerships with other agencies and service uses. The partnership was particularly in areas such as multi-professional training, service delivery, continuation of health and social services for families, and referrals. One way of achieving closer cooperation among the various agencies involved in child protection work is through the establishment of 'multidisciplinary' or interagency teams or meetings (61). Most of the literature emphasizes the efficiency of this multidisciplinary approach to case consultation and its positive effect on service delivery (61).

There are several guides to the development and implementation of a multidisciplinary child protection team. One model is case consultation teams. These teams focus on case conferences, service development, and work to enhance interagency collaborations (61). Another model is treatment teams, often in hospitals, which collaborate on treatment plans for abused children and their families. They may also provide some long-term case management (62). A third model is resource development teams. These address the issue of child maltreatment through public education and advocacy. Members may be professionals working in the field or other citizens (63). Their program strengthens natural support networks through self-help groups and skills training sessions. The literature also describes mixed model teams that combine the above functions.

Child maltreatment in all its manifestations constitutes a diagnostic and therapeutic problem to all hospital personnel caring for children and adolescents. To optimise practical procedures and to ensure child protection independent of decisions made by any single person, several Austrian hospitals have formed child protection teams or child abuse and neglect teams. In 1999, the Federal Ministry for the Environment, Youth and Family published a recommendation to install Child Protection Team (CPT) in all paediatric departments in Austria and provided a set of guidelines to assist CPT in carrying out their work in paediatric hospitals. These guidelines currently form the constitutional basis of CPT in 68% of all Austrian paediatric hospitals. The CPT team comprises the following professionals groups: paediatricians, paediatric surgeons, a child and adolescent psychiatrics, psychologists, psychotherapists, nurses, a social worker and a secretary. The CPT is available only to inpatient and was founded principally as a tool to provide support to the staff on the individual wards of the departments involved. Inpatient data from CPT functioning in hospitals are relatively scarce in the literature. The detailed data about the functioning and effectiveness of CPT are available only from the USA and Canada. Unfortunately, in its current form the function of CPTs lacks a suitable quality assurance structure (both qualitative and financial-structural), as has also been documented in US CPTs. An improvement in this could ensure a better detection of maltreatment, a more appropriate handling of the whole problem and guaranteed protection of the children concerned.

CORE ACTIVITIES

Nurses and paediatrician are often the first contact of children who are abused and neglected, and their education provides them with a broad base in assessment, planning, implementing and evaluating health care and nursing care in holistic way. They are responsible for primary, secondary and tertiary level of protection. The bulk of the responsibility in identifying and managing child maltreatment therefore lies with the health care teams.

There are many indicators that could help health professionals to identify the children at risk of maltreatment. These include inconsistent history, delay in seeking attention, parent-child interaction, and mismatch in history and examination. However, there has been a lack of clarity about the purpose and appropriate use of indicators of concern. For example, in Emergency department (ED), ED physicians limited their documentation to a single presenting complaint, and it was difficult to be certain that a particular indicator was looked for and not found (e.g., whether the child had an unclothed examination or only the symptomatic limb was examined). The documentation of childhood injuries in the ED is inadequate, making any assessment of abuse difficult. On review of the medical record, there was high percentage of children who had one or more indicators that merited further analysis before a diagnosis of accident could be assigned; however, only 0.9% of children were referred to further examination. The poor referral rate in ED suggests that ED and orthopaedic staff are unaware of the significance of the indicators of maltreatment.

In a study conducted in United Kingdom (64), it has been found that a large number of the protocols in ED department included long lists of signs and symptoms of abuse with no guidance on how to use these. Those with practical value included a short checklist, with clear guidelines on what to do if concerns were identified. Some indicators were very specific (for example, children under 1 year with a fracture, burn or scale), while others were more descriptive (for example, the parents behaviour gives rise to concern). One included recognised risk factors (for example, teenage parents, low income, or prematurity) as well as signs and symptoms, but gave no indicator on how these were to be interpreted.

Tertiary protection in the Australian and New Zealand context consists of medical follow-up for children entering the child protection system, and monitoring of the development and behavioural progress in these children beyond 6 months, involvement of preventative child protection programmes which include programs on high-risk families with young infants and child protection research (65). Most paediatricians who are doing tertiary protection may also get involved in the advocacy for the child for services through joining in multidisciplinary meetings, and participate with other child protection agency stake-holders in decisions aimed to achieve the best child protection outcomes (65).

The management of maltreated children has a number of options. For both sexual and physical abuse, cognitive-behavioural therapy (CBT) has dominated as the treatment with the most empirical validation. Parent training, in which parents are taught how to behaviourally specify goals for change, to track target behaviours, to positively reinforce pro-social conduct, and to punish or ignore their children's aversive behaviours have also been extended to include coping skills, self-control skills, communication skills training and psycho-education (66). Some interventions have been developed specifically for children who have been physically abused. These include peer training, a school-based intervention that uses pro-social peers to help children who are withdrawn to develop social skills (67). For children up to five years of age, a therapeutic child development program has been developed to provide an intensive milieu of services, such as nutrition, health care, developmental therapies, and case management, provided by responsive adults (68).

Group treatment has been a typical modality of intervention for sexual abuse given its cost effectiveness and potential to reduce stigma. The theoretical orientations of group therapy have varied widely and include most commonly eclectic treatment models comprising various combinations of the following components: psycho-education regarding sexual abuse and sexual abuse prevention, exploration of the abuse experience, exploration of feelings, art therapy, play therapy, role plays, problem solving, puppet work, writing exercises, and behaviour management (69, p.674).

SERVICE DELIVERY MODEL FOR CHILD PROTECTION

Based on the evidence from the literature review it is recommended that every health district and hospital have formal surveillance and accountability procedures or a clinical governance framework to improve quality and safety. To succeed, these frameworks must: 1) devolve governance and performance monitoring to the level of clinical units or departments where care is provided and whose staff bears the ultimate responsibility; 2) feature practice-relevant, data-driven agendas that actively seek involvement and innovation on the part of practising clinicians, and; 3) require hospital executives, clinical governance units and quality improvement coordinators to sponsor and support quality and safety activities within units. A relevant action plan should be developed for improving quality and safety and implement the clinical governance framework incorporating work force development and early identification and intervention into the implementation plan (70). This plan may include;

- Develop service delivery capacity: health service districts, hospitals and its departments should develop delivery capacity in relation to facilities, staffing, and management.
- Develop district and department governance procedures: The governance structure and procedure should be developed from the state government executive to the district and health area managers level. This procedure should inform practice based framework and be implemented to the hospitals and districts.
- Professional training provision in child safety: Health department, universities, specialty collages, and medical societies should collaborate in forging new training programmes and career paths that focus on optimizing quality and safety. A key reform is to enable doctors, nurses and allied health professionals to more effectively undertake high-order bedside tasks that require specialised training by devolving and distracting, low-order clerical and non-clinical procedural tasks to appropriately trained assistants. In times of future shortages of specific groups of skilled clinicians, professional boundaries will need some renegotiation in situations where evidence confirms that tasks previously considered as the exclusive province of one type of practitioner can be safely carried out by other groups.
- Develop multi-disciplinary teamwork: Interdisciplinary team activities should be developed to reduce the risk of harm of children. Education and training should be provided to train multidisciplinary team's safety procedures, team skills and communication skills.
- Establish clinical orientation procedures: All hospital departments should provide all newly appointed clinicians and nurses with a multidisciplinary orientation and information package that outlines departmental policies and procedures and personnel roles and responsibilities.

- Develop clinical care coordination procedures: All hospital departments should have clear procedures for (1) clinical handover between shifts for all disciplines and between different care teams, (2) accessing information and advice from external caregivers (e.g., general practitioner and specialists) with regards to the suspicion of children who are abused and neglected, (3) recording clinical information arising from emergency and paediatric department clinics, case conference and consultant visits and conveying it to others who need to know, and (4) transferring structured child information (clinic identification and assessment and community referrals) to general practitioners and other clinicians involved in the clinical care.

- Implement early identification and early intervention practices: The health system is often the only infrastructure that reaches children younger than three years and therefore can initiate programmes to promote early development and prevent risks. In new born infant health check and health visits program, early detection of child abuse and neglect should be one of paediatricians' and nurses' tasks. Once children are identified to be at risk of potential harm referrals to relevant early intervention program should be made. The parenting program (e.g., Triple P parenting program) should be made available in clinical and community settings. The educational system can promote child development by supporting comprehensive programmes for early child development. If the programmes are of high quality, have family involvement, and when needed provide health care and food supplementation or micronutrients, evidence suggests that disparities among the most disadvantaged children can be reduced before school entry. Linking early development programmes administered through the health system with programmes in the educational system increases the likelihood of building intervention follow-up for children at risk. To increase coverage of early child development programmes and improve their quality and effectiveness, better advocacy strategies, coordination mechanisms, and improved policy are needed. Research is required on approaches to delivering feasible effective child protection programmes at scale and on the effects of synergies on child outcomes.

- Implement pre and in-service training for health professional's development: Training local frontline health and social services professionals, and providing support and consultation in child protection is needed. Health professionals who were trained with knowledge and skills increase the rate of detection of child abuse and neglect (70). Due to the key role that nurses have in protecting children, specialist training in child protection needs to be provided to all nurses including those who do not work directly with children. They need to be able to access information on child protection issues as required. Many nurses work either directly with children or indirectly in settings where children may be present (e.g., in private homes or in clinics where children accompany parents who are service users). This includes district nurses, community psychiatric nurses, and nurses working in the fields of learning disability and addiction. If they are to effectively contribute to the child protection agenda, they need at least some basic training about child protection, particularly around identifying children at risk and responding to any cases of suspected or alleged abuse of children. For new staff, participation in such training could be incorporated into their induction program, especially if an on-line training package is developed to provide basic knowledge about child protection issues.

REFERENCES

[1]   Dunne MP, Purdie DM, Cook MD, Boyle FM, Najman JM. Is child sexual abuse declining? Evidence from a population-based survey of men and women in Australia. Child Abuse Negl 2003;27(2): 141-52.

[2]   Mazza D, Dennerstein L, Garamszegi CV, Dudley EC. The physical, sexual and emotional violence history of middle-aged women: a community-based prevalence study. Med J Aust 2001;175(4): 199-201.

[3]   Moore EE, Romaniuk H, Olsson CA, Jayasinghe Y, Carlin JB, Patton GC. The prevalence of childhood sexual abuse and adolescent unwanted sexual contact among boys and girls living in Victoria, Australia. Child Abuse Negl 2010;34(5):7-.

[4]   Najman JM, Dunne MP, Purdie DM, Boyle FM, Coxeter PD. Sexual abuse in childhood and sexual dysfunction in adulthood: an Australian population-based study. Arch Sex Behav 2005;34(5):517-26.

[5]   Cohen RA, Paul RH, Stroud L, Gunstad J, Hitsman BL, McCaffery J, et al. Early life stress and adult emotional experience: an international perspective. Int J Psychiatr Med 2006;36(1):35-52.

[6]   Price-Robertson R, Smart D, Bromfield L. Family is for life: How childhood experiences within the family help or hinder the lives of young adults. Fam Matters 2010;85:7-17.

[7]   Straus MA, Savage SA. Neglectful behavior by parents in the life history of university students in 17 countries and its relation to violence against dating partners. Child Maltreat 2005;10(2):124-35.

[8]   Rosenman S, Rodgers B. Childhood adversity in an Australian population. Soc Psychiatry Psychiatr Epidemiol 2004;39(9):695-702.

[9]   Commission for Children and Young People and Child. Commission for Children and Young People and ChildGuardian Act 2000. Brisbane: Commission for Children and Young People and Child, 2001 Reprinted as in force on 1 July 2008. Report No.

[10]   Flaherty EG, Sege R. Barriers to physician identification and reporting of child abuse. Pediatr Annu 2005;34:349-56.

[11]   Gunn VL, Hickson GB, Cooper WO. Factors affecting pediatricians' reporting of suspected child maltreatment. Ambulent Pediatr 2005;5(96-101).

[12]   Hoyle P. The promise of clinical governance. Royal Australasian College of Medical Administrator, 2006.

[13]   Braithwaite J, Travaglia JF. An overview of clinical governance policies, paractices and initiatives. Aus Health Rev2008;32(1).

[14]   Australian Council of Health Care Standards (ACHS). National report on health services accreditation performance. Accessed 2013 Mar 10. URL: www.achs.org.au.

[15]   Scott IA, Poole PJ, Jayathissa S. Improving quality and safety of hospital care: a reappraisal and an agenda for clinically relevant reform. Int Med J 2008;38:44-55.

[16]   O'Conner N, Paton M. Governance of and governance by: implementing a clinical governance framework in an area mental health service. Australasian Psychiatr 2008;16(2):69-73.

[17]   Cowan J. Children and young people: reviewing practice and policies. Clin Governance Int J 2008;13(1):73-8.

[18]   Department of Health. The nursing, midwifery and health visiting contribution to health and health care. London: Department Health, 1993.

[19]   Hogan H, Basnett I, McKee M. Consultant's attitudes to clinical governance: Barriers and incentives to engagement. Public Health 2007;121:614-22.

[20]   Blumenthal D, Kilo C. A report card on continuous quality-improvement. Milbank Q 1998;76(625-648).

[21]   Locock L. Redesigning health care: New wine from old bottles. J Health Service Res Policy. 2003;8:120-2.

[22]   Morrison P, Heineke J. Why do health practitioners resist quality management. Quality Progress 1992;25:51-5.

[23]   Johnstone M, Kanitsaki O. Patient safety and the integration of graduate nurses into effective organisational clinical risk management systems and processes: An Australian study. Organizational Manage Health Care 2008;17(2):162-73.

[24]   Swerissen H, Jordan L. Clinical governance in community health care settings: Evidence and issues. Aust J Primary Health 2005;11(2):26-31.

[25]   Crisp BR, Lister PG. Nurses' perceived training needs in chldr protection issues. Health Educ 2006;106(5):381-99.

[26]   Laming L. The Victoria Climbie Inquiry: Report of an inquiry by Lord Laming. London: HMSO, 2003.

[27]   Hammond H. Child protection inquiry into the circumstances surrounding the death of Kennedy McFarlane. Edinburgh: Dumfries Galloway Child Protection Committee, 2001.

[28]   Lupton C, Khan P, North N, Lacy D. The role of health professionals in the Child Protection process. Portsmouth: Social Services Research Unit, University Portsmouth, 2000 21.

[29]   Royal College of Nursing. Child protection. Every nurse's responsibility. London: RCN, 2003.

[30]   Quin G, Evans R. Accident and emergency department access to the child protection register: a questionnaire survey. EMJ 2002;19:136-7.

[31]   Powell C. Child protection: The crucial role of hte children's nurse. Paediatr Nurs 1997;9(9):13-6.

[32]   Thoebald S. Child protection. Why continuing education for nurses is important. Pediatr Nurs 2000;12(3):6-7.

[33]   Murray T. Child protection neglected in pediatric training. Med Post 2002;38(25):1.

[34]   Gunn VL, Hickson GB, Cooper WO. Factors affecting pediatricians' reporting of suspected child maltreatment. Ambulent Pediatr 2005;5:96-101.

[35]   Kendall-Tackett K, Lyon T, Taliaferrro G, Little L. Why child maltreatment researchers should include children's disability status in their maltreatment studies. Child Abuse Negl 2005;29:147-51.

[36]   Wilson SL, Kuebli JE, Hughes HM. Patterns of maternal behavior among neglectful families: implications for research and intervention. Child Abuse Negl 2005;29:985-1001.

[37]   Korbin JE. Neighborhood and community connectedness in child maltreatment research. Child Abuse Negl 2003;27:137-40.

[38]   Sedlack AJ, Bdroadhurst DD. Third national incidece study of child abuse and neglect: final report. Washington, DC: US Department Health Human Services, 1996.

[39]   Dubowitz H. Preventing child gengecta nd physical abuse: A role for pediatricians. Pediatr Rev 2002;23:191-6.

[40]   Kelly A. A public health nursing perspective. In: Fergusson H, Kenny P, eds. Behalf of the child: Child welfare, child protection and the Child Care Act 1991. Bublin: AA Farmar, 1995:186-202.

[41]   Gilligan R. Irish child care services-Policy, practice and provision. Dublin: Institute Public Administration, 1991.

[42]   Burke TP. Survey of the workload of public health nurses. Dublin, Ireland: Institute Community Health Nursing, 1986.

[43]   NSW Department of Health. Child Protection Service Plan 2004-2007. In: Health NDo, editor: NSW Department of Health 2004; 2004.

[44]   Queensland Health. Strategic Policy Framework for Children's and Young People's Health 2002-2007. Brisbane, QLD: Queensland Health, 2002.

[45]   Gough D, Bell M. Providing services for children and young People who have experienced sexual abuse. Child Abuse Rev 2005;14:1-3

[46]   Johnson Z, Howell F, Molloy B. Community mothers programme: randomised contorlled trial of non-professional interveniton in parenting. BMJ 1993;306:1449-52.

[47]   Cowley S, J. BR. Resources revisited: salutogenesis from a lay perspective. J Adv Nurs 1999;29:994-1004.

[48]   Greenwalt BC, Sklare G, Portes P. The therapeutic treatment provided in cases involving physical child abuse: A description of current practices. Child Abuse Negl 1998;22(1):71-8.

[49]   Choy S. The psychological perspective. In: Untalan FF, Mills CS, eds. Interdisciplinary perspectives in child abuse and neglect. New York: Praeger, 1992.

[50]   Graziano AM, Mills JR. Treatment for abused children: When is a partial solution acceptable? Child Abuse Negl 1992;16:217-28.

[51] White JC. The role of the social worker. In: Bross DC, Michaels LF, eds. Foundations of child advocacy: Legal representation of the maltreated child. Longmont, CO: Bookmakers Guild, 1987:61-70.

[52] Elmer E, Schultz BS. Social work evaluation and family assessment. In: D.C. Bross DC, Krugman RD, Lenherr MR, Rosenberg DA, Schmitt BD, ed. The new child protection team handbook. New York: Garland, 1988:136-49.

[53] Tomison AM, ed. Interagency collaboration and communication in child protection cases: some findings from an Australian case tracking study. Paper presented at the Fifth ISPCAN Asian Conference on Child Protection; 26-28 November, 1999; Hong Kong: National Child Protection Clearing House, Australian Institute of Family Studies.

[54] Campbell KA, Bogen DL, Berger RP. The other children. A survey of child abuse physicians on the medical evaluation of children living with a physically abused child. Arch Pediatr Adolesc Med 2006;160:1241-6.

[55] Tomison A, Poole L. Preventing child abuse and neglect: Findings from an Australian audit of prevention programs. Melbourne, Australia: Australian Institute Family Studies, 2000.

[56] Darlington Y, Feeney JA. Collaboration between mental health and child protection services: Professionals' perceptions of best practice. Child Youth Serv Rev 2008;30(2):187-98.

[57] Bailey S. Confidentiality and young people: Myths and realities. In: Cordess C, editor. Confidentiality and mental health. London: Jessica Kingsley, 2001:71-84.

[58] Morrison T. Partnership and collaboration: Rhetoric and reality. Child Abuse Negl 1996;20(2):127-40.

[59] Pietsch J, Short L. Working together: Families in which a parent has a mental illness: Developing 'best practice' for service provision and interagency collaboration. Melbourne, Australia: Mental Health Research Institute, 1998.

[60] Mizrahi T, Rosenthal BB. Complexities of coalition building: Leaders' successes, strategies, struggles, and solutions. Social Work 2001;46(1):63-78.

[61] Crocker D. Innovative models for rural child protection teams. Child Abuse Negl 1996;20(3):205-11

[62] Gentry T, Brisbane FL. The solution for child abuse rests with the community. Children Today 1982:22-4.

[63] Miller JL, Whittaker JK. Social services and social support: blended programs for families at risk of child maltreatment. Child Welfare 1988;67.(2):161-74.

[64] Sidebotham P, Biu T, Goldsworthy L. Child protection procedures in emergency departments. Emergency Med J 2008;24:831-5.

[65] Cruickshanks P, Skellern C. Role of the tertiary child protection paediatrician: Expert and advocate. J Paediatr Child Health 2007;43:34-9.

[66] Kolko DJ. Clinical monitoring of treatment course in child physical abuse: psychometric characteristics and treatment comparisons. Child Abuse Negl1996;20:23-43.

[67] Fantuzzo JW, Wray L, Hall R, Goins C, Azar S. Parent and social-skills training for mentally retarded mothers identified as child maltreaters. Am J Mental Defic 1986;91:135-40.

[68] Moore E, Seattle WA, Armsden G, Seattle W, Gogerty PL. A twelve-year follow-up study of maltreated and at-risk children who received early therapeutic child care. Child Maltreat 1998;3(1): 3-16.

[69] Deare JR. A meta-analytic investigation of group treatment outcomes for sexually abused children. Child Abuse Negl 1997;21(7):669-80.

[70] Cerezo MA, Pons-Salvador G. Improving child maltreatment detection systems: a large-scale case study involving health, social services, and school professionals. Child Abuse Negl 2004;28(11):1153-69.

In: Public Health Yearbook 2013
Editor: Joav Merrick

ISBN: 978-1-63321-095-0
© 2014 Nova Science Publishers, Inc.

Chapter 39

MANAGING OCCUPATIONAL STRESS INJURY IN POLICE SERVICES: A LITERATURE REVIEW

*Christine Randall[1] and Nicholas Buys, PhD[1,2]**

[1]School of Human Services and Social Work, Griffith University,
Parkland, Gold Coast, Australia
[2]Griffith Health Institute, Griffith University, Parkland, Gold Coast, Australia

ABSTRACT

Occupational stress is an increasingly significant economic and social burden in Australia, yet its impact is not being adequately addressed, particularly in emergency services organisations, such as police services. Management of workplace stress injury is therefore a priority, requiring integration of effective occupational rehabilitation systems to prevent and mitigate this condition at an organisational level. This literature review describes the specific issues associated with occupational stress in police services. Findings of the review indicate that attention is required to the job and organisational characteristics of police services, stress management processes, training and knowledge, and the police culture and organisational climate. These issues contribute to stress and create barriers to rehabilitation within police services. Recommendations for addressing occupational stress in police organisations are provided, with a focus on developing and maintaining effective prevention and rehabilitation processes.

Keywords: Occupational stress, police services, stress management

INTRODUCTION

Stress in the work context is a significant issue given the economic impact on employers and society. The median cost for a mental disorders claim in Australia was calculated at $18,000 in 2008-09, whilst the median cost for all serious workers' compensation claims during the

---

* Corresponding author: Professor Nicholas Buys, PhD, School of Human Services and Social Work, Griffith University, Australia. Email: n.buys@griffith.edu.au.

same period was $7,700 (1). There are considerable indirect and hidden costs associated with stress injury (2). For example, workplace stress significantly affects employee productivity, absenteeism, and presenteeism with an estimated overall cost of over $10 billion per year (2-4). Hidden costs are also associated with staff turnover, the impact of stress on physical health, such as cardiovascular disease and musculoskeletal disorders, and the consequences for families and society. The direct and indirect costs of stress suggest that employers need to manage this condition in the workplace to ensure their businesses remain competitive.

In Australia, employers have a legal obligation to prevent and manage workplace injuries. This includes the provision of safe work environments, workers' compensation insurance and rehabilitation assistance (5-7). Employers must also adhere to health and safety legislation, regulations and codes of practice (8,9). Those employers that manage and reduce occupational injury and disease beyond legislative demands can reduce insurance premiums, and improve productivity and company image (5,10,11). Numerous studies have identified workplace interventions as key to recovery and successful return to work, recognising that work environment factors, such as work tasks and work organisation, social relationships and organisational culture, are significant in work disability (12-16). A favourable work environment is particularly important when returning workers with mental health issues to the workplace (12).

Addressing workplace stress injury is particularly relevant in front line emergency services, such as police services. Personal and other service occupations have the highest frequency of workers' compensation claims for occupational diseases and up to 75% of these claims are for mental disorders. Police services, corrective services and fire brigade services account for 84% of the mental disorders claims in the personal and other services occupational categories, (1), making these public order and safety occupations a primary concern for mental disorder claims. Police officers and emergency service personnel in particular face operational stressors (17,18), and these stressors are significantly added to or moderated by workplace factors (19,20), necessitating an organisational response to injury.

ORGANISATIONAL RESPONSE TO INJURY: WORKPLACE REHABILITATION

One response to managing the direct and indirect costs of occupational stress injury to organisations is to develop effective occupational rehabilitation systems to both prevent and manage injuries (21). Occupational rehabilitation is a process aimed at maintaining and/or restoring injured workers' functional effectiveness via appropriate and timely services (22, 23). Effective occupational rehabilitation includes immediate interventions after injury with the aim of returning injured workers back to the same workplace as early and safely as possible (5,24,25). Six essential components of successful return to work rehabilitation programs have been identified that include centralized coordination of return to work, individual psychological and occupational interventions, workplace-based interventions, work accommodations, contact between the stakeholders and concerted action (13).

While the focus of much rehabilitation literature has been on individual clinical and psychological factors associated with return to work, addressing these is not necessarily the most effective approach for promoting return to work outcomes (12-15). Whilst clinical treatment may reduce symptoms, the impact on return to work outcomes is limited unless combined with other interventions within a systems approach that acknowledges the interaction between the injured worker and health care, the work environment and the compensation system (12-14,16). Work environment factors, such as work tasks and work organisation, social relationships and organisational culture, are now recognised as significant in work disability, and numerous studies have identified workplace interventions as key to recovery and successful return to work (12-16).

Although a favourable work environment is particularly important when returning workers with mental health issues to the workplace (12), workplace interventions also have to be feasible in practice (15,16). Studies have found that implementation of return to work programs within organisations requires active participation from key stakeholders, such as injured workers and their supervisors. (15,16). Stakeholder involvement factors include interactions between all participants, including compensation, health care and the work context, recognising the multi-causality of work disability beyond the initial injury (12,13, 16). Contemporary approaches to occupational rehabilitation, such as disability management, emphasise the seamless transition from prevention to post-injury rehabilitation and the involvement of stakeholders (21,26-28). Disability management is focused on employers and takes a systematic approach to the integration of prevention, claims management, early intervention and return to work case management (26), and has been highlighted as an effective occupational rehabilitation model, especially when applied within large organisations (21,26,28-30). Injured workers are actively involved in their rehabilitation programs and are encouraged to have input into the development of return to work goals and plans, participate in stakeholder meetings, and contribute their work experience to the design of work accommodations. Injured workers are further empowered with information about their medical condition/s and company policies (26). This approach has been shown to achieve improvements in return to work outcomes, productivity and employee satisfaction, as well as saving on costs associated with absenteeism (26, 31, 32). Large companies with successful disability management programs provide training and support for supervisors and financial incentives for departments to encourage local ownership of temporary work disability (31,32). Supervisors, union representatives and co-workers are also actively involved in both prevention and rehabilitation processes (26). Despite the promises of a disability management approach, minimal research has been undertaken into the application of disability management policies and practices (28) and the implementation of disability management principles in organisations (30). In particular there is little published information on effective interventions in the area of occupational stress (33). Clearly there is a need for more focus on the specific needs and cultures of Australian organisations in addressing occupational rehabilitation issues.

OCCUPATIONAL STRESS

Stress and psychological injuries are of significant concern to employers due to increased workers compensation costs, (6,30,34), and to employees given its impact on job satisfaction and quality of life (19,20,35). Physical health is also affected by chronic stress, increasing the risk of other occupational injuries to both the stressed individual and co-workers (36).

Organisationally focused approaches to stress are thought to potentially benefit more employees than individually focused approaches (33), which are often now questioned in terms of their effectiveness to manage occupational stress (34,37,38). Different understandings of stress focus on different solutions, such as treating individuals or adjusting environments. Contemporary perspectives are more multidimensional than either the traditional psycho-medical or the stressor and strain model, taking ecological or systemic approaches (39). Ecologically, humans are viewed as living systems within environmental systems with psychological and social factors influencing each other (39).

In the work context, stress is best understood as a process influenced by several factors where stressors interact with an individual's capacities resulting in strain if the stressors exceed the resources (30,40). Work stress definitions are often confused by the different uses of the term stress to also denote 'stressors' (the demands), as well as 'strain' (the negative outcome of stress) (30). Perceived work stress is the extent to which a person feels strain in relation to their work. Demanding jobs that lack individual control over the work and flexibility are considered most stressful (34,41,42). However, the assumption that stress is inherently negative or that it should be completely avoided is inaccurate (43). For example positive stress that does not exceed capacity can optimise productivity, while an ongoing lack of demands to challenge an individual can lead to long term dissatisfaction and be perceived as stressful (30). Frequent work stress is most strongly associated with problems for both individuals and organisations (41). Furthermore, strain resulting from work, personal and social stressors can impact on workers and are therefore considered in work stress studies (44).

INDIVIDUAL VERSUS ORGANISATIONAL FACTORS

Given that occupational stress is recognised as the incompatibility between individual capacity and organisational demands (30,40,44-46), it is important to address the both individual and organisational causes of stress in the workplace (12,47-49). Focusing on getting a stressed worker better, only to return the worker to the same stressful workplace is clearly ineffective and therefore requires co-operation from organisational stakeholders (12). Conducting the rehabilitation process from within the workplace allows the needs of the stressed individual to be addressed in the context of simultaneous reduction in workplace stressors demonstrating the employer's commitment to the wellbeing of all workers.

Individual factors contributing to stress include those that determine ability to cope with stressors, such as personality traits and coping styles (39,50). For example, personality and locus of control have been found to affect ability to cope with interpersonal stressors (51). People with internal locus of control believe that they can influence the outcomes of a situation, whereas people with an external locus of control do not believe in their ability to control an event. Kenny (50) explores coping in the context of development from early childhood to adulthood, stating that attachment processes and other developmental experiences influence the adult personality and ability to cope with stress. Personal life stressors and life changes, such as the death of a family member, birth of a child, moving house or financial problems also generate stress that may affect ability to cope in the work context (18).

Interventions focussed on individual factors emphasise teaching individuals to control stress responses; these include behavioural self-control (52), biofeedback (53), meditation and abdominal breathing (54), progressive visualisation and cognitive processing (55). These interventions aim to decrease stress reactions by controlling thought, physiological and behavioural responses to stressors (52,53,55). Established interventions, such as cognitive behavioural therapy and psychoanalysis, have common features such as progressive visualisation and relaxation, cognitive processing, and shifting to more positive feelings and more positive behaviours (55).

Given the value of work in modern society, the amount of time spent at work and the current changes that are affecting the nature of work, it is not surprising that work stress appears to be increasing (56). Three broad 'causes' of organisational stress have been identified as job-induced (e.g., work overload), organisationally-induced (e.g., communication problems) and change-induced (e.g., new supervisor) (4,57). Occupational stress and rehabilitation are impacted by organisational culture and climate, particularly in terms of how members of that organisation behave and expect others to behave (58,59). It is now clear from research that organisational climate cannot be ignored in efforts to reduce the fiscal and human costs of occupational stress (47,58). Improving the climate (and eventually the culture) of an organisation requires supportive leadership, peer support, and a shared understanding of goals and experiences, which contributes to a positive work environment conducive to good mental health and employee motivation (47,58). Further, Bell et al. (47) suggested strategies that address organisational culture (accepting and addressing the effects of trauma), workload (adequate variety and appropriate distribution), work environment (safety and comfort), job specific education, group support (social support and debriefing opportunities), supportive supervision, and resources for self-care (counselling, support groups or other resources).

CREATING HEALTHY ORGANISATIONS

Given the significance of organisational factors in occupational stress, it has been proposed that the management of stress involves the creation of 'healthy organisations', which are defined as ones which recognise that health is more than the absence of stress and other ill health and therefore create an environment which facilitates good health and positive emotions (60). Healthy organisations re-focus responsibility for the health of employees to the organisation and give more control to workers by encouraging their participation in change management, job re-design, open communication, and understanding of the political or economic constraints within which the organisation operates (61). This demonstrates organisational commitment to the worker, facilitating worker commitment to the organisation. It is therefore suggested that healthy organisations are those that adopt appropriate methods of job-person matching or job design that facilitates the expertise and needs of workers; managing and rewarding performance; informing and involving workers; and supporting lifestyle and family needs of workers (60,61). According to Schurman and Israel, any organisational intervention must be specific to the context rather than 'off-the-shelf'. The intervention must engage relevant people in direct learning activities that allow them to understand stress processes in their organisation at a systemic level and should involve participants in the development of change strategies (62). Improving health and safety in a large organisation also requires good communication, a detailed analysis of needs and implementation at a systemic level with support from all areas of the organisation (57).

POLICE CONTEXT

Over the past two decades, occupational stress literature has increasingly recognised the impact of organisational factors, such as organisational culture, on stress-related issues in policing. While police officers face operational stressors, such as occupational exposure to body fluids (17), critical incidents and violence (18), these stressors are significantly added to or moderated by organisational factors (19,20). For example, the development of PTSD, which is the most frequently investigated consequence of trauma in police officers (18), has been found to be most affected by the work environment (18,41,63).

Police stress is linked with health problems, antisocial behaviour and suicidal ideation (41,64). Causes of occupational stress for police officers include: 1) organisational factors, such as the paramilitary structures; 2) operational issues associated with tasks such as protecting people, rescuing traumatised people, role conflicts and dangerous work; 3) external systems, such as the criminal justice system, and public perceptions, including media coverage and; 4) personal life stressors (18). Critical incidents are defined as adverse events which may result in a range of symptoms from exhaustion to symptoms of progressing mental illness (63). These have been linked with post-traumatic stress disorder (PTSD) symptoms in police officers, including measurable physical and physiological symptoms (18,20,63). Indeed, police officers are exposed to a high degree of work stress in the form of critical incidents and 'disasters', such as intentional violence against humans, and studies have therefore linked police work to conditions such as "vicarious traumatization, secondary traumatic stress, traumatic counter-transference, burnout, and compassion fatigue" (18).

The situation of workplace stress for police is more complex than the stress relating to critical incidents, thereby requiring attention to a range of psychological, organisational and operational factors. Police work stressors are often described as organisational (such as lack of recognition) and operational (such as dealing with the public) (18,63). Psychological characteristics such as an external locus of control and negative affect have been linked to increased occupational stress experiences in correctional officers (65). Similarly, ineffective coping mechanisms, such as avoidance, are strongly related to perceived work stress and health outcomes, such as anxiety and burnout in police officers (41). In addition to the individual factors linked with poor mental health outcomes, police officers have complex work environments, including inadequate equipment, unsuitable co-workers, unfair workload distribution, inadequate supervision, unclear work roles, and shift work (41,63).

According to Mayhew (19), health and safety risks in policing include critical incidents, such as death, homicide and assault on police officers. However, this list of risks also includes organisational factors such as stress and fatigue due to staff shortages, limited job control, staff conflict, autocratic management, unfair performance appraisal, workers' compensation tribunal hearings and police culture (19), as well as poor relationships and lack of internal communication (20,66). Numerous studies indicate that work environment stress, rather than critical incidents, best predict perceived stress, PTSD symptoms and other health problems

(41,63). Work environment stressors include a lack of consultation and communication, inadequate control and excessive workloads, and poor levels of support (63). Organisational stressors and the negative public image of the police have also been found to magnify the impact of critical incidents faced by police officers (67). Outside of the workplace, negative life events, including work-family conflict, and past trauma also contribute to PTSD symptoms (63).

Mental health problems, including PTSD symptoms, in police officers have been linked to four factors: 1) regular exposure to traumatic events; 2) an individual's previous exposure to trauma; 3) "negative life events" outside of work; and 4) "routine work environment stress" (63). Maguen et al. acknowledge that policing is stressful and results in both physical and psychological symptoms. They examined the links between 'routine work environment stress' and PTSD symptoms utilising several measures of the four factors listed above to assess 180 recruits and reassess them after 12 months on the job. They found that the fourth factor (routine work environment stress) was most closely linked to PTSD symptoms. Work environment stressors affecting PTSD symptoms included dysfunctional equipment, routine operational hassles, work role ambiguity, poor interpersonal relationships with co-workers and discrimination (63).

There is a strong association between policing work and traumatic stress and burnout (18,20,63). There are also behavioural impacts of chronic stress among police officers, including suicide, drug and alcohol abuse, absenteeism and premature retirement, all of which occur at significantly higher rates than in other occupational groups (19,68). These findings have prompted research and discussion focused on addressing these risks in the police context. For instance, social support has been found to protect against the development of burnout and traumatisation conditions in police (18), and this extends to social support from the workplace. A supportive work environment protects police officers from developing PTSD symptoms and other mental health problems, by providing a compassionate context within which critical incidents are processed. Workplace cohesion and morale and strong leadership improve role clarity and job engagement and protects against the effects of stress (63). Furthermore, the workplace mediates between negative life events outside of work and PTSD symptoms. It was therefore concluded that whilst the organisation cannot control critical incidents and negative life events, it can provide the environment to buffer against the impacts of these factors (63). Prior trauma was also dismissed as a significant predictor of PTSD, suggesting that the focus should be on optimising the work environment rather than assessing previous traumatic events in police recruits lives (63).

OCCUPATIONAL REHABILITATION CHALLENGES
IN POLICE ORGANISATIONS

Police organisations need to address the complex issue of occupational stress due to the psychological, physical and behavioural impact of this occupational illness on individuals and their organisation. However, despite the significant body of evidence implicating organisational factors in the cause of occupational stress in policing, prevention activities (such as initial and ongoing police training) have continued to focus on operational dangers, leaving police officers ill prepared for organisational stressors (20,66). This imbalance between the evidence about causes of mental health conditions in police work and the interventions focused on treating individuals, rather than changing the organisational environment, has been echoed by other stress research (18,41). Accordingly, Gershon et al. (41) recommend a multi-layered approach, aimed at improving coping mechanisms in officers (shifting from avoidant and negative coping strategies to cognitive problem-solving strategies), as well as addressing modifiable stressors such as organisational unfairness and job dissatisfaction. They also describe innovative strategies implemented by some progressive police organisations that include provision of specific cognitive problem solving skills programs, Alcoholics Anonymous groups, couples' counselling retreats, peer support programs, changes to organisational structure, improved training programs and critical incident management systems (41).

Prevention and rehabilitation processes are likely to be affected by the police personality and culture. Police working personalities are developed in the context of the paramilitary organisational culture, the divided organisational subcultures (officers and staff) and the nature of their duties (69,70). These working personalities have been found to include characteristics such as natural suspicion (of outsiders and management), increased alertness to danger, solidarity with other serving officers and bravery (71-73). In the policing context, injury or disease translates to no longer being an active serving officer, no longer being seen as brave and not being able to stand alongside colleagues in the face of danger; these 'signs of weakness' stand in direct contrast to the accepted behaviour of police officers. In summary, the contextual and process issues described above suggest that solutions need to be sought in both overt processes and policies, and less tangible interpersonal factors concerning organisational culture, climate, characteristics and understandings about stress.

ADDRESSING OCCUPATIONAL STRESS IN POLICE ORGANISATIONS

Consistent with an ecological focus on addressing occupational stress in police the following recommendations reflect the complex nature of this condition. Changes to the organisational culture of police services, from the prevailing 'macho'/ paramilitary environment, would positively impact on injury prevention and early intervention efforts, encouraging members to remain positively engaged with their organisations. Research from the past 20 years indicates that organisational climate cannot be ignored in efforts to reduce the fiscal and human costs of occupational stress (47,58). Addressing the punitive culture of police organisations is necessary to prevent general bullying, particularly of injured and recovering workers. Organisational culture is often a cause of police officers' hesitation in reporting stress related issues, which limits the organisation's capacity to respond to problems and implement effective and early secondary prevention and rehabilitation. Improving the climate (and eventually the culture) of an organisation requires supportive leadership, peer support, and a shared understanding of goals and experiences, which contributes to a positive work environment conducive to good mental health and employee motivation (47, 58). Trust is an important issue in organisational culture, and is built upon a shared identity between supervisors and supervisees and ongoing co-operation between them (74).

Consistent with a disability management approach to managing injury, staff at all levels of the organisation should be involved in strategy development and supporting health, wellbeing and rehabilitation initiatives. Lack of worker involvement in these areas reduces the potential for prevention and rehabilitation (75), with failures to develop healthy organisations attributed to the fact that change was not managed with the participation of the workers (62). Healthy organisations re-focus the responsibility for health to the organisation, but simultaneously give more control to workers by encouraging their participation in change management, job re-design, open communication, and understanding of the political or economic constraints within which the organisation operates (60,61).

Dissemination of information to promote understanding about prevention and rehabilitation within the police service is critical to successful rehabilitation initiatives. This includes: (a) information about the prevention and rehabilitation of physical and psychological injury and illness for specific members of the organisation; (b) supervisors to be more informed about stress issues, prevention and rehabilitation to undertake their role in making decisions and providing support for staff; (c) clearer boundaries between industrial relations issues and rehabilitation; (d) better understanding by injured workers of rehabilitation procedures, and the roles of support staff; and (e) more information and support for the families of injured and stressed officers.

Organisations must adopt a more holistic and comprehensive understanding of psychological issues, including personal stressors. This is consistent with research that showed whilst both individual and organisational factors influenced the development of vicarious trauma, the focus of intervention remained on affected individuals (47). Practically useful website information designed for officers, including flow charts, contact details and useful links, should be provided and regularly promoted to all stakeholders so they are more informed and confident in the rehabilitation process. Supervisors need to training to detect early signs of stress to prevent the escalation of mental health issues to dangerous levels, as well as understanding and supporting different coping mechanisms. People in support roles need knowledge and skills to effectively manage rehabilitation, including advanced people management and communication skills. It is important that there are clear requirements and processes for all stakeholders when injured workers returned to the workplace. Advice to injured workers about what to expect during the return to work process and education for others in that workplace allows for more realistic expectations and more positive return to work experiences. Resources for self-care, such as counselling, support groups or other resources, have also been identified as important to maintaining wellbeing within an organisation (47).

A critical component of occupational rehabilitation for police officers is the availability of systematic debriefing processes that are automatically initiated and adequately resourced to prevent subsequent psychological issues. Research suggests that a supportive work environment protects police officers from developing PTSD symptoms and other mental health problems, by providing a compassionate context within which critical incidents are processed. Workplace cohesion and morale and strong leadership improve role clarity and job engagement and protects against the effects of stress (63). Furthermore, the workplace mediates between negative life events outside of work and PTSD symptoms.

Interventions are required at each stage of the occupational rehabilitation process from pre-injury through to maintenance of the return to work. There are several potential improvements to be made to develop more proactive and strategic injury and illness prevention initiatives. A feature of a comprehensive disability management approach to occupational stress is the ongoing data collection and evaluation of the common causes of stress, injury and attrition to improve prevention systems and strategies for serving officers. Upon identifying a problematic area for injuries and illness, the issues should be followed up and addressed in consultation with local managers. Simpson (4) recommends systematic organisational assessment of risks considering all levels, including the whole organisation, work groups and individuals, to effectively address organisational needs.

As a pre-injury strategy organisations should develop a detailed understanding of job factors and organisational characteristics that can be used to counteract the sometimes unavoidable operational risk factors associated with policing, particularly those causing mental illness, such as PTSD. Reducing work environment stressors and improving organisational support mechanisms reduces the development of serious mental illness, despite the operational risks. Further, improving training and knowledge for key stakeholders and providers may stem the escalation of stress, reduce the impact of injury and improve the outcomes of rehabilitation. A better awareness of stress and injury management processes for all stakeholders can improve the social structures and actions of officers to increase trust in the organisation and understanding about prevention and rehabilitation, thereby reducing the negative influence of stigma. Increased awareness requires time, resources and genuine interest in training to create a context where individuals feel more comfortable in reporting stress and participating in rehabilitation processes. Providing occupational rehabilitation awareness training can therefore have a broad and far reaching impact on injury prevention and rehabilitation outcomes in the organisation.

Injury and illness reporting processes are affected by the organisational climate, trust issues, as well as understanding of stress and rehabilitation processes. The needs and experiences of injured and ill individuals therefore need to take precedence over formal procedures to increase officers' willingness to seek help for stress or other issues impacting work capacity. Training to recognise stress and strategies to compensate for geographic isolation are required to identify absences and initiate earlier rehabilitation. Once a rehabilitation need is identified, stakeholders need simple clear processes to fast track reporting and initiate support, especially when there is no workers' compensation claim to guide the process. To achieve an increase in the rate of reporting of stress and other illness, strategies have to be approached in a supportive manner and be combined with making leaders more accountable for their people management skills and preparing the leaders of the future for this aspect of the role. Non-judgemental support and information about processes, such as lodging a workers' compensation claim, encourages people to report stress symptoms and obtain early assistance.

Effective systems for early identification of stress and wellbeing issues can prevent injuries. Absenteeism management strategies include identifying non-consecutive absence patterns that might point to early signs of stress, training for supervisors to identify and respond to issues before they escalate, and improved secondary prevention systems, including risk management and debriefing after traumatic incidents. These changes require a shift in the prevailing social structures that expect police officers to get on with the job regardless of what they have experienced. If the damage is psychological, individuals should receive appropriate care and treatment, such as mental health first aid. People in support and supervisory roles need work structures that allow them to get to know staff to be able to detect potential stress and rehabilitation issues, and respond before early signs of stress escalate to serious psychological injury.

An effective approach for responding to injury is the removal of the distinction between compensable and non-compensable cases, streamlining processes and clarifying responsibilities for responding to injury, and focusing on achieving optimal outcomes and addressing individual needs. Both external and internal factors influence organisations, creating tension between people and processes. Whilst compensable cases tend to have some clear processes driven by the workers' compensation authority, they create complexities in other organisational processes, such as the transition from the workers' compensation decision to internal support mechanisms. At the initial contact with the absent individual, an increased focus on addressing needs will reduce the risk of a non-compensable case being dismissed as needing no support at all. Similarly, when a workers' compensation claim is rejected by the insurer internal support options should still be considered, because a workers' compensation claim may be rejected based on eligibility criteria even if the individual needs support for an illness that affects their ability to work. For example, a drop in the number of mental stress claims has been linked to jurisdictions tightening up on what is accepted, thereby reducing claim numbers but not the incidence of stress (76,77). More proactive intervention outside of the claims process and would increase officers' trust in the organisation that they will be looked after following injury.

Streamlining processes and clarifying responsibilities for responding to injury, illness and absence is important to facilitate intervention and is required to increase trust in the organisation, increase local ownership of rehabilitation, and improve rehabilitation outcomes. This should include simplifying processes for interaction with external stakeholders like the workers' compensation authority and streamlining processes to initiate early intervention. Responding processes need to be focused on achieving optimal outcomes and addressing individual needs. The initial direct contact with the affected member needs to be early to gain an overview of the affected officer's needs and achieve a successful return to work. This requires minimal barriers to reporting. Injured workers need to be directly involved in communication throughout the rehabilitation process. Promoting individual ownership of rehabilitation has been established as important (26), and includes mechanisms encouraging feedback about support processes. Good communication with the absent officer early in the process helps them to understand issues, processes, roles and responsibilities, and promotes their constructive participation in the rehabilitation process. Early and effective contact with the absent individual is an opportunity to re-establish or maintain the occupational bond, address tensions and reduce stressors (30). If the initial contact is delayed or ineffective due to lack of time or excessive focus on paperwork, the whole rehabilitation process is jeopardised.

Intervention processes need to be focused on well-established principles of effective rehabilitation, especially for people with mental health problems. For instance, a holistic bio-psychosocial approach with multidisciplinary input, cognitive behavioural therapy and organisational interventions has been found to be effective in improving mental health and promoting successful return to work (78). Provided specific organisational needs are addressed, appropriate individual interventions are provided and stakeholder participation strategies are effectively implemented, well integrated return to work programs have been found to be effective for a range of conditions (12-16). Investing in rehabilitation interventions is cost effective because it promotes return to work outcomes and reduces compensation costs. Interventions aimed at return to work focus on job accommodations, including modified work tasks and work organisation (12,13). Creative approaches to finding return to work options for people requiring suitable duties are enhanced by easily accessible job descriptions and involving injured employees in decision making. Van Oostrom et al. (15) found that facilitating injured workers and supervisors to develop their own consensus-based solutions to return to work barriers is effective in identifying obstacles and practical solutions. The roles of supervisors and co-workers in a successful return to work process are vital, especially when mental health problems are involved, but these stakeholders often lack the knowledge and skills required to fulfil this role effectively, jeopardising the return to work outcome (12). As the return to work process is quite dependent on support from supervisors, they need to be well informed. Other stakeholders in the workplace, such as co-workers and supervisors, also need information about the return to work process to be able to accommodate the limitations prescribed on suitable duties plans. A favourable work environment is particularly important when returning workers with mental health issues to the workplace (12).

Return to work maintenance needs attention to achieve complete resolution of issues. In some cases the organisation should be more flexible about rehabilitation goals if permanently modified duties make the return to work more sustainable. For psychological and serious injuries there is a particular need for procedural mechanisms to ensure return to work maintenance and resolution of issues. Such mechanisms include systems to detect a re-emergence of health issues early and to restart the rehabilitation process quickly to ensure continued work functioning. Long-term monitoring, especially for psychological illnesses, is beneficial. In particular, all stakeholders within the workplace need to have an understanding of the long-term nature of mental health issues to support long-term return to work maintenance.

CONCLUSION

It is evident in Australia that there are ongoing challenges for the management of workplace stress stemming from workers' compensation and organisational systems. Rising costs associated with workplace injury and illness, especially as a result of mental stress, indicate the need for research that focuses on the specific occupational rehabilitation needs and practices of large organisations, taking into account the complex interactions between individual and organisational factors. In policing organisations, there is a particular need to consider the organisational climate and culture and to address these with input from all levels of the organisation. While effective processes and policies are important, interpersonal factors concerning organisational culture, climate, characteristics and understandings about stress need to be understood and managed. Effective organisational communication is required to address both interpersonal and organisational issues and achieve a balance between the two. Creating a healthy organisational environment capable of identifying and addressing the needs of officers, improving the organisational climate to increase reporting of health concerns, and responding to and addressing injury or illness with a focus on individual needs will contribute to achieving more sustainable return to work outcomes. Effective occupational rehabilitation systems in police services therefore require insight into interpersonal factors and organisational processes to address established social structures and the actions of officers, as well as the interactions between them.

REFERENCES

[1]   Safe Work Australia. Compendium of workers' compensation statistics Australia 2009-10. In: Section DA, editor. Canberra: Safe Work Australia, 2012:111.

[2]   Jauregui M, Schnall PL. Work, psychosocial stressors, and the bottom line. In: Schnall PL, Dobson M, Rosskam E, eds. Unhealthy work: causes, consequences, cures. Critical approaches in the health social sciences series. Amityville, NY: Baywood, 2009:153-67.

[3]   Working Carers Gateway. Managing stress in the workplace Lismore: NSW Health, 2010. Accessed 2013 Mar 10. URL: http://www.workingcarers.org.au/work/1149-managing-stress-at-work-for-employers-and-employees.

[4]   Simpson B. Occupational stress: Assessing the risk, addressing the hazard. In: Barrett T, Cameron D, eds. Safe business, good business A practical guide to occupational safety, health and insurance in Australasia, 2 ed. Guildford, Western Australia: Vinyard Publishing, 2004:151-69.

[5]   WorkCover Queensland. Insurance Brisbane: WorkCover Queensland, 2012. Accessed 2013 Mar 10. URL: http://www.workcoverqld.com.au/insurance.

[6]   Biggs HC. Occupational concerns and workplace well-health. Work 2009;32(1):1-3.

[7]   Department of Industrial Relations Queensland. What are your obligations? General information, 2005.

[8]   Department of Justice and Attorney-General. What are your obligations? General information. [Government website]. The State of Queensland, 2010. Accessed 2013 Mar 10. URL: http://www.deir. qld.gov.au/workplace/rights/yourobligation/info/index.htm.

[9]   National Research Centre for Occupational Health and Safety Regulation. About occupational health and safety regulation in Australia [University website]. Canberra: Australian National University, 2002. funded by WorkCover NSW, WorkSafe Victoria and Workplace Health and Safety Queensland]. Accessed 2013 Mar 10. URL: http://ohs.anu.edu.au/ohs/index.php.

[10]   CCH Occupational Health and Safety. Workplace rehabilitation manual Safety COH, editor. North Ryde, NSW: CCH Australia, 1990.

[11]   NOHSC. The cost of work-related injury and illness for Australian employers, workers and the community. Canberra: NOHSC, Commonwealth of Australia, 2004.

[12]   Briand C, Durand M-J, St-Arnaud L, Corbière M. Work and mental health: Learning from return-to-work rehabilitation programs designed for workers with musculoskeletal disorders. Int J Law Psychiatry 2007;30(4-5):444-57.

[13]   Briand C, Durand M-J, St-Arnaud L, Corbière M. How well do return-to-work interventions for musculoskeletal conditions address the multicausality of work disability? J Occup Rehabil 2008;18(2):207-17.

[14]   Wald J, Taylor S. Work impairment and disability in Posttraumatic Stress Disorder: A review and recommendations for psychological injury research and practice. Psychol Inj Law 2009;2(3):254-62.

[15]   van Oostrom S, van Mechelen W, Terluin B, de Vet H, Anema J. A participatory workplace intervention for employees with distress and lost time: A feasibility evaluation within a Randomized Controlled Trial. J Occup Rehabil 2009;19(2):212-22.

[16]   Tjulin Å, Edvardsson Stiwne E, Ekberg K. Experience of the implementation of a multi-stakeholder return-to-work programme. J Occup Rehabil 2009;19(4):409-18.

[17]   Wald J. The psychological consequences of occupational blood and body fluid exposure injuries. Disabil Rehabil 2009;31(23):1963-9.

[18]   Patterson GT. Mental stress and workers' compensation claims among police officers. J Workplace Rights 2009;14(4):441-55.

[19]   Mayhew C. Occupational health and safety risks faced by police officers. Canberra: Australian Institute of Criminology, 2001.

[20]   Stinchcomb J. Searching for stress in all the wrong places: Combating chronic organisational stressors in policing. Pol Prac Res 2004;5(3):259-77.

[21]   Harder H, Scott L. Comprehensive disability management. Edinburgh: Elsevier, 2005.

[22]   WorkCover NSW. Glossary. 2003.

[23]   NOHSC. Uniform guidelines for accreditation of rehabilitation providers. Canberra: Australian Government Publishing Service, 1995.

[24]   Harrison K, Allen S. Features of occupational rehabilitation systems in Australia: A map through the maze. Work 2003;21(2):141-52.

[25]   WorkCover NSW. Workers compensation and injury management fact sheet 2: Injury management and return-to-work programs. In: WorkCoverNSW, ed. Gosford, NSW: WorkCover NSW; no date.

[26]   Buys N, Randall C. Disability management: A global response to disability in the workplace. In: Marshall C, Kendall E, Banks M, Gover RM, eds. Disabilities: Insights from across fields and around the world. Westport, CT: Praeger, 2009: 129-44.

[27]   Smith D. Implementing disability management: A review of basic concepts and essential components. Empl Assist Quart 1997;12(4):37-50.

[28]   Westmorland M, Buys N. Disability management in a sample of Australian self-insured companies. Disabil Rehabil 2002;24(14):746-54.

[29]   Shrey D. Disability management in industry: the new paradigm in injured worker rehabilitation. Disabil Rehabil 1996;18(8):408-14.

[30]   Kendall E, Muenchberger H. Stress at work: Using a process model to assist employers to understand the trajectory. Work 2009;32(1):19-25.

[31]   Ceniceros R. Disability accommodation programs cut costs. Business Insurance 2010;44(33):24.

[32]   McDonald C. Integrated disability management fuels power company's comp claim success. National Underwriter PC 2010;114(29):12-3, 27.

[33]   Caulfield N, Chang D, Dollard MF, Elshaug C. A review of occupational stress interventions in Australia. Int J Stress Manage 2004;11(2):149-66.

[34]   Kompier M, Taris T. Psychosocial risk factors and work-related issues: state of the art and issues for future research. In: Antoniou A-S, Cooper C, eds. Research companion to organizational health psychology. New horizons in management. Cheltenham, UK: Edward Elgar Publishing, 2005:59-69.

[35]   Graves W. Police cynicism: Causes and cures. FBI Law Enforc Bull 1996;65:16-20.

[36]   Dollard M. Introduction: Context, theories and intervention In: Dollard M, Winefield A, Winefield H, eds. Occupational stress in the service professions London: Taylor Francis, 2003:1-42.

[37]   Dick P. The social construction of the meaning of acute stressors: A qualitative study of the personal accounts of police officers using a stress counselling service. Work Stress 2000;14(3):226-44.

[38]   Hart PM, Cotton P. Conventional wisdom is often misleading: police stress within an organisational health framework. In: Dollard MF, Winefield AH, Winefield HR, eds. Occupational stress in the service professions. London: Taylor Francis, 2003:103–41.

[39]   Kenny D, McIntyre D. Constructions of occupational stress: nuisances, nuances or novelties. In: Antoniou A-S, Cooper C, eds. Research companion to organizational health psychology. New horizons in management. Cheltenham, UK: Edward Elgar Publishing, 2005:20-58.

[40]   Gordon DR, Schnall PL. Beyond the individual: Connecting work environment and health. In: Schnall PL, Dobson M, Rosskam E, eds. Unhealthy work: Causes, consequences, cures. Critical approaches in the health social sciences. New York: Baywood, 2009:1-15.

[41]   Gershon RRM, Barocas B, Canton AN, Li X, Vlahov D. Mental, physical, and behavioral outcomes associated with perceived work stress in police officers. Crim Justice Behav 2009;36(3):275-89.

[42]   Spooner-Lane R, Patton W. Determinants of burnout among public hospital nurses. Aust J Adv Nurs 2007;25(1):8-16.

[43]   Nelson D, Simmons B. Eustress and attitudes at work: a positive approach. In: Antoniou A-S, Cooper C, editors. Research companion to organizational health psychology. New horizons in management. Cheltenham, UK: Edward Elgar Publishing, 2005:102-10.

[44]   Kendall E, Muenchberger H. Stressors and supports across work and non-work domains: The impact on mental health and the workplace. Work 2009;32(1):27-37.

[45]   Diamantopoulou A. Europe under stress. Work Stress 2002;5:3.

[46]   Humphrey J. Job Stress. Needman Heights, MA: Allyn Bacon, 1998.

[47]   Bell H, Kulkarni S, Dalton L. Organizational prevention of vicarious trauma. Fam Society 2003;84(4):463-70.

[48]   Giga SI, Cooper CL, Faragher B. The development of a framework for a comprehensive approach to stress management interventions at work. Int J Stress Manage 2003;10(4):280-96.

[49]   La Montagne AD. Evaluation of occupational stress interventions: An overview. National Occupational Health and Safety Commission Symposium on the OH&S implications of stress, 12 December 2001; Melbourne: National Occupational Health Safety Commission, 2001.

[50]   Kenny D. Psychological foundations of stress and coping: A developmental perspective. In: Kenny DT, Carlson JG, McGuigan FJ, Sheppard JL, eds. Stress and health: Research and clinical applications. Australia: Harwood Academic, 2000:73-104.

[51]   Hahn SE. The effects of locus of control on daily exposure, coping and reactivity to work interpersonal stressors: a diary study. Pers Individ Dif 2000;29(4):729-48.

[52]   McGuigan FJ. Why might stress management methods be effective? In: Kenny DT, Carlson JG, McGuigan FJ, Sheppard JL, eds. Stress and health: research and clinical applications. Australia: Harwood Academic, 2000:151-61.

[53]   McKee MG, Kiffer JF. Biofeedback and stress. In: Kenny DT, Carlson JG, McGuigan FJ, Sheppard JL, eds. Stress and health: research and clinical applications. Australia: Harwood Academic, 2000:163-78.

[54]   Stoyva J. Stress management: What can we learn from the meditative disciplines? In: Kenny DT, Carlson JG, McGuigan FJ, Sheppard JL, eds. Stress and health: research and clinical applications. Australia: Harwood Academic, 2000:179-93.

[55]   Sheppard JL. Behavior change following affect shift: A model for the treatment of stress disorders. In: Kenny DT, Carlson JG, McGuigan FJ, Sheppard JL, eds. Stress and health: research and clinical applications. Australia: Harwood Academic, 2000:195-222.

[56]   Szymanski EM. Disability, job stress, the changing nature of careers, and the career resilience portfolio. Rehabil Couns Bull 1999;42:279-84.

[57]   Kendall E, Murphy P, Bursnall S, O'Neill V. Containing the costs of occupational stress: A new approach to identifying, defining, preventing and managing stress in the workplace. Perth: Workcover WA, 2001.

[58]   Cotton P. Developing an optimal organisational climate. Towards safest workplaces II, March 2004: ComCare; 2004.

[59]   Muchinsky P. Psychology applied to work: An introduction to industrial and organisational psychology, 5th ed. Pacific Grove CA: Brookes/Cole, 1997.

[60]   Cartwright S, Cooper C. The role of organizations in promoting health and wellbeing. In: Cartwright S, Cooper C, eds. Innovations in stress and health. Basingstoke: Palgrave Macmillan, 2011:153-72.

[61]   Henry J. The healthy organization. In: Antoniou A-S, Cooper C, eds. Research companion to organizational health psychology. New horizons in management. Cheltenham, UK: Edward Elgar Publishing, 2005:382-92.

[62]   Schurman S, Israel B. Redesigning work systems to reduce stress: A participatory action research approach to creating change. In: Murphy L, Hurrell J, Sauter S, Keita G, eds. Job Stress Interventions. Washington, DC: American Psychological Association, 1995.

[63]   Maguen S, Metzler TJ, McCaslin SE, Inslicht SS, Henn-Haase C, Neylan TC, et al. Routine work environment stress and PTSD symptoms in police officers. J Nerv Ment Dis 2009;197(10):754-60.

[64]   Collins PA, Gibbs ACC. Stress in police officers: a study of the origins, prevalence and severity of stress-related symptoms within a county police force. Occup Med 2003;53(4):256-64.

[65]   Botha C, Pienaar J. South African correctional official occupational stress: the role of psychological strengths. J Crim Justice 2006;34(1):73-84.

[66]   Kop N, Euwema M, Schaufeli W. Burnout, job stress and violent behaviour among Dutch police officers. Work Stress 1999;13(4):326-40.

[67]   Brown J, Fielding J, Grover J. Distinguishing traumatic, vicarious and routine operational stressor exposure and attendant adverse consequences in a sample of police officers. Work Stress 1999;13(4):312-25.

[68]   Anshel MH, Robertson M, Caputi P. Sources of acute stress and their appraisals and reappraisals among Australian police as a function of previous experience. J Occup Org Psych 1997;70(4):337-56.

[69] Parsons D, Jesilow P. In the same voice: Women and men in law enforcement. Santa Ana, CA: Seven Locks Press, 2001.

[70] Perez DW, Shtull PR. Police research and practice: An American perspective. Police Pract Res 2002;3(3):169-87.

[71] Skolnick J. A sketch of the police officer's "working personality". In: Hancock B, Sharp PM, eds. Criminal justice in America: Theory, practice and policy. Upper Saddle River, NJ: Prentice Hall, 1996.

[72] Kappeler VE, Sluder RD, Alpert GP. Forces of deviance: Understanding the dark side of policing. Prospect Heights, IL: Waveland Press, 1994.

[73] Prenzler T. Is there a police culture? Aust J Public Admin 1997;54(4):47-56.

[74] Dirks K, Skarlicki D. Trust in leaders: Existing research and emerging issues. In: Kramer R, Cook K, eds. Trust and distrust in organizations: Dilemmas and approaches. New York: Russell Sage Foundation, 2004:21-40.

[75] O'Donnell C. Motor accident and workers' compensation insurance design for high quality health outcomes and cost containment. Disabil Rehabil 2000;22:88-96.

[76] Safe Work Australia. Compendium of workers' compensation statistics Australia 2008–09. In: Section DA, ed. Canberra: Safe Work Australia, 2011.

[77] Safe Work Australia. Work-related injuries in Australia, 2005–06: Factors affecting applications for workers' compensation Canberra: Commonwealth of Australia, 2009.

[78] Campbell J, Wright C, Moseley A, Chilvers R, Richards S, Stabb L. Avoiding long-term incapacity for work: Developing an early intervention in primary care. Exeter, UK: Peninsula Medical School, Primary Care Research Group, 2007.

In: Public Health Yearbook 2013
Editor: Joav Merrick

ISBN: 978-1-63321-095-0
© 2014 Nova Science Publishers, Inc.

Chapter 40

USING THE ILLINOIS TEST OF PSYCHOLINGUISTIC ABILITY TO ASSESS VISUAL AND AUDITORY ABILITIES IN CHINESE CHILDREN WITH LEARNING DIFFICULTIES

Jing Sun, PhD[*1] *and Nicholas Buys, PhD*[2]

[1]School of Medicine and Griffith Health Institute, Griffith University,
Gold Coast Campus, Parkland, Australia
[2]School of Human Services and Social Work, and Griffith Health Institute,
Griffith University, Parkland, Gold Coast, Australia

ABSTRACT

There is ample evidence to indicate that children with learning difficulties have visual-perceptual and auditory ability deficits. The aim of the study was to investigate whether the deficits in visual-perceptual and auditory abilities also exist in Chinese children in the schools. One-hundred-forty nine students aged 6 to 10 years who attended Child Growth and Development Clinics at Capital Institute of Pediatrics, Beijing, China were invited to attend the study, and 54 children who had no learning difficulties and had normal neurological development were randomly selected from the local schools as the control group. The results showed significant lower scores in visual-perceptual and auditory abilities in the study group than control group. To prevent children's learning difficulties, health promotion focusing on visual-perceptual and auditory abilities should be mandatory for children who have learning difficulties, even in the absence of neurological impairments and with normal general intelligence development.

Keywords: Learning difficulties, visual ability, auditory ability, Illinois Test of Psycholinguistic Ability

* Correspondence: Jing Sun, PhD, School of Medicine, Griffith University and Griffith Health Institute, Griffith University, Gold Coast Campus, Parkland, Q4222 Australia. E-mail: j.sun@griffith.edu.au

INTRODUCTION

Although children with learning disabilities are often regarded as a heterogeneous group, they often have difficulties in processing information using their visual-perceptual and auditory abilities. Their visual and auditory abilities are related to the academic performance of students with learning disabilities (1). Research on the relationship of visual and auditory abilities to learning disabilities is often associated with the constructs of comprehension, memory, association, and integration of visual and auditory abilities, and visual and verbal expression (1-3). Mammarella (3) and colleagues found children with learning difficulties had spatial working memory deficits compared to normal matched counterparts. A recent study by Menghini and colleagues (4) found children with dyslexia had difficulties not only in comprehension and phonological coding, but also visual spatial working memory. Other studies found the occurrence of learning difficulties in children in reading, maths and written language was related to the deficits of spatial-visual abilities (5). Despite ample findings of visual and auditory deficits in children with learning difficulties, there are no studies that have assessed these deficits in Chinese children with learning difficulties. This study explores the characteristics of visual and auditory abilities among Chinese children with learning disabilities.

METHODS

One hundred and forty five children with learning difficulties, 103 male (69.1%) and 42 female (31.9%), were recruited from Child Growth and Development Clinics at the Affiliated Children's Hospital in Capital Institute of Pediatrics in Beijing, China. The subjects were referred for evaluation by teachers because of their low academic performance, behavioral and/or learning problems. Subjects with known neurological disorders including epilepsy, traumatic brain injury, and neurological impairments were excluded from the study. The criteria for the inclusion of children as subjects in the study group were: 1) the children's school achievement was below the 10% percentile based on grade level, 2) the children's level or intelligence was within the normal range or above average and 3) there were no visual and hearing impairments (examined by the neurologists at Children's Hospital of Capital Institute of Pediatrics, Beijing, China). All children were from families of Han ethnic origin and from middle to low socio-economic levels. Fifty two children aged 6 to 10 years who had normal academic achievement and normal intelligence scores on the Wechsler Intelligence Test were randomly chosen from children from grades one to four from a local primary school as the comparison group. The informed consents were obtained from parents of the participating children. The ethical clearance to conduct the study was approved by the research board of the Capital Institute of Pediatrics, Beijing, China.

Measures

The ITPA subtests were used to assess visual and auditory abilities of the children (6, 7). These subtests are designed to assess fundamental abilities underlying learning process by sampling three dimensions, i.e., two channels of communication (auditory-vocal, visual-motor), psycholinguistic processes (reception, association, expression), and levels of organization (representational, automatic). The ITPA consists of 10 subtests, including Auditory Reception, Visual Reception, Auditory Association, Visual Association, Verbal Expression, Manual Expression, Grammatical Closure, Visual Closure, Auditory Sequential Memory, and Visual Sequential Memory. The reliability and validity of ITPA test is high with internal consistency coefficients range from .60-.96, with a median of .88 (7). Information regarding demographic data including age, gender, type of family, living condition was collected using a questionnaire. Information relating to parental education methods, parity, child's sleeping status, type of delivery, size of accommodation, birth weight, and time length of lack of oxygen was also collected.

Statistical methods

Comparisons of differences between study and control groups on demographic variables, family functioning, disease history, birth status, were conducted using Chi-square for the categorical variables, and t test for continuous variables. An independent sample t test was used to compare the difference between study and control groups in visual-perceptual and auditory abilities. To explore the correlation between visual and auditory abilities, a Pearson correlation test was used. For all statistical tests, statistical significance was accepted as at probability (P value) level less than 0.05.

RESULTS

Table 1 demonstrates that there are significant differences between study and control groups in gender, parental education methods, and living conditions. There were more boys in the study group than control group, and more parents in the study groups used 'simple, rigid and autocratic', and 'inconsistent' education methods. In addition, there were more children in the study group living in apartments than those in the control group. There were no significant differences in child ages, disease history, birth status, parity, sleeping status, type of delivery, size of accommodation, birth weight, and time length of lack of oxygen.

Table 1. Comparison of demographic factors between study and control group

Variables	Normal child (N= 54)	Child with learning disability (N= 149)	Chi-square value	P
	N (%)	N (%)		
Gender				
Female	24 (48.0%)	44 (29.9%)	5.39	0.02
Male	26 (52.0%)	103 (70.1)		
Type of family				
Single parent	1 (2.0%)	3 (2.1%)	4.80	0.30
Nuclear family	23 (46.0%)	82 (56.6%)		
Big family with grandparents	18 (36.0%)	37 (25.5%)		
Big family which had more than two Nuclear family	5 (10.0)	7 (4.8%)		

Table 1. (Continued)

Variables	Normal child (N= 54)	Child with learning disability (N= 149)	Chi-square value	P
	N (%)	N (%)		
Grandparent living with grandchildren	3 (6.0%)	16 (11.0%)		
Method of education of parents				
Over protective, spoiling, lenient and superseding	3 (6.1%)	22 (15.1%)	15.92	0.001
Simple, rigid and autocratic	5 (10.2%)	30 (20.5%)		
Democratic, patient and teach with skill and patience	22 (44.9%)	26 (17.8%)		
Inconsistent methods	19 (38.8%)	68 (46.6%)		
Accommodation Type				
House	26 (54.2%)	44 (30.8%)	8.47	0.004
Apartment	22 (45.8 %)	99 (69.2%)		
Child sleep with parent				
Independent sleeping	9 (18.8%)	35 (24.0%)	2.94	0.23
sleep with somebody	22 (45.8%)	47 (32.2%)		
sleep with parents	17 (35.4%)	64 (43.8%)		
Prenatal Diseases				
Yes	4 (8.5%)	11 (8.0%)	0.01	0.92
No	43 (91.5%)	126 (92.0%)		
Prenatal diseases				
1	5 (38.5%)	20 (40.8%)	7.28	0.20
2	0 (0.0%)	2 (4.1%)		
3	3 (23.1%)	16 (32.7%)		
4	3 (23.1%)	5 (10.2%)		
8	2 (15.3%)	1 (2.0%)		
10	0 (0.0%)	5 (10.2%)		
Gravida				
1	36 (78.3%)	90 (72.0%)	0.96	0.81
2	8 (17.4%)	28 (22.4%)		
3	2 (4.3%)	6 (4.8%)		
4	0 (0.0%)	1 (0.8%)		
Parity				
1	43 (100.0%)	116 (96.7%)	1.47	0.48
2	0 (0.0%)	3 (2.5%)		
3	0 (0.0%)	1 (0.8%)		
Full term				
Yes	44 (97.8)	134 (94.4%)	0.87	0.35
No	1 (2.2%)	8 (5.6%)		
Type of delivery				
Vaginal	34 (72.3%)	86 (60.6%)	2.65	0.45
Surgery	11 (23.5%)	42 (29.6%)		
Assistance by equipment	1 (2.1%)	9 (6.3%)		
Induced by equipment	1 (2.1%)	5 (3.5%)		
Lack of oxygen in delivery				
Yes	5 (12.5%)	15 (11.9%)	0.01	0.92
No	35 (87.5%)	111 (88.1%)		
Age M(SD)	7.88 (1.18)	8.06 (1.78)	0.63	0.53
Size of Accommodation for each person in a family M(SD)	9.37 (9.03)	12.17 (17.36)	1.06	0.29

Variables	Normal child (N= 54)	Child with learning disability (N= 149)	Chi-square value	P
	N (%)	N (%)		
Birth weight M(SD)	3187.73 (460.31)	3289.73 (612.69)	1.02	0.31
Time length of lacking oxygen M(SD)	10.07 (16.74)	2.13 (2.10)	-1.56	0.15

Table 2. Comparison in visual and auditory abilities between children with learning difficulties and normal children

Variables	Normal child (n=50) M (S D)	Child with learning disability (n=149) M (S D)	t	P
Visual reception	37.67 (9.05)	39.77 (9.84)	1.34	0.18
Auditory reception	22.21 (6.96)	19.33 (6.62)	**2.66**	**0.008**
Visual memory	18.04 (5.31)	16.03 (7.62)	1.76	**0.008**
Auditory memory	35.89 (14.27)	35.40 (9.93)	0.27	0.79
Auditory Association	28.20 (8.33)	29.08 (8.29)	0.65	0.52
Visual Association	25.22 (8.52)	24.21 (9.07)	0.70	0.49
Visual Closure	34.79 (10.19)	29.46 (11.08)	**3.04**	**0.003**
Grammar	22.12 (5.94)	21.34 (8.17)	0.62	0.54
Manual expression	27.21 (4.57)	26.01 (6.79)	1.14	0.26
Verbal Expression	22.29 (6.26)	20.16 (6.41)	**2.06**	**0.04**
Total auditory ability	26.00 (6.00)	23.75 (4.99)	**2.58**	**0.01**
Total visual ability	28.52 (6.11)	25.51 (6.09)	**2.92**	**0.004**
Visual and auditory Memory	26.96 (8.10)	24.27 (6.23)	**2.45**	**0.02**
visual and auditory Closure	28.34 (7.45)	23.86 (7.90)	**3.48**	**0.001**
Visual and auditory association	26.60 (7.71)	25.18 (6.96)	1.21	0.23
Visual and auditory reception	29.83 (6.92)	28.12 (6.44)	1.60	0.11
Visual and auditory Expression	24.81 (4.25)	21.60 (4.76)	**4.14**	**0.001**

Table 3. Association between visual and auditory abilities

Groups	Abilities		1	2	3	4	5	6	7	8	9
Learning difficulties	1. visual reception:		1.00								
	2. Auditory reception	R	0.44	1.00							
		P	0.00								
	3. Visual memory	R	0.41	0.42	1.00						
		P	0.00	0.00							
	4. Auditory Association	R	0.50	0.55	0.61	1.00					
		P	0.00	0.00	0.00						
	5. Auditory memory	R	0.33	0.24	0.44	0.50	1.00				
		P	0.00	0.00	0.00	0.00					
	6. Visual Association	R	0.40	0.42	0.41	0.57	0.27	1.00			

Table 3. (Continued)

Groups	Abilities		1	2	3	4	5	6	7	8	9
		P	0.00	0.00	0.00	0.00	0.00				
	7. Visual Closure	R	0.52	0.46	0.53	0.63	0.40	0.50	1.00		
		P	0.00	0.00	0.00	0.00	0.00	0.00			
	8. Verbal Expression	R	0.55	0.48	0.56	0.62	0.31	0.48	0.49	1.00	
		P	0.00	0.00	0.00	0.00	0.00	0.00	0.00		
	9. grammar	R	0.57	0.52	0.60	0.72	0.48	0.56	0.61	0.62	1.00
		P	0.00	0.00	0.00	0.00	0.00	0.00	0.00	0.00	
	10. Manual expression	R	0.50	0.49	0.51	0.56	0.39	0.52	0.53	0.54	0.54
		P	0.00	0.00	0.00	0.00	0.00	0.00	0.00	0.00	0.00
Normal children	1. visual reception:		1.00								
	2. Auditory reception	R	**0.51**	1.00							
		P	0.00								
	3. Visual memory	R	**0.32**	0.23	1.00						
		P	0.02	0.11							
	4. Auditory Association	R	**0.51**	**0.47**	**0.49**	1.00					
		P	0.00	0.00	0.00						
	5. Auditory memory	R	**0.38**	**0.34**	0.20	**0.56**	1.00				
		P	0.01	0.01	0.15	0.00					
	6. Visual Association	R	**0.62**	**0.64**	**0.30**	**0.68**	**0.36**	1.00			
		P	0.00	0.00	0.03	0.00	0.01				
	7. Visual Closure	R	**0.49**	**0.54**	**0.54**	**0.78**	**0.52**	**0.65**	1.00		
		P	0.00	0.00	0.00	0.00	0.00	0.00			
	8. Verbal Expression	R	**0.33**	0.22	0.22	0.18	-0.16	**0.40**	0.16	1.00	
		P	0.02	0.11	0.11	0.20	0.27	0.00	0.26		
	9. grammar	R	**0.53**	**0.39**	**0.57**	**0.77**	**0.62**	**0.59**	**0.63**	**0.25**	1.00
		P	0.00	0.01	0.00	0.00	0.00	0.00	0.00	0.08	
	10. Manual expression	R	**0.69**	**0.53**	**0.33**	**0.61**	**0.50**	**0.55**	**0.61**	**0.24**	**0.61**
		P	0.00	0.00	0.02	0.00	0.00	0.00	0.00	0.10	0.00

Table 2 demonstrates the difference between study and control groups in visual and auditory abilities. There were statistical significant differences between the two groups in auditory comprehension, visual memory, visual closure, and verbal expression, and also in total auditory and visual abilities scores.

There were no differences between the two groups in auditory memory, auditory association and visual association, grammar, and manual expression. Table 3 presents results concerning associations among visual ability and auditory abilities in the study and control groups. The results show that the learning difficulty group showed a different correlation pattern from the normal children group. In the learning difficult group, five components of visual abilities and auditory abilities are significantly interrelated, and all visual ability components are significantly inter-correlated with auditory abilities components. In the normal children group, visual abilities are significantly inter-correlated. Most components of auditory abilities are significantly inter-correlated except the relationship between verbal expression to auditory reception, auditory association, and auditory working memory. Most components of visual abilities are statistically inter-correlated with components of auditory abilities with the exception of the relationship of visual memory and auditory reception, and the relationship of verbal expression to visual memory and visual closure.

DISCUSSION

This study indicates that poor visual and auditory abilities are significantly related to learning difficulties, and parental education method and gender are also significant predictors of learning difficulties. The significant difference between the study and control groups in visual and auditory abilities, and significant associations between visual and auditory abilities in the study group suggest that children with learning difficulties may have problems processing information using their visual sensory and auditory sensory channels in a coordinated and integrative manner. These findings, which are consistent with published studies (1,2), may be due to children with learning difficulties lack coordination and integration of visual comprehension of written materials, visual-motor, visual processing, and visual working memory. (8). Children with learning difficulties also had additional deficits in auditory comprehension, and verbal expression of information.

It is noted that children with learning difficulties have lower scores in visual working memory but not in verbal working memory, suggesting that poor academic performance and information processing abilities may be related to subtle neurological development deficits in the brain. Spatial working memory ability is governed by the prefrontal lobe of the brain. Deficits in working memory in children with learning difficulties may indicate their poor development in specific abilities and these abilities are linked to problems with neurological development in the prefrontal lobe (3).

Children with learning difficulties in the present study did not have perinatal antecedents. All children in the study group had normal birth weight. They also did not differ from normal children in disease history, age, sleeping status, size of accommodation that they lived, and delivery type when they were born. The statistically significant difference between the learning difficulty and normal children groups in parental education method and living status suggest that 'simple, rigid and autocratic', 'inconsistent' education methods, and living in an apartment may restrict and limit the opportunities for them to develop sufficient self-esteem and confidence, and 'normal' visual spatial and auditory abilities (9).

The limitations of this study include the small number of children in the control group that may have led to a bias in results. The study was conducted in the clinical setting, which may limit the generalisability of the conclusions to the school community setting. Future studies should examine the interplay between visual-auditory abilities, family and school environment, and neurological characteristics, so intervention strategies can be developed that target groups of children with specific deficits and environments. It is recommended that the prevention of learning difficulties should focus on the development of adequate visual and auditory abilities including comprehension, perception, association and coordination, expression in school aged children. Health promotion programs should coordinate and promote both visual and auditory ability development in children at an early age to prevent deficits that impact subsequent academic performance.

REFERENCES

[1]   Girbau D, Schwartz RG. Phonological working memory in Spanish-English bilingual children with and without specific language impairment. J Commun Disord 2008;41(2):22.

[2]   Torrioli MG, Frisone MF, Bonvini L, Luciano R, Pasca MG, Lepori R, et al. Perceptual-motor, visual and cognitive ability in very low birthweight preschool children without neonatal ultrasound abnormalities. Brain Dev 2000;22(3):163-8.

[3]   Mammarella IC, Lucangeli D, Cornoldi C. Spatial working memory and arithmetic deficits in children with nonverbal learning difficulties. J Learn Disabil 2010;43(5):455-68.

[4]   Menghini D, Carlesimo GA, Marotta L, Finzi A, Vicari S. Developmental dyslexia and explicit long-term memory. Dyslexia 2010;16(3):213-25.

[5]   Goldstein DJ, Britt TW. Visual-motor coordination and intelligence as predictors of reading, mathematics, and written language ability. Percept Mot Skills 1994;78(3 Pt 1):819-23.

[6]   Belford B, Blumergh M. Factor analytic study of the revised Illinois test of Psycholinguistic Abilities (ITPA). Percept Mot Skills 1975;40:153-4.

[7]   Kirk SA. Summaries of research on the revised Illinois Test of Psycliolinguistic Abilities. Tucson, AZ: University Arizona, 1972.

[8]   Jongmans M, Mercuri E, de Vries L, Dubowitz L, Henderson SE. Minor neurological signs and perceptual-motor difficulties in prematurely born children. Arch Dis Child Fetal Neonatal Ed 1997;76(1):F9-14.

[9]   Lahane S, Shah H, Nagarale V, Kamath R. Comparison of self-esteem and maternal attitude between children with learning disability and unaffected Siblings. Indian J Pediatr 2012 Nov 22.

Submitted: April 08, 2013. *Revised:* May 22, 2013. *Accepted:* May 30, 2013.

In: Public Health Yearbook 2013
Editor: Joav Merrick

ISBN: 978-1-63321-095-0
© 2014 Nova Science Publishers, Inc.

Chapter 41

RELATIONSHIP BETWEEN RESILIENCE AND QUALITY OF LIFE IN CHINESE UNDERGRADUATE UNIVERSITY STUDENTS

Jing Sun, PhD[*1] *and Nicholas Buys, PhD*[2]
[1]School of Medicine and Griffith Health Institute, Griffith University,
Gold Coast campus, Parkland, Australia
[2]School of Human Services and Social Work, and Griffith Health Institute,
Griffith University, Parkland, Gold Coast, Australia

ABSTRACT

This study aims to investigate the relationship between resilience and quality of life (QOL) amongst undergraduate students across nine Beijing universities in China. A two stage cluster randomly selected sample and study design was used. There were 2,700 students were invited to attend to the study, and 2,046 students responded to the survey with high response rate of 75.8 percent.

A standardised QOL questionnaire was used to assess university students perceived physical, mental health of QOL. Standardised resilience scales were used to determine their association with QOL. Multivariate linear regression analysis was used to analyse the association of QOL to resilience and social capital while demographic variables including age and gender were adjusted in the model. There were 26 percent of variances explained by resilience for physical health and 27.7 percent explained for mental health of QOL. The strongest explanatory variables in determining QOL were primarily focused on the individual's perception of self in the context of being a student (sense of self-acceptance, sense of autonomy, purpose of life, and personal growth) and also based on their involvement in the wider population (environmental mastery, and relations with others). These results suggest that resilience is an important factor to determine their QOL when they develop their ability to cope university life and be prepared to transit to the adult life.

* Correspondence: Jing Sun, PhD, School of Medicine, Griffith University and Griffith Health Institute, Griffith University, Gold Coast Campus, Parkland, Q4222 Australia. E-mail: j.sun@griffith.edu.au

Keywords: Quality of life, resilience, university students, China

INTRODUCTION

Quality of life (QOL) in undergraduate students has become an important clinical and community concern internationally (refs). QOL is most commonly construed as a multidimensional construct. The most commonly used definition of QOL is based on World Health Organization's (WHO's) definition of health including physical, mental components (1-3). QOL is defined by the WHOQOL Group (1994) as: "A person's perception of his / her position in life within the context of the culture and value systems in which they live, and in relation to their goals, expectations, standards, and concerns" (4). Poor QOL can result in poor academic performance and negative employment outcome.

University students face a range of stressors in their university life: for example, academic pressures, financial problems, and employment concerns. This can all affect their QOL. This situation is exemplified in Chinese university students as most undergraduate students are single children who are characterised as self-centered, with poor communication skills and capacity for self-regulation (5,6). Resilience has been found an important factor affecting QOL (1-3). Resilience is defined as the capacity of individuals, schools, families and communities to cope successfully with everyday challenges including life transitions, times of cumulative stress and significant adversity or risk. Typically, resilient individuals have high self-esteem, internal locus of control, optimism and clear aspirations, reflectiveness and problem solving capacity, respect for the autonomy of themselves and others, healthy communication patterns, and the capacity to seek out friends and environmental supports. These factors can prevent negative outcomes, as resilient individuals tend to have higher self-esteem, positive relations with others and an improved outlook on their life (7-9).

In China, the challenge has never been greater to raise children who are able to stand their ground amid growing educational, social and economic pressures, and increasing adolescent and youth mental disorders such as depression, eating disorders and other antisocial behaviours including drug abuse (10). The term the term "resilience" has been typically applied to youth who have overcome difficult situations such as abuse, neglect, poverty or school failure and gone on to become satisfied, productive and successful adults (5-7). But more recently, it has been recommended that schools, universities and educators can learn to help all youth to develop a "resilient mind-set."

Stress and adversity are an inevitable part of life in university students and therefore it makes sense to introduce resilience building strategies to youth in university. Resiliency promotion programs for youth have existed since the 1970's and have focused primarily on building self-esteem, increasing school readiness and supporting interpersonal relationships. Most promotion efforts, however, have tended to overlook the importance of multiple strategies that involve educational and social processes in the development of resilience, handling of stress and dealing with adversity to promote a good QOL. However, one of the neglected issues in research on QOL is adolescence, in particular among university youth in China. University youth is marked by biological, social role, and psychological changes, especially in rapid social and economic change times in China, and how they adapt to these changes can impact their transition into adulthood. If the additional stress of study impedes their development and successful transition, it is important to learn if this can be altered or buffered by promoting their resilience level. Despite the important role that resilience play in QOL in university students, there is limited research has explored the relationship between resilience and QOL in university students in China.

The primary hypothesis developed to guide this study framework was that a sense of resilience is significantly related to high level of QOL among Chinese university students'. It is postulated that positive scores in resilience will be significant indicators of QOL in the university. Deviations (i.e., negative or insignificant regression coefficients) from this trend in resilience would presumably result in a negative or insignificant impact on the QOL of university students. The aim of this study was therefore to determine the health-related QOL of university students, and how it is affected by the presence of resilience characteristics.

METHODS

Two stage stratified randomly selected sampling was implemented at both university and individual student levels. There were nine university in Beijing from eligible 59 universities were randomly selected first then students were randomly selected from each of the nine universities. Survey method was used and a survey was administered during normal class hours. In total, 2,700 students were invited to take part in the study, and 2,046 students completed the survey with high response rate of 75.8%. The majority of students were freshmen and second year students. Written informed consent was obtained from the participating students. Ethical clearance was obtained from the human ethics committee at the Peking University, China.

Measures

Self-reported questionnaire were included in the survey instrument. These questionnaires include Chinese versions of the original standardised scales. Demographic characteristics included age, gender, place of origin, family income, and university year level.

Quality of Life measures: The World Health Organisation Quality of Life brief questionnaire (WHOQOL) was used to assess QOL in university students. For the purpose of this paper, two components of QOL were measured: physical and mental health. The WHOQOL-BREF is considered to be suitable for the current study because of its proven value as a cross-culturally valid and reliable instrument and its ease of completion with only 26 questions. A further advantage is that normative data are also available for the children population represented in the survey (with indications of sex differences and age trends), together with information of the scale of differences to be expected between 'well' people drawn from community settings and 'ill' people, with a wide range of existing health problems, drawn from health care contexts. Detailed normative data has recently been published by the Chinese WHOQOL group (11). The QOL scale has a good reliability with Cronbach Alpha level of more than 0.70 (12)

Respondents were asked to choose from four possible responses in a Likert format, where 1 is "very disatisfied" and 5 is "very satisfied". Scores range from 0 to 100 for each dimension of QOL after the scores were standardised, with higher scores reflecting greater levels of satisfaction of life. A score of less than 75 is suggestive of the lower than average score in either physical or mental health, as it was strongly associated with major depression (13).

Resilience: The resilience questionnaire developed by Ryff and Keyes (14) was used to measure six aspects of resilience. This includes: self-acceptance, the establishment of quality ties to others, a sense of autonomy in thought and action, the ability to manage complex environments to suit personal needs and values, the pursuit of meaningful goals and a sense of purpose in life, and continued growth and development as a person. The resilience questionnaire has six components and each component has 14 questions and 84 questions in total. The scale uses a five-point Likert scale asking 1 is strongly disagree to 5 is strongly agree, and participants only need to select one answer among the five choices. A higher score indicates a higher level of resilience for each component. Resilience scale has good reliability and validity (14).

Statistical analysis

All data were analysed using SPSS package version 22.0. Descriptive statistics (means and standard deviations) of resilience and QOL scores are presented. Both bivariate (unadjusted) and multivariate (adjusted) linear regression was used to determine the possible relation of the explanatory variables, resilience and QOL in Chinese university students, the outcome variable. The confounding demographic information variables were used in the adjusted multivariate model to explain the significance of resilience on four main components physical health, psychological health, social functioning and environmental health of QOL.

Linear regression analyses using both bivariate and multivariate were performed for each QOL component. Confounding factors including age, gender, family socioeconomic status, university academic ranking, previous living condition, year of university were controlled in the analysis. Significance level was determined at $p < 0.05$ (2-tailed) for all multiple linear regression analyses.

RESULTS

There were 2,700 students initially invited to participate in the study, with a final sample of 2,046, representing a high response rate of 75.8%. Of this sample 62.2% were males, 37.8% females, with ages ranging from 16 to 31 years old (Mean age = 19, SD = 1). Sixty-seven percent of the participants were first-year students, 18.5% second-year students, 11.0% third-year students and 3.2% fourth-year students (Table 2). Names of the university institution published in the website based on the Thompson Reuter index, with their ranking and stratified sample sizes (n) and percentage (%) are shown in Table 1 below. Equivalent sample sizes at both university rank, and within-university level was obtained.

Table 1. Nine Beijing universities of varying rank and number of sample sizes for each university

University ranking and number/percentage of students sampled	*n*	*%*
Excellent level		
1	288	14.1
2	195	9.5
3	179	8.7
Total	662	32.3
Good level		
1	283	13.8
2	239	11.7
3	184	9.0
Total	706	34.5
Average level		
1	216	10.6
2	244	11.9
3	218	10.7
Total	678	33.2

Table 2. Sample demographics at individual and family level with individual health perception of each participant

Variable	N (%)
University rank	
Top	662 (32.40)
Medium	706 (34.50)
Low	678 (33.10)
Family structure	
Double parents	1689 (82.60)
Single parent	357 (17.40)
Persons living together	
2	169 (8.30)
3	1043 (51.00)
4	611 (29.90)
5	174 (8.50)
6-11	49 (2.40)
Age group	
16-20 years	1760 (86.00)
21-30 years	286 (14.00)
Gender	
Male	1273 (62.20)
Female	773 (37.80)
Years in university	
1	578 (28.3)
2	478 (23.4)
3	425 (20.8)

Table 2. (Continued)

Variable	N (%)
4	565(27.6)
Income group	
Less than 10,000	586 (28.60)
10,000-29,999	830 (40.60)
30,333-59,999	353 (17.30)
60,000 and above	277 (13.50)
City living	
Capital city	738 (36.10)
Small city	413 (20.20)
Rural	895 (43.70)
Health status	
Very bad	43 (2.10)
Normal	527 (25.80)
Good	769 (37.60)
Very good	523 (25.60)
Excellent	184 (9.00)
Whether have health problem	
Yes	502 (24.5)
No	1544 (75.5)

Table 3. Descriptive statistics in QOL and resilience

	Mean	SD	Range	Skewness	Kurtosis
Quality of Life					
Physical Health	47.32	15.65	0-100	0.21	0.20
Psychological Health	49.38	16.30	0-100	0.21	-0.05
Resilience					
Autonomy	50.22	4.91	30-75	0.83	2.80
Environmental mastery	51.10	5.46	24-80	0.88	2.31
Personal growth	52.15	8.47	27-82	1.16	1.12
Positive relations	52.45	8.02	31-84	1.45	1.88
Purpose in life	51.47	5.83	24-80	1.00	2.96
Self-acceptance	50.98	5.65	28-77	1.12	2.28

Information in regard to family background was also collected with 82% of individuals coming from two-parent households, and the average student living with 3-4 family members. Mean family income was 10,000-29,000 Chinese Yuan and the geographical location of residence indicated a significant portion of students came from rural areas (43.7%), with 36.1% from the capital city, and 20.2% from other urban cities. Almost a quarter (24.1%) of individuals stated they had an existing health problem, but when asked of perceived health condition, 25.8% stated they were normal, 37.6% had good health and 34.6% believed they had very good or excellent health. Only 2.1% of respondents stated they had very poor health.

Descriptive analysis result for QOL and resilience

Total scores of QOL and resilience were analysed using descriptive statistics prior to linear regression (see table 3). QOL total scores means ranged from 47.32 (physical health) to 49.38 (psychological health) within observed range = 0-100. Resilience mean values remained fairly constant in each resilience factor, ranging from 50.22 to 52.45. All resilience and QOL measure have normal distribution with skewness and kurtosis are within accepted range of -3 to +3.

Multiple linear regression results

Linear regression was implemented to identify the possible relationship that resilience had on four QOL factors: physical health, psychological health. Comparisons in statistical analysis were also made between unadjusted bivariate analysis and subsequent adjusted multivariate analysis to quantify the possible impact of demographic information into a QOL model.

Table 4 indicates that resilience significantly related to physical health of QOL. These effects are significant even when confounding factors including gender, university academic ranking, family structure, geographic living before they came to university, and health status.

DISCUSSION

This study investigated the relationship between resilience and QOL. All possible confounding factors, demographics, was investigated in an adjusted multivariate model and compared with the original crude bivariate model. Results indicate a positive and significant correlation between QOL and the resilience in both crude unadjusted and multivariate adjusted models, thus supporting the original hypothesis. In this study 24% of the sample reported a number of physical health problems, a substantial number that is of concern as low resilience can exacerbate physical health problems.

Resilience has a significantly positive relationship with physical health of QOL even when confounding factors were controlled in the multiple regression model. The six components of resilience scale were all significantly related to physical health of QOL. The relationship between self-acceptance and physical health indicates that with an increasing level of self-acceptance there is an increasing level of positive attitude towards self-appearance, positive feelings and confidence in managing physical health. The finding of an association between positive relations with others and physical health suggests that the presence of warm, satisfying and trusting relationships with self and others assists in dealing with physical health issues. Sense of autonomy is related to physical health, indicating that individuals rating high on this characteristic are able to self-determine and independently deal with bodily pain and disease issues. The relationship between environmental mastery and physical health suggests that with an increasing level of sense of mastery individuals are able to manage environmental support, and control resources when they deal with any physical illness.

Table 4. Linear regression for resilience and social capital (for QoL: physical health)

Variable	Crude model			Adjusted model		
	B (CI)	SE	P value	B (CI)	SE	P value
Resilience						
Autonomy	0.16 (0.03–0.29) *	0.07	0.02	0.17 (0.05–0.29) **	0.06	0.01
Environment mastery	0.53 (0.39–0.66) ***	0.07	<0.001	0.34 (0.21–0.46) ***	0.07	<0.001
Personal growth	0.29 (0.18–0.39) ***	0.05	<0.001	0.17 (0.08–0.27) ***	0.05	<0.001
Positive relations	0.30 (0.18–0.41) ***	0.06	<0.001	0.20 (0.09–0.30) ***	0.06	<0.001
Purpose in life	-0.10(-0.24-0.02)	0.07	0.05	-0.12 (-0.23–0.00)*	0.06	0.05
Self-acceptance	0.31 (0.16–0.45) ***	0.07	<0.001	0.24 (0.11–0.38) ***	0.07	<0.001
University rank				-0.50 (-1.19-0.19)	0.35	0.15
Family structure				-1.75 (-3.35–-0.15) *	0.82	0.03
Sex				0.69 (-0.48-1.86)	0.60	0.25
Years in university				-0.89 (-1.63–-0.16)	0.38	0.02
City living				0.61 (-0.03-1.25)	0.33	0.06
Health condition				1.86 (1.27-2.46)	0.30	<0.001
Persons living together				-0.16 (-0.84-0.52)	0.35	0.65
Income group				-0.28 (-0.85-0.30)	0.29	0.344
	$R^2 = 24.10\%$, df = 6			$R^2 = 26.00\%$, df = 22		

* $p<.05$, ** $p < 0.01$, *** $p < 0.001$.

Table 5. Linear regression for resilience and social capital (for QoL: psychological health)

Variable	Crude model			Adjusted model		
	B (CI)	SE	P value	B (CI)	SE	P value
Resilience						
Autonomy	0.16 (0.02-0.30)*	0.07	0.02	0.16 (0.04-0.29)**	0.06	0.01
Environmental mastery	0.49 (0.35-0.64)***	0.07	<0.001	0.28 (0.14-0.41)***	0.07	<0.001
Personal growth	0.19 (0.08-0.29)***	0.05	<0.001	0.08(-0.01-0.18)*	0.05	0.04
Positive relations	0.21 (0.10-0.33)***	0.06	<0.001	0.12(0.01-0.23)*	0.06	0.03
Purpose in life	0.31 (0.18-0.44)***	0.07	<0.001	0.31 (0.18-0.43)***	0.06	<0.001
Self-acceptance	0.43 (0.28-0.58)***	0.08	<0.001	0.38 (0.24-0.52)***	0.07	<0.001
University rank				-0.17(-0.88-0.54)	0.36	0.63
Family structure				0.01(-1.64-1.66)	0.84	0.99
Sex				0.28(-0.92-1.49)	0.61	0.65
Years in university				-0.88(-1.64-0.12)*	0.39	0.02
City living				-0.38(-1.04-0.28)	0.34	0.26
Health condition				1.39(0.77-2.00)***	0.31	<0.001
Persons living together				0.13(-0.57-0.83)	0.36	0.72
Income group				0.46(-0.14-1.05)	0.30	0.13
	R^2 = 26.70%, df = 6			**R^2 = 27.7%, df = 22**		

* $p<.05$, ** $p < 0.01$, *** $p < 0.001$.

The relationship between sense of directedness and physical health indicates the beliefs that give life meaning are important for university students to deal with and manage physical health towards positive development. The relationship between personal growth and physical health suggests that having a sense of improvement or expansion over time, and feels interested in life encourages students to actively s to manage and control their physical health.

The significant relationship between all components of resilience and mental health suggest that resilience is predictive of mental health status of university students. This is consistent with the findings of previous research; low level of resilience can contribute to psychological distress and depression (15). Our findings also indicate that personal level characteristics such as sense of self-acceptance, sense of autonomy, purpose of life personal growth, and environmental related characteristics such as environmental mastery and relations with other were associated with mental health status. This is because decreasing levels of resilience decrease the opportunities to develop individual self-esteem and coping strategies through external supports, and, more importantly, hinders the capacity of the individual to buffer and cope stressful situations (16,17). The study has two limitations. First, the study is a cross-sectional study so the interpretation of the causal relationship between resilience and QOL need to be treated with caution. Second, the study used the self-reported measure to assess QOL so the results may be viewed as subjective. Further research should be conducted to include other settings and cities in China as there may be differences between students in metropolitan Beijing and students at universities located in rural and remote areas. A prospective study design is recommended for the next stage of the study to determine the causal relationship between resilience and QoL, and more objective measures such as anthropometry and biomedical methods used to measure physical and mental health status of the university students.

In conclusion, resilience has been found significantly related to physical and mental health in university students. It is recommended that university health promotion policies and activities focus on the development programs to enhance resilience of university students to prevent the development of physical and mental health problems and thereby facilitate students' academic work and successful transition to adult life.

REFERENCES

[1]   Drukker M, Kaplan C, Feron F, Os JV. Children's health-related quality of life, neighborhood socio-economic deprivation and social capital. A contextual analysis. Soc Sci Med 2003;57:825-41.
[2]   Jirojanakul P, Skevington SM, Hudson J. Predicting young children's quality of life. Soc Sci Med 2003;57:1277-88.
[3]   Lawford J, Eiser C. Exploring links between the concepts of Quality of Life and Resilience. Pediatr Rehabil 2001;4(1):209-16.
[4]   WHOQOL Group. Thg World Health Organization quality of life assessment (WHOQOL): Development and general psyhcometric propterties. Soc Sci Med 1998;46(12):1569-85.
[5]   Sun J, Stewart D. Age and gender effects on resilience in children and adolescents. Pediatr Rehabil 2007;9(4):16-25.
[6]   Sun J, Stewart D, Yuan BJ, Zhang SH. Validation of General Health Questionnaire-30 in parents with primary school children. Compr Psychiatry 2011, in press.
[7]   Masten A, Best KM, Garmezy N. Resiliency and development: Contributions from the study of children who overcome adversity. Dev Psychopathol 1991;2:425-44.

[8]   Rutter M. Psychosocial resilience and protective mechanisms. In: Rolf J, Masten A, Cicchetti D, Nuechterlein K, Weintraub S, eds. Risk and protective factors in the development of psychopathology. New York: Cambridge University Press, 1990.

[9]   Sun J, Stewart D. Development of population based resilience measures in the primary school setting. Health Educ 2007;107(6):575-99.

[10]   Sun J, Buys N, Wang XC. Depressive symptoms, family Functioning, university environment, and social support: a population based study in university students in Beijing China. Int J Psychol Behav Sci 2011;1(1):41-7.

[11]   Skevington SM, Lotfy M, O'Connell KA, Group W. The World Health Organization's WHOQOL-BREF quality of life assessment: psychometric properties and results of the international field trial. A report from the WHOQOL group. Qual Life Res 2004;13(2):299-310.

[12]   WHO. WHOQoL-OLD. Geneva: World Health Organization, 2006.

[13]   Kroenke K, Outcalt S, Krebs E, Bair MJ, Wu J, Chumbler N, et al. Association between anxiety, health-related quality of life and functional impairment in primary care patients with chronic pain. Gen Hosp Psychiatry 2013, in press.

[14]   Ryff C, Keyes C. The structure of psychological well-being revisited. J Pers Soc Psychol 1995;69:719-27.

[15]   Gerber M, Kalak N, Lemola S, Clough PJ, Perry JL, Pühse U, et al. Are adolescents with high mental toughness levels more resilient against stress? Stress Health 2013;29(2):164-71.

[16]   Jia-Yan P. A resilience-based and meaning-oriented model of acculturation: A sample of mainland Chinese postgraduate students in Hong Kong. Int J Intercult Relat 2011;35(5):592-603.

[17]   Malti T, Noam GG. The hidden crisis in mental health and education: the gap between student needs and existing supports. New Dir Youth Dev 2008(120):13-29.

Submitted: April 07, 2013. *Revised:* May 16, 2013. *Accepted:* May 29, 2013.

In: Public Health Yearbook 2013
Editor: Joav Merrick

ISBN: 978-1-63321-095-0
© 2014 Nova Science Publishers, Inc.

Chapter 42

VALIDATION OF SHARED DECISION MAKING QUESTIONNAIRE IN THE DENTAL ENCOUNTER

Jessica Peters, BA, BOralH[1],
Jing Sun[*], PhD[2], and Florian Mack, PhD[1],

[1]School of Oral Health and Dental Science, Griffith University,
Centre for Medicine and Oral Health, Southport, Australia
[2]School of Medicine and Griffith Health Institute, Griffith University,
Gold Coast campus, Parkland, Australia

ABSTRACT

Communication within the dental encounter is paramount to successful clinical outcomes. This study examined the concept of shared decision-making (SDM) in patients who have received treatment for a single missing tooth. Method: A cross sectional study design was used for the study. Patients were recruited from a university dental clinic and a private dental practice. Exploratory factor analysis was used to identify the dimensions of patient's SDM, their level of dental knowledge and their treatment satisfaction. Results: Exploratory factor analysis showed that 9 factors were extracted from the questionnaire. Overall, the 9 factor structure had a high level of reliability for each individual dimension. Of the 108 participants, only 26.5% were exposed to SDM. Independent sample t tests showed that there was no significant difference between the SDM group and comparison group on levels of denture knowledge, post treatment functional and economic satisfaction. However, a significant difference was seen in regards to knowledge of other treatment alternatives and post treatment aesthetic/social satisfaction, with the SDM group reporting higher levels. Conclusions: The results suggest that a 9 factor solution can be used to assess the patient's experience in the dental encounter. In regards to the use of SDM in the dental encounter, further research is required using a larger sample size from an increased number of dental practices. However, SDM is an important component of clinical dental practice and should be further explored in clinical dentistry.

---

[*] Correspondence: Jing Sun, PhD, School of Medicine, Griffith University and Griffith Health Institute, Griffith University, Gold Coast Campus, Parkland, Q4222Australia. E-mail: j.sun@griffith.edu.au

Keywords: Shared decision-making, reliability, validity

INTRODUCTION

Patient participation in medical decision-making is receiving increasing emphasis (1). Over the decades there has been a profound change in the clinician patient relationship (2). This change is represented by a shift from the paternalistic model (doctor decides, patient complies without any explanations) to the informative model (doctor provides information, patient decides) (1,3). This paradigm shift has resulted in an increased focus on shared decision-making between doctors and patients. The informative model gives patients the opportunity to participate in decisions by expressing his or her preferences among alternative treatment options (2). When selecting a treatment for a specific medical condition, there is rarely one treatment that is clearly superior to others (1). Given the variety of treatment options for most medical problems, the responsibility for choosing a treatment should be shared by both the clinician and the patient and thus a shared decision making (SDM) process should be employed (1).

SDM is defined as an approach in which the clinician and patient go through all phases of the decision making process together (1). SDM transcends the legal obligation of informed consent, which does not necessarily involve the shared discussion of treatment options, benefits and risks (4). When SDM is employed, information is provided about the health problem, the possible treatment options and consequences of the treatments are discussed, and together the clinician and patient consider how these fit with the patients preferred outcomes (1). After the options are considered, a treatment decision is made based on mutual agreement (5).

In order for SDM to be successfully achieved, certain criteria need to be obtained (5). Firstly, the doctor needs to provide an environment in the consultation where patient participation is encouraged and patients must feel that their contributions are valued (1). The goals of the patient and their desired treatment outcome must be discussed in the consultation (5). Individual patients vary in their preferences for health states, tolerances for pain and discomfort and future needs (5). Obtaining this information from the patient is crucial to selecting the most appropriate treatment option for an individual patient (5). Finally a critical characteristic of SDM is to provide the patients with sufficient information, including treatment alternatives and their possible consequences (6). This is to ensure that the patient is not making a decision in the face of avoidable ignorance (7).

Elwyn et al. (7) developed a three stage model of SDM that can act as a guide to skill development in routine clinical practice. The first stage, *introducing choice,* is to inform patients that options exist. The second stage, *option talk,* involves exploring the patient's existing knowledge, clarifying any incorrect knowledge that the patient may have and clearly outlining the pros and cons of the alternative treatment options (7). The final stage of the model is *decision talk,* which explores the need to either defer a decision or make an immediate decision (7). Allowing time for this is a cornerstone for effective SDM because patients often need to take the time to discuss their options with others in a form of deliberation process (7-9).

The concept of SDM has been thoroughly explored in clinical medicine. Numerous studies have reported improvements in patient satisfaction, treatment adherence, quality of life, and well-being when patients are more involved in their treatment choice (5, 6, 10-12).

Similar to medicine, many dental problems have a variety of treatment options. It therefore follows that the responsibility for choosing the most suitable treatment should be shared by both the dentist and the patient thereby employing the SDM approach. However, little research on SDM was found in the dental literature. Therefore, an aim of this study was to examine whether dental professionals are engaging in SDM with their patients.

While the concept of SDM has little presence in the dental literature, studies have sought to determine what the patient values in the dental encounter. It is evident that patients are less concerned with the technical competency of the dentist (13). Rather, patients view the communication skills of the dentist as most important (13, 14). For example, a study completed by Sbaraini et al. (13) examined patient's experiences of dental care in Australia. They concluded that patients want a dentist who is caring and supportive, who listens to their concerns and takes time to explain treatment options and procedures. Patient's valued dentists who made them aware of the options, educated them about how to maintain a healthy mouth, and supported and reassured them frequently during visits (13). Research has also examined the factors that predict patient satisfaction after the dental encounter. Factors identified include; cost, convenience, technical competence with the largest factor being interpersonal skills of the dentist (14). This is consistent with literature from the medical field indicating that the most important predictor of patient satisfaction is the quality of the doctor-patient relationship (2,4,15). With the most important predictor of patient satisfaction being the ability of the dentist to communicate, it is postulated that dental patients would value SDM in the dental encounter. It is proposed that the use of SDM in the dental encounter is an effective way to enhance dental knowledge in dental patients and to achieve a high level of post treatment satisfaction among dental patients.

In the medical literature, it has been argued that SDM is especially applicable to long-term health decisions and when the intervention requires more than one session (6). Many dental procedures fit these criteria, for instance, the treatment of missing teeth. The three key treatment modalities available for the replacement of missing teeth include; removable partial denture (RPD), fixed partial denture (FPD) and implant supported crown (16). There are both advantages and disadvantages associated with each treatment modality and this is well outlined within the literature (17). No matter which treatment option is selected, several appointments are required and the final choice will have a long-term impact on the patient. The purpose of this study was to develop a questionnaire to examine SDM in patients who have received dental treatment for a single missing tooth, with two specific aims in mind. Firstly, this study aims to determine if patients who have experienced SDM will have a higher level of knowledge of the treatment alternatives. Secondly, this study attempts to determine if patients who have experienced SDM will have a greater sense of treatment satisfaction.

METHODS

A cross sectional study design was used to collect data from dental patients who either visited the Griffith University dental clinic or a private dental practice in Tasmania. Data was collected in December 2012 to February 2013.

Participants

Participants used in this study were patients who had received treatment for a single tooth gap. A single tooth gap is defined as a gap resulting from a single missing tooth that is bordered by one or more natural teeth on either side (18). Participants may have had multiple missing teeth; however the presence of a single tooth gap was required. Two inclusion criteria were used when selecting participants for this study. Participants must have received treatment for a single missing tooth and the treatment must have already been completed. Participants were selected from either the Griffith University dental clinic in Queensland or a private dental practice in Tasmania. Patients who had received this type of treatment were identified using computer records. The total sample comprised 109 patients; all whom had either received a removable partial denture, fixed partial denture or implant supported crown to replace their missing tooth. Ethics approval was obtained from the Griffith University Human Research Ethics Committee (reference no. D0H/27/12/HREC). Edentulous patients (patients will all their teeth missing), patients with no missing teeth, patients with missing wisdom teeth only and patients with multiple missing teeth in a row, were excluded from the study.

Research tools

A questionnaire was developed by the researchers to assess the patient's overall treatment experience. The questionnaire included 107 items that examined the patient's dental habits and history, the number of missing teeth prior to treatment, the types of treatment modalities discussed with them, the patient's knowledge of treatment alternatives, the recommendations provided by the dentist, and the final treatment choice. Post treatment satisfaction was assessed on four different levels including; functional, aesthetic, social and economic satisfaction following dental treatment. Items were scored on a 2 point scale (1, yes; 0, no) or on a 6 point scale (5, strongly agree; 4, agree; 3, somewhat agree; 2, somewhat disagree; 1, disagree; 0, strongly disagree). The knowledge questions were scored based on a semantic scale ranging from 1 to 7.

Exposure to SDM was assessed by examining whether treatment alternatives were provided to the patient. Patients who were presented with all three treatment modalities were assigned to the SDM group. If the patient was only given two treatment options or simply told what treatment was best without exploring alternatives, it was assumed that SDM was not utilized and these patients were assigned to the comparison group. Demographic factors were also collated including; age, gender, income, place of residence, level of education, family and general health status. Information regarding whether or not the patient's treatment was covered by private health insurance or whether or not the patient received government assistance for their dental treatment was also collated.

Data collection

Patients who had received treatment for a single tooth gap were approached in both the private dental practice and the university dental clinic. These participants were provided with an information sheet outlining the purpose of the study and the study procedure.

Statistical analysis

Data analysis was completed using SPSS version 21.0. Statistical analysis was conducted on unweighted data. A principle component analysis was conducted to investigate the subscales structure within the questionnaire. Varimax rotation was considered appropriate for the current study, which uses an orthogonal rotation method that minimizes the number of variables that has high loadings on each factor. Exploratory factor analysis was used to extract the factor structure of the questionnaire. Pearsons correlation bivariate analysis was completed to ensure each factor was not highly correlated and represented an independent factor. Reliability was assessed from analyses of internal consistency using Cronbach α. Independent t tests were conducted to examine differences in satisfaction and knowledge between the SDM group and the comparison group.

Exploratory factor analysis

Exploratory factor analysis for the developed questionnaire was undertaken. The results are presented in table 1. Further analysis using the Scree test showed that nine factors could be meaningfully extracted (see figure 1). This nine factor solution can be considered as a relatively adequate representation of the data.

RESULTS

One hundred-nine participants completed the survey with 100% response rate. Of these participants, 48.6% were aged between 45-64 years, while 45.9% were aged 65 years and above and only 5.5 % aged between 25-44 years. Among the respondents, 65 (59.6%) were female. Education levels indicated that 39.4 % had tertiary education, 14.7 % had diploma/Training and Further Education, 44.0 % had secondary education and only 1.8 % had primary education level. When looking at place of residence, 82 (75.9%) were from metropolitan/city area, 21 (19.4%) from a semi-rural area and 5 (4.6%) from a rural area. In terms of family status, 84 (77.1%) were living in a relationship/partnership and 25 (22.9%) were single. When looking at average household income, 32% of participants reported earning $37,000 or less, 34.9% reported $37,001-$80,000, 28.3% reported $80,001-$180,000, and 4.7% reported $180,001 and over per year. Although, 109 participants completed the survey, 106 participants answered all 107 items.

Table 1. Principle component analysis for ninefactor structure

	Post treatment aesthetic/ social satisfaction	Knowledge of other treatment modalities	Pre-treatment self esteem	Procedural factors	Oral health beliefs	Pre-treatment functioning	Post treatment functional satisfaction	Denture knowledge	Post treatment economic satisfaction
95. After the replacement of my missing tooth I am happier with how my mouth looks.	**.873**	-.007	.057	-.071	.162	-.040	.031	-.033	-.013
94. After the replacement of my missing tooth I feel more confident.	**.872**	.039	.143	.054	.198	.017	.092	-.068	.083
99. After the replacement of my missing tooth I feel more comfortable smiling.	**.855**	.097	.121	-.074	.189	-.059	.008	.019	.097
97. After the replacement of my missing tooth I now enjoy meeting new people.	**.808**	.092	.269	.050	.028	-.096	.159	.131	.067
96. After the replacement of my missing tooth I feel better about myself.	**.800**	.069	.111	.056	.076	.044	.176	.025	.203
98. After the replacement of my missing tooth I now enjoy speaking in public.	**.735**	.170	.299	.044	-.006	-.126	.152	.182	.044
80. A major reason for the replacement of my missing tooth was my appearance.	.441	-.020	.302	-.086	.213	-.104	.030	.075	-.342
71. Did you know how an implant was inserted before your treatment?	.109	**.895**	-.017	-.102	.053	.138	-.067	.072	-.122
70. Did you know what an implant looked like before your treatment?	.030	**.885**	-.137	.030	.073	-.186	.152	.081	.115
72. Did you know how to clean an implant before your treatment?	.100	**.878**	-.031	-.116	.047	.169	-.005	.036	-.149
68. Did you know how a bridge was constructed before your treatment?	.125	**.874**	.012	-.079	.033	.183	-.089	.092	.002
69. Did you know how to clean a bridge before your treatment?	.045	**.852**	-.119	.050	.106	-.102	.132	.065	.068
67. Did you know what a bridge looked like before your treatment?	.022	**.805**	-.161	.016	.088	-.185	.189	.161	.045
73. Damage to the surrounding teeth through drilling was a factor that influenced my final treatment choice.	-.058	.451	.210	.420	.015	.142	-.026	.096	.143
88. Before my treatment I did not like meeting new people.	.135	-.099	**.886**	.188	-.057	.031	.032	.057	.014
90. Before my treatment I felt that people were staring at my missing tooth.	.232	.034	**.860**	.107	-.094	.041	-.074	.005	.014
86. Before my treatment I did not feel good about myself.	.116	-.032	**.854**	.108	.032	.168	.042	-.137	.101
85. Before my treatment I lacked confidence.	.088	-.109	**.854**	.162	-.061	.064	-.011	.114	.013
89. Before my treatment I did not like speaking in public.	.099	-.056	**.852**	.174	.079	.148	.043	-.089	-.012
87. Before my treatment I was unhappy with how my mouth looked.	.312	-.129	**.701**	.021	.047	.141	-.055	.078	-.133
77. The amount of pain I associated with each procedure influenced my final treatment choice.	-.017	-.099	.141	**.875**	.024	.058	.063	-.023	.010
76. I experience fear/anxiety towards dental treatment and this influenced my final treatment choice.	.032	-.117	.019	**.806**	.069	.133	.023	.025	-.014
78. The amount of discomfort I associated with each procedure influenced my final treatment choice.	-.003	-.176	.100	**.800**	.041	.126	-.021	.039	-.065

	Post treatment aesthetic/ social satisfaction	Knowledge of other treatment modalities	Pre-treatment self esteem	Procedural factors	Oral health beliefs	Pre-treatment functioning	Post treatment functional satisfaction	Denture knowledge	Post treatment economic satisfaction
74. Duration of the treatment was a factor that influenced my final treatment choice.	-.041	.159	.218	.650	-.251	.013	.043	-.015	.091
79. The materials that are used in each procedure were a factor that influenced my final treatment choice.	-.090	-.016	.001	.612	-.208	.041	-.161	-.018	-.301
75. Cost of the treatment was a factor that influenced my final treatment choice.	.112	.120	.202	.612	.035	.042	-.129	-.024	-.027
104. I believe that good teeth are important for my general health.	.158	.069	-.112	-.039	.846	-.015	.152	.090	.035
106. I believe that good teeth are important for eating and chewing.	.022	.094	-.059	-.083	.781	.055	.065	.059	.085
103. I believe that someone with all their teeth looks better than someone with missing teeth.	.020	.025	.087	-.089	.764	-.077	.074	.106	-.031
107. I believe good teeth are important for maintaining nutrition.	.228	.132	-.018	.076	.673	.008	-.053	.074	.054
102. I believe that good teeth are important for my appearance	.412	-.030	.104	.044	.648	-.216	-.032	.085	-.034
105. I believe that missing or decayed teeth are a sign of poor health.	.352	.255	-.050	-.007	.360	.176	-.120	.050	.227
84. Before my treatment I found it difficult to eat crunchy vegetables.	.023	.058	.139	.169	-.046	.882	.128	-.036	-.008
82. Before my treatment I found it difficult to eat crunchy fruit.	.004	-.002	.182	.110	-.010	.878	.175	.026	-.065
83. Before my treatment I found it difficult to eat cooked meat.	-.139	.004	.183	.186	-.092	.846	.151	.051	.039
81. A major reason for the replacement of my missing tooth was my ability to eat and chew.	-.239	.042	.023	.014	.023	.468	.278	-.062	-.214
91. After the replacement of my missing tooth I can now eat crunchy fruit.	.118	.048	-.001	-.057	.030	.191	.903	-.035	.095
93. After the replacement of my missing tooth I can now eat crunchy vegetables.	.184	.120	.001	-.078	.067	.177	.900	-.006	.107
92. After the replacement of my missing tooth I can now eat cooked meat.	.193	.053	-.015	-.018	.101	.216	.858	.071	.105
66. Did you know how to clean a denture before your treatment?	.039	.119	.040	.033	.099	.021	-.010	.929	.116
65. Did you know how to use a denture before your treatment?	.028	.208	-.022	.004	.126	.012	.057	.926	-.010
64. Did you know what a denture looked like before your treatment?	.116	.115	.008	-.020	.167	-.033	-.027	.878	-.057
101. I believe that I paid too much for my treatment (reversed).	.102	-.080	.021	-.133	.026	-.044	.146	-.021	.786
100. I believe that I received value for the cost of my dental treatment.	.232	.070	.027	-.019	.135	-.114	.113	.079	.771

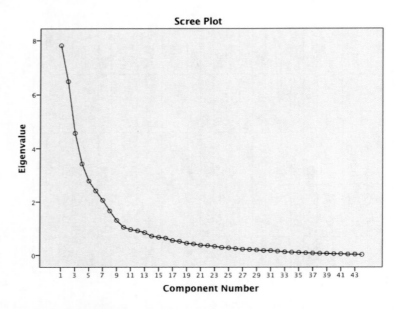

Figure 1. Nine factor extraction Scree plot based on factor analysis.

Table 2. Inter-correlation between the nine factors obtained from factor analysis

	Post treatment physical and social satisfaction	Post treatment functional satisfaction	Post treatment economic satisfaction	Denture knowledge	Knowledge of other treatment modalities	Pre-treatment self esteem	Pre-treatment functioning	Procedural factors	Oral health beliefs
Post treatment physical and social satisfaction									
Post treatment functional satisfaction	.248*								
Post treatment economic satisfaction	.212*	.177							
Denture knowledge	.185	.020	.084						
Knowledge of other treatment modalities	.160	.085	0.26	.276**					
Pre-treatment self esteem	.408**	.063	.019	-.007	-.151				
Pre-treatment functioning	-.029	.230*	-.059	.011	.029	.284**			
Procedural factors	.056	-.046	-.149	.056	-.003	.305**	.263**		
Oral health beliefs	.400**	.097	.215*	.235*	.173	.052	-.089	-.094	

** Correlation is significant at the 0.01 level (2-tailed).

Dental characteristics of participants

Seventy-nine (72.5%) participants received private health insurance for their dental treatment whereas 21 (19.3%) received government assistance for their dental treatment. Eighteen (16.3%) participants from the total sample reported that they had previously been treated for gum disease. In regards to the number of missing teeth, 38 (34.9%) had only 1 missing tooth, 26 (24.1%) had 2-3 missing teeth and 45 (41.7%) had more than 3 missing teeth. When looking at the location of the missing tooth, 69 (63.3%) participants indicated that their missing tooth was located at the front of their mouth, with 74 (67.9%) participants indicating that their missing tooth could be seen when they smiled. The most commonly reported cause of tooth loss was; decay (35.8%), trauma (26.6%), cracked tooth (17.4%) and failed dental treatment (16.5%). Eight (7.3%) participants were unsure of the cause of their missing tooth. When looking at how long the patient waited before seeking treatment, 70 (64.2%) sought treatment immediately, 9 (8.3%) sought treatment within one year, 11 (10.1%) sought treatment within 1-3 years and, 19 (17.4%) waited more than 3 years for treatment. Finally, when looking at the final treatment choice, 41 (37.6%) participants received a fixed dental prosthesis, 32 (29.4%) participants received a chrome cobalt denture, 11 (10.1%) participants received an acrylic denture, and 27 (24.8%) participants received an implant retained crown.

Grouping of participants

Whether or not alternative treatment options were discussed with patients by their dentist was examined. It was found that only 29 (26.6%) participants were presented with all three treatment options and could subsequently be assigned to the SDM group. Twenty-one (19.3%) participants were presented with two treatment options, 57 (52.3%) participants were presented with one treatment option and two (1.8%) were not presented with any treatment options. These participants were assigned to the comparison group.

Factor analysis

The Exploratory Factor Analysis derived a nine component solution from the factor analysis (see table 1). Factor 1 [Items 79, 93, 94, 95, 96, 97, 98] indicated the respondent's level of post treatment aesthetic and social satisfaction. For example: after the replacement of my missing tooth; I feel more confident, I am happier with how my mouth looks, and I feel more comfortable smiling. Factor 2 was knowledge of the two other treatment modalities; implant retained crown and FPD. This was assessed using items 66, 67, 68, 69, 70, and 71. Pre-treatment self-esteem was the third factor, which included 6 items 84, 85, 86, 87, 88 and 89. For example; before my treatment I did not like meeting new people, I felt that people were staring at my missing tooth, I lacked confidence and I did not feel good about myself. Factor 4 represented the degree in which procedural factors impacted on the patient's treatment choice. This was measured using items 72, 73, 74, 75, 76, 77, and 78. The fifth factor comprised the oral health beliefs of the patient. This was measured using 5 items 101, 102, 103, 105, and 106 such as: I believe that; good teeth are important for general health, maintaining nutrition, and eating and chewing. Factor 6 included items 81, 82, and 83, which measured pretreatment masticatory functioning. Factor 7 included 3 items, which measured patient's satisfaction with post treatment masticatory functioning [90, 91, 92]. The eighth factor expressed the patient's level of denture knowledge, which was assessed using items 63, 64, and 65. The ninth and final factor was post treatment economic satisfaction. This was measured using item 99 and 100. Pearsons correlation bivariate analysis was completed to ensure each factor was not highly correlated (correlation < .85) and therefore represented an independent concept (see table 2). All of the nine factors identified were normally distributed except for post treatment functional satisfaction. Therefore, non-parametric tests were applied to the analysis of this factor.

The variance explained for the nine factors were 11.73%, 11.57%, 11.03%, 8.43%, 7.58%, 6.92%, 6.45%, 6.20%, and 4.02% respectively. The total variance explained by the nine factors was 73.93%.

Reliability

The overall reliability level of the questionnaire was relatively high with a Cronbach α level of .86. Table 3 indicates that the subscales based on the 9 extracted factors were generally found to be reliable with levels ranging from .67 to .95.

Discriminant validity of SDM questionnaire

An independent sample t-test was conducted to compare the SDM group and the comparison group on knowledge of treatment alternatives and treatment satisfaction (see table 4). In regards to denture knowledge, there was no significant difference between the two groups (p value .918). There was however a significant difference between the SDM group and the comparison group on level of knowledge of other treatment modalities (p value .020), with the SDM group showing a higher level of knowledge. When looking at treatment satisfaction, no significant difference was found between the SDM group and the comparison group on levels of post treatment functional satisfaction (p value .842 see table 5) or post treatment economic satisfaction (p value .755). There was however a significant difference between the SDM group and the comparison group on levels of post treatment aesthetic/social satisfaction (p value .031) with the SDM group showing a higher level of satisfaction.

DISCUSSION

Exploratory factor analysis in the current study showed a nine factor solution. A process was undertaken in order to reach the conclusion that nine factors were required. For the first factor analysis model, factor loading of less than 0.4 were suppressed and 10 factors were extracted based on Eigenvalue more than one. For the second factor analysis model, nine factors were selected. In comparison to the first model, the nine factors generated from the second factor analysis, better reflected the meaning of clustered questions. In the nine factor analysis item 72 and 101 cross loaded on two factors. These items were subsequently placed with the factor that best represented that particular dimension. These questions had high content validity and explained 73.93% of the total variance.

Table 3. Reliability correlations, Cronbach α

Questionnaire	Reliability correlations, Cronbach α (9 factors)
Total score	.86
Post treatment aesthetic/social satisfaction	.92
Post treatment functional satisfaction	.95
Post treatment economic satisfaction	.67
Denture knowledge	.93
Knowledge of other treatment modalities	.95
Pretreatment self esteem	.93
Pretreatment functioning	.86
Procedural factors	.82
Oral health beliefs	.77

Table 4. Differences in dental knowledge and treatment satisfaction between the SDM group and the comparison group

Variables	Group		*t*	P value
	SDM group (n= 29) Mean (SD)	Comparison group (n= 79) Mean (SD)		
Knowledge				
Denture knowledge	15.03 (6.17)	15.18 (6.89)	-.103	.918
Knowledge of other treatment modalities	22.09 (13.67)	15.94 (12.13)	2.41	.020
Satisfaction				
Post treatment aesthetic/social satisfaction	26.28 (7.12)	22.47 (9.91)	2.20	.031
Post treatment economic satisfaction	6.97 (2.06)	7.12 (2.52)	-.314	.755

Table 5. Differences in post treatment functional satisfaction

Group	Median	Min, Max	Z score	P value
SDM group	12.00	.00, 15.00	-.200	.842
Comparison group	13.00	.00,15.00		

Among the nine extracted factors, the first factor was titled post treatment aesthetic and social satisfaction. This covered the patient's satisfaction with the appearance of their treatment and whether this had a positive impact on their social interaction. Factor two covered the patient's knowledge of the implant and bridge treatment modalities. The third factor, the pre-treatment self-esteem factor, described the impact their missing tooth had on how the patient perceived themselves, their appearance and their interaction within social situations. Factor 4 was the procedural factor, which described the impact the different aspects of the specific dental procedures had on the patient's treatment choice. The fifth factor, the oral health belief factor described how important the patient believed oral health is, its importance in maintaining nutrition and its impact on general health. Factor 6 was pre-treatment functioning, which described the masticatory functioning of the patient prior to the replacement of their missing tooth. Functional satisfaction was the seventh factor, which referred to the patient's perceived improvement in masticatory functioning after the completion of their dental treatment. Factor 8 covered the patient's knowledge of the denture treatment option. The ninth and final factor, the post treatment economic satisfaction factor, described whether or not the patient believed that they received value for the cost of their dental treatment. SPSS was used to determine the validity and reliability of the questionnaire.

A Cronbach α level of .86 was obtained indicating that the overall reliability level of the questionnaire was relatively high. The 9 extracted factors were also found to be reliable with levels ranging from .67 to .95.

These questions had high content validity and explained 73.93% of the total variance. This questionnaire was developed to assess communication in the dental encounter. More specifically, the researchers aimed to utilize the questionnaire to determine if dentists were engaging in SDM with their patients. The researchers also aimed to determine if those patients who experienced SDM as identified in the questionnaire had a higher knowledge of treatment alternatives and a higher sense of treatment satisfaction. The questionnaire showed good level of discriminant validity that it can sensitively differentiate the difference between the SDM group and comparison group in post treatment aesthetic and social satisfaction. That is, the SDM group had a significantly higher sense of post treatment aesthetic and social satisfaction than the comparison group. The SDM questionnaire can also differentiate the SMD group and comparison group in regards to the knowledge of other treatment modalities, with the SDM group having a higher level of knowledge than the comparison group. This result is consistent with other studies that indicate that effective SDM can be measured by examining the patient's overall knowledge of treatment options (19).

The results indicated that only 26.6% of participants were exposed to SDM. In regards to knowledge, no significant difference was seen between the two groups with respect to denture knowledge. This may be because the denture treatment modality is more widely known amongst the general population. Consequently, SDM is not required to provide sufficient knowledge of this treatment modality.

No difference was seen on other levels of satisfaction. While several studies have highlighted the link between SDM and increased satisfaction, other studies suggest otherwise (19). It has been suggested that when clinicians display uncertainty and do not specifically recommend a treatment option for the patient, satisfaction can be decreased (19). This is because the provision of treatment options and the uncertainty as to which treatment option to select can overwhelm and confuse patients (19). The use of satisfaction as the most appropriate outcome measure of an effective decision making process has subsequently been questioned (20).

Limitations

This study was limited to patients from a private dental practice and a university dental clinic in Australia. In order to better understand the dental encounter and the use of SDM within dental practice, a large sample size from a broad range of dental practices should be utilized and in addition to this, this study only examined the decision making process involved in a single tooth replacement. Exploring the decision making process of other clinical situations may further aid in understanding the decision making process in the dental encounter. Finally, this study focused on a single treatment decision. In order to gain better insight into the use of SDM within clinical dentistry, examination of the complete dental encounter from the initial consultation to completion of treatment, to long- term post treatment maintenance, may be required.

CONCLUSION

This study was the first to explore the use of SDM in clinical dental practice in regards to single tooth replacement. A questionnaire was developed and a nine factor structure was derived using the present sample. This suggests that a nine factor solution can be used to assess the decision making process in the dental encounter. In regards to examining the prevalence of SDM and its ability to improve patient's knowledge and satisfaction, further research is required using a large sample size from an increased number of dental practices. This study highlights the importance of SDM in dental practice and provides direction for further research into SDM in clinical dentistry.

REFERENCES

[1]   Frosch DL, Kaplan RM. Shared decision making in clinical medicine: past research and future directions. Am J Prev Med 1999;17(4):85-94.

[2]   Butalid L, Verhaak PFM, Boeije HR, Bensing JM. Patients' views on changes in doctor-patient communication between 1982 and 2001: A mixed-methods study. BMC Fam Pract 2012;13:80.

[3]   Benbassat J, Pilpel D, Tidhar M. Patients' preferences for participation in clinical decision making: a review of published surveys. Behav Med 1998;24(2):81-8.

[4]   Matthias MS, Salyers MP, Frankel RM. Re-thinking shared decision-making: Context matters. Patient Educ Couns 2013, in press.

[5]   Charles C, Gafni A, Whelan T. Shared decision-making in the medical encounter: what does it mean? (or it takes at least two to tango). Soc Sci Med 1997;44(5):681-92.

[6]   Joosten EAG, DeFuentes-Merillas L, de Weert GH, Sensky T, van der Staak CPF, de Jong CAJ. Systematic review of the effects of shared decision-making on patient satisfaction, treatment adherence and health status. Psychother Psychosom 2008;77(4):219-26.

[7]   ElwynG, Frosch D, Thomson R, Joseph-Williams N, Lloyd A, Kinnersley P, et al. Shared decision making: a model for clinical practice. J Gen Intern Med 2012;27(10):1361-7.

[8]   Epstein RM, Street RLJr. Shared mind: communication, decision making, and autonomy in serious illness. Ann Fam Med 2011;9(5):454-61.

[9]   Elwyn G, Miron-Shatz T. Deliberation before determination: the definition and evaluation of good decision making. Health Expect 2010;13(2):139-47.

[10]   Montgomery AA, Harding J, Fahey T. Shared decision making in hypertension: the impact of patient preferences on treatment choice. Fam Pract 2001;18(3):309-13.

[11]   Towle A, Godolphin W. Framework for teaching and learning informed shared decision making. BMJ 1999;319(7212):766-71.

[12]   Savage R, Armstrong D. Effect of a general practitioner's consulting style on patients' satisfaction: a controlled study. BMJ 1990;301(6758):968-70.

[13]   Sbaraini A, Carter SM, Evans RW, Blinkhorn A. Experiences of dental care: What do patients value? BMC Health Serv Res 2012;12:177.

[14]   Newsome PR, Wright GH. A review of patient satisfaction: 2. Dental patient satisfaction: An appraisal of recent literature. Br Dent J 1999;186(4 Spec No): 166-70.

[15]   Crow R, Gage H, Hampson S, Hart J, Kimber A, Storey L et al. The measurement of satisfaction with healthcare: implications for practice from a systematic review of the literature. Health Technol Assess 2002;6(32):1-244.

[16]   Al-Quran FA, Al-Ghalayini RF, Al-Zu'bi BN. Single-tooth replacement: factors affecting different prosthetic treatment modalities. BMC Oral Health 2011;11:34.

[17]   Hebel K, Gajjar R, Hofstede T. Single-tooth replacement: bridge vs. implant-supported restoration. J Can Dent Assoc 2000;66(8):435-8.

[18]   MackF, Samietz SA, Mundt T, Proff P, Gedrange T, Kocher T, et al. Prevalence of single-tooth gaps in a population-based study and the potential for dental implants--data from the Study of Health in Pomerania (SHIP-0). J Craniomaxillofac Surg 2006;34(Suppl 2):82-5.

[19]   Politi MC, Clark MA, Ombao H, DizonD, Elwyn G. Communicating uncertainty can lead to less decision satisfaction: a necessary cost of involving patients in shared decision making? Health Expect 2011;14(1):84-91.

[20]   Sepucha K, Ozanne E, Silvia K, Partridge A, Mulley AG Jr. An approach to measuring the quality of breast cancer decisions. Patient Educ Couns 2007;65(2):261-9.

In: Public Health Yearbook 2013
Editor: Joav Merrick

ISBN: 978-1-63321-095-0
© 2014 Nova Science Publishers, Inc.

Chapter 43

ASSOCIATION OF SHARED DECISION MAKING TO KNOWLEDGE AND TREATMENT SATISFACTION IN DENTAL PATIENTS

*Jessica Peters, BA, Boral[1], Jing Sun, PhD[*2], and Florian Mack, PhD[1]*

[1]School of Oral Health and Dental Science, Griffith University, Centre for Medicine and Oral Health, Southport, Australia
[2]School of Medicine and Griffith Health Institute. Griffith University, Logan Campus, Meadowbrook, Australia

ABSTRACT

Shared decision making (SDM) is an approach in which the clinician and patient go through all stages of the decision making process together. The use of SDM has been thoroughly explored in clinical medicine, however little research has examined SDM in dentistry. This study examined the use of SDM in patients who have received treatment for missing teeth. Method: A cross sectional study design was used to assess patients from a university dental clinic and a private dental practice. Patients were required to complete the SDM questionnaire. Results: Of the 144 participants, only 29.9% were exposed to SDM. The results of multiple linear regression suggested that the provision of SDM in the dental encounter, led to an increase in patient's knowledge of treatment alternatives and post treatment aesthetic/social satisfaction. However, the provision of SDM in the dental encounter did not lead to an increase in denture knowledge, post-treatment functional satisfaction or post-treatment economic satisfaction. Multiple linear regressions also identified pre-treatment self-esteem, oral health beliefs and attitudes and pre-treatment masticatory functioning as factors that mediate the relationship between SDM and the outcome variables. Conclusion: Decision-making in dentistry and the outcomes of dental treatment is a multifocal complex process.

[*] Correspondence: Jing Sun, PhD, School of Medicine, Griffith University and Griffith Health Institute, Griffith University, Gold Coast Campus, Parkland, Q4222Australia. E-mail: j.sun@griffith.edu.au

Keywords: Shared decision-making, tooth replacement, communication, patient knowledge, treatment satisfaction

INTRODUCTION

Research has highlighted shared decision making (SDM) as a method to facilitate a strong clinician patient relationship (1,2). SDM is an approach in which the clinician and patient go through all phases of the decision making process together (1). When SDM is employed, information is provided about the health problem, the possible treatment options and consequences of the treatments are discussed, and together the clinician and patient consider how these fit with the patient's preferred outcomes (1). After all the options are considered, a decision is made based on mutual agreement (3).

The concept of SDM has been thoroughly explored in the medical literature with many benefits reported (2,4-12). Such benefits include improvements in; treatment adherence, patient knowledge, quality of life, satisfaction, general health and wellbeing. It is however evident that little research has examined SDM in the dental encounter (13). With many benefits reported in clinical medicine, it is proposed that dental patients would benefit greatly if SDM was implemented in the dental encounter. This study subsequently seeks to examine SDM in the dental encounter. More specifically, this study seeks to examine the use of SDM in patients who have received treatment for missing teeth and determine if SDM leads to increased knowledge and satisfaction.

This study will provide evidence of the benefits obtained when SDM is employed in dentistry, specifically in patients seeking treatment for missing teeth. It is hoped that this study will demonstrate that similar benefits can be obtained when SDM is used in the dental setting as reported in the medical setting. This study will demonstrate that involving patients in the decision making process is critical in achieving successful clinical outcomes, with particular emphasis on increased dental knowledge and treatment satisfaction. This study is particularly important, as the use of SDM in dentistry has not yet been fully explored.

While this study seeks to demonstrate the importance of SDM in the dental encounter, it is recognized that multiple factors are at play. Mediating factors are expected to influence the relationship between SDM and dental knowledge and SDM and treatment satisfaction. These factors include: procedural factors, pre-treatment masticatory functioning, pre-treatment self-esteem and oral health beliefs/attitudes. These factors will be included in the current study. The aim of this study is to examine SDM in patients who have received dental treatment for missing teeth and to determine if SDM leads to increased dental knowledge and treatment satisfaction. This study also aims to identify factors that mediate the relationship between SDM and dental knowledge and SDM and treatment satisfaction. Specifically, the following objectives of the study will be examined: 1) To determine participants level of knowledge of dental treatment options via the implementation of the SDM questionnaire, 2) To determine participants level of post treatment satisfaction via the implementation of the SDM questionnaire, 3) To compare the SDM group and the comparison group on levels of knowledge of dental treatment options and post treatment satisfaction using linear regression and 4) To explore the mediating effects of procedural factors, oral health beliefs/attitudes, pre-treatment masticatory functioning, and pre-treatment self-esteem on the relationship between SDM and dental knowledge and SDM and satisfaction using linear regression.

The hypotheses of the study

- Patients who have experienced SDM have a higher level of knowledge of dental treatment options.
- Patients who have experienced SDM do not have a higher level of knowledge of dental treatment options.
- Patients who have experienced SDM have a greater sense of post treatment satisfaction.
- Patients who have experienced SDM do not have a greater sense of post treatment satisfaction.
- Procedural factors, oral health beliefs/attitudes, pre-treatment masticatory functioning, and pre-treatment self-esteem mediate the relationship between SDM and dental knowledge and SDM and treatment satisfaction.
- Procedural factors, oral health beliefs/attitudes, pre-treatment masticatory functioning, and pre-treatment self-esteem do not mediate the relationship between SDM and dental knowledge and SDM and treatment satisfaction.

METHODS

A cross sectional study design was used to collect data from patients who either visited the Griffith University dental clinic or a private dental practice. Data was collected from December 2012 to May 2013. Patients who have received treatment for a tooth gap were invited to attend the study. A tooth gap is a gap resulting from a missing tooth that is bordered by one or more natural teeth on either side (14). Participants may have multiple missing teeth; however the presence of a tooth gap with either a single or double span is required. Two inclusion criteria were used. Participants must have received treatment for missing teeth and the treatment must have been completed. Participants were selected from the Griffith University dental clinic in Queensland and a private dental practice in Tasmania. Patients were identified via computer records. Informed consent has been obtained from both facilities. There were 144 dental patients invited to attend the study and all of them agreed to participate in the study with 100% response rate. Ethical approval has been obtained through Griffith University Ethics Committee.

Measures

A questionnaire has been developed to assess SDM in patients who have received treatment for missing teeth. A pilot study has been completed and necessary adjustments were made. The questionnaire includes 107 items. Items are scored on either a 2 point scale (1, yes; 0, no) or on a 6 point scale (5, strongly agree; 4, agree; 3, somewhat agree; 2, somewhat disagree; 1, disagree; 0, strongly disagree). When asked about treatment alternatives, patients must rank their level of knowledge from 1 to 7. The reliability and validity of the SDM questionnaire has been established.

A Cronbach α level of .86 was obtained indicating that the overall reliability of the questionnaire is high. The SDM questionnaire demonstrates high content validity (explaining 73.93% of the total variance) and discriminant validity (ability to distinguish the SDM group from the comparison group).

Outcome variables

Knowledge
The participant's knowledge of treatment alternatives was assessed using eight questions (question 64- 72). Three questions are present for each of the three treatment modalities and patients are required to rank their level of knowledge from 1 to 7. For example; did you know what an implant looked like before the completion of your treatment?

Treatment satisfaction
Treatment satisfaction is assessed on four levels; functional, aesthetic, social and economic satisfaction. Three items (90-92) assess functional satisfaction, which measure the patient's satisfaction with their post treatment masticatory functioning. For example: after the replacement of my missing tooth I can now eat crunchy fruit. Item 94-96 assess aesthetic satisfaction. This includes: after the replacement of my missing tooth I am happier with how my mouth looks. Social satisfaction is measured using items 96-99. For example: after the replacement of my missing tooth I now enjoy meeting new people. Economic satisfaction is measured using item 100 and 101. For example: I believe that I received value for the cost of my dental treatment.

Mediating variables
The questionnaire also examines procedural factors, oral health beliefs/attitudes, pre-treatment masticatory functioning and the patient's pre-treatment self-esteem. These factors may mediate the relationship between the independent and outcome variables.

Confounding factors
Demographic factors, which may confound the relationship between SDM and knowledge and SDM and satisfaction, will also be collated. This includes; age, gender, income, place of residence, level of education, family and general health status. Whether the patient's treatment was covered by private health insurance or government assistance will also be collated.

Procedure of data collection
Patients were approached in both the private and public dental clinics. They were provided with an information sheet outlining the purpose of the study and the study procedure. If patients agreed to participate they were provided with the questionnaire. Data was entered into SPSS.

Statistical analysis

SPSS version 22.0 was used to analyse the data. Factor analysis, Chi-Square and multiple linear regression analysis were used to analyse the data.

Factor analysis, reliability and validity of the SDM questionnaire

Statistical analysis was conducted on unweighted data. A principle component analysis was conducted to investigate the subscales structure within the questionnaire. Varimax rotation was considered appropriate for the current study, which uses an orthogonal rotation method that minimizes the number of variables that have high loadings on each factor. Exploratory factor analysis was used to extract the factor structure of the questionnaire. Pearsons correlation bivariate analysis was completed to ensure each factor was not highly correlated and represented an independent concept. Reliability was also assessed from analyses of internal consistency using Cronbach α. A normality check was completed, and non-parametric tests applied to any factor that was not normally distributed.

Chi squared bivariate analysis

Chi squared bivariate analysis was completed to examine the differences between the SDM group and comparison group on demographic factors. Demographic factors that were included in the chi squared analysis were: age, gender, place of residency, level of education, income, general health, family status, and whether or not the patient received private health or government assistance for their dental treatment. If a significant difference was found the confounding factors were included in the multivariate analysis.

Multiple linear regressions

Multiple linear regressions were run to test the relationship between SDM and the dependent variables dental knowledge and treatment satisfaction. Three models were run for each linear regression in order to test the three research hypotheses.

H_1: Patients who have experienced SDM have a higher level of knowledge of dental treatment options.

To test hypothesis one, the multiple linear regression model was used to examine the relationship between the independent variable SDM and the dependent variable knowledge of dental treatment options. Confounding factors identified from the chi-squared analysis were controlled in the model.

H_2: Patients who have experienced SDM have a greater sense of post treatment satisfaction.

To test hypothesis two, the multiple linear regression model was used to examine the relationship between the independent variable SDM and the dependent variable treatment satisfaction. Confounding factors identified from the chi-squared analysis were controlled in the model.

H₃: Procedural factors, oral health beliefs/attitudes, pre-treatment masticatory functioning, and pre-treatment self-esteem mediate the relationship between SDM and dental knowledge and SDM and treatment satisfaction.

To test hypothesis three, the mediating factors were imputed into a separate block to see if they influence the relationship between the independent and dependent variables. Confounding factors identified from the chi-squared analysis were controlled in the model. The level of significance to test research hypotheses is $p<0.05$.

RESULTS

The demographic characteristics of the sample are depicted in table 1 below. One hundred and forty four participants completed the survey with 100% response rate. Of these participants, 50.0% were aged between 45-64 years, while 44.4% were aged 65 years and above and only 5.6 % aged less than 44 years. Among the respondents, 82 (56.9%) were female. Education levels indicated that 42.4 % had tertiary education, 16.0 % had diploma/training and further education, 40.3 % had secondary education and only 1.4 % had primary education level. When looking at place of residence, 107 (74.8%) were from metropolitan/city area, 30 (21.0%) from a semi-rural area and 6 (4.2%) from a rural area. In terms of family status, 107 (74.8 %) were living in a relationship/partnership and 36 (25.0%) were single. When look at average household income, 30.4% of participants reported earning $37,000 or less, 34.8% reported $37,001- $80,000, 29.0% reported $80,001- $180,000, and 5.8% reported $180,001 and over per year.

Dental characteristics of the sample

As seen in table 2 below, 105 (72.9%) participants received private health insurance for their dental treatment whereas 27 (18.8%) received government assistance for their dental treatment. Thirty (20.8%) participants from the total sample reported that they had previously been treated for gum disease. In regards to the number of missing teeth, 52 (36.1%) had only 1 missing tooth, 35 (24.5%) had 2-3 missing teeth and 56 (39.2%) had more than 3 missing teeth. When looking at the location of the missing teeth, 89 (61.8%) participants indicated that their missing tooth was located at the front of their mouth, with 98 (68.1%) participants indicating that their missing tooth could be seen when they smiled. The most commonly reported cause of tooth loss was; decay (34.7%), trauma (27.8%), cracked tooth (18.8%) and failed dental treatment (17.4%). Nine (6.3%) participants were unsure of the cause of their missing tooth. When looking at how long the patient waited before seeking treatment, 88 (61.1%) sought treatment immediately, 15 (10.4%) sought treatment within one year, 13 (9.0%) sought treatment within 1-3 years and, 30 (20.8%) waited more than 3 years for treatment. Finally, when looking at the final treatment choice, 48 (33.3%) participants received a fixed dental prosthesis, 39 (27.1%) participants received a chrome cobalt denture, 14 (9.7%) participants received an acrylic denture, and 45 (31.3%) participants received an implant-retained crown.

Table 1. Demographic characteristics of the sample

Categorical Variable	N (%)
Age	
>44 years	8 (5.6%)
45- 64 years	72 (50.0%)
65 years and over	64 (44.4%)
Gender	
Male	62 (43.1%)
Female	82 (56.9%)
Education level	
Primary education	2 (1.4%)
Secondary education	58 (40.3%)
Diploma/Tafe	23 (16.0%)
Tertiary education	61 (42.4%)
Place of residency	
Metropolitan/city area	107 (74.8%)
Semi-rural area	30 (21.0%)
Rural area	6 (4.2%)
Family status	
Living in a relationship/partnership	107 (74.8%)
Single	36 (25.0%)
Household income	
<$37,000	42 (30.4%)
$37,001- $80,000	48 (34.8%)
$80,001- $180,000	40 (29.0%)
>$180,001	8 (5.8%)

Grouping of participants

Whether or not alternative treatment options were discussed with patients by their dentist was examined. It was found that only 43 (29.9%) participants were presented with all three treatment options and could subsequently be assigned to the SDM group. Twenty-five (17.7%) participants were presented with two treatment options, 73 (51.8%) participants were presented with one treatment option and two (1.4%) participants were not presented with any treatment options. These participants were assigned to the comparison group.

Dependent and mediating variables
The mean and standard deviation of the dependent and mediating variables are presented in table 3 below. As all variables are normally distributed (see table 4), presentation of the mean and standard deviation is most appropriate.

Factor analysis

Factor analysis needed to be completed on the SDM questionnaire before the hypothesis could be tested and the relationship between SDM and dental knowledge and SDM and treatment satisfaction could be determined. Factor analysis was completed on the items in the SDM questionnaire in order to classify the variables into more meaningful categories.

Table 2. Dental characteristics of participants

Variable	N (%)
Private health insurance	
Yes	105 (72.9%)
No	39 (27.1%)
Government assistance	
Yes	27 (18.8%)
No	117 (81.3%)
Gum Disease	
Yes	30 (20.8%)
No	114 (79.2%)
Number of missing teeth before treatment	
Only one missing tooth	52 (36.1%)
2-3 missing teeth	35 (24.5%)
> 3 missing teeth	56 (39.2%)
Location of missing tooth	
Front	89 (61.8%)
Middle	48 (33.3%)
Back	36 (25.0%)
Can your missing tooth be seen when you smile	
Yes	98 (68.1%)
No	46 (31.9%)
Cause of tooth Loss	
Trauma/accident	40 (27.8%)
Tooth decay	50 (34.7%)
Gum disease	10 (6.9%)
Root resorption	7 (4.9%)
Failed dental treatment	25 (17.4%)
Tooth never formed	9 (6.3%)
Tooth was impacted	9 (6.3%)
Cracked tooth	27 (18.8%)
Unsure	9 (6.3%)
How long the tooth was missing before seeking treatment	
< 3 months	88 (61.1%)
3-6 months	11 (7.6%)
6 months -1 year	4 (2.8%)
1-3 years	13 (9.0%)
> 3 years	30 (20.8)
Final treatment choice	
CrCo RPD	39 (27.1%)
Acrylic RPD	14 (9.7%)
Implant supported crown	45 (31.3%)
FPD	48 (33.3%)

The Exploratory Factor Analysis derived a nine component solution from the factor analysis (see appendix 1). Pre-treatment self-esteem was the first factor, which included 7 items 80, 85, 86, 87, 88, 89 and 90. For example; before my treatment I did not like meeting new people, and I did not feel good about myself. Factor 2 was knowledge of the two other treatment modalities; implant retained crown and FPD. This was assessed using items 67, 68,

69, 70, 71, 72 and 73. Factor 3 [items 94, 95, 96, 97, 98, 99] indicated the respondent's level of post treatment aesthetic and social satisfaction. For example: after the replacement of my missing tooth I feel more confident. Factor 4 represented the degree in which procedural factors impacted on the patient's treatment choice. This was measured using items 74, 75, 76, 77, 78 and 79. The fifth factor comprised the oral health beliefs/attitudes of the patient. This was measured using items 102, 103, 104, 106, and 107 such as: I believe that good teeth are important for general health. Factor 6 included items 81, 82, 83, and 84, which measured pretreatment masticatory functioning. Factor 7 measured patient's satisfaction with post treatment masticatory functioning [91,92,93]. The eighth factor expressed the patient's level of denture knowledge, which was assessed using items 64, 65, and 66. The ninth and final factor was post treatment economic satisfaction. This was measured using item 100 and 101.

Pearson's correlation bivariate analysis

Pearson's correlation bivariate analysis was completed to ensure each factor was not highly correlated (correlation $< .85$) and therefore represented an independent concept (see table 5). The variance explained by the nine factors were 11.28%, 11.15%, 11.10%, 8.03%, 7.51%, 7.08%, 6.40%, 6.04%, and 3.96% respectively. The total variance explained by the 9 factors was 72.54%.

Table 3. Mean and standard deviation of the dependent and mediating variables

Dependent Variables	Mean (SD)
Knowledge of treatment alternatives	19.40 (13.15)
Denture knowledge	15.00 (6.50)
Post- treatment aesthetic/social satisfaction	24.05 (8.81)
Post-treatment functional satisfaction	12.37 (3.57)
Post-treatment economic satisfaction	7.17 (2.39)
Mediating Variables	**Mean (SD)**
Procedural factors	6.90 (6.21)
Pre-treatment masticatory functioning	11.15 (5.67)
Pre-treatment self esteem	13.79 (9.59)
Oral health beliefs/attitudes	23.05 (2.47)

Reliability of the SDM questionnaire

The overall reliability level of the questionnaire was relatively high with a Cronbach α level of 0.860. Table 6 below indicates that the subscales based on the 9 extracted factors were generally found to be reliable with levels ranging from 0.798 to 0.954.

Table 4. Skewness and kurtosis of dependent and mediating variables

Variable	Skewness (standard error)	Kurtosis (standard error)
Knowledge of treatment alternatives	0.791 (0.206)	-0.638 (0.408)
Denture knowledge	-0.682 (0.205)	-0.985 (0.407)
Post- treatment aesthetic/social satisfaction	-0.554 (0.205)	-0.869 (0.407)

Jessica Peters, Jing Sun and Florian Mack

Table 4. (Continued)

Variable	Skewness (standard error)	Kurtosis (standard error)
Post-treatment functional satisfaction	-1.813 (0.206)	0.076 (0.410)
Post-treatment economic satisfaction	-0.568 (0.206)	-0.627 (0.408)
Procedural factors	1.134 (0.206)	1.569 (0.408)
Pre-treatment masticatory functioning	-0.195 (0.207)	-1.002 (0.411)
Pre-treatment self esteem	0.634 (0.207)	-0.652 (0.411)
Oral health beliefs/attitudes	-1.203 (0.206)	0.745 (0.408)

Table 5. Inter-correlation between the nine factors obtained from factor analysis

	Post treatment physical and social satisfaction	Post treatment functional satisfaction	Post treatment economic satisfaction	Denture knowledge	Knowledge of other treatment modalities	Pre-treatment self esteem	Pre-treatment functioning	Procedural factors
Post treatment physical and social satisfaction	.258**	0.161						
Post treatment functional satisfaction	0.117	0.035	0.114					
Post treatment economic satisfaction	.197*	0.036	-0.007	.292**				
Denture knowledge	.463**	0.072	0.128	-0.015	-0.128			
Knowledge of other treatment modalities	0.019	.196*	-0.103	-0.024	0.021	.272**		
Pre-treatment self esteem	0.011	-0.065	-0.117	0.05	-0.044	.205*	.191*	
Pre-treatment functioning	.379**	0.118	.209*	.219**	0.132	0.117	-0.067	-0.072

** Correlation is significant at the 0.01 level (2-tailed).

Chi-Squared test

For the current study, a Chi-squared test was used to describe the demographic characteristics of the SDM group and the comparison group and to compare the differences between them. The results are presented in table 7 below.

Table 6. Reliability correlations, Cronbach α

Questionnaire	Reliability correlations, Cronbach α (9 factors)
Total score	0.860
Pre-treatment self esteem	0.913
Knowledge of other treatment modalities	0.918
Post treatment aesthetic/social satisfaction	0.916
Procedural factors	0.806
Oral health beliefs	0.798
Pre-treatment functioning	0.850
Post treatment functional satisfaction	0.954
Denture knowledge	0.914
Post treatment economic satisfaction	0.695

Table 7. Chi-squared analysis to identify confounding factors

Variable	Group		χ^2	P value
	Comparison group N(%)	SDM group (%)		
Age			3.262	0.353
<25	1 (100%)	0 (0%)		
25-44	3 (42.9%)	4 (57.1%)		
45- 64	50 (69.4%)	22 (30.6%)		
>64	47 (46.5%)	17 (39.5%)		
Gender			4.070	**0.044****
Male	38 (61.3%)	24 (38.7%)		
Female	63 (76.8%)	19 (23.2%)		
Place of residency			1.081	0.583
Metropolitan	78 (72.9%%)	29 (27.1%)		
Semi-rural	19 (63.3%)	11 (36.7%)		
Rural	4 (66.7%)	2 (33.3%)		
Level of education			0.403	0.940
Primary	1 (50.0%)	1 (50.0%)		
Secondary	41 (70.7%)	17 (29.3%)		
Diploma/tafe	16 (69.6%)	7 (30.4%)		
Teriary	43 (70.5%)	18 (29.5%)		
Family status			0.120	0.729
Single	26 (72.2%)	10 (27.8%)		
Living in a relationship/partnership	74 (69.2%)	33 (30.8%)		
Household income			3.589	0.464
0-18,200	3 (75.0%)	1 (25.0%)		
18,201-37,000	30 (78.9%)	8 (21.1%)		
37,001-80,000	34 (70.8%)	14 (29.2%)		
80,001- 180,000	24 (60.0%)	16 (40.0%)		
>180,000	5 (62.5%)	337.5%)		
General health			4.756	0.191
Poor	2 (100%)	0 (0%)		
Good	47 (73.4%)	17 (26.6%)		
Very good	32 (60.4%)	21 (39.6%)		
Excellent	20 (80.0%)	5 (20.0%)		
Private health insurance			0.070	0.791
Yes	73 (69.5%)	32 (30.5%)		
No	28 (71.8%)	11 (28.2%)		
Government assistance			0.246	0.620
Yes	20 (74.1%)	7 (25.9%)		
No	81 (69.2%)	36 (30.8%)		

**P< 0.05.

The demographic factor of gender was significance ($p= 0.044$). This indicates that there is not equal distribution between the comparison group and the SDM group in regards to this variable. Gender is therefore a confounding factors that has the potential to influence the relationship between the independent and dependent variables. Gender will subsequently be included in the multiple linear regression. A non-significant result ($p>0.05$) was found for the variables of age, place of residency, education, family status, household income, general health, private health insurance and government assistance. This indicates that these variables are represented equally in both the SDM group and the comparison group.

Multiple linear regression

From factors analysis, the dependent variable knowledge was broken down into two factors; denture knowledge and knowledge of treatment alternatives. The dependent variable treatment satisfaction was broken down into; post treatment aesthetic/social satisfaction, post treatment functional satisfaction and post treatment economic satisfaction. Subsequently, linear regression was run for each of the five dependent variables produced from factor analysis. Three models were run for each of the five dependent variables.

The relationship between SDM and knowledge of treatment alternatives
As demonstrated in table 8 below, SDM had a positive relationship with knowledge of treatment alternatives. That is, the provision of SDM in the dental encounter, lead to an increase in knowledge of treatment alternatives. SDM had a regression coefficient value of 6.501 (95% CI: 1.763, 11.238) demonstrating a significant positive influence of knowledge of treatment alternatives ($p=0.008$).

Table 8. The relationship between SDM and knowledge of treatment alternatives

Predictor Variable	Regression coefficient (95% CI)	P value
SDM	6.501 (1.763, 11.238)	0.008**

Table 9. The influence of SDM, mediating factors and confounding factors on knowledge of treatment alternatives

Predictor variable	Regression coefficient (95% CI)	P value
Independent variable		
SDM	5.903 (1.057, 10.749)	**0.017****
Mediating factors		
Pre-treatment self esteem	0.243 (-0.003, 0.489)	**0.050****
Procedural factors	-0.102 (-0.465, 0.262)	0.581
Oral health beliefs/attitudes	1.161 (0.159, 2.164)	**0.024****
Pre-treatment functioning	-0.171 (-0.647, 0.306)	0.480
Confounding factors		
Gender	-3.029 (-8.064, 2.005)	0.236

** $P< 0.05$.
Correlation coefficient (R): 0.343.
Adjusted R squared: 0.075.
ANOVA F value: 2.792**.

Table 9 below, displays the influence SDM had on knowledge of treatment alternatives, when the mediating factors and confounding factor gender were also considered. Even when including the mediating and confounding factors, SDM still had a significant positive influence on knowledge of treatment alternatives (p=0.017).

This level of significance was however slightly lower, when these additional factors were included. When looking at the influence the mediating factors had on knowledge of treatment alternative, it appears that pre-treatment self-esteem (p= 0.050) and oral health beliefs/attitudes (p= 0.024) were significant mediators of the relationship between SDM and knowledge of treatment alternatives. Pre-treatment self-esteem had a regression coefficient value of 0.243 (95% CI: -0.003, 0.489) demonstrating a significant positive mediating relationship. That is, as the pre-treatment self-esteem of the patient increased, knowledge of treatment alternatives also increased. A significant mediating effect was also seen for oral health beliefs/attitudes with a regression coefficient of 1.161 (95% CI: 0.159, 2.164) demonstrating a significant positive mediating influence on knowledge of treatment alternatives. That is, as the oral health belief/attitudes of the patient increased, knowledge of treatment alternatives also increased. The mediating factors; pre-treatment functioning and procedural factors, as well as the confounding factor gender did not appear to be strong mediators in the relationship between SDM and knowledge of treatment alternatives as indicated by non-significant p values.

The ANOVA F ratio for the model was 2.792. This was statistically significant with a p value <0.05. This indicates that the prediction of the X/Y relationship was significant. The adjusted R-squared value was 0.075. This suggests that 7.5% of the variance in knowledge of treatment alternatives is explained by SDM, the mediating factors and the confounding factor gender.

Relationship between SDM and denture knowledge
As demonstrated in table 10 below, SDM did not appear to be a strong predictor of denture knowledge (p=0.644).

As demonstrated in table 11 below, even when taking into account the influence of mediating and confounding factors, SDM still was not found to be a strong predictor of denture knowledge (p= 0.664). That is, the provision of SDM in the dental encounter, did not lead to an increase in denture knowledge. When looking at the mediating factors, pre-treatment self-esteem (p=0.579), procedural factors (p=0.490), and pre-treatment functioning (p=0.961) did not significantly mediate the relationship between SDM and denture knowledge. The mediating factor oral health beliefs/attitudes was however significant (p= 0.020) with a regression coefficient of 0. 612 (95% CI: 0.100, 1.125). As the regression coefficient was positive it was suggested that as the oral health beliefs/attitudes of the patient increased, the denture knowledge of the patient also increased. Finally, gender (p= 0.737) was not found to significantly predict denture knowledge.

Table 10. The relationship between SDM and denture knowledge

Predictor Variable	Regression coefficient (95% CI)	P value
SDM	0.564 (-1.847, 2.976)	0.644

The ANOVA F ratio for the model was 0.213. This was not statistically significant. The adjusted R-squared value was 0.019. This suggests that only 1.9% of the variance in denture knowledge is explained by SDM, the mediating factors and the confounding factor gender.

Relationship between SDM and post-treatment aesthetic/social satisfaction

As demonstrated in table 12 below, SDM had a positive relationship with post-treatment aesthetic/social satisfaction. SDM had a regression coefficient value of 3.873 (95% CI: 0.752, 6.993) demonstrating a significant positive influence on post-treatment aesthetic/social satisfaction (p=0.015). That is, the provision of SDM in the dental encounter, lead to an increase in post treatment aesthetic/social satisfaction.

Table 11. The influence of SDM, mediating factors and confounding factors on denture knowledge

Predictor variable	Regression coefficient (95% CI)	P value
Independent variable		
SDM	0.544(-1.931, 3.020)	0.664
Mediating factors		
Pre-treatment self esteem	0.033 (-0.090, 0.162)	0.579
Procedural factors	0.065 (-0.121, 0.251)	0.490
Oral health beliefs/attitudes	0.612 (0.100, 1.125)	**0.020****
Pre-treatment functioning	-0.012 (-0.211, 0.201)	0.961
Confounding factors		
Gender	0.438 (-2.135, 3.010)	0.737

**P< 0.05.
Correlation coefficient (R): 0.252.
Adjusted R squared: 0.019.
ANOVA F value: 0.213.

Table 13 below, displays the influence SDM had on post-treatment aesthetic/social satisfaction, when the mediating factors and confounding factor gender were also considered. As shown in table 13, even when examining the influence of the mediating and confounding factors, SDM still had a significant positive influence on post-treatment aesthetic/social satisfaction (p=0.023). This level of significance was however slightly lower, when these additional factors were also included. When looking at the influence the mediating factors had on the relationship between SDM and post-treatment aesthetic/social satisfaction, it appears that pre-treatment self-esteem (p<0.001) and oral health beliefs/attitudes (p<0.001) demonstrated a significant effect. Pre-treatment self-esteem had a regression coefficient value of -0.413 (95% CI: -0.546, -0.275) demonstrating a significant negative relationship. That is, when the pre-treatment self-esteem of the patient decreased, the post-treatment aesthetic/social satisfaction increased. A significant predictive effect was also seen for oral health beliefs/attitudes with a regression coefficient of 1.258 (95% CI: 0.703, 1.814) demonstrating a significant positive influence on post-treatment aesthetic/social satisfaction. That is, as the oral health belief/attitudes of the patient increased, post-treatment aesthetic/social satisfaction also increased. The mediating factors pre-treatment functioning and procedural factors, as well as the confounding factor gender did not appear to influence the relationship between SDM and knowledge of treatment alternatives as indicated by non-significant p values.

The ANOVA F ratio for the model was 12.227. This was statistically significant with a p value <0.001. This indicates that the prediction of the X/Y relationship was significant. The adjusted R-squared value was 0.336. This suggests that 33.6% of the variance in post treatment aesthetic/social satisfaction is explained by SDM, the mediating factors and the confounding factor gender.

Table 12. The relationship between SDM and post treatment aesthetic/social satisfaction

Predictor Variable	Regression coefficient (95% CI)	P value
SDM	3.873 (0.752, 6.993)	**0.015****

Table 13. The influence of SDM, mediating factors and confounding factors on post-treatment aesthetic/social satisfaction

Predictor variable	Regression coefficient (95% CI)	P value
Independent variable		
SDM	3.123 (0.437, 5.809)	**0.023****
Mediating factors		
Pre-treatment self esteem	-0.413 (-0.546, -0.275)	**<0.001*****
Procedural factors	-0.154 (-0.355, 0.047)	0.132
Oral health beliefs/attitudes	1.258 (0.703, 1.814)	**<0.001*****
Pre-treatment functioning	0.107 (-0.156, 0.371)	0.423
Confounding factors		
Gender	-2. 363 (-5.154, 0.427)	0.096

**P< 0.05 ***P< 0.001.
Correlation coefficient (R): 0.605.
Adjusted R squared: 0.336.
ANOVA F value: 12.227***.

Relationship between SDM and post-treatment functional satisfaction

As demonstrated in table 14 SDM did not appear to be a strong predictor of post-treatment functional satisfaction (p=0.134).

As demonstrated in table 15 even when taking into account the influence of mediating and confounding factors, SDM still was not found to be a strong predictor of post treatment functional satisfaction (p= 0.216). That is, the provision of SDM in the dental encounter, did not lead to an increase in post treatment functional satisfaction. The mediating factor pre-treatment functioning had a regression coefficient value of -0.160 (95% CI: -0.283, -0.037) demonstrating a significant negative relationship (p= 0.011). That is, pre-treatment functioning was shown to mediate the relationship between SDM and post treatment functional satisfaction. As the regression coefficient was negative it is suggested that as the pre-treatment functioning of the patient decreased, the post treatment functional satisfaction increased. The other mediating factors: pre-treatment self-esteem (p=0.870), procedural factors (p=0.087) and oral health beliefs/attitudes (p=0.141) did not influence the relationship between SDM and post-treatment functional satisfaction. Finally, gender (p= 0.751) did not significantly predict post-treatment functional satisfaction.

Table 14. The relationship between SDM and post treatment functional satisfaction

Predictor Variable	Regression coefficient (95% CI)	P value
SDM	0.945 (-0.293, 2.183)	0.134

Table 15. The influence of SDM, mediating factors and confounding factors on post-treatment functional satisfaction

Predictor variable	Regression coefficient (95% CI)	P value
Independent variable		
SDM	0.791 (-0.467, 2.049)	0.216
Mediating factors		
Pre-treatment self esteem	-0.005 (-0.069, 0.058)	0.870
Procedural factors	-0.082 (-0.176, 0.012)	0.087
Oral health beliefs/attitudes	0.195 (-0.065, 0.455)	0.141
Pre-treatment functioning	-0.160 (-0.283, -0.037)	**0.011****
Confounding factors		
Gender	-0.210 (-1.517, 1.098)	0.751

**$P < 0.05$.
Correlation coefficient (R): 0.310.
Adjusted R squared: 0.053.
ANOVA F value: 2.248**.

The ANOVA F ratio for the model was 2.248. This was statistically significant with a *p* value <0.05. This indicates that the prediction of the X/Y relationship was significant. The adjusted R-squared value was 0.053. This suggests that 5.3% of the variance in post treatment functional satisfaction is explained by SDM, the mediating factors and the confounding factor gender.

Relationship between SDM and post-treatment economic satisfaction

As demonstrated in table 16 below, SDM did not appear to be a strong predictor of post treatment economic satisfaction ($p=0.681$).

As demonstrated in table 17 below, even when taking into account the influence of mediating and confounding factors, SDM still was not found to be a strong predictor of post treatment economic satisfaction ($p= 0.724$). That is, the provision of SDM in the dental encounter, did not lead to an increase in post treatment economic satisfaction. When looking at the mediating factors, pre-treatment self-esteem ($p=0.043$) did have a significant mediating effect (95% CI: -0.090, 0.001) on the relationship between SDM and post treatment economic satisfaction. This is represented by a negative regression coefficient, which indicates that as the pre-treatment self-esteem of the patient decreased, their post treatment economic satisfaction increased. All of the other mediating factors, procedural factors ($p=0.189$), oral health beliefs/attitudes ($p=0.111$) and pre-treatment functioning ($p=0.419$) as well as gender ($p= 0.795$) did not significantly influence the relationship between SDM and denture knowledge.

Table 16. The relationship between SDM and post treatment economic satisfaction

Predictor Variable	Regression coefficient (95% CI)	P value
SDM	-0.182 (-1.057, 0.692)	0.681

Table 17. The influence of SDM, mediating factors and confounding factors on post-treatment economic satisfaction

Predictor variable	Regression coefficient (95% CI)	P value
Independent variable		
SDM	-0.159 (-1.050, 0.731)	0.724
Mediating factors		
Pre-treatment self esteem	-0.044 (-0.090, 0.001)	**0.043****
Procedural factors	-0.044 (-0.111, 0.022)	0.189
Oral health beliefs/attitudes	0.149 (-0.035, 0.333)	0.111
Pre-treatment functioning	0.036 (-0.052, 0.123)	0.419
Confounding factors		
Gender	-0.210 (-1.045, 0.802)	0.795

**P< 0.05.
Correlation coefficient (R): 0.268.
Adjusted R squared: 0.028.
ANOVA F value: 1.625**.

The ANOVA F ratio for the model was 1.625. This was statistically significant with a *p* value <0.05. This indicates that the prediction of the X/Y relationship was significant. The adjusted R-squared value was 0.028. This suggests that 2.8% of the variance in post treatment economic satisfaction is explained by SDM, the mediating factors and the confounding factor gender.

DISCUSSION

Exploratory factor analysis in the current study showed a 9 factor solution, suggesting that 9 factor can be used to assess the patient's experience in the dental encounter specifically relating to the treatment of missing teeth. The Cronbach α level of 0.86 indicated that the overall reliability level of the questionnaire was high. The 9 extracted factors were also found to be reliable with levels ranging from 0.798 to 0.954. These questions had high content validity and explained 72.54% of the total variance. Subsequently it is concluded that the SDM questionnaire is a valid and reliable measure of SDM in patients who have received treatment for missing teeth.

SDM and knowledge

The results of linear regression suggested that the provision of SDM in the dental encounter was associated with increased knowledge of treatment alternatives. This result is consistent with other studies that indicate that effective SDM can be measured by examining the patient's overall knowledge of treatment options (15). However, SDM was not associated with increased denture knowledge. This finding may be explained by the fact that the denture treatment modality is more widely known amongst the general population. It is possible that SDM is not required for this type of knowledge to be obtained.

APPENDIX 1. PRINCIPLE COMPONENT ANALYSIS FOR NINE-FACTOR STRUCTURE

	Pre-treatment self esteem	Knowledge of other treatment modalities	Post treatment social/ aesthetic satisfaction	Procedural factors	Oral health beliefs	Pre-treatment functioning	Post treatment functional satisfaction	Denture knowledge	Post treatment economic satisfaction
Before my treatment I did not like meeting new people.	**.877**	-.073	.165	.168	-.012	.077	.008	.066	.089
Before my treatment I did not feel good about myself.	**.861**	-.069	.138	.097	.066	.165	.029	-.073	.098
Before my treatment I felt that people were staring at my missing tooth.	**.850**	-.042	.251	.100	-.054	.020	-.030	-.040	.052
Before my treatment I did not like speaking in public.	**.850**	-.098	.135	.136	-.034	.104	-.012	.100	.079
Before my treatment I lacked confidence.	**.820**	-.072	.142	.078	.007	.233	.000	-.145	.147
Before my treatment I was unhappy with how my mouth looked.	**.720**	-.093	.310	.029	.036	.153	-.021	.027	-.162
A major reason for the replacement of my missing tooth was my appearance.	**.434**	-.013	.225	-.122	.225	-.235	.159	.155	-.244
Did you know how an implant was inserted before your treatment?	-.046	**.878**	.105	-.059	.010	.085	-.003	.080	-.213
Did you know how to clean an implant before your treatment?	-.009	**.877**	.126	-.064	-.010	.105	-.042	.102	-.093
Did you know how a bridge was constructed before your treatment?	-.109	**.873**	.078	-.018	.101	-.104	.092	.067	.172
Did you know what an implant looked like before your treatment?	-.033	**.865**	.106	-.084	-.014	.114	.055	.043	-.221
Did you know how to clean a bridge before your treatment?	-.084	**.837**	.068	.027	.109	-.059	.076	.113	.159
Did you know what a bridge looked like before your treatment?	-.177	**.766**	.015	-.052	.138	-.152	.161	.134	.097
Damage to the surrounding teeth through drilling was a factor that influenced my final treatment choice.	.081	**.410**	-.105	.391	.103	.182	-.179	.058	.161

	Pre-treatment self esteem	Knowledge of other treatment modalities	Post treatment social/ aesthetic satisfaction	Procedural factors	Oral health beliefs	Pre-treatment functioning	Post treatment functional satisfaction	Denture knowledge	Post treatment economic satisfaction
After the replacement of my missing tooth I feel more confident.	.192	.068	**.858**	.045	.167	.002	.123	-.073	.059
After the replacement of my missing tooth I feel better about myself.	.174	.082	**.827**	.033	.088	.077	.137	.015	.189
After the replacement of my missing tooth I now enjoy meeting new people.	.285	.109	**.825**	-.002	.039	-.020	.066	.122	.092
After the replacement of my missing tooth I feel more comfortable smiling.	.181	.079	**.822**	-.132	.166	-.100	.064	.038	.063
After the replacement of my missing tooth I am happier with how my mouth looks.	.128	-.022	**.809**	-.115	.179	-.101	.160	-.058	-.076
After the replacement of my missing tooth I now enjoy speaking in public.	.329	.160	**.736**	-.009	.049	-.013	.054	.149	.071
I believe that missing or decayed teeth are a sign of poor health.	-.050	.244	**.413**	.068	.390	.134	-.110	-.061	.165
The amount of pain I associated with each procedure influenced my final treatment choice.	.147	-.107	-.042	**.870**	.024	.080	.057	-.065	.069
The amount of discomfort I associated with each procedure influenced my final treatment choice.	.038	-.130	-.008	**.812**	.047	.134	.019	.003	.050
I experience fear/anxiety towards dental treatment and this influenced my final treatment choice.	.110	-.164	-.011	**.797**	.045	.132	-.008	.025	-.037
Duration of the treatment was a factor that influenced my final treatment choice.	.095	.185	-.035	**.692**	-.240	.001	-.016	.000	.044
Cost of the treatment was a factor that influenced my final treatment choice.	-.111	-.053	-.082	**.567**	-.152	-.030	-.149	.100	-.178
The materials that are used in each procedure were a factor that influenced my final treatment choice.	.183	.070	.064	**.533**	.107	.045	-.055	.011	-.131
I believe that good teeth are important for my general health.	-.084	.053	.093	.006	**.865**	-.020	.148	.117	.016

Appendix 1. (Continued)

	Pre-treatment self esteem	Knowledge of other treatment modalities	Post treatment social/ aesthetic satisfaction	Procedural factors	Oral health beliefs	Pre-treatment functioning	Post treatment functional satisfaction	Denture knowledge	Post treatment economic satisfaction
I believe that good teeth are important for eating and chewing.	.002	.060	.031	-.094	**.753**	.113	.083	.033	.078
I believe that someone with all their teeth looks better than someone with missing teeth.	.036	.025	.053	-.065	**.725**	-.086	.032	.157	.007
I believe good teeth are important for maintaining nutrition.	.016	.161	.208	.100	**.690**	.014	-.030	-.002	.003
I believe that good teeth are important for my appearance.	.153	-.071	.345	-.017	**.642**	-.235	-.044	.132	.031
Before my treatment I found it difficult to eat crunchy fruit.	.167	-.040	.054	.105	-.046	**.886**	.120	.023	-.047
Before my treatment I found it difficult to eat crunchy vegetables.	.201	.022	.056	.124	-.050	**.879**	.067	-.033	.011
Before my treatment I found it difficult to eat cooked meat.	.212	-.016	-.032	.149	-.096	**.869**	.079	.032	.004
A major reason for the replacement of my missing tooth was my ability to eat and chew.	-.002	.085	-.180	.022	.109	**.528**	.128	-.050	-.175
After the replacement of my missing tooth I can now eat crunchy fruit.	.020	.056	.092	-.054	.042	.128	**.930**	-.009	.071
After the replacement of my missing tooth I can now eat crunchy vegetables.	.015	.086	.158	-.077	.046	.118	**.925**	.011	.088
After the replacement of my missing tooth I can now eat cooked meat.	-.021	.083	.193	-.029	.091	.136	**.874**	.084	.088
Did you know how to use a denture before your treatment?	-.013	.193	-.003	.050	.121	.004	.075	**.921**	.054
Did you know how to clean a denture before your treatment?	.026	.131	.009	.059	.093	.011	-.009	**.915**	.153
Did you know what a denture looked like before your treatment?	-.011	.146	.104	-.020	.161	-.047	.014	**.842**	-.116
I believe I paid too much reversed	.108	-.084	.120	-.105	.013	-.054	.121	.049	**.792**
I believe that I received value for the cost of my dental treatment.	.109	.054	.251	-.030	.168	-.152	.134	.048	**.733**

The oral health beliefs and attitudes of a patient were a significant predictor for both knowledge of treatment modalities and denture knowledge. This is consistent with research that suggests that patients with strong oral health beliefs are more motivated to understand their oral health conditions and how their health status can be improved (16). Finally, self-esteem was a significant mediator in the relationship between SDM and knowledge of other treatment modalities. It was found that patients with low self-esteem prior to dental treatment had lower knowledge of treatment options following treatment. This is consistent with research that suggests that low self-esteem and psychological dysfunction can hinder an individual's ability to retain new information (17).

SDM and post -treatment satisfaction

This study demonstrated that the provision of SDM in the dental encounter was associated with an increase in post treatment aesthetic/social satisfaction. This finding supports Swanson et al. who concluded that involving patients in treatment decisions and providing a thorough explanation, leads to increased satisfaction (18). However in the current study, SDM was not associated with increased post treatment economic or functional satisfaction.

When looking at the influence the mediating factors had on post treatment satisfaction, the pre-treatment self-esteem of the patient was found to be significantly related to post treatment aesthetic/social satisfaction and post treatment economic satisfaction. It was found that patients with low self-esteem prior to dental treatment, reported higher levels of aesthetic/social satisfaction and economic satisfaction following treatment. The presence of missing teeth can negatively impact on a patients psychological and social functioning and may act as a barrier to personal and social success (19,20). Patients with greater psychosocial impairment attributed to unfavourable dentition, have greater clinical outcomes following prosthodontics rehabilitation and this is supported in the current study (21).

The oral health beliefs of the patient were found to be significantly related to post treatment aesthetic/social satisfaction. This suggests that the oral health beliefs of a patient can impact their treatment outcomes. The current study subsequently supports researchers who suggest that patients with strong oral health beliefs are more likely to appreciate the changes obtained following treatment and report greater levels of satisfaction (22).

Finally, the pre-treatment functioning of a patient was found to be significantly related to post treatment functional satisfaction. The results of the linear regression suggested that patients with impaired masticatory functioning prior to treatment, reported greater post treatment functional satisfaction. The results of the current study are consistent with studies that suggest that patients with greater functional impairment prior to treatment will have greater clinical outcomes following prosthodontics rehabilitation (21).

Limitations

There are a number of limitations for this study. Selection bias may have been present in the current study, as it did not have blind selection. Random sampling would be a method to overcome selection bias. Allocation to the SDM group and the comparison group was based upon participants recognising the use of SDM in the interaction with their dentist and reporting this in the questionnaire. Some measurement bias may have been present if patients failed to indicate that SDM had been used if in fact it had. Finally, analysis bias may have occurred when entering data into SPSS. However, cleaning the data would help overcome this bias. In order to reduce the occurrence of random error, increasing the sample size is required.

As data is only collected from two dental clinics, the generalizability of the results is limited. The researchers made every effort to improve this by selecting patients who had received different treatment options for their missing teeth and participants from a wide range of backgrounds. The fact that the study included both private and public dental patients does improve the generalizability of the results. However, in order to improve the generalizability of these results and to gain a better insight into the use of SDM in dentistry a large sample size from a broader range of dental practices should be utilized. In addition to this, this study only examines SDM in tooth replacement. Exploring SDM in other clinical situations may further aid in understanding the decision-making process in the dental encounter.

CONCLUSION

In conclusion it is evident that decision-making in dentistry and the outcomes of dental treatment is a complex process and multiple factors are at play. While SDM is important in achieving favourable treatment outcomes, it is suggested that further research is required examining the interaction of patient factors with SDM. Perhaps the use of SDM in combination with encouraging patients to have strong oral health beliefs and attitudes and helping to improve patients self-esteem would aid in achieving more successful clinical outcomes including patient's dental knowledge and patient satisfaction.

REFERENCES

[1]   Frosch DL, Kaplan RM. Shared decision making in clinical medicine: past research and future directions. Am J Prev Med 1999;17(4):285-94.
[2]   Joosten EA, DeFuentes-Merillas L, de Weert GH, Sensky T, van der Staak CP, de Jong CA. Systematic review of the effects of shared decision-making on patient satisfaction, treatment adherence and health status. Psychother Psychosom 2008;77(4):219-26.
[3]   Charles C, Gafni A, Whelan T. Shared decision-making in the medical encounter: what does it mean? (or it takes at least two to tango). Soc Sci Med 1997;44(5):681-92.
[4]   Adams JR, Drake RE, Wolford GL. Shared decision-making preferences of people with severe mental illness. Psychiatr Serv 2007;58(9):1219-21.
[5]   Clever SL, Ford DE, Rubenstein LV, Rost KM, Meredith LS, Sherbourne CD, et al. Primary care patients' involvement in decision-making is associated with improvement in depression. Med Care 2006;44(5):398-405.
[6]   Deyo RA, Cherkin DC, Weinstein J, Howe J, Ciol M, Mulley AG, Jr. Involving patients in clinical decisions: impact of an interactive video program on use of back surgery. Med Care 2000;38(9):959-69.
[7]   Gattellari M, Butow PN, Tattersall MH. Sharing decisions in cancer care. Soc Sci Med 2001;52(12):1865-78.
[8]   Greenfield S, Kaplan S, Ware JE, Jr. Expanding patient involvement in care. Effects on patient outcomes. Ann Intern Med 1985;102(4):520-8.

[9]   Hamann J, Cohen R, Leucht S, Busch R, Kissling W. Shared decision making and long-term outcome in schizophrenia treatment. J Clin Psychiatry 2007;68(7):992-7.

[10]   Morgan MW, Deber RB, Llewellyn-Thomas HA, Gladstone P, Cusimano RJ, O'Rourke K, et al. Randomized, controlled trial of an interactive videodisc decision aid for patients with ischemic heart disease. J Gen Intern Med 2000;15(10):685-93.

[11]   Ruland CM, White T, Stevens M, Fanciullo G, Khilani SM. Effects of a computerized system to support shared decision making in symptom management of cancer patients: preliminary results. J Am Med Inform Assoc 2003;10(6):573-9.

[12]   van Roosmalen MS, Stalmeier PF, Verhoef LC, Hoekstra-Weebers JE, Oosterwijk JC, Hoogerbrugge N, et al. Impact of BRCA1/2 testing and disclosure of a positive test result on women affected and unaffected with breast or ovarian cancer. Am J Med Genet Part A 2004;124A(4):346-55.

[13]   Johnson BR, Schwartz A, Goldberg J, Koerber A. A chairside aid for shared decision making in dentistry: a randomized controlled trial. J Dent Educ 2006;70(2):133-41.

[14]   Mack F, Samietz SA, Mundt T, Proff P, Gedrange T, Kocher T, et al. Prevalence of single-tooth gaps in a population-based study and the potential for dental implants--data from the Study of Health in Pomerania (SHIP-0). J Craniomaxillofac Surg 2006;34(Suppl 2):82-5.

[15]   Politi MC, Clark MA, Ombao H, Dizon D, Elwyn G. Communicating uncertainty can lead to less decision satisfaction: a necessary cost of involving patients in shared decision making? Health Expect 2011;14(1):84-91.

[16]   Broadbent JM, Thomson WM, Poulton R. Oral health beliefs in adolescence and oral health in young adulthood. J Dent Res 2006;85(4):339-43.

[17]   Whitesell NR, Mitchell CM, Spicer P. A longitudinal study of self-esteem, cultural identity, and academic success among American Indian adolescents. Cultur Divers Ethnic Minor Psychol 2009;15(1):38-50.

[18]   Swanson KA, Bastani R, Rubenstein LV, Meredith LS, Ford DE. Effect of mental health care and shared decision making on patient satisfaction in a community sample of patients with depression. Med Care Res Rev 2007;64(4):416-30.

[19]   Chen P, Yu S, Zhu G. The psychosocial impacts of implantation on the dental aesthetics of missing anterior teeth patients. Br Dent J 2012;213(11):E20.

[20]   Kerosuo H, Hausen H, Laine T, Shaw WC. The influence of incisal malocclusion on the social attractiveness of young adults in Finland. Eur J Orthodont 1995;17(6):505-12.

[21]   Ozhayat EB. Influence of self-esteem and negative affectivity on oral health-related quality of life in patients with partial tooth loss. Community Dent Oral Epidemiol 2012.

[22]   Reifel NM, Rana H, Marcus M. Consumer Satisfaction. Adv Dent Res 1997;11(2):281-90.

In: Public Health Yearbook 2013
Editor: Joav Merrick

ISBN: 978-1-63321-095-0
© 2014 Nova Science Publishers, Inc.

Chapter 44

IMPACT OF STRESS ON DEPRESSION AND ANXIETY IN DENTAL STUDENTS AND PROFESSIONALS

Christine Farrelly[1], Jing Sun, PhD[2] and Florian Mack, PhD[1]*

[1]School of Oral Health and Dental Science, Griffith University, Centre for Medicine and
Oral Health, Southport, Australia
[2]School of Medicine, Griffith Health Institute. Griffith University, Logan Campus,
Meadowbrook, Australia

ABSTRACT

Recent evidence has highlighted stress and poor mental health as risk factors for further physical and psychological illness. Dental students have frequently been shown to suffer higher prevalence of stress and psychological dysfunction, though few studies use relevant comparison groups when reporting these measures. The study aims to examine the difference in psychological dysfunction between dental students and students in other disciplines. Questionnaires were distributed to cohorts of dental students, undergraduate students and dental professionals around Australia. The DASS-21 was used to assess all participants' depression and anxiety and a modified version of the Dental Environmental Stress Questionnaire (DES) called the Student Environmental Stress (SES) Scale was used to assess students stress only. Demographic details for all participants were also collected. Dental students were significantly more stressed than dentists, and there were also significant difference between anxiety and depression between the three groups. Dental students only had significantly higher scores on one aspect of the extracted SES components. Linear regression showed a consistent significant relationship between student stress and all aspects of psychological dysfunction. The results of this study indicate that dental students do suffer higher psychological stress then dentists in the workforce. It also demonstrates the stress levels of dental students had higher level stress than undergraduate students in other discipline in academic study. The relationship between high student stress and psychological dysfunction enforces the importance of employing stress reduction program in the context of Australian universities and in particular dental students' academic program.

---

* Corresponding author: Jing Sun, PhD, and Griffith Health Institute and School of Medicine, Griffith University, Griffith University, Gold Coast Campus, Parklands, QLD, 4222 Australia. Email: j.sun@griffith.edu.au.

Keywords: Stress, anxiety, depression, dental students, students, Dentist, dental professional

INTRODUCTION

Mental health and its impact on an individual's physical and psychological morbidity is important public health issue (1). Researchers have suggested a causal link between mental strains and an increased risk of morbidity (2), so early intervention is paramount. It has been well documented in the literature that dental students suffer from high levels of stress throughout their education (3). Associations between specific dental stressors and enhanced anxiety and depressive symptomology have also been demonstrated (4,5). A recent review by Alzahem (6) indicated that the major sources of stress faced by dental students were living accommodation factors, personal factors, educational environment factors, academic factors and clinical factors. It can be seen in the review that many of the major sources of stress for dental students can actually be relevant to most university students. Issues relating to these factors may be pertinent to most undergraduates and mental health issues faced by undergraduate students have also often been demonstrated in the literature (7,8). In past research though, psychological issues faced by dental students often lacked a representative comparison group (9).

It is a common conception among the general population that Dentists have one of the highest rates of suicide of any profession and a number of articles have been written about this apparent phenomenon with conflicting reports (10,11). Irrefutable though, are the high levels of stress faced by Dentists and this has been well documented for many years (12,13). How does the mental health of dental professionals compare to their university years though? A review of the literature found that studies comparing these cohorts were rare (14). A comparison of Dentists mental health with a cohort of dental students would help to determine if any theme of psychological dysfunction pertinent in University dissipates after graduation or if those in the dental industry are destined to be perpetually under strain.

The methodology of the proposed study allows for investigation into the correlation between mental health and personal factors and offers important contribution to mental health research. The use of novel self-report measures will allow the relationship between student stress and mental health to be explored. To the knowledge of the researchers, the proposed measures have yet to be employed in dental students or dental professionals and the correlations between these measures will help in understanding the relationship between stress and mental health in these cohorts.

This study aims to provide a meaningful reflection of the mental health of dental students by recruiting a sample of undergraduate students as a realistic baseline. It is postulated that the true levels of stress may in fact be altered when a general student population is included. Overall, the study will provide information regarding the mental health issues affecting dental students and dental professionals in Australia. If a relationship between student stress and psychological dysfunction is found, it will provide evidence that stress is detrimental to a student's health. Practically, it will provide a focus for policy-makers within the University environment to develop intervention and prevention programs tailored to the needs of specific students. This will allow for mental health issues faced by future students to be prevented before they lead to physical and psychological morbidity.

The present study will ask the following research questions; Are dental students more stressed, depressed and anxious than dental professionals and other undergraduate students? And are perceived student stressors and coping mechanisms associated with mental health?

To answer the research questions, specific aims have been developed for the study. The overall study aims are to compare the difference between dental students and professionals in psychological problems and to examine the association between stress, coping strategies and mental health in students and dental professionals in Australia. To answer the research questions and in accordance with the aims of the study the following hypotheses have been developed:

H_1: There are differences in the stress, anxiety and depression levels among dental students, undergraduate university students and dental professionals.

H_2: Dental students have higher perceived student stress than other undergraduate students.

H_3: Higher perceived student stress is associated with higher levels of psychological dysfunction.

METHODS

Study design and sample

Cross sectional study design was used for the study. Participants were sampled from a population of students attending University's in Queensland, primarily around the South East region. A quota sampling method was used, defining university students and dental students as the subgroups of interest and convenience sampling of each subgroup took place. Students were approached while at university and participation was completely voluntary. Any undergraduate students who were selected will be invited to attend this study. Students who were at post graduate level, on exchange program, were under the age of 17 due to consent issues, and external students due to difficulty in contact for this study were not invited to attend the study.

Dental Professional sample were approached from the wider community and Universities around Australia in attempts to achieve a representative sample population for comparability and generalizability. The sampling strategy was similar to the strategy employed to recruit the students, with convenience sampling of the accessible subpopulation. Surveys were handed out in person to Dentists in the southeast Queensland region and were collected immediately or returned to the researchers via mail. Questionnaires also were mailed out to Dentists working in other parts of Australia where prior permission has first been sought. All Dentists and Dental Specialists were invited to fill out the questionnaire, though Dental Assistants and Dental Hygienists who were not included in the study.

Informed consent was obtained from student sample and dental professionals, and ethics approval was obtained from Griffith University Ethics Committee (DOH/04/13/HREC).

Measures

DASS-21 (15)

The major variables of interest in the current study include levels of stress, anxiety and depression as measured by the DASS-21. The DASS-21 is a shortened version of a self-report questionnaire (DASS-42) developed by Australian Psychologists (15). The measure consists of seven questions specific for each measure and asks for symptoms experienced over the past week. Responses are scored on a four point Likert Scale from '0 = did not apply to me at all' to '3 = applied to me very much, or most of the time' (See Appendix 1). Depression, anxiety and stress scores can be described as normal, mild, moderate, severe or extremely severe depending on participants' total score for each item. The DASS-21 is a reliable and valid self-report measure that has been successfully employed previously in a variety of clinical and non-clinical samples (16, 17). Studies have found that the shortened version has advantages over the 42-item version, including a cleaner factor structure and smaller inter-factor correlations (18). Psychometric properties of the shortened scale have been verified in numerous studies and the questionnaire has been determined to have discriminate and construct validity and excellent internal consistency (18-21). The scale has shown to effectively differentiate between diagnostic groups and show correlations with other existing measures for similar constructs (18, 20).

Modified Dental Environmental Stress Questionnaire – Student Environmental Stress Questionnaire

In order to also gain a greater insight into the perceived sources of stress specifically faced by students, a modified version of the Dental Environmental Stress (DES) Scale will be used (22). The original scale developed by Garbee et al. (22) has been used successfully and consistently to measure perceived sources of stress in Dental Students and other professional students numerous times, both in its original format and modified versions (4, 9, 23, 24). For the proposed study, some items on the DES were modified in a similar way to those utilized by Murphy, Grey and colleagues (9). In order to pertain information regarding to stressors that may be faced by all undergraduate students, the questions were revised so that they applied to both groups. The survey was first reduced to thirty items after omitting questions relating specifically to patient and clinical responsibilities. Secondly, the questions that pertained specifically to Dentistry were altered to reflect a general university environment. For example, a question on the original DES that asked, "lack of confidence to be a successful dentist" became "lack of confidence to be a successful graduate (See appendix 2 for omitted and altered questions). It was ensured that the essential purpose of the question remained intact and the altered questions were reviewed and approved by the researchers to ensure their face validity as predictors of undergraduate stress. The 30 remaining questions asked students to indicate the level of stress associated with each item on a Likert Scale of '1= not stressful' to '4= very stressful' and fifth option indicating the question was irrelevant. The questionnaire was termed the Students Environmental Stress (SES) Scale.

Coping and demographics

The participants surveyed will also be asked about the coping strategies they use in times of stress, both positive and negative. Additional demographic and socio-economic variables were also collected in the survey questionnaire. This included general data on age, income and living arrangements. Specific demographics relating to students and dental professionals were also asked.

Statistical analysis

The statistical package for social sciences (SPSS) will be used for data processing and data analyses. Dimension reduction of the DASS-21 will completed based previous models of the instrument and factor analysis of the modified DES will be conducted to condense the data and allow for ease of interpretation. Validity will be determined for each measure by determining Cronbachs alpha for each sub-population in the study. A chi-square test will be undertaken to present the demographic data and to determine any differences between the groups in these factors. Comprehensive analysis of the data will depend on the specific hypotheses under investigation.

Hypothesis 1: Dental students have higher stress, anxiety and depression levels than other undergraduate university students and dental professionals.

To test the first hypothesis, a multivariate analysis of variance (MANOVA) or equivalent non-parametric test will be carried out to determine any differences in the dependent variable, psychological disturbance among the grouping variable which is participants profession (Dentist, dental student or undergraduate student).

Hypothesis 2: Dental students have higher perceived stress than other undergraduate students.

An Independent samples t-test will be carried out to determine differences in student stress between dental students and other undergraduate students.

Hypothesis 3: Higher perceived student stress is associated with higher psychological distress.

A multiple linear regression model will be used to determine the relationship between the independent variable, students' perceived stress from the SES with the dependent variable, and students' scores on the DASS-21. The influence of demographic variables and other factors will also be determined by including them as confounding variables in the analysis.

The level of significance to test the hypotheses for the current study was set $p > 0.05$.

RESULTS

Statistical assumption check

The analytical assumptions for the current study depended on the hypothesis being tested and statistical test being carried out. Firstly the data was checked to identify and outliers or invalid values. It was found that one participant's data (ID 30) contained an outlier in the DASS-21 measure; this was checked and corrected. Assumptions were met for the dimension reduction for both measures (DASS-21 and SES Scale) and Factor Analyses were carried out. The

DASS-21 data was reduced in accordance with previous psychometric analyses (18, 20) and the components and their internal reliability is shown below in Appendix 1. Factor analysis for the SES scale yielded four components, with a Bartlett's test of sphericity was significant (p<0.001) and the measure of sampling adequacy was 0.786, which is sufficient.

Assumptions for Pearson's correlation were met as data was entered as a Likert scale and are linearly related to one another. Data was also checked for extreme outliers. A Pearson's Correlation was carried out on the factors for each measure to confirm that they were not highly correlated. Each measure was below 0.80 confirming independence of components for both the DASS-21 and the SES Scale.

The three groups included in the analysis are dental professionals, dental students, and undergraduate students and each are sufficiently independent of each other. The dependent variables included are depression, anxiety and stress and were normally distributed as shown by skewness and kurtosis between -3 and +3. Levene's test of variance was completed and it was determined that homogeneity of variance in the groups could be assumed for the measure of stress only. The measures of anxiety and depression had a p-value below 0.05 and therefor the assumption for a MANOVA could not be met for these measures. Due to this assumption of variance not being met, a non-parametric test must be used, Kruskal-Wallis in this case. Kruskal-Wallis test uses median instead of means and determines rank differences between the groups as an extension of a Mann-Whitley test.

The two groups being tested in the t-test are dental students and undergraduate students and the dependant variable is perceived stress on a student stress scale. For the t-test, the dependant variable had to be normally distributed. This was checked by determining that the skewness and kurtosis for the four factors discovered by means of factor analysis were all within the range of -3 to 3. As they were, a t-test is a suitable analysis. Variance within the groups was determined by Levene'e test for Equality of Variances, and t-values and significance were determined accordingly.

For the final statistical model, multiple linear regression analysis, the relationship between student stress and psychological dysfunction is approximately linear as demonstrated by a scatter plot (data not shown).

It is an assumption while running a multiple linear regression model that the DV is normally distributed. In the case of the current study the DV's are stress, anxiety or depression as measured by the DASS-21. These are normally distributed as shown in Appendix 4. The IV's are continuous in regards to student stress levels, so they may be entered directly into the regression model. Categorical confounding factors and coping mechanisms need to be transformed to be included in the regression.

Descriptive analysis results

After cleaning the data the final sample contained valid data from 153 participants. In regards to the explanatory variable, data was collected from 78 Dental Students, 54 undergraduate students and 21 Dental professionals.

The median age of the entire sample was 22 years (17-68). Within in the sample, 86 (55.1%) were females and 70 (44.9%) were males. The majority of the sample were non-smokers (90.5%) and 72% said that they drank alcohol. The demographic and descriptive statistics for categorical data for the entire sample are shown below in Tables 1 to 3.

Table 1. Overall demographics for the sample

Demographic Variable	N (%)
Gender	
Male	70 (45.8)
Female	83 (54.2)
Living arrangement	
Living alone	6 (3.6)
Share house	70 (45.8)
Living with Family	56 (36.6)
Living with Partner	21 (13.7)
Income	
1-5999	61 (39.9)
6000-19999	57 (37.3)
20000-59999	17 (11.1)
60000-99999	4 (2.6)
100000 +	14 (9.2)
Smoking	
No	134 (90.3)
Former	6 (4.1)
Yes	8 (5.4)
Alcohol	
No	42 (28)
Yes	108 (72)

Table 2. Student demographics

Demographic Variable	N (%)
Year of study	
1st	34 (26.6)
2nd	28 (21.9)
3rd	15 (11.7)
4th	25 (19.5)
5th	26 (20.3)
Study load	
Full time	124 (96.9)
Part time	4 (3.1)
GPA	
0-3.9	3 (2.7)
4-4.9	11 (9.7)
5-5.9	36 (31.9)
6-7	63 (55.8)
Prior study	
Secondary	58 (45.3)
Diploma/TAFE	7 (5.5)
Incomplete bachelors	43 (33.6)
Bachelors	15 (11.7)
Postgraduate	5 (3.9)

Table 3. Dental professional demographics

Dentists demographic characteristics	N (%)
How long employed	
1-5	4 (20)
6-10	2 (10)
over 10	14 (70)
Completion of degree	
Australia	14 (73.7)
Overseas	5 (26.3)
Role in dental field	
Principal dentist	2 (10.5)
General dentist	10 (52.6)
Specialist	7 (36.8)

There are three groups in the current study. In addition to the entire samples descriptive statistics shown above, the demographics for each group are presented below in Table 4.

In order to describe the outcome variables, the average scores on the DASS-21 for each group are shown below in Table 5. In regards to students and their stressors, the average values are shown in Table 6. Potential confounding factors are determined by means of a Chi-square test for categorical variables or by ANOVA or t-test for continuous variables. Descriptive statistics for continuous and potentially confounding factors are shown below in Table 7. The Chi-square analysis for determining confounding factors among categorical variables is shown in Table 8.

Table 4. Cohort Demographics

Sample Variables	Dentist N (%)	Dental student N (%)	Student N (%)	Total N (%)
Gender				
Male	12 (17.1)	28 (40)	30 (42.9)	70 (45.8)
Female	9 (10.8)	50 (60.2)	24 (28.9)	83 (54.2)
Living arrangement				
Living alone	1 (16.7)	3 (50)	2 (33.3)	6 (3.6)
Share house	0	50 (71.4)	20 (28.6)	70 (45.8)
Living with Family	11 (19.6)	16 (28.6)	29 (51.8)	56 (36.6)
Living with Partner	9 (42.9)	9 (42.9)	3 (14.3)	21 (13.7)
Income				
1-5999	0	37 (60.7)	24 (39.3)	61 (39.9)
6000-19999	0	32 (56.1)	25 (43.9)	57 (37.3)
20000-59999	3 (17.6)	9 (52.9)	5 (29.4)	17 (11.1)
60000-99999	4 (100)	0	0	4 (2.6)
100000 +	14 (100)	0	0	14 (9.2)
Smoking				
No	17 (12.7)	68 (50.7)	49 (36.6)	134 (90.3)
Former	2 (33.3)	2 (33.3)	2 (33.3)	6 (4.1)
Yes	1 (12.5)	6 (75)	1 (12.5)	8 (5.4)
Alcohol				
No	5 (11.9)	18 (42.9)	19 (45.2)	42 (28)
Yes	15 (13.9)	59 (54.6)	34 (31.5)	108 (72)

Table 5. Psychological dysfunction as measured by DASS-21

	Cohort		
	Dentist	**Student**	**Dental Student**
Depression	3.9 (4.2)	10.52 (9.41)	9.95 (9.45)
Anxiety	3.2 (3.87)	7.67 (7.07)	9.5 (8.66)
Stress	9.62 (6.47)	13.37 (9.8)	16.75 (9.98)

Table 6. Perceived Student stress scores as measured by the SES Scale

	Student group	
	Undergraduate student	**Dental student**
Home and relationship	5.96 (4.99)	6.02 (5.8)
School and faculty	12.86 (4.06)	18.5 (5.43)
Finance and future	12.07 (3.63)	13.4 (4.22)
Time and workload	18.75 (4.22)	18.61 (5.42)

Table 7. Continuous variables among the cohorts- Age and leisure activities

	Dentist M (SD)	**Undergraduate Student M (SD)**	**Dental student M (SD)**
Age ** **	43.53 (13.7)	20.57 (4.8)	23.05 (3.6)
Gym/Working out	2.3 (1.8)	2.6 (2.7)	2.6 (1.8)
Team/Individual sport** **	0.52 (1.03)	1.33 (2.05)	2.7 (1.8)
Catching up with friends	1.9 (1.16)	1.33 (2.06)	2.7 (1.85)
Leisure activities: Beach/shopping ** **	1.67 (1.56)	1.87 (1.68)	1.1 (1.2)
Movie/TV	0.4 (0.58)	1.07 (1.6)	1.12 (1.46)
Music	0.95 (1.6)	1.3 (2.27)	1.26 (2.34)
Studying **	0.95 (1.6)	1.37 (2.27)	1.2 (2.3)
Sleeping	7.1 (1.3)	7.3 (1.45)	7.1 (1.2

** $p < 0.05$ between three groups.

** $p < 0.05$ between student and dental student.

Table 8. Chi-square test to determine confounding factors between the three groups

Sample Variables	Dentist N (%)	Dental student N (%)	Student N (%)	Total	x^2	p-value
Gender					6.24	.044
Male	12 (17.1)	28 (40)	30 (42.9)	70 (45.8)		
Female	9 (10.8)	50 (60.2)	24 (28.9)	83 (54.2)		
Living arrangement					43.43	p<0.001
Living alone	1 (16.7)	3 (50)	2 (33.3)	6 (3.6)		
Share house	0	50 (71.4)	20 (28.6)	70 (45.8)		
Living with Family	11 (19.6)	16 (28.6)	29 (51.8)	56 (36.6)		
Living with Partner	9 (42.9)	9 (42.9)	3 (14.3)	21 (13.7)		
Income					132.59	p<0.001
1-5999	0	37 (60.7)	24 (39.3)	61 (39.9)		
6000-19999	0	32 (56.1)	25 (43.9)	57 (37.3)		
20000-59999	3 (17.6)	9 (52.9)	5 (29.4)	17 (11.1)		
60000-99999	4 (100)	0	0	4 (2.6)		
100000 +	14 (100)	0	0	14 (9.2)		

Table 8. (Continued)

Sample Variables	Dentist N (%)	Dental student N (%)	Student N (%)	Total	x^2	p-value
Smoking					**4.33**	0.363
No	17 (12.7)	68 (50.7)	49 (36.6)	134 (90.3)		
Former	2 (33.3)	2 (33.3)	2 (33.3)	6 (4.1)		
Yes	1 (12.5)	6 (75)	1 (12.5)	8 (5.4)		
Alcohol					**2.53**	0.283
No	5 (11.9)	18 (42.9)	19 (45.2)	42 (28)		
Yes	15 (13.9)	59 (54.6)	34 (31.5)	108 (72)		

An ANOVA showed that there was a significant difference between the groups for team or individual sports, leisure activities, studying and age. (Data not shown). In relation to hypothesis three, which focuses specifically on students, a t-test revealed that there were significant difference between student groups in leisure activities, team/individual sport and age (data not shown). Also in regards to hypothesis three, a separate Chi-square test needed to be carried out comparing categorical demographics among the student groups only. This test revealed that there were significant differences among these groups in the factors of 'Gender', 'Prior study', 'GPA', 'Year of study' and 'Living arrangement'. Results are also shown in Table 8.

Associations between potential confounding variables and both outcome variables

Factor analysis was firstly completed to reduce the data so hypothesis testing could be carried out. The results of factor analysis and their reliability are shown in Appendix 1 and 2 for the two measures used. Pearson's Correlation was also carried out to determine that none of the variables used were too highly correlated; the results of this analysis are shown in Appendix 3. After these analyses were carried out it was then possible to explore the associations between potential confounding variables and outcome and explanatory variables.

Within the current study, there is the possibility that certain demographic factors may be under or overexpressed in certain cohorts. If this is the case, these variables are referred to as confounding factors, as they may confound the relationship between the variables and elicit unwanted effects. These factors should therefore be included in relevant statistical analyses. The confounding factors within the current study depend on the variable type and the specific hypothesis.

The categorical demographic data among the three groups that may have an influence on the first hypothesis are shown below in table 8. The Chi-square analysis revealed that there were disproportionate amounts of males and females among the three groups (x^2=6.241, p=0.044). It was also found that more students lived in share houses when compared to Dentists (x^2=43.433, p<0.001) and that Dentists earned significantly more money (x^2=132.595, p<0.001). Smoking and alcohol use were similar throughout the three groups. A one-way ANOVA was used to determine if there were significant differences in the continuous variables between the three groups (see table 7 above). It was found that the Dental professional group was significantly older than both the dental student and undergraduate student group (p<0.05). There were significant differences between the three groups in the amount of times per week they engaged in team or individual sports and leisure activities such as shopping (p<0.05). Also, not surprisingly there was a significant difference between Dental Professionals and both student groups in how often they studied (p<0.05).

The second hypothesis explores the bivariate relationship between undergraduate students and dental students in regards to their stress levels. The potential categorical confounding factors are again revealed by Chi-square test and shown in Table 9 below. It was found that males and females where not distributed evenly between the groups (x^2=5.006, p=0.032). Significantly more dental students were found to be in later years of study (x^2=66.026, p<0.001) and they also had higher GPA's (x^2=44.924, p<0.001). Prior study was also disproportionate between the groups (x^2=29.037, p<0.001) as was living arrangement (x^2=15.977, p=0.001), though income and study load were similarly distributed. Continuous variables that were also significantly different have been revealed via a t-test and are shown above in Table 7. The amount of times per week the students engage in team sports and leisure activities like beach or shopping is significantly different (p<0.05) and dental students are also significantly older (p<0.05).

The effect of confounding variables can only be specifically revealed when running certain analyses. In the case of the statistical analyses used to address the first two hypotheses, confounding factors can be identified via a Chi-square test, though any effect they elicit cannot be statistically tested as they can't be inserted into the model. However, in the case of the linear regression model in the current study, which explores the relationship between student stress and psychological dysfunction, the influence of confounding factors may actually be measured. Confounding factors identified through Chi-square analysis (Table 9) or t-test (Table 7) may be entered directly into the model and it may be seen if these factors influence the relationship between the IV and the DV. This is a great advantage of a multiple linear regression model. The confounding factors identified between undergraduate students and dental students are mentioned above; gender, year of study, GPA, prior study and living arrangement were the categorical variables that have to be transformed before entering them into the regression. The continuous confounding factors of age, team sports and leisure activities can be directly entered in the model.

The linear regression models, which explore associations between potential confounding factors and both outcome and explanatory variables, are shown below in Table 13 to 15. The first linear regression (Table 13) explores the association between student stress and depression. Higher stress was significantly related to depression with a regression coefficient of 0.130 (95% CI= 0.073-0.186) (p<0.001). It was found the confounding factors of age (regression coefficient -0.274, 95% CI= -0.554-0.006) and living with family (regression coefficient -2.491, 95% CI= -4.446—0.536) had a significant protective effect on the relationship between student stress and depression levels (p<0.05). All other confounding factors were not significant. Table 14 demonstrates that student stress predicts anxiety with a regression coefficient of 0.138 (95% CI= 0.088-0.188) with a significance of p<0.001. It can be seen that confounding factors do not have any significant influence on the relationship. Finally Table 15 explores the predictive relationship between student stress and psychological stress. It shows that student stress significantly predicts psychological stress with a regression coefficient of 0.137 (95% CI= 0.088-0.186) (p<0.001). In regards to confounding factors, it can be seen that student stress is more predictive of psychological stress for females, with a regression coefficient of 2.914 (95%CI=1.296-4.533) (p<0.05). However, engaging in leisure activities has a significant negative relationship (p<0.05), indicating a protective influence on the student stress-psychological stress relationship (Regression coefficient -0.559, 95%CI= -1.066- -0.051). No other confounding factors reached significance.

Confounding factors results

A Chi Square test was completed to determine if any categorical demographic variables were confounding factors. The results of the Chi-square are shown in Table 8 for the entire sample and in Table 9 for determining confounding factors pertinent to the linear regression models.

A t-test was completed to test hypothesis two regrading differences between dental students and undergraduate students in student stress factors. It was found that dental students had significantly higher stress in regards to school and faculty (t=-6.337, p<0.001). All other stressors were not significant (p>0.05) between the groups, indicating that the students felt similar amounts of perceived stress toward home and relationship, finance and future and time and workload. The results are shown in Table 10 below.

A MANOVA and Kruskal-Wallis ANONVA were completed to test hypothesis one: there are differences in the stress, anxiety and depression levels among dental students, undergraduate university students and dental professionals. It was found that there were significant differences in the levels of stress between dental students and dental professionals, yielding an F ratio of 5.3 (p<0.01) (Table 11). Also it was found that there were significant differences in anxiety (x^2= 12.823, P=0.002) and depression (x^2 = 10.737, p=0.005) among all three groups, as shown in Table 12 below.

Linear regression models were run to determine the relationship between perceived student stress and aspects psychological dysfunction, namely depression, anxiety and stress. It was found that higher student stress score was positively associated with depression, (regression coefficient = 0.130, 95% CI= 0.073-0.186), anxiety (regression coefficient = 0.138, 95% CI= 0.088-0.188) and psychological stress (regression coefficient = 0.137, 95% CI= 0.088-0.186) and all associates were significant to p<0.001.

Table 9. Chi-square test to determine confounding factors between the student groups

Student variables	Dental student N (%)	Student N (%)	Total	x^2	p-value
Gender				5.006	0.032
Male	28 (48.3)	30 (51.7)	58		
Female	50 (67.6)	24 (32.4)	74		
Year of study				66.026	p<0.001
1st	2 (5.9)	32 (94.1)	34		
2nd	17 (60.7)	11 (39.3)	28		
3rd	11 (73.3)	4 (26.7)	15		
4th	21 (84)	4 (16)	25		
5th	26 (100)	0	26		
Study load				.380	0.538
Full time	74 (59.7)	50 (40.3)	124		
Part time	3 (75)	1 (25)	4		
GPA				44.924	p<0.001
0-3.9	0	3 (100)	3		
4-4.9	0	11 (100)	11		

Student variables	Dental student N (%)	Student N (%)	Total	x^2	p-value
5-5.9	19 (52.8)	19 (52.8)	36		
6-7	56 (88.9)	7 (11.1)	63		
Prior study				29.037	<0.001
Secondary	24 (41.4)	34 (58.6)	58		
Diploma/TAFE	1 (14.3)	6 (85.7)	7		
Incomplete bachelors	36 (83.7)	7 (16.3)	43		
Bachelors	13 (86.7)	2 (13.3)	15		
Postgraduate	3 (60)	2 (40)	5		
Income				0.423	0.809
1-5999	37 (60.7)	24 (39.3)	61		
6000-19999	32 (56.1)	25 (43.9)	57		
20000-59999	9 (64.3)	5 (35.7)	14		
60000-99999	0	0			
Living arrangement				15.977	0.001
Living alone	3 (40)	2 (40)	5		
Share house	50 (71.4)	20 (28.6)	70		
Living with Family	16 (35.6)	29 (64.4)	45		
Living with Partner	9 (75)	3 (25)	12		

Table 10. Differences in student stress between undergraduate students and dental students

Variable	Student group		t	p-value
	Dental student	Undergraduate student		
	Mean (SD)	Mean (SD)		
Home and relationship	6.03 (5.8)	6.15 (5.035)	0.130	0.897
School and faculty	18.5 (5.4)	12.8 (4.11)	-6.337	<0.001***
Finance and future	13.4 (4.2)	12 (3.6)	-1.971	0.051
Time and workload	18.6 (5.4)	18.4 (4.1)	-0.241	0.810

Table 11. Comparing stress between Dentist, Undergraduate student and Dental student. (Parametric variables) (N=152)

	Dentist (21)	Undergraduate student (54)	Dental student (77)	F	Post hoc.
Stress	9.6 (6.4)	13.37 (9.8)	16.75 (9.98)	5.3**	Dental student > Dentist **

**p<0.01.

Table 12. Kruskal-Wallis Test for determining differences in anxiety and depression between the groups (non-parametric variables) (N= 152)

	Dentist (n=21) Median (min,max)	Undergraduate student (n=54) Median (min,max)	Dental student (n=77) Median (min,max)	x^2	p-value
Anxiety	2 (0,14)	7 (0,28)	6 (0,36)	12.823	0.002
Depression	4 (0,14)	8 (0,34)	8 (0,40)	10.737	0.005

Results on prevalence of mental health symptoms and the association between student stress and mental health

The small confidence intervals indicate the accuracy of the association. The influence of confounding factors that were determined via Chi-square and t-test are described above and are also included in the models. The addition of the confounding factors did not alter the significance of the relationship between student stress and any aspect of psychological dysfunction. The Adjusted R^2 values for each model demonstrate that the variance accounted for by student stress and the confounders for each of the aspects of depression, anxiety and stress was 26.9%, 26.1% and 34.4% consecutively. This is an adequate amount of variance explained by the factors in each case. The results are shown below in Tables 13 to 15.

Table 13. Student stress as predictor of depression

Predictor variables	Regression coefficient (95% CI)	p-value
Student stress	0.130 (0.073-0.186)	**<0.001**
Age	-0.274 (-0.554-0.006)	**0.050**
Gender	0.594 (-1.263-2.452)	0.527
Individual/team sports	-0.303 (-0.877-0.271)	0.297
Leisure activities	-0.519 (-1.102-0.064)	0.080
Low GPA	1.744 (-0.956-4.445)	0.203
Later year of study	-1.446 (-3.316-0.424)	0.128
Prior tertiary study	-0.899 (-3.142-1.344)	0.428
Living with family	-2.491 (-4.446—0.536)	**0.013**

Correlation coefficient (R)= .587.
Adjusted R^2 = .269.
ANOVA F value = 4.577***.

Table 14. Student Stress as predictor of anxiety

Predictor variables	Regression coefficient (95% CI)	p-value
Student stress	0.138 (0.088-0.188)	**<0.001**
Age	-0.066 (-0.322-0.190)	0.609
Gender	1.344 (-0.303-2.991)	0.108
Team/individual sports	0.036 (-0.467-0.538)	0.889
Leisure activities	-0.180 (-0.691-0.331)	0.487
High GPA	-0.010 (-2.363-2.343)	0.993
Later year of study	-1.331 (-2.997-0.335)	0.116
Prior tertiary study	-0.326 (-2.281-1.629)	0.741
Living with family	-0.914 (-2.636-0.809)	0.295

Correlation coefficient (R)= 0.582.
Adjusted R^2 = 0.261.
ANOVA F value = 4.378***.

Table 15. Student Stress as predictor of psychological stress on DASS

Predictor variables	Regression coefficient (95% CI)	p-value
Student stress	0.137 (0.088-0.186)	**<0.001**
Age	-0.028 (-0.273-0.216)	0.819
Gender	2.914 (1.296-4.533)	**0.001**
Team/individual sports	0.151 (-0.305-0.652)	0.550
Leisure activities	-0.559 (-1.066- -0.051)	**0.031**
High GPA	-1.184 (-4.20400.506)	0.112
Lower year of study	-0.267 (-1.905-1.371)	0.747
Prior tertiary study	-1.277 (-3.253-0.700)	0.203
Living with family	-1.736 (-2.888-0.529)	0.174

Correlation coefficient (R)= 0.642.
Adjusted R^2 = 0.344.
ANOVA F value = 6.046***.
(For the above linear regressions *** indicates significance at the <0.001 level.).

DISCUSSION

The current study endeavoured to gauge the levels of stress, anxiety and depression of dental students, using dentists and undergraduate students as relevant comparison groups. The levels of internal reliability of the DASS-21 questionnaire were similar to previous studies, indicating the consistency of the current sample (16).

In regards to the first hypothesis, which attempts to explore differences in psychological dysfunction between the three study groups, it was found that the hypothesis was partially supported. Dental students were significantly more stressed than dentists, though no significant difference was found with their comparison to undergraduate students. It was also found that there were significant difference between the groups for anxiety and depression. These results support the literature that suggests that dental students are under high amounts of psychological strain compared to dentists and other students (9,14).

From the results, the second hypothesis was also partially supported. Dental students were found to have significantly higher levels of stress regards to school and faculty. This may be due to the intense practical involvement of many parts of Dental School, when compared to a general university cohort. Dental students have the added pressure of learning practical clinical skills throughout their education, on top of an already heavy theoretical workload. The other factors all displayed a non-significant relationship between the groups. This finding demonstrates that university students actually share high levels of perceived stress, regardless of degree choice demonstrating the influence of the environmental factors associated with stress (2). This is supported by other studies of university students (7).

The results of this study also support the third hypothesis. Higher student stress is consistently associated with all aspects of psychological dysfunction. Firstly a strong predictive relationship was found between higher student stress and higher levels of depression. A protective influence of increasing age and living with family is evident in the stress-depression relationship in students. The protective effect of age is in accordance with other studies that suggest that age correlates negatively with depression (25). The apparent protective effect of living with family may suggest that increased family support is helpful in helping a student deal with stress issues so they don't led to depressive symptoms. Students stress also had a strong significant relationship with anxiety. The results showed that no confounding factors elicited a significant effect indicating an extremely predictive relationship between heightened student stress and high levels of anxiety.

Finally, the relationship between student stress and psychological stress was shown to be significantly positive also. Gender also showed a significant positive relationship, indicating that females who are under stress were more likely to show symptoms of psychological stress. This is an interesting finding and may be possibly due to the influence of employed coping strategies. This is obviously an important issue for future investigations. It was also demonstrated that leisure activities such as shopping and going to the beach had a negative influence on the student stress-psychological stress relationship. This demonstrates the importance of 'switching off' and taking time out, so not to let perceived stress take its toll on and manifest as psychological symptoms.

Limitations

There are a number of limitations for the study. Shortfalls in any study may occur during sampling, data entry or within the actual study design itself. Selection bias may have been present in the current study. Though all efforts were made to include a wide range of participants, random sampling of participants from a sampling frame is the best way to reduce this type of error. Measurement bias of the self-report instrument may also have been present, though validity and reliability of the questionnaires has been verified in the current study as shown in appendix 1 and 2. There may also have been some response bias amongst the participants in the current study. Anonymity of the questionnaires attempted to keep this phenomenon to a minimum. Analysis bias involved in entering of data in SPSS is also a possibility in the current study. This may have skewed any final results, though checking and cleaning the data attempts to control this potential bias. It is also important to remember the possible influence of confounding factors in regards to the first two hypotheses. They cannot be directly entered into the models so their influence is unknown. The results should be interpreted with caution and in future, attempts at random sampling will hopefully ensure the demographic factors are similar between the groups.

Within the current study, data is only collected form a sub-sect of Australian dental and student populations and the generalizability of the results is limited. Efforts were made to represent all individuals within the cohort populations, though the sample will always be subject to sampling error (standard error). To improve generalizability of future results and to gain a better insight into student stress and mental health, a larger sample size from a broader range of universities and dental practices should be utilised. If possible, random sampling should also be employed. This reduces the standard error and may further aid in understanding psychological dysfunction in students and dental professionals.

CONCLUSION

In conclusion, it is apparent that dental students do suffer higher levels of stress in their university years than their graduates in the workplace. They also suffer higher levels of perceived stress in some factors, though it is made apparent in the study that the general university cohort is also suffering elevated levels of student stress and psychological dysfunction. A student's stress is strongly predictive of psychological dysfunction and this makes the implementation of stress reduction instruction an imperative part of tertiary education. Measures to reduce stress should be introduced and students should be educated in the importance of stress management in order to reduce the risk of physical and psychological morbidity. From the results of this investigation, future studies may now implement a randomised control trial to investigate the effects of an intervention program to combat psychological dysfunction in students.

ACKNOWLEDGMENTS

Special thanks are due to all the students and staff at Griffith University Dental School and the dental clinics that took part. The authors would also like to thank Mrs S Peters for her continuous encouragement and help with sampling of the Dental professional population.

REFERENCES

[1]   Cohen S, Janicki-Deverts D, E. MG. Psychological stress and disease. JAMA 2007;298(14):1685-7.
[2]   McEwen BS. Protective and damaging effects of stress mediators. N Engl J Med 1998;338(3):171-9.
[3]   Polychronopoulou A, Divaris K. Dental students' perceived sources of stress: a multi-country study. J Dent Educ 2009;73(5):631-9.
[4]   Gorter R, Freeman R, Hammen S, Murtomaa H, Blinkhorn A, Humphris G. Psychological stress and health in undergraduate dental students: fifth year outcomes compared with first year baseline results from five European dental schools. Eur J Dent Educ 2008;12(2):61-8.
[5]   Naidu RS, Adams JS, Simeon D, Persad S. Sources of stress and psychological disturbance among dental students in the West Indies. J Dent Edu 2002;66(9):1021-30.
[6]   Alzahem AM, van der Molen HT, Alaujan AH, Schmidt HG, Zamakhshary MH. Stress amongst dental students: a systematic review. Eur J Dent Edu 2011;15(1):8-18.
[7]   Bayram N, Bilgel N. The prevalence and socio-demographic correlations of depression, anxiety and stress among a group of university students. Soc Psychiatry Psychiatr Epidemiol 2008;43(8):667-72.
[8]   Hamaideh SH. Stressors and reactions to stressors among university students. Int J Soc Psychiat 2011;57(1):69-80.
[9]   Murphy RJ, Gray SA, Sterling G, Reeves K, DuCette J. A comparative study of professional student stress. J Dent Edu 2009;73(3):328-37.
[10]   Alexander RE. Stress-related suicide by dentists and other health care workers. Fact or folklore? J Am Dent Assoc 2001;132(6):786-94.
[11]   Sancho FM, Ruiz CN. Risk of suicide amongst dentists: myth or reality? Int Dent J 2010;60(6):411-8.
[12]   Ayers KM, Thomson WM, Newton JT, Rich AM. Job stressors of New Zealand dentists and their coping strategies. Occup Med (Lond) 2008;58(4):275-81.
[13]   Myers HL, Myers LB. 'It's difficult being a dentist': stress and health in the general dental practitioner. Br Dent J 2004;197(2):89-93.

[14]   Newbury-Birch D, Lowry RJ, Kamali F. The changing patterns of drinking, illicit drug use, stress, anxiety and depression in dental students in a UK dental school: a longitudinal study. Br Dent J 2002;192(11):646-9.

[15]   Lovibond SH, Lovibond PF. Manual for the Depression Anxiety Stress Scales. 2nd ed. Sydney: Sydney Psychology Foundation, 1995.

[16]   Bentley MA, Crawford JM, Wilkins JR, Fernandez AR, Studnek JR. An Assessment of Depression, Anxiety, and Stress Among Nationally Certified EMS Professionals. Prehosp Emerg Care 2013, Epub 2013 Feb19.

[17]   Tully PJ, Zajac IT, Venning AJ. The structure of anxiety and depression in a normative sample of younger and older Australian adolescents. J Abnorm Child Psychol 2009;37(5):717-26.

[18]   Antony MM, Bieling PJ, Cox BJ, Enns MW, Swinson RP. Psychometric properties of the 42-item and 21-item versions of the Depression Anxiety Stress Scales in clinical groups and a community sample. Psychol Assessment 1998;10(2):176-81.

[19]   Gloster AT, Rhoades HM, Novy D, Klotsche J, Senior A, Kunik M, et al. Psychometric properties of the Depression Anxiety and Stress Scale-21 in older primary care patients. J Affect Disord 2008;110(3):248-59.

[20]   Henry JD, Crawford JR. The short-form version of the Depression Anxiety Stress Scales (DASS-21): construct validity and normative data in a large non-clinical sample. Br J Clin Psychol 2005;44(Pt 2):227-39.

[21]   Sinclair SJ, Siefert CJ, Slavin-Mulford JM, Stein MB, Renna M, Blais MA. Psychometric evaluation and normative data for the depression, anxiety, and stress scales-21 (DASS-21) in a nonclinical sample of U.S. adults. Eval Health Prof 2012;35(3):259-79.

[22]   Garbee WH, Jr., Zucker SB, Selby GR. Perceived sources of stress among dental students. J Am Dent Assoc 1980;100(6):853-7.

[23]   Sanders AE, Lushington K. Sources of stress for Australian dental students. J Dent Educ 1999;63(9):688-97.

[24]   Westerman GH, Grandy TG, Ocanto RA, Erskine CG. Perceived sources of stress in the dental school environment. J Dent Educ 1993;57(3):225-31.

[25]   Christensen H, Jorm AF, Mackinnon AJ, Korten AE, Jacomb PA, Henderson AS, et al. Age differences in depression and anxiety symptoms: a structural equation modelling analysis of data from a general population sample. Psychol Med 1999;29(2):325-39.

In: Public Health Yearbook 2013
Editor: Joav Merrick

ISBN: 978-1-63321-095-0
© 2014 Nova Science Publishers, Inc.

Chapter 45

EFFECT OF GREEN TEA CONSUMPTION ON OBESITY AND HYPERTENSION: A SYSTEMATIC REVIEW PROTOCOL

Saman Khalesi[1], Jing Sun, PhD[1] and Nicholas Buys, PhD[2]*

[1]School of Public Health and Griffith Health Institute, Griffith University,
Gold Coast campus, Parkland, Australia
[2]School of Human Services and Social Work, and Griffith Health Institute,
Griffith University, Parkland, Gold Coast, Australia

ABSTRACT

Green tea is a healthy drink and evidence of its positive effect on both obesity and hypertension is emerging. This review protocol is concerned with the efficacy of green tea consumption in improving health status of people with obesity and hypertension. Interventional randomized or non-randomized studies, as well as cross sectional studies, with a focus on the effect of green tea consumption on obesity and/or hypertension will be identified. Literature will be searched by two authors independently through PubMed, Medline, Scopus and Cochrane library. All articles from January 2003 to end of May 2013, which meet the inclusion/exclusion criteria, will be studied. Human studies analyzing the effect of green tea consumption on either obesity or hypertension or both, or respective indicators (oriental tea, anthropometry, abdominal fat, central fat, body mass index, blood lipid profile, metabolic syndrome, high blood pressure, systolic blood pressure and diastolic blood pressure, waist circumference and waist hip ratio) will be included. Study of indicators will only be included, if the endpoint data reports an association or correlation with obesity and/or hypertension. Only studies with focus on green tea, oriental tea or green tea extract or its catechins will be included. Studies with artificial catechins or catechins from sources other than green tea will not be included. Search terms will include green tea, *Camellia sinensis*, green tea extract, green tea catechins, green tea supplements with obesity, overweight, abdominal fat, central fat,

---

* Corresponding author: Saman Khalesi, Griffith Health Institute and School of Public Health, Gold Coast Campus, Parkland, Q4222 Australia. Email: saman.khalesitaharoom@griffithuni.edu.au.

metabolic syndrome, hypertension, blood pressure, anthropometry, waist circumference, waist/hip ratio and blood lipid profile.

Keywords: Green tea, hypertension, obesity

INTRODUCTION

Obesity has become one of the world's most epidemic diseases with more than 1.4 billion people either obese or overweight (1). Obesity is now the fifth leading risk of all death in the world and a main cause of cardiovascular disease, diabetes, and stroke (1). Obesity is characterized by a body mass index (BMI) of 30 or more and overweight by a BMI of more than 25 and less than 30 (2). In Australia three out of five adults are either overweight or obese and the prevalence of obesity among males, 18 years and older, increased from 57.5% in 2001 to 62.8% in 2007-08 and among females, 18 years and older, increased from 42.2% in 2001 to 47.6% in 2007-08 (3). Hypertension, another epidemic disease, is also a major cause of cardiovascular disease and stroke. In the United States (US) the prevalence of hypertension among people 18 years and older was 28.6% in 2009-2010(4). There have been some recent advances in the treatment of hypertension. However, approximately two thirds of hypertensive people in the US have not controlled their high blood pressure levels (5). In 2005, 14% of people age 45-54 and 41% of those over 75 had hypertension in Australia (6).

Tea is the most frequently consumed beverage around the world after water (7). There is increasing evidence to demonstrate that green tea may have an effect on preventing hypertension and obesity. Green tea is made from the steamed and dried leaves of the *Camellia sinensis* plant. It is a widely consumed beverage containing healthy phenolic components, which have anti-oxidative effects on the body. Numerous studies have been published on green tea and its health benefits on lipid profile (8,9) blood glucose level (10), and cancer (11,12). The effectiveness of green tea in improving hypertension or weight reduction and management, along with other complications, has been investigated in both animal and human studies (13-15). However, there is no systematic review of the literature summarizing the association between green tea and obesity and hypertension. The present study aims to undertake this review as a step towards a future intervention study.

Study objectives

The primary aim of this systematic review is to summarize and examine literature on the association between green tea consumption and obesity and hypertension at population level. Following this it is expected that green tea consumption may be found to have effect on lowering blood pressure level and body weight and improvement of blood lipid profile.

Study questions

In this systematic review the following questions are addressed:

1. Does green tea have an impact on reducing obesity? If so, is the effect significant?
2. Does green tea have an impact on reducing hypertension? If so, is the effect significant? What is the optimal intake of green tea consumption to provide the greatest impact on obesity and/or hypertension?

METHOD AND DESIGN

To address the study aim and questions a comprehensive literature search will be undertaken. Human trials that assess the effect of green tea on obesity or hypertension will be reviewed, including randomized parallel interventions and uncontrolled before-and-after studies. The reporting of the review will follow the "Preferred Reporting Items for Systematic Reviews and Meta-Analysis: the PRISMA statement" (16). All methodologies in studies reviewed will be assessed using the validated quality checklist developed by Downs and Black (17).

Search methods

Literature on green tea consumption and its impact, for the period January 2003 to the end of May 2013, will be identified using electronic databases of Medline, PubMed, Scopus and Cochrane Library (CENTERAL). Grey literature (publications issued by government, academia and industry or uncontrolled by commercial publishing interests) (18) will be searched through the OpenGrey database. Search terms are detailed in Table 1.

Database searches, scanning and screening of articles will be undertaken independently by two authors. Both authors will follow the eligibility criteria to include or exclude articles.

Table 1. Search Terms

Search String	AND
Green tea	Obesity
Camellia sinensis	Hypertension
Catechins	Overweight
Green tea extract	Body Mass Index
Green tea supplement Oriental tea	Abdominal fat Central fat Waist circumference Waist hip ratio
	Anthropometry
	Metabolic syndrome
	Blood lipid profile
	Blood pressure Triglyceride Serum cholesterol Blood glucose High density lipoprotein Low density lipoprotein

In case of any disagreement, the matter will be resolved through discussion. A third author will be involved in decision making if consensus cannot be reached between the first two reviewers. All combination of search terms would be considered and run through the search engine. All article citations related to the search combination would be saved through EndNote, regardless of duplications, for further screening. Screening of saved articles will begin by removing duplicates and reviewing the titles at first stage and going through the abstract and complete article at next stages. Choosing articles would be by considering eligibilities and inclusion criteria.

Eligible studies

All human randomized interventional studies which address green tea consumption with obesity or hypertension or both would be included. Only literature published in English language will be considered. Human trials which focus on green tea consumption or its catechins, extract or supplements will be studied. Artificial catechins or catechins extracted from sources other than green tea will be excluded. Studies of the effect of green tea on lipid profile will only be included if the reported end point data is on obesity and/or hypertension or the findings show correlations or associations between consumption and obesity and/or hypertension. Studies which fail to address the dosage and frequency of green tea consumption or fail to mention intervention period will be excluded. The number of excluded studies and the reasons of exclusion will be noted.

Data extraction

Data will be extracted by the two reviewers from the included articles. In the case of any missing data, vague results or needs for complementary data, the corresponding author of the article will be contacted to clarify the information. For the dosage of green tea the preferential unit of reporting is gram of green tea. Units of dosage other than gram of green tea (e.g., milliliter, milligram, or number of cups), would be calculated to the nearest approximate gram of solid green tea. The intended data to be extracted from articles is mention in the table 2.

Table 2. Components of data extraction

Intended data to be extracted form articles
• General information of the paper (title, authors, publication details, year of publication, etc.)
• Study type (randomized controlled trials, cohort, etc.)
• Population characteristics (demographic, geographical settings, size of population, health status, etc.)
• Intervention characteristics (location, length of study, dosage and frequency of green tea consumption, number of dropouts, etc.)
• Eligibility (inclusion and exclusion criteria of the study)
• Result and outcome (changes, mean differences, odd ratio, *p*-value, etc.)
• Follow up data (period, results, if available)
• Adverse effect (if applicable) • Limitations (if applicable) • Important notes or conclusions of authors

Table 3. The measuring sections and items to assess articles' quality of methodology

Measuring sections	Measuring items
Reporting	Clear hypothesis, aim and objective Clear described main outcomes Clear described characteristics of patients Clear described of intervention Clear described confounder distribution among groups Clear described main outcomes Provided estimates of random variability in data of main outcome Reported adverse events of the intervention Described characteristics of patients lost to follow-up Reported actual probability value for main outcome
External validity	Subjects asked to participate represented the entire population of recruitment Subjects actually participated represented the entire population of recruitment Study treatment environment represented the entire population treatment environment
Internal validity-bias	Study attempted to blind study the subject through intervention Study attempted to blind those measuring main outcomes **Clear in using "data dredging", if applicable** Analysis adjusted for different length of follow-up, if applicable Appropriate statistical approaches to assess outcomes Reliable compliance with the intervention Accurate outcome measures
Internal validity-confounding (selection bias)	Participants in different groups recruited from same population Participants in different groups recruited over the same time period Randomization of participants into study groups Concealed randomization until completion of recruitment Adequate adjusted confounding in the analysis Accounted losses of patients to follow-up
Power	Sufficient power of study to detect clinically important effect, when the probability of chance is less than 5%

Methodology quality assessment

The quality of eligible articles, in case of their methodology, will be assessed using a 32-score quality checklist developed by Downs and Black (17). The checklist was developed for both randomized controlled trials and non-randomized studies. To interpret the scoring system we will follow the method used by Harrison et al. (19), where scores higher than 12 would be considered good quality papers. Data may be considered from papers with lower scores if the number of selected articles is inadequate. The scoring scale developed by Downs and Black (17) consists of 27 items with total of 32 scores. The sections and items to be assessed in each article are mentioned in Table 3. The scoring will be carried out by both reviewers.

Data analysis methods

Data will be presented in tabular and narrative form. Information on year, setting, population, intervention, outcome and quality of studies will be presented in tables. Outcome measures of Relative risk (RR) or odds ratio (OR) of included studies with confidence interval of 95%, with or without green tea consumption, will be reported in tables as well. Where necessary, an attempt to calculate the quantity of missed value will be made. A footnote will document how the value is calculated.

Reporting of results

The results of the systematic review will be reported following guidelines set by the Preferred Reporting Items for Systematic Review (PRISMA) study group (16). All papers extracted data will be presented in tables. Odds ratio, *p*-value and mean differences of included studies will be presented in tables as well. A narrative comparative approach will discuss the finding of each paper and the similarities/differences of the results of selected papers will be discussed. Finally the guideline for green tea interventions and possible improving effect on obesity and hypertension will be discussed.

Expected outcomes and significance of study

Through this study we expect to understand the effect of green tea consumption on improvement of health status of people with obesity and/or hypertension. It is anticipated that a correlation between dosage of green tea consumption and its effectiveness and correlation between length of green team consumption and its effectiveness will be found. Moreover, the best method of consuming green tea (as tea, supplement or extract) as well as the most influenced age group and gender would be expected from this review. As the secondary outcome we anticipate finding any association between green tea consumption and or indicators (blood lipid profile, waist circumference and etc.).

Although green tea has been used in many interventional studies and clinical trials for treatment of obesity and hypertension, the effectiveness of the green tea usage and the dosage related information is not clear. This systematic review of literature may provide reliable information on green tea consumption for practitioners or researchers dealing with obesity and hypertension. It may be helpful for dieticians planning diets for obese or hypertensive patients as well. Moreover, it can provide a guideline for industries dealing with green tea extract or supplements to improve obesity or hypertensive conditions.

ETHICS AND DISSEMINATION

Our systematic review is to evaluate the effectiveness of green tea on obesity and hypertension base on reviewing literature and previous studies. As no primary data collection or intervention would be undertaken, ethical clearance will not be required. The review protocol however, has been registered with the International Prospective Register of Systematic Review (PROSPERO) with registration number CRD42013004720. The result of the review will be submitted for publication in peer reviewed journals. This study will begin in June, 2013, with reporting of study findings by September, 2013.

LIMITATIONS

The limitations of this systematic review will be as follow: 1) publications will be restricted to those English, thereby potentially limiting the range of studies reviewed; 2) if any essential data is missing, the corresponding author will be contacted. However poor or incomplete reports of study design, patient population, and intervention may impact the quality of interpretation of findings (20); 3) as a review will include a wide range of studies, there will not be any homogeneity between populations in term of patient demographic variables, diet or other characteristics. Although this may affect the generalization of our interpretations, we will attempt to differentiate our reporting base on various characteristics.

REFERENCES

[1]   Obesity and overweight. Fact sheet n°311 [database on the Internet]. WHO 2012.

[2]   Obesity: preventing and managing the global epidemic. Report of a WHO consultation report series 894 [database on the Internet]. WHO 2000.

[3]   Gender Indicators. cat no.4125.0 [database on the Internet]. ABS 2012.

[4]   Ogden CL, Carroll MD, Kit BK, Flegal KM. Prevalence of obesity in the United States, 2009-2010. Washington, DC: US Department of Health and Human Services, Centers for Disease Control and Prevention, National Center for Health Statistics, 2012.

[5]   Hajjar I, Kotchen JM, Kotchen TA. Hypertension: trends in prevalence, incidence, and control. Annu Rev Public Health 2006;27(1):465-90.

[6]   Australia Bureau of Statistics, Australia, 2004-05. cat. no.4364.0 [database on the Internet]. ABS 2006.

[7]   Schneider C, Segre T. Green tea: potential health benefits. Am Fam Physician 2009;79(7):591-4.

[8]   Erba D, Riso P, Bordoni A, Foti P, Biagi PL, Testolin G. Effectiveness of moderate green tea consumption on antioxidative status and plasma lipid profile in humans. J Nutr Biochem 2005;16(3):144.

[9]   Maron DJ, Lu GP, Cai NS, Wu ZG, Li YH, Chen H, et al. Cholesterol-lowering effect of a theaflavin-enriched green tea extract: a randomized controlled trial. Arch Intern Med 2003;163(12):1448.

[10]   Maruyama K, Iso H, Sasaki S, Fukino Y. The association between concentrations of green tea and blood glucose levels. J Clin Biochem Nutr 2009;44(1):41.

[11]   Mu LN, Lu QY, Yu SZ, Jiang QW, Cao W, You NC, et al. Green tea drinking and multigenetic index on the risk of stomach cancer in a Chinese population. Int J Cancer 2005;116(6):972-83.

[12]   Sun C-L, Yuan J-M, Koh W-P, Mimi CY. Green tea, black tea and breast cancer risk: a meta-analysis of epidemiological studies. Carcinogenesis 2006;27 (7):1310-5.

[13]   Antonello M, Montemurro D, Bolognesi M, Di Pascoli M, Piva A, Grego F, et al. Prevention of Hypertension, Cardiovascular Damage and Endothelial Dysfunction with Green Tea Extracts. Am J Hypertens 2007;20(12):1321-8.

[14]   Auvichayapat P, Prapochanung M, Tunkamnerdthai O, Sripanidkulchai B-o, Auvichayapat N, Thinkhamrop B, et al. Effectiveness of green tea on weight reduction in obese Thais: A randomized, controlled trial. Physiol Behav 2008;93(3):486-91.

[15]   Nagao T, Hase T, Tokimitsu I. A green tea extract high in catechins reduces body fat and cardiovascular risks in humans. Obesity 2007;15(6):1473-83.

[16]   Moher D, Liberati A, Tetzlaff J, Altman DG. Preferred reporting items for systematic reviews and meta-analyses: the PRISMA statement. Ann Intern Med 2009;151(4):264-9.

[17]   Downs SH, Black N. The feasibility of creating a checklist for the assessment of the methodological quality both of randomised and non-randomised studies of health care interventions. J Epidemiol Community Health 1998;52(6):377-84.

[18]   Bowling A. Research methods in health: investigating health and health services. Maidenhead: Open University Press, 2009.

[19]   Harrison RA, Siminoski K, Vethanayagam D, Majumdar SR. Osteoporosis-Related Kyphosis and Impairments in Pulmonary Function: A Systematic Review. J Bone Miner Res 2007;22(3):447-57.

[20]   Glasziou P, Meats E, Heneghan C, Shepperd S. What is missing from descriptions of treatment in trials and reviews? BMJ (Clinical research ed) 2008;336(7659):1472-4.

SECTION FIVE – ACKNOWLEDGMENTS

In: Public Health Yearbook 2013
Editor: Joav Merrick

ISBN: 978-1-63321-095-0
© 2014 Nova Science Publishers, Inc.

Chapter 46

ABOUT THE EDITOR

Joav Merrick, MD, MMedSci, DMSc, is professor of pediatrics, child health and human development affiliated with Kentucky Children's Hospital, University of Kentucky, Lexington, United States and the Division of Pediatrics, Hadassah-Hebrew University Medical Center, Mount Scopus Campus, Jerusalem, Israel, the medical director of Health Services, Division for Intellectual and Developmental Disabilities, Ministry of Social Affairs and Social Services, Jerusalem, the founder and director of the National Institute of Child Health and Human Development. Numerous publications in the field of pediatrics, child health and human development, rehabilitation, intellectual disability, disability, health, welfare, abuse, advocacy, quality of life and prevention. Received the Peter Sabroe Child Award for outstanding work on behalf of Danish Children in 1985 and the International LEGO-Prize ("The Children's Nobel Prize") for an extraordinary contribution towards improvement in child welfare and well-being in 1987.

Contact:
Office of the Medical Director,
Division for Intellectual and Developmental Disabilities,
Ministry of Social Affairs,
POBox 1260, IL-91012 Jerusalem, Israel.
E-mail: jmerrick@zahav.net.il

In: Public Health Yearbook 2013

ISBN: 978-1-63321-095-0

Editor: Joav Merrick

© 2014 Nova Science Publishers, Inc.

Chapter 47

ABOUT THE NATIONAL INSTITUTE OF CHILD HEALTH AND HUMAN DEVELOPMENT IN ISRAEL

The National Institute of Child Health and Human Development (NICHD) in Israel was established in 1998 as a virtual institute under the auspicies of the Medical Director, Ministry of Social Affairs and Social Services in order to function as the research arm for the Office of the Medical Director. In 1998 the National Council for Child Health and Pediatrics, Ministry of Health and in 1999 the Director General and Deputy Director General of the Ministry of Health endorsed the establishment of the NICHD.

MISSION

The mission of a National Institute for Child Health and Human Development in Israel is to provide an academic focal point for the scholarly interdisciplinary study of child life, health, public health, welfare, disability, rehabilitation, intellectual disability and related aspects of human development. This mission includes research, teaching, clinical work, information and public service activities in the field of child health and human development.

Service and academic activities

Over the years many activities became focused in the south of Israel due to collaboration with various professionals at the Faculty of Health Sciences (FOHS) at the Ben Gurion University of the Negev (BGU). Since 2000 an affiliation with the Zusman Child Development Center at the Pediatric Division of Soroka University Medical Center has resulted in collaboration around the establishment of the Down Syndrome Clinic at that center. In 2002 a full course on "Disability" was established at the Recanati School for Allied Professions in the Community, FOHS, BGU and in 2005 collaboration was started with the Primary Care Unit of the faculty and disability became part of the master of public health course on "Children and society". In the academic year 2005-2006 a one semester course on "Aging with disability" was started as part of the master of science program in gerontology in our collaboration with the Center for Multidisciplinary Research in Aging. From 2011 teaching medical second, fourth and six year medical students at Hadassah-Hebrew University Medical Center, Jerusalem.

Research activities

The affiliated staff have over the years published work from projects and research activities in this national and international collaboration. In the year 2000 the International Journal of Adolescent Medicine and Health and in 2005 the International Journal on Disability and Human development of Freund Publishing House (London and Tel Aviv), in the year 2003 the TSW-Child Health and Human Development and in 2006 the TSW-Holistic Health and Medicine of the Scientific World Journal (New York and Kirkkonummi, Finland), all peer-reviewed international journals were affiliated with the National Institute of Child Health and Human Development. From 2008 also the International Journal of Child Health and Human Development (Nova Science, New York), the International Journal of Child and Adolescent Health (Nova Science) and the Journal of Pain Management (Nova Science) affiliated and from 2009 the International Public Health Journal (Nova Science) and Journal of Alternative Medicine Research (Nova Science).

National collaboration

Nationally the NICHD works in collaboration with the Faculty of Health Sciences, Ben Gurion University of the Negev; Department of Physical Therapy, Sackler School of Medicine, Tel Aviv University; Autism Center, Assaf HaRofeh Medical Center; National Rett and PKU Centers at Chaim Sheba Medical Center, Tel HaShomer; Department of Physiotherapy, Haifa University; Department of Education, Bar Ilan University, Ramat Gan, Faculty of Social Sciences and Health Sciences; College of Judea and Samaria in Ariel and in 2011 affiliation with Center for Pediatric Chronic Illness and Center for Down Syndrome, Department of Pediatrics, Hadassah-Hebrew University Medical Center, Mount Scopus Campus, Jerusalem.

International collaboration

Internationally with the Department of Disability and Human Development, College of Applied Health Sciences, University of Illinois at Chicago; Strong Center for Developmental Disabilities, Golisano Children's Hospital at Strong, University of Rochester School of Medicine and Dentistry, New York; Centre on Intellectual Disabilities, University of Albany, New York; Centre for Chronic Disease Prevention and Control, Health Canada, Ottawa; Chandler Medical Center and Children's Hospital, Kentucky Children's Hospital, Section of Adolescent Medicine, University of Kentucky, Lexington; Chronic Disease Prevention and Control Research Center, Baylor College of Medicine, Houston, Texas; Division of Neuroscience, Department of Psychiatry, Columbia University, New York; Institute for the Study of Disadvantage and Disability, Atlanta; Center for Autism and Related Disorders, Department Psychiatry, Children's Hospital Boston, Boston; Department of Paediatrics,

Child Health and Adolescent Medicine, Children's Hospital at Westmead, Westmead, Australia; International Centre for the Study of Occupational and Mental Health, Düsseldorf, Germany; Centre for Advanced Studies in Nursing, Department of General Practice and Primary Care, University of Aberdeen, Aberdeen, United Kingdom; Quality of Life Research Center, Copenhagen, Denmark; Nordic School of Public Health, Gottenburg, Sweden, Scandinavian Institute of Quality of Working Life, Oslo, Norway; Centre for Quality of Life of the Hong Kong Institute of Asia-Pacific Studies and School of Social Work, Chinese University, Hong Kong.

Targets

Our focus is on research, international collaborations, clinical work, teaching and policy in health, disability and human development and to establish the NICHD as a permanent institute in Israel in order to conduct model research and together with the four university schools of public health/medicine in Israel establish a national master and doctoral program in disability and human development at the institute to secure the next generation of professionals working in this often non-prestigious/low-status field of work. For this project we need your support. We are looking for all kinds of support and eventually an endowment.

SUPPORT FOR OUR WORK

In the United States

In the United States the Israel Foundation for Human Development was created in order to support the work of the National Institute of Child Health and Human Development in Israel. It is possible to send donations to the Israel Foundation for Human Development Inc, which is a recognized tax-exempt organization in the United States (charitable non-for-prifit organization with 501c (3) tax exempt number 56-230-6116). Checks for the Foundation in the United States can be send to Israel Foundation for Human Development Inc., President Arlene Feldman, 2 Lawrence Street, New Hyde Park, New York 11040. Phone: 516-352-3596. E-mail: AFeldman@FarrellFritz.com

Contact in Israel

Professor Joav Merrick, MD, MMedSci, DMSc
Medical Director, Division for Mental Retardation
Ministry of Social Affairs, POBox 1260
IL-91012 Jerusalem, Israel
E-mail: jmerrick@zahav.net.il

INDEX

B

C

D

E

G

I

N

O

P

Q

R

S

V

W

X

Y

Z

β